Analysis and Evaluation of
Conceptual Models of Nursing

Analysis and Evaluation of Conceptual Models of Nursing

Third Edition

Jacqueline Fawcett, PhD, FAAN
Professor
University of Pennsylvania
School of Nursing
Philadelphia, Pennsylvania

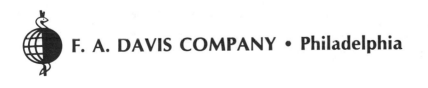

F. A. DAVIS COMPANY • Philadelphia

F. A. Davis Company
1915 Arch Street
Philadelphia, PA 19103

Printed in the United States of America

Last digit indicates print number: 10 9 8 7 6 5 4

Publisher, Nursing: Robert G. Martone
Production Editor: Marianne Fithian
Cover Design: Donald B. Freggens, Jr.

As new scientific information becomes available through basic and clinical research, recommended treatments and drug therapies undergo changes. The author(s) and publisher have done everything possible to make this book accurate, up to date, and in accord with accepted standards at the time of publication. The authors, editors, and publisher are not responsible for errors or omissions or for consequences from application of the book, and make no warranty, expressed or implied, in regard to the contents of the book. Any practice described in this book should be applied by the reader in accordance with professional standards of care used in regard to the unique circumstances that may apply in each situation. The reader is advised always to check product information (package inserts) for changes and new information regarding dose and contraindications before administering any drug. Caution is especially urged when using new or infrequently ordered drugs.

Library of Congress Cataloging-in-Publication Data

Fawcett, Jacqueline.
　　Analysis and evaluation of conceptual models of nursing / Jacqueline Fawcett. — 3rd ed.
　　　　p.　　cm.
　　Includes bibliographical references and index.
　　ISBN 0-8036-3411-0 (alk. paper)
　　1. Nursing models.　2. Nursing models—Evaluation.　I. Title.
　　[DNLM: 1. Models, Nursing.　WY 100 F278a 1995]
　　RT84.5.F38　1995
　　610.73'01'1 — dc20
　　DNLM/DLC
　　for Library of Congress　　　　　　　　　　　　　　　　　94-10087
　　　　　　　　　　　　　　　　　　　　　　　　　　　　　　　CIP

Preface

The third edition of this book, like the previous two editions, was written for all nurses and nursing students who are interested in the development of nursing knowledge and the use of that knowledge to guide nursing research, education, administration, and practice. This edition represents an ongoing attempt to clarify the continuing confusion between conceptual models and theories that remains in the nursing literature. To that end, the third edition continues to focus on the global formulations of nursing knowledge that are called *conceptual models of nursing*, with additional discussion of grand theories and middle-range theories that have been derived from the conceptual models.

The continuing centrality of conceptual models of nursing to all nursing activities is attested to by the voluminous international literature that has appeared since the first edition of this book went to press. Furthermore, the many conferences on conceptual models of nursing and nursing theories held throughout the United States and abroad over the years have attracted thousands of nurses and nursing students.

The continuing evolution of conceptual models of nursing is reflected in the revisions for the third edition of this book. Chapter 1 presents a revised and detailed discussion of the components of the structural hierarchy of contemporary nursing knowledge. Emphasis is placed on the distinctions among the components, which include the metaparadigm, philosophies, conceptual models, theories, and empirical indicators. The section on world views has been revised to present a new, more parsimonious schema. The discussion of how conceptual models guide nursing research, nursing education, nursing administration, and nursing practice has been expanded to include an overview of the construction of conceptual-theoretical-empirical structures for research, education, administration, and practice.

Chapter 2 presents a revised framework for analysis and evaluation of conceptual models of nursing that reflects my continuously evolving understanding of the structural hierarchy of nursing knowledge. The discussion of the social utility, social congruence, and social significance of conceptual models has been revised to reflect my increased understanding of methods for determining the credibility of conceptual models of nursing, with emphasis placed on both informal and formal methods of evaluating their social significance.

Chapters 3 through 9 present systematic analyses and objective evaluations of the most recent versions of works by Dorothy Johnson, Imogene King, Myra Levine, Betty Neuman, Dorothea Orem, Martha Rogers, and Callista Roy. Each of those chapters has been completely rewritten to reflect the revised framework for analysis and evaluation of conceptual models of nursing and to incorporate the most recent refinements in each conceptual model. A special feature of Chapters 3 through 9 is the discussion of strategies for the implementation of each conceptual model that have been successfully used in clinical agencies. Each chapter also includes a comprehensive review of virtually all of the published literature dealing with the use of the conceptual model in nursing research, nursing education, nursing administration, and nursing practice. In addition, several of the chapters contain an expanded analysis of the theories that have been derived from the conceptual model.

A continuing hallmark of Chapters 3 through 9 is the care that was taken to present an accurate account of the conceptual model as it was developed by its author rather than to draw from secondary analyses and other interpretations of the author's work. Each of those chapters includes many direct quotes from the model author's original works. The quotations reflect the author's writing style and the language customs at the time of publication of the particular book or journal article; pronouns have not been altered to reflect current nonsexist language. Readers are encouraged to use this book in combination with the original source material for each conceptual model, which is identified in the accompanying bibliography.

Other works that might fit this book's definition of a conceptual model were not included in this edition. The works that are included continue, in my opinion, to be the major representatives of conceptual models in the contemporary nursing literature. In fact, several of the other most frequently cited works fit this book's definition of a grand theory or a middle-range theory. Readers who are interested in understanding the content of other conceptual models are encouraged to use the framework for analysis and evaluation of conceptual models that is presented in Chapter 2. Readers who are interested in understanding the content of nursing theories are encouraged to use the framework for analysis and evaluation of nursing theories that is presented in my companion text, *Analysis and Evaluation of Nursing Theories* (also published by F. A. Davis). My sincere hope is that both books will stimulate readers to continue their study of conceptual models and nursing theories and to adopt explicit conceptual-theoretical-empirical structures for their nursing activities.

Chapter 10 has been completely revised. The discussion now centers on the value of using an explicit conceptual model to guide nursing practice and the substantive and process elements of implementing conceptual model–based nursing practice.

Each chapter of the book presents a list of key terms or key concepts, which are defined and discussed in the chapter. Each chapter also includes a comprehensive bibliography of all relevant literature that could be located through hand and computer-assisted searches of an extensive list of nursing books and journals. The vast amount of literature precluded a continuation of the annotated bibliographies. Instead, the citations are divided into relevant sections. The sections for Chapters 3 through 9 are primary sources, commentary, research, doctoral dissertations, master's theses, education, administration, and practice. The citations to doctoral dissertations and master's theses are limited to those that could be retrieved from *Dissertation Abstracts International* and *Master's Abstracts International*. All books, book chapters, journal articles, and abstracts were closely examined to determine their direct relevance to the particular conceptual model. The bibliographies for all chapters contain citations to a variety of opinions that are not always in agreement with the positions taken in this book. In particular, some of the citations contain different interpretations of the content of conceptual models and critiques that do not present what I regard as accurate or appropriate judgments about the conceptual models. Those citations are included in the interest of the reader's exposure to the debate and dialogue about conceptual models and other components of contemporary nursing knowledge. I continue to be indebted to the model authors and to my students and colleagues for the many citations of relevant publications they shared with me.

Most chapters also include tables and diagrams that highlight, summarize, or expand certain narrative points. Of special note are the tables in Chapters 3 through 9 that summarize the nursing process format for each conceptual model. Chapter 1 includes a new diagram of the structural hierarchy of contemporary nursing knowledge. Chapter 10 contains one diagram depicting the translation of the structural hierarchy for nursing practice and another diagram depicting the process of perspective transformation. Chapter 4 (King's General Systems Framework), Chapter 6 (Neuman's Systems Model), and Chapter 9 (Roy's Adaptation Model) also include diagrams developed by the model authors to illustrate the components of their conceptual models.

The Appendix for this edition has been expanded to include not only lists of audio and video productions with their distribution sources but also strategies for computer-based searches of the literature and a list of societies devoted to the advancement of particular conceptual models.

Chapters 1 and 2 should be read before the remainder of the book. Those two chapters provide the background that facilitates understanding of the place for conceptual models of nursing in the structural hierarchy of contemporary nursing knowledge, as well as the framework used for the analysis and evaluation of each conceptual model. Chapter 10 may be read at any time. That chapter should be of special interest to clinicians and administrators who are interested in strategies for the application of conceptual models in the real world of nursing practice.

The writing of the third edition of this book was a consuming, stimulating, and growth-enhancing experience. Its preparation is due to many people. First, I continue to be indebted to Dorothy Johnson, Imogene King, Myra Levine, Betty Neuman, Dorothea Orem, Martha Rogers, and Callista Roy, whose ongoing efforts to continuously refine the knowledge base for the discipline of nursing made this edition possible. My conversations and written communications with those nursing pioneers has greatly enhanced my understanding and appreciation of all the obstacles they have overcome to share their visions of nursing with us.

I am also indebted to my students and colleagues at the University of Pennsylvania, and at other universities where I have been privileged to serve as a visiting faculty member or to present a paper, for their support, intellectual challenges, and constructive criticism.

My gratitude to my husband, John S. Fawcett, is boundless. His unconditional love, support, and understanding throughout the many long days of the summer of 1993 that I spent at the computer is greatly appreciated. I appreciate, too, his planning of outings to see a movie or go on a picnic so that I had a break from the writing. I am also grateful to Captain Linda J. Lee, Captain Douglas K. Lee, Clara E. Lee, and Rachel M. Lee, of the Schooner *Heritage*, for the relaxed yet exciting sailing along the coast of Maine and the time away from the telephone and the mail that contributed to the completion of this edition of the book.

Finally, I continue to be indebted to Robert G. Martone, Ruth DeGeorge, Herbert J. Powell, Jr., and Marianne Fithian of F. A. Davis Company, for their encouragement and the time spent discussing the content and design of this edition.

Jacqueline Fawcett

Credits

Contents

Chapter 1 **Conceptual Models and Contemporary Nursing Knowledge** **1**

Chapter 2 **Analysis and Evaluation of Conceptual Models of Nursing** **51**

Chapter 3 **Johnson's Behavioral System Model** **67**

Chapter 4 **King's General Systems Framework** **109**

Chapter 5 **Levine's Conservation Model** **165**

Chapter 6 **Neuman's Systems Model** **217**

Chapter 7 **Orem's Self-Care Framework** **277**

Chapter 8 **Rogers' Science of Unitary Human Beings** **375**

Chapter 9 **Roy's Adaptation Model** **437**

Chapter 10 **Implementing Conceptual Models in Nursing Practice** **517**

Appendix **Resources for Conceptual Models of Nursing** **547**

Index **555**

CHAPTER

1

Conceptual Models and Contemporary Nursing Knowledge

This chapter lays the groundwork for the remainder of the book. Here, conceptual models are defined and placed in the structural hierarchy of contemporary nursing knowledge. The other components of the hierarchy—metaparadigm, philosophies, theories, and empirical indicators — are then defined, and the relationship of each of those components to conceptual models is discussed. Special emphasis is placed on the distinctions between conceptual models and theories and the need to use these two knowledge components in different ways. The chapter concludes with a discussion of the conceptual-theoretical-empirical systems of nursing knowledge required for scientific and professional activities.

The key terms used in this chapter are listed below. Each term is defined and described in the chapter.

KEY TERMS

CONCEPTUAL MODELS	Reciprocal Interaction World View
Concepts	Simultaneous Action World View
Propositions	Categories of Nursing Knowledge
METAPARADIGM	THEORIES
Person	Grand Theories
Environment	Middle-Range Theories
Health	EMPIRICAL INDICATORS
Nursing	CONCEPTUAL-THEORETICAL-
PHILOSOPHIES	EMPIRICAL SYSTEMS OF
Reaction World View	NURSING KNOWLEDGE

CONCEPTUAL MODELS

Conceptual models have existed since people began to think about themselves and their surroundings. They now exist in all areas of life and in all disciplines. Indeed, everything that a person sees, hears, reads, and experiences is filtered through the cognitive lens of some conceptual frame of reference (Lachman, 1993).

The term **conceptual model** is synonymous with the terms conceptual framework, conceptual system, paradigm, and disciplinary matrix. A conceptual model is defined as a set of abstract and general concepts and the propositions that integrate those concepts into a meaningful configuration (Lippitt, 1973; Nye & Berardo, 1981).

Concepts are words that describe mental images of phenomena. The concepts of a conceptual model are so abstract and general that they are neither directly observed in the real world nor limited to any particular individual, group, situation, or event. Adaptive system is an example of a conceptual model concept (Roy & Andrews, 1991). It can refer to several types of systems, including individuals, families, groups, communities, and entire societies.

Propositions are statements that describe or link concepts. The propositions of a conceptual model are also so abstract and general that they are not amenable to direct empirical observation or test. Some propositions are general descriptions or definitions of the conceptual model concepts. Because conceptual model concepts are so abstract, not all of them are defined, and those that are defined typically have broad definitions. Definitional propositions for conceptual model concepts, therefore, do not state how the concepts are empirically observed or measured, and they should not be expected to do so. Adaptation level, for example, is broadly defined as "a changing point that represents the person's ability to respond positively in a situation" (Roy & Andrews, 1991, p. 4).

Other propositions state the relationships between conceptual model concepts in a general manner. They are exemplified by the following statement: Changes in environmental stimuli are associated with changes in adaptation level (Roy & Andrews, 1991).

The concepts and propositions of each conceptual model often are stated in a distinctive vocabulary. One model, for example, uses the terms stimuli and adaptation level (Roy & Andrews, 1991), and another uses the terms resonancy, helicy, and integrality (Rogers, 1990). Furthermore, the meaning of each term usually is connected to the unique focus of the conceptual model. Thus, the same or similar terms may have different meanings in different conceptual models. For example, adaptation is defined as a response to stimuli in one model (Roy & Andrews, 1991) and as a way in which the person and the environment become congruent over time in another model (Levine, 1991).

The vocabulary of each conceptual model should not be considered jargon. Rather, the terminology used by the author of each conceptual model is the result of considerable thought about how to convey the meaning of that particular perspective to others (Biley, 1990). Furthermore, as Akinsanya (1989) points out, "Every science has its own peculiar terms, concepts and principles which are essential for the development of its knowledge base. In nursing, as in other sciences, an understanding of these is a prerequisite to a critical examination of their contribution to the development of knowledge and its application to practice" (p. ii).

Conceptual models evolve from the empirical observations and intuitive insights of scholars and/or from deductions that creatively combine ideas from several fields of inquiry. A conceptual model is inductively developed when generalizations about specific observations are formulated and is deductively developed when specific situations are seen as examples of other more general events. For example, much of the content of the Self-Care Framework was induced from Orem's observations of "the constant elements and relationships of nursing practice situations" (Orem & Taylor, 1986, p. 38). In contrast, Levine (1969) indicated that she deduced the Conservation Model from "ideas from all areas of knowledge that contribute to the development of the nursing process" (p. viii).

Functions of Conceptual Models

A conceptual model provides a distinctive frame of reference and "a coherent, internally unified way of thinking about . . . events and processes" (Frank, 1968, p. 45) for its adherents that tells them how to observe and interpret the phenomena of interest to the discipline. Each conceptual model, then, presents a unique focus that has a profound influence on our perceptions. The unique focus of each model is an approximation or simplification of reality that includes only those concepts that the model author considers relevant and as aids to understanding (Lippitt, 1973; Reilly, 1975). Thus, certain aspects of the phenomena of interest to a discipline are regarded as particularly relevant, and other aspects are ignored. For example, Neuman's (1989) Systems Model focuses on preventing the deleterious impact of stressors, whereas Orem's (1991) Self-Care Framework emphasizes enhancing the person's self-care capabilities and actions. Note that Neuman's model does not deal with self-care, and Orem's does not focus on the impact of stressors.

Each conceptual model also provides a systematic structure and a rationale for the scholarly and practical activities of its adherents, who comprise a subculture or community of scholars within a discipline (Eckberg & Hill, 1979). More specifically, each conceptual model gives direction to the search for relevant questions about phenomena and suggests solutions to practical problems. Each one also provides general criteria for knowing when a problem has been solved. Those features of a conceptual model are illustrated in the following example. The Roy Adaptation Model focuses on adaptation of the person to environmental stimuli and proposes that management of the most relevant stimuli leads to adaptation (Roy & Andrews, 1991). Here, a relevant question might be: What are the most relevant stimuli in a given situation? Anyone interested in solutions to problems in adaptation would focus on the various ways of managing stimuli. Also, one would be led to look for manifestations of adaptation when seeking to determine if the problem has been solved.

Furthermore, conceptual models of nursing "provide [explicit] philosophical and pragmatic orientations to the service nurses provide patients—a service which only nurses can provide—a service which provides a dimension to total care different from that provided by any other health professional" (Johnson, 1987, p. 195). Conceptual models of nursing provide explicit orientations not only for nurses but also for the general public. They identify the purpose and scope of nursing and provide frameworks for objective records of the effects of nursing. Johnson (1987) explained, "Conceptual models specify for nurses and society the mission and boundaries of the profession. They clarify the realm of nursing responsibility and accountability, and they allow the practitioner and/or the profession to document services and outcomes" (pp. 196–197).

Historical Evolution of Conceptual Models of Nursing

Conceptual models are not really new to nursing, as they have existed since Nightingale (1859) first advanced her ideas about nursing. Most early conceptualizations of nursing, however, were not presented in the formal manner of models. It remained for the Nursing Development Conference Group (1973, 1979), Johnson (1974), Riehl and Roy (1974, 1980), and Reilly (1975) to explicitly label various perspectives of nursing as conceptual models.

Peterson (1977) and Hall (1979) linked the proliferation of formal conceptual models of nursing with interest in conceptualizing nursing as a distinct discipline and the concomitant introduction of ideas about nursing theory. Meleis (1991) reached the same conclusion in her historiography of nursing knowledge development. Readers who are especially interested in the progression of nursing knowledge are referred to her excellent work, because a comprehensive historic review is beyond the scope of this book.

The works of several nurse scholars currently are recognized as conceptual models. Among the best known are Johnson's Behavioral System Model, King's General Systems Framework, Levine's Conservation Model, Neuman's Systems Model, Orem's Self-Care Framework, Rogers' Science of Unitary Human Beings, and Roy's Adaptation Model (Johnson, 1980, 1990; King, 1971, 1990; Levine, 1969, 1991; Neuman, 1989; Neuman & Young, 1972; Orem, 1971, 1991; Rogers, 1970, 1990; Roy, 1976; Roy & Andrews, 1991).

The development of conceptual models of nursing and labeling them as such is an important advance for the discipline. Reilly's (1975) comments help to underscore this point.

> We all have a private image (concept) of nursing practice. In turn, this private image influences our interpretation of data, our decisions, and our actions. But can a discipline continue to develop when its members hold so many differing private images? The proponents of conceptual models of practice are seeking to make us aware of these private images, so that we can begin to identify commonalities in our perceptions of the nature of practice and move toward the evolution of a well-ordered concept. (p. 567)

Johnson (1987) also pointed out that nurses always use some frame of reference for their activities and explained the drawbacks of implicit frameworks. She stated,

> It is important to note that some kind of implicit framework is used by every practicing nurse, for we cannot observe, see, or describe, nor can we prescribe anything for which we do not already have some kind of mental image or concept. Unfortunately, the mental images used by nurses in their practice, images developed through education and experience and continuously governed by the multitude of factors in the practice setting, have tended to be disconnected, diffused, incomplete and frequently heavily weighted by concepts drawn from the conceptual schema used by medicine to achieve its own social mission. (p. 195)

Conceptual models of nursing, then, are the formal presentations of some nurses' private images of nursing. The proponents of nursing models maintain that use of a conceptual model facilitates communication among nurses and provides a systematic approach to nursing research, education, administration, and practice.

THE METAPARADIGM

Now that conceptual models have been defined and their functions have been described, they may be placed within the structural hierarchy of contemporary nursing knowledge. As can be seen in Figure 1–1, conceptual models actually are the third component in the hierarchy; the first component is the **metaparadigm.**

The metaparadigm of any discipline is made up of global concepts that identify the phenomena of interest to a discipline and global propositions that state the relationships among those phenomena (Kuhn, 1977). The metaparadigm is the most abstract component in the structural hierarchy of contemporary nursing knowledge and "acts as an encapsulating unit, or framework, within which the more restricted . . . structures develop" (Eckberg & Hill, 1979, p. 927).

The concepts and propositions of a metaparadigm are admittedly extremely global and provide no definitive direction for such activities as research and clinical practice. That is to be expected because the meta-

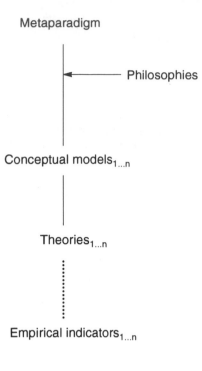

Metaparadigm

Philosophies

Conceptual models$_{1...n}$

Theories$_{1...n}$

Empirical indicators$_{1...n}$

FIGURE 1-1. The structural hierarchy of contemporary nursing knowledge.

paradigm "is the broadest consensus within a discipline. It provides the general parameters of the field and gives scientists a broad orientation from which to work" (Hardy, 1978, p. 38). Thus, the functions of a metaparadigm are to summarize the intellectual and social missions of a discipline and place a boundary on the subject matter of that discipline (Kim, 1989). The functions of a metaparadigm are reflected in the following four requirements (Fawcett, 1992):

1. The metaparadigm must *identify a domain that is distinctive from the domains of other disciplines.* That requirement is fulfilled only when the concepts and propositions represent a unique perspective for inquiry and practice.

2. The metaparadigm must *encompass all phenomena of interest to the discipline in a parsimonious manner.* That requirement is fulfilled only if the concepts and propositions are global and if there are no redundancies in concepts or propositions.

3. The metaparadigm must *be perspective-neutral.* That requirement is fulfilled only if the concepts and propositions do *not* represent a specific perspective, that is, a specific paradigm or conceptual model, or a combination of perspectives.

4. The metaparadigm must *be international in scope and substance.*

That requirement, which is a corollary of the third requirement, is fulfilled only if the concepts and propositions do not reflect particular national, cultural, or ethnic beliefs and values.

The Metaparadigm of Nursing

The phenomena of interest to nursing are represented by four central concepts: *person, environment, health,* and *nursing. Person* refers to the recipient of nursing, including individuals, families, communities, and other groups. *Environment* refers to the person's significant others and physical surroundings, as well as to the setting in which nursing occurs, which ranges from the person's home to clinical agencies to society as a whole. *Health* is the person's state of well-being, which can range from high-level wellness to terminal illness. *Nursing* refers to the definition of nursing, the actions taken by nurses on behalf of or in conjunction with the person, and the goals or outcomes of nursing actions. Nursing actions typically are viewed as a systematic process of assessment, labeling, planning, intervention, and evaluation.

The relationships among the metaparadigm concepts are described in four propositions (Donaldson & Crowley, 1978; Gortner, 1980). The first proposition links the person and health; it states that *the discipline of nursing is concerned with the principles and laws that govern the life-process, well-being, and optimal functioning of human beings, sick or well.*

The second proposition emphasizes the interaction between the person and the environment; it states that *the discipline of nursing is concerned with the patterning of human behavior in interaction with the environment in normal life events and critical life situations.*

The third proposition links health and nursing; it declares that *the discipline of nursing is concerned with the nursing actions or processes by which positive changes in health status are effected.*

The fourth proposition links the person, the environment, and health; it asserts that *the discipline of nursing is concerned with the wholeness or health of human beings, recognizing that they are in continuous interaction with their environments.*

The version of the metaparadigm presented here represents an extension and elaboration of the original metaparadigm of nursing published several years ago (Fawcett, 1984b). One difference is the addition of a description of each of the four metaparadigm concepts. Another difference between the earlier and current versions is the formalization of themes into propositions. Still another difference is the addition of the fourth proposition. The current version of the metaparadigm meets the four requirements cited previously.

In particular, the four metaparadigm concepts are generally regarded as the central or domain concepts of nursing (Flaskerud & Halloran, 1980; Jennings, 1987; Wagner, 1986). They are a modification of four concepts induced from the conceptual frameworks of baccalaureate programs accredited by the National League for Nursing. The original concepts were *man, society, health,* and *nursing* (Yura & Torres, 1975). *Man* was changed to *person* to avoid gender-specific language, and *society* was changed to *environment* to more fully encompass phenomena of relevance to the person (Fawcett, 1978). Additional support for the centrality of the four metaparadigm concepts comes from the successful use of those concepts as a schema for analysis of the content of conceptual models of nursing and nursing theories (Fawcett, 1989, 1993; Fitzpatrick & Whall, 1989; Marriner-Tomey, 1994).

The metaparadigm propositions provide a unique perspective of the concepts that helps to distinguish nursing from other disciplines. The first three propositions represent recurrent themes identified in the writings of Florence Nightingale and many other nursing scholars and clinicians of the nineteenth and twentieth centuries. Donaldson and Crowley (1978) commented that "these themes suggest boundaries of an area for systematic [i]nquiry and theory development with potential for making the nature of the discipline of nursing more explicit than it is at present" (p. 113). The fourth proposition, according to Donaldson and Crowley (1978), "evolves from the practical aim of optimizing of human environments for health" (p. 119).

Taken together, the four concepts and four propositions identify the unique focus of the discipline of nursing and encompass all relevant phenomena in a parsimonious manner. Furthermore, the concepts and propositions are perspective-neutral because they do not reflect a specific paradigm or conceptual model. Moreover, the metaparadigm concepts and propositions do not reflect the beliefs and values of any one country or culture and, therefore, are international in scope and substance.

Proposals for Alternative Metaparadigm Concepts and Propositions

The version of the nursing metaparadigm previously presented should not be regarded as premature closure on explication of phenomena of interest to the discipline of nursing. Indeed, it is anticipated that modifications in the metaparadigm concepts and propositions will be offered as the discipline of nursing evolves. Modifications must, however, fulfill the four requirements for a metaparadigm identified earlier in this chapter. To date, the various proposals for alternatives to the four metaparadigm concepts and propositions have not fulfilled one or more of the requirements.

One modification that already has been suggested is that the term *client* replace *person* (Newman, 1983). *Client,* however, reflects a particular view of the *person* and, therefore, is not a perspective-neutral concept. In fact, the term *client* is used to represent the *person* in only two conceptual models of nursing (King, 1990; Neuman, 1989). Consequently, the suggested modification does not fulfill the third requirement for a metaparadigm.

Another modification that has been proposed is the elimination of the concept *nursing* from the metaparadigm (Conway, 1985, 1989). Conway claimed that *nursing* represents the discipline or the profession and is not an appropriate metaparadigm concept because it creates a tautology. Similarly, Meleis (1991) commented, "It would be an instance of tautological conceptualizing to define nursing by all the concepts and then include nursing as one of the concepts" (p. 101). Kolcaba and Kolcaba (1991), however, rejected the charge of a tautology. They noted that inasmuch as the metaparadigm concept *nursing* stands for nursing activities or actions, a tautology is not created.

Conway (1985) did not offer a substitute metaparadigm concept to represent the actions or activities of nurses. Consequently, her proposal to eliminate *nursing* from the metaparadigm does not encompass all phenomena of interest to the discipline of nursing. Furthermore, Conway offered no justification for the uniqueness of a discipline dealing with the *person, environment,* and *health.* Her proposal, therefore, does not fulfill the first and second requirements for a metaparadigm.

Other scholars view *nursing* as a distinct phenomenon of interest to the discipline. Kim (1987) identified *nursing* as a component of two domains of nursing knowledge. She regarded *nursing* as the central feature of the *practice domain* and as an essential component of the *client-nurse domain.* In addition, Barnum (1994) identified *nursing acts* as a commonplace, that is, a topic addressed by most nursing theories. Finally, King (1984) found that *nursing* was a central concept in the philosophies of nursing education of several nursing education programs. That finding suggests that the concept *nursing* is a discipline-wide phenomenon and, therefore, must be included in the metaparadigm.

A potential modification in the metaparadigm is the exclusion of the concept *environment.* Barnum (1994) did not include *environment* in her list of nursing commonplaces. She did, however, point out that "a complete theory of nursing [is one that contains] context, content, and process [and that] context is the environment in which the nursing act takes place" (p. 21). Thus, Barnum's view of *environment* as a metaparadigm concept is unclear. If Barnum meant to exclude *environment,* her modification would not fulfill the second requirement for a metaparadigm.

Another potential modification in the metaparadigm is the exclusion of the concept *health.* Kim (1987) identified four domains of nursing knowledge. The *client domain* is concerned with the client's development, problems, and health care experiences. The *client-nurse domain* focuses on encounters between client and nurse and the interactions between the two in the process of providing nursing care. The *practice domain* emphasizes the cognitive, behavioral, and social aspects of nurses' professional actions. The *environment domain* takes in the time, space, and quality variations of the client's environment.

Hinshaw (1987) pointed out that Kim's work does not include the concept *health*, and asked: "Is health a strand that permeates each of the . . . domains . . . rather than a major separate domain?" (p. 112). Kim (personal communication, October 31, 1986) has indicated that the *client domain* could encompass *health*.

Kim's failure to explicitly identify *health* in her proposal creates a void in an otherwise informative explication of the discipline of nursing. Thus, her proposal does not fulfill the second requirement for a metaparadigm.

Two additional suggested modifications center on proposals for additional metaparadigm concepts. Meleis (1991) maintained that the domain of nursing knowledge encompasses seven central concepts: *nursing client, transitions, interaction, nursing process, environment, nursing therapeutics,* and *health.* She proposed that

> the nurse interacts (interaction) with a human being in a health/illness situation (nursing client) who is in an integral part of his sociocultural context (environment) and who is in some sort of transition or is anticipating a transition (transition); the nurse/patient interactions are organized around some purpose (nursing process, problem solving, or holistic assessment) and the nurse uses some actions (nursing therapeutics) to enhance, bring about, or facilitate health (health). (p. 101)

The inclusion of *nursing process, nursing therapeutics,* and *interactions* in Meleis' proposal represents a redundancy that can be avoided by use of the single concept, *nursing.* Moreover, the inclusion of *transitions* reflects a particular perspective of human life. Thus, Meleis' proposal for the central concepts of nursing, although meritorious, does not meet the second and third requirements for a metaparadigm.

King's (1984) review of the philosophies of a representative sample of National League for Nursing accredited nursing education programs in the United States revealed nine concepts. The concepts are: *man, health, environment, social systems, role, perceptions, interpersonal relations, nursing,* and *God.* King found that all nine concepts were not evident, however, in the philosophies of all the schools included in the sample. She recommended that the most frequently cited concepts could represent the domain of nursing. Those concepts are: *man, health, role,* and *social systems.*

King's proposal falls short of meeting all requirements for a metaparadigm. First, the inclusion of *role* and *social systems* reflects a sociological orientation to nursing. Second, the elimination of *environment* and *nursing* results in a narrow view of the domain. Moreover, the elimination of *environment* and *nursing* leaves a list of concepts more closely aligned with the discipline of social work (Ben-Sira, 1987) than with nursing. Thus, her proposal does not meet the first, second, and third requirements for a metaparadigm.

Three other suggested modifications in the version of the metaparadigm presented in this chapter are more radical than rewording, adding, or eliminating a concept. One proposal calls for a new metaparadigm proposition that would replace the four propositions given earlier in this chapter. Newman and associates (1991) claimed that the focus of the discipline of nursing is summarized in the following statement: "Nursing is the study of caring in the human health experience" (p. 3). In a later publication, they asserted that "the theme of caring is sufficiently dominant, when combined with the theme of the human health experience, to be considered as the focus of the discipline" (Newman et al., 1992, p. vii).

Despite those authors' claims to the contrary, their proposition represents just one frame of reference for *nursing* and for *health*. In fact, Newman and associates (1991) ended their initial treatise by maintaining that caring in the human health experience can be most fully elaborated only through a unitary-transformative perspective.

Moreover, although the authors offered their proposition as a single statement that integrates "concepts commonly identified with nursing at the metaparadigm level" (p. 3), and although they identified the metaparadigm concepts as *person, environment, health,* and *nursing,* their proposition does not include *environment.* In an attempt to clarify their position, Newman and associates (1992) later stated, "we view the concept of environment as inherent in and inseparable from the integrated focus of caring in the human health experience" (p. vii). Despite that clarification, the substitute proposition does not meet the second and third requirements for a metaparadigm because it is neither sufficiently comprehensive nor perspective-neutral.

Another proposal comes from Malloch and associates (1992), who suggested a revision of the statement by Newman and associates (1991). Their focus statement is: "Nursing is the study and practice of caring within contexts of the human health experience" (p. vi). Malloch and associates maintained that their statement extends the focus of the discipline to *nursing* practice and incorporates the environment by the use of the term *contexts.* They noted that *environment* "includes, but is not limited to, culture, community, and ecology" (p. vi). Moreover, they claimed that the use of the term *caring* brings unity to the metaparadigm concepts of *person, environment, health,* and *nursing.* Apparently, they do not regard *caring* as a particular perspective of *nursing.* Although this substitute proposition is sufficiently comprehensive, it does not meet the third requirement for a metaparadigm because it is not perspective-neutral.

Still another proposal calls for the elimination of the four metaparadigm concepts and propositions and the substitution of the concepts of *human care, environmental contexts,* and *well-being (health)* and a proposition asserting the centrality of *caring* to the discipline of nursing. Leininger (1990) claimed that "human care/caring [is] the central phenomenon and essence of nursing" (p. 19), and Watson (1990) maintained that "human caring needs to be explicitly incorporated into nursing's meta-paradigm" (p. 21). Even more to the point, Leininger (1991a) maintained: "Care is the essence of nursing and the central, dominant, and unifying focus of nursing" (p. 35). On the basis of that position, Leininger (1988, 1991c) rejected the metaparadigm concepts of person and nursing. She commented,

> The author rejects the idea that nursing and person explain nursing, for one cannot explain nor predict the same phenomenon one is study-ing. Nursing is the phenomenon to be explained. Moreover, person, per se, is not sufficient to explain nursing as it fails to account for groups, families, social institutions, and cultures. (1988, p. 154) The concepts of person and nursing are quite inappropriate. Person is far too limited and nursing cannot be logically used to explain and predict nursing. The latter is a redundancy and a contradiction to explain the same phenome-non being studied by the same concept. (1991c, p. 152)

In another publication, Leininger (1991a) continued to reject the metaparadigm concept of person, and she apparently rejected environment and health as well. She stated,

> From an anthropological and nursing perspective, the use of the term person has serious problems when used transculturally, as many non-Western cultures do not focus on or believe in the concept person, and often there is no linguistic term for person in a culture, family and institutions being more prominent. While environment is very impor-tant to nursing, I would contend it is certainly not unique to nursing, and there are very few nurses who have advanced formal study and are prepared to study a large number of different types of environments or ecological niches worldwide. [The metaparadigm] concepts had serious problems except for that of health. Again, as a concept health is not distinct to nursing although nursing plays a major role in health attain-ment and maintenance—many disciplines have studied health. (pp. 39–40)

In her discussions, Leininger failed to acknowledge that an earlier discussion of the metaparadigm concept person indicated that that con-cept can refer to any entity that is a recipient of nursing actions, including individuals, families, and other types of groups, communities, and socie-ties (Fawcett, 1984a). Furthermore, in her 1991a publication, Leininger did not acknowledge that the point of the inclusion of the concept envi-ronment in the metaparadigm is to provide a context for the person, to indicate that the recipient of nursing actions is surrounded by and inter-acts with other people and the social structure (Fawcett, 1984a). In fact, she neither acknowledged her own previously published statement that "Care should be central to [the] nursing metaparadigm and supported by the concepts of health and environmental contexts" (Leininger, 1988, p. 154), nor acknowledged her statement in the same book that "In the very near future, one can predict that the current concepts of person, environ-ment, health, and nursing will no longer be upheld. Instead, human care, environmental contexts, and well being (or health) will become of major interest to most nurse researchers and new theorists" (Leininger, 1991b, p. 406). Moreover, Leininger has not acknowledged that the inclusion of the concept *nursing* in the metaparadigm was not to create a tautology but rather to serve as a single-word symbol of all nursing actions and activities taken on behalf of or in conjunction with the person, family, community, or other entity (Fawcett, 1984a).

In addition, both Leininger and Watson failed to acknowledge that although the term *caring* is included in several conceptualizations of the discipline of nursing (Morse et al., 1990), it is not a dominant theme in every conceptualization and, therefore, does not represent a discipline-wide viewpoint. In fact, caring reflects a particular view of nursing and a particular kind of nursing (Eriksson, 1989). Furthermore, as Swanson (1991) pointed out, although there may be "characteristic behavior patterns that are universal expressions of nurse caring . . . caring is not uniquely a nursing phenomenon" (p. 165). Caring behaviors, moreover, may not be generalizable across national and cultural boundaries (Mandelbaum, 1991). Also, as Rogers (1992) asserted, "as such, caring does not identify nurses any more than it identifies workers from another field. Everyone needs to care" (p. 33).

In summation, Leininger's discussions about the metaparadigm tend to be contradictory, and she fails to acknowledge that her ideas could be readily incorporated into the widely cited metaparadigm concepts of *person, environment, health,* and *nursing.* More specifically, *person* already refers to collectives as well as to individuals, *environment* already is viewed as context, *health* already refers to a broad spectrum of states that includes well-being, and *nursing* can be viewed as directed toward human care. Thus, her proposal clearly does not meet the first, third, and fourth requirements for a metaparadigm.

Conceptual Models and the Metaparadigm

Most disciplines have a single metaparadigm but multiple conceptual models, as indicated by the subscript notation, 1 . . . n, in Figure 1–1. The models are derived from the metaparadigm and, therefore, incorporate the most global concepts and propositions in a more restrictive, yet still abstract manner. Each conceptual model, then, provides a different view of the metaparadigm concepts. As Kuhn (1970) explained, although adherents of different models are looking at the same phenomena, "in some areas they see different things, and they see them in different relations to one another" (p. 150). The acceptance of multiple conceptual models is an outgrowth of the recognition of the value of diverse perspectives for a discipline (Moore, 1990; Nagle & Mitchell, 1991). For example, nursing now has at least seven different conceptual models, and Nye and

Berardo (1981) identified 16 different conceptual models of the family derived from the metaparadigm of sociology.

As with conceptual models and metaparadigms of other disciplines, the conceptual models of nursing represent various paradigms derived from the metaparadigm of the discipline of nursing. Thus, it is not surprising that each defines the four metaparadigm concepts differently and links those concepts in diverse ways.

Examination of conceptual models of nursing reveals that *person* usually is identified as an integrated bio-psycho-social being but is defined in diverse ways, such as an adaptive system (Roy & Andrews, 1991), a behavioral system (Johnson, 1990), a self-care agent (Orem, 1991), or an energy field (Rogers, 1990). *Environment* frequently is identified as internal structures and external influences, including family members, the community, and society, as well as the person's physical surroundings. The environment is seen as a source of stressors in some models (Neuman, 1989) but as a source of resources in others (Rogers, 1990). *Health* is presented in various ways, such as a continuum from adaptation to maladaptation (Roy & Andrews, 1991), a dichotomy of behavioral stability or instability (Johnson, 1990), or a value identified by each cultural group (Rogers, 1990). The conceptual models also present descriptions of the concept of *nursing*, usually by defining nursing and then specifying goals of nursing actions and a nursing process. The goals of nursing action frequently are derived directly from the definition of health given by the model. For example, a nursing goal might be to assist people to attain, maintain, or regain the system stability (Neuman, 1989).

The nursing process described in each model emphasizes assessing the person's health status, setting goals for nursing action, implementing nursing actions, and evaluating the person's health status after nursing intervention. The steps of the process, however, frequently differ from model to model. Later chapters in this book present detailed descriptions of several conceptual models of nursing and discuss the connections between the concepts of each model.

PHILOSOPHIES

The **philosophy** is the second component in the structural hierarchy of contemporary nursing knowledge (Figure 1–1). A philosophy may be defined as a statement of beliefs and values (Kim, 1989; Seaver & Cartwright, 1977). More specifically, philosophies are statements about what people assume to be true in relation to the phenomena of interest to a discipline (Christensen & Kenney, 1990) and what they believe regarding the development of knowledge about those phenomena. An example of a philosophical statement is "The individual . . . behaves purposefully, not in a sequence of cause and effect" (Roy, 1988, p. 32).

Philosophies encompass ethical claims about what the members of a discipline should do, ontological claims about the nature of human beings and the goal of the discipline, and epistemic claims dealing with how knowledge is developed (Salsberry, 1991).

Ethical claims about nursing are summarized in the dominant collective philosophy of humanism (Gortner, 1990), which emphasizes "humanistic (moral) values of caring and the promotion of individual welfare and rights" (Fry, 1981, p. 5). Ontological and epistemic claims about nursing are summarized in three contrasting world views: *reaction, reciprocal interaction,* and *simultaneous action* (Fawcett, 1993). Those three world views emerged from an analysis of four existing sets of world views: mechanism and organicism (Ackoff, 1974; Reese & Overton, 1970); change and persistence (Hall, 1981, 1983; Thomae, 1979; Wells & Stryker, 1988); totality and simultaneity (Parse, 1987); and particulate-deterministic, interactive-integrative, and unitary-transformative (Newman, 1992). The different world views lead to different conceptualizations of the metaparadigm concepts, different statements about the nature of the relationships among those concepts (Altman & Rogoff, 1987), and different ways to generate and test knowledge about the concepts and their connections.

World Views

The *reaction world view* (Table 1–1) contains elements of the mechanistic, persistence, totality, and particulate-deterministic world views. The metaphor for the reaction world view is the compartmentalized human being. The person is viewed as the sum of discrete biological, psychological, sociological, and spiritual parts. The person is regarded as inherently at rest, responding in a reactive manner to external environmental stimuli. Behavior is considered a linear chain of causes and effects, or stimuli and reactions. Change occurs only when the person must modify behaviors to survive. Consequently, stability is valued. Threats to stability are, however, predictable and controllable if enough is known about the stimuli that would force a change. Knowledge is developed only about quantifiable phenomena that can be isolated, defined in a concrete manner, and measured by objective instruments.

The *reciprocal interaction world view* (Table 1–2) is a synthesis of elements from the organismic, simultaneity, totality, change, persistence,

TABLE 1–1. **THE REACTION WORLD VIEW**

Humans are bio-psycho-social-spiritual beings.
Human beings react to external environmental stimuli in a linear, causal manner.
Change occurs only for survival and as a consequence of predictable and controllable antecedent conditions.
Only objective phenomena that can be isolated, defined, observed, and measured are studied.

From Fawcett, J. (1993). From a plethora of paradigms to parsimony in world views. *Nursing Science Quarterly, 6,* 58, with permission.

TABLE 1–2. **THE RECIPROCAL INTERACTION WORLD VIEW**

Human beings are holistic.
Parts are viewed only in the context of the whole.
Human beings are active.
Interactions between human beings and their environments are reciprocal.
Reality is multidimensional, context-dependent, and relative.
Change is a function of multiple antecedent factors.
Change is probabilistic and may be continuous or may be only for survival.
Both objective and subjective phenomena are studied through quantitative and qualitative methods of inquiry.
Emphasis is placed on empirical observations, methodological controls, and inferential data analytic techniques.

From Fawcett, J. (1993). From a plethora of paradigms to parsimony in world views. *Nursing Science Quarterly, 6*, 58, with permission.

and interactive-integrative world views. The metaphor for the reciprocal interaction world view is the holistic, interacting human being. The person is viewed as an integrated, organized entity who is not reducible to discrete parts. Although parts of the human being are acknowledged, they have meaning only within the context of the whole person. The person is regarded as inherently and spontaneously active. The person and the environment interact in a reciprocal manner. Changes in behavior occur throughout life as the result of multiple factors within the individual and within the environment. At times, changes are continuous. At other times, persistence or stability reigns, and change occurs only to foster survival. The probability of change at any given time can only be estimated. Knowledge development focuses on both objective phenomena and subjective experiences and is accomplished by means of both quantitative and qualitative methodologies. Multiple dimensions of experience are taken into account, the context of the person-environment interaction is considered, and the product of knowledge development efforts is regarded as relative to historical time and place. Emphasis is always placed on empirical observations within methodologically controlled situations, and data are analyzed objectively by means of inferential statistics.

The *simultaneous action world view* (Table 1–3) combines elements of the organismic, simultaneity, change, and unitary-transformative world views. The metaphor for the simultaneous action world view is the unitary human being, who is regarded as a holistic, self-organized field. The human being is more than and different from the sum of parts and is recognized through patterns of behavior. The person-environment interchange is a mutual, rhythmical process. Changes in patterns of behavior occur continuously albeit unpredictably as the human being evolves. Although the patterns are sometimes organized and sometimes disorganized, change is ultimately in the direction of increasing organization of behavioral patterns. Knowledge development emphasizes personal be-

TABLE 1-3. **THE SIMULTANEOUS ACTION WORLD VIEW**

Unitary human beings are identified by pattern.
Human beings are in mutual rhythmical interchange with their environments.
Human beings change continuously and evolve as self-organized fields.
Change is unidirectional and unpredictable as human beings move through stages of organization and disorganization to more complex organization.
Phenomena of interest are personal knowledge and pattern recognition.

From Fawcett, J. (1993). From a plethora of paradigms to parsimony in world views. *Nursing Science Quarterly, 6,* 58, with permission.

coming through recognition of patterns. The phenomena of interest are, therefore, the person's inner experiences, feelings, values, thoughts, and choices.

Categories of Nursing Knowledge

Ontological claims about nursing are also reflected in different broad *categories of knowledge*, which represent the diverse approaches found in adjunctive disciplines and in nursing. Categories of knowledge from adjunctive disciplines include *developmental, systems,* and *interaction* approaches (Johnson, 1974; Reilly, 1975; Riehl & Roy, 1980). Categories of knowledge mentioned in the nursing literature are *needs* and *outcomes* (Meleis, 1991); *client focused, person-environment focused,* and *nursing therapeutics focused* (Meleis, 1991); *humanistic* and *energy fields* (Marriner-Tomey, 1989); and *intervention, substitution, conservation, sustenance,* and *enhancement* (Barnum, 1994).

The various categories of knowledge are "different classes of approaches to understanding the person who is a patient, [so that they] not only call for differing forms of practice toward different objectives, but also point to different kinds of phenomena, suggest different kinds of questions, and lead eventually to dissimilar bodies of knowledge" (Johnson, 1974, p. 376). Each category, then, emphasizes different phenomena and leads to different questions about the nurse-patient situation. Consequently, each category fosters development of a different body of knowledge about the person, the environment, health, and nursing.

Development

The *developmental* category of knowledge, which has its origins in the discipline of psychology, emphasizes processes of growth, development, and maturation. Emphasis is also placed on identification of actual and potential developmental problems and delineation of intervention strategies that foster maximum growth and development of people and their environments.

The major thrust of the developmental approach is change, with the assumption made "that there are noticeable differences between the states of a system at different times, that the succession of these states implies the system is heading somewhere, and that there are orderly processes that explain how the system gets from its present state to wherever it is going" (Chin, 1980, p. 30). Following from the assumption of change are the characteristics of direction, identifiable state, form of progression, forces, and potentiality.

The developmental approach postulates that changes are directional and that the individuals, groups, situations, and events of interest are headed in some direction. Chin (1980) outlined the direction of change as: "(a) some goal or end state (developed, mature), (b) the process of becoming (developing, maturing), or (c) the degree of achievement toward some goal or end state (increased development, increase in maturity)" (p. 31).

The characteristic of identifiable state refers to the different states of the person seen over time. Those states frequently are termed stages, levels, phases, or periods of development. Such states may be quantitatively or qualitatively differentiated from one another. As Chin (1980) points out, shifts in state may be either small, nondiscernible steps that eventually are recognized as change, or sudden, cataclysmic changes.

Developmental change, according to Chin (1980), is possible through four different forms of progression. First, unidirectional development may be postulated, such that "once a stage is worked through, the client system shows continued progression and normally never turns back" (p. 31). Second, developmental change may take the form of a spiral, so that although return to a previous problem may occur, the problem is dealt with at a higher level. Third, development may be seen as "phases which occur and recur . . . where no chronological priority is assigned to each state; there are cycles" (p. 32). Fourth, development may take the form of "a branching out into differentiated forms and processes, each part increasing in its specialization and at the same acquiring its own autonomy and significance" (p. 32).

The developmental approach also postulates the existence of forces, defined by Chin (1980) as "causal factors producing development and growth" (p. 32). Those forces may be viewed as a natural component of the person undergoing change, a coping response to new situations and environmental factors that leads to growth and development or as internal tensions within the person that at some time reach a peak and cause a disruption that leads to further growth and development.

The developmental approach further postulates that people have the inherent potential for change. Potentiality may be overt or latent, triggered by internal states or certain environmental conditions. The characteristics of the developmental category of knowledge are listed in Table 1–4.

TABLE 1–4. **CHARACTERISTICS OF THE DEVELOPMENTAL APPROACH**

Growth, development, and maturation
Change
Direction of change
Identifiable state
Form of progression
Forces
Potentiality

Systems

The *systems* category of knowledge, which originated in the disciplines of biology and physics, treats phenomena "as if there existed organization, interaction, interdependency, and integration of parts and elements" (Chin, 1980, p. 24). The systems approach emphasizes identification of actual and potential problems in the function of systems and delineation of intervention strategies that maximize efficient and effective system operation. The focus of the systems approach, then, is the examination of the system, its parts, and their relationships at a given time. In contrast to the developmental approach, change is of secondary importance in the systems approach.

The major features of the systems approach are the system and its environment. Hall and Fagen (1968) defined system as "a set of objects together with relationships between the objects and between their attributes" (p. 83). They defined environment as "the set of all objects a change in whose attributes affect the system and also those objects whose attributes are changed by the behavior of the system" (p. 83). When viewing any particular phenomenon, the designation of what is system and what is environment depends on the situation. Thus, a system could be the person whose parts are body organs and whose environment is the family. The system also might be the community, whose parts are families and whose environment is the state in which the community is located.

Systems are open or closed. An open system "maintains itself in a continuous inflow and outflow, a building up and breaking down of components, [whereas a closed system is] "considered to be isolated from [its] environment" (Bertalanffy, 1968, p. 39). Moreover, open systems continuously import energy in a process called negative entropy or negentropy, so that the system may become more differentiated, more complex, and more ordered. Conversely, closed systems exhibit entropy, such that they move toward increasing disorder.

According to Bertalanffy (1968), all living organisms are open systems. Although closed systems therefore do not exist in nature, it sometimes is convenient to view a system as if it had no interaction with its environment (Chin, 1980). The artificiality of that view, however, must be taken into account.

Important characteristics of the systems approach are boundary; tension, stress, strain, and conflict; equilibrium and steady state; and feedback. Boundary refers to the line of demarcation between a system and its environment. The placement of the boundary must take all relevant system parts into account. Thus, boundary is "the line forming a closed circle around selected variables, where there is less interchange of energy . . . across the line of the circle than within the delimiting circle" (Chin, 1980, p. 24). Boundaries may be thought of as more or less permeable. The greater the boundary permeability, the greater the interchange of energy between the system and its environment.

Tension, stress, strain, and conflict are terms that refer to the forces that alter system structure. Chin (1980) explained that the differences in system parts, as well as the need to adjust to outside disturbances, lead to different amounts of tension within the system. He further noted that internal tensions arising from the system's structural arrangements are called the stresses and strains of the system. Conflict occurs when tensions accumulate and become opposed along the lines of two or more components of the system. Change then occurs to resolve the conflict.

Systems are assumed to tend to move toward a balance between internal and external forces. Chin (1980) explained that "when the balance is thought of as a fixed point or level, it is called 'equilibrium.' 'Steady state,' on the other hand, is the term . . . used to describe the balanced relationship of parts that is not dependent upon any fixed equilibrium point or level" (p. 25). Bertalanffy (1968) maintained that steady state, which also is referred to as a dynamic equilibrium, is characteristic of living open systems. He further commented that the steady state is maintained by a continuous flow of energy within the system and between the system and its environment.

The flow of energy between a system and its environment is called feedback. Chin (1980) described feedback as a series of outputs and inputs across the system-environment boundary. He claimed that systems

> are affected by and in turn affect the environment. While affecting the environment, a process we call output, systems gather information about how they are doing. Such information is then fed back into the system as input to guide and steer its operations. (p. 27)

The feedback process works so that as open systems interact with their environments, any change in the system is associated with a change in the environment, and vice versa. The characteristics of the systems category of knowledge are listed in Table 1–5.

Interaction

The *interaction* category of knowledge, which stems from the discipline of sociology, emphasizes social acts and relationships between peo-

TABLE 1–5. **CHARACTERISTICS OF THE SYSTEMS APPROACH**

Integration of parts
System
Environment
Open and closed systems
Boundary
Tension, stress, strain, conflict
Equilibrium and steady state
Feedback

ple. The focus, therefore, is on identification of actual and potential problems in interpersonal relationships and delineation of intervention strategies that promote optimal socialization.

The interaction approach is derived primarily from symbolic interactionism, which "sees human beings as creatures who define and classify situations, including themselves, and who choose ways of acting toward and within them" (Benoliel, 1977, p. 110). Symbolic interactionism "postulates that the importance of social life lies in providing the [person] with language, self-concept, role-taking ability, and other skills" (Heiss, 1976, p. 467). The major characteristics of the interaction approach are perception, communication, role, and self-concept.

The person's perceptions of other people, the environment, situations, and events—that is, the awareness and experience of phenomena—depend on meanings attached to those phenomena. The meanings, or definitions as they sometimes are called, determine how the person behaves in a given situation. Thus, the key data to be gathered when working in the context of the interaction approach are the person's perceptions, that is, his or her definition of the situation. Heiss (1981) explained,

> The fact that an other is, in fact, kindly or cruel may not be very significant. The fact that we define him or her as one or the other is important, because—regardless of the facts—we will act on that belief. (p. 3)

The person's perceptions are derived from social interactions with others. People may adopt fully, modify, or reject others' definitions of phenomena, but they are always influenced in some way by others. This is especially so when the other is significant to the person.

During social interactions, people communicate with one another. Communication is through language, "a system of significant symbols" (Heiss, 1981, p. 5). Communication, therefore, involves the transfer of arbitrary meanings of things from one person to another. Thus, people must communicate with one another to find out each other's perceptions of the particular situation.

Communication is important in learning roles, which are "prescriptions for behavior which are associated with particular actor-other combinations. They are the ways we think people of a particular kind ought to act toward various categories of others" (Heiss, 1981, p. 65). Each person has many different roles, each one providing a behavioral repertoire. We adopt the behaviors associated with a given role, when, through communication, we determine that a given role is called for in a particular situation.

The person's ability to perform roles, and to perform them according to self-imposed and societal standards, influences self-concept. "The self-concept is the individual's thoughts and feelings about himself" (Heiss, 1981, p. 83). An important aspect of self-concept is self-evaluation, which refers to "our view of how good we are at what we think we are" (Heiss, 1981, p. 83).

An especially important feature of the interaction approach is the emphasis on the person as an active participant in interactions. People are thought to actively evaluate communication from others, rather than passively accept their ideas. Moreover, they actively set goals on the basis of their perceptions of the relevant factors in a given situation. The characteristics of the interaction category of knowledge are listed in Table 1-6.

Other Categories

Other categories of nursing knowledge have been identified in recent years. The little that has been written about those approaches is summarized below, and their characteristics are listed in Table 1-7.

NEEDS AND OUTCOMES. The needs and outcomes categories were developed by Meleis (1991), who also included an interaction category in her classification of schools of nursing thought. The needs category focuses on nurses' functions and consideration of the patient in terms of a hierarchy of needs. When patients cannot fulfill their own needs, nursing care is required. The function of the nurse is to provide the necessary action to help patients meet their needs. The needs category reduces the human being to a set of needs, and nursing, to a set of functions. Nurses are

TABLE 1-6. **CHARACTERISTICS OF THE INTERACTION APPROACH**

Social acts and relationships
Perception
Communication
Role
Self-concept

TABLE 1–7. **CHARACTERISTICS OF OTHER CATEGORIES OF
NURSING KNOWLEDGE**

Category	Characteristics
Needs	Nursing as set of functions to help patients meet their needs
Outcomes	Outcomes of nursing care
Client-focused	Comprehensive nursing perspective of the client
Person-environment-focused	Relationship between clients and their environment
Nursing therapeutics	What nurses shoud do under what circumstances
Humanistic	Nursing as art and science
Energy fields	Energy
Intervention	Manipulation of patient or environmental variables to effect change
Substitution	Provision of substitutes for lost or impaired patient capabilities
Conservation	Preservation of beneficial aspects of patient's situation
Sustenance	Helping patient endure insults to health
Enhancement	Improvement of quality of patient's existence

portrayed as the final decision makers for nursing care. The *outcomes* category was not well described by Meleis (1991), who commented only that emphasis is placed on the outcomes of nursing care and comprehensive descriptions of the recipient of care.

CLIENTS, PERSON-ENVIRONMENT INTERACTION, AND NURSING THERAPEUTICS. Meleis (1991) identified a second classification scheme that included the categories of *client*, *person-environment interaction*, and *nursing therapeutics*, as well as the category of interactions. The *client* category refers to a comprehensive focus on the client as viewed from a nursing perspective. The *person-environment* category emphasizes a focus on the relationship between clients and their environments. The *nursing therapeutics* category deals with a focus on what nurses should do and under what circumstances they should act.

HUMANISTIC AND ENERGY FIELDS CATEGORIES. Marriner-Tomey (1989) identified two other categories, the *humanistic* and *energy fields*. Her classification scheme also included an interpersonal relationships category, which is similar to the interaction category already discussed in this chapter. Marriner-Tomey mentioned that the *humanistic* category views nursing as an art and science, and she implied that the *energy field* category incorporates the concept of energy. Of interst is the fact that Marriner-Tomey (1994) neither retained her classification scheme in the third edition of her book, nor provided an explanation for that omission.

INTERVENTION, SUBSTITUTION, CONSERVATION, SUSTENANCE, AND ENHANCEMENT. Barnum (1994) developed a substantially different classification scheme for categories of nursing knowledge. The scheme is based on "the character of the nursing act in relation to the patient" (p. 211). The *intervention* category emphasizes the nurse's professional actions and decisions and regards the patient as an object of nursing rather than a participant in nursing care. Agency, or action, rests with the nurse, who makes the care decision and manipulates selected patient or environmental variables to bring about change.

The *substitution* category focuses on provision of substitutes for patient capabilities that cannot be enacted or have been lost. Agency rests with the patient, in that the patient exercises his or her will and physical control to the greatest possible extent. In contrast, the *conservation* category emphasizes preservation of beneficial aspects of the patient's situation that are threatened by illness or actual or potential problems. That category bridges the polarity of agency seen in the intervention and substitution categories in that agency rests with nurses, but they act to conserve the existing capabilities of the patient.

The *sustenance* category emphasizes helping the patient endure insults to health. The focus is on supporting the patient and building psychological and physiological coping mechanisms. The *enhancement* category regards nursing as a way to improve the quality of the patient's existence following a health insult.

Conceptual Models, Philosophies, and the Metaparadigm

As can be seen in Figure 1–1, philosophies do not follow directly in line from the metaparadigm of the discipline, and they do not directly precede conceptual models. Rather, the metaparadigm of a discipline identifies the phenomena about which philosophical claims are made. The unique focus and content of each conceptual model then reflect the philosophical claims. For example, a philosophy may make the claim that all people are equal. That philosophical claim would be reflected in a conceptual model that depicts the nurse and the patient as equal partners in health care (Kershaw, 1990).

THEORIES

The next component in the structural hierarchy of nursing knowledge is the **theory** (Figure 1–1). A theory is less abstract than its parent conceptual model but more abstract than the empirical indicators that operationalize the theory concepts. Theories are made up of relatively specific and concrete concepts and propositions that purport to account for or organize some phenomena (Barnum, 1994).

Theories vary in scope; that is, they vary in the relative level of concreteness and specificity of their concepts and propositions. Theories that are broadest in scope are called *grand theories*. These theories are made up of rather abstract and general concepts and propositions that cannot be generated or tested empirically. Indeed, grand theories are developed through thoughtful and insightful appraisal of existing ideas or creative intellectual leaps beyond existing knowledge. Examples of grand theories in nursing include Leininger's (1991a) theory of culture care diversity and universality, Newman's (1986) theory of health as expanding consciousness, and Parse's (1981, 1992) theory of human becoming.

The fact that grand theories are less abstract than conceptual models is illustrated by Parse's theory, which was derived in part from Rogers' (1970) conceptual model. Rogers' conceptual model is a frame of reference for all of nursing, whereas Parse's theory limits the domain of interest to the lived experience of health. The concepts of Parse's theory, like all grand theory concepts, are rather abstract. They are human becoming, meaning, rhythmicity, and cotranscendence. The propositions also are rather abstract. For example, one nonrelational proposition describes meaning as follows: "Structuring meaning multidimensionally is cocreating reality through the languaging of valuing and imaging" (Parse, 1981, p. 69). A relational proposition links all four concepts: "[Human becoming] is structuring meaning multidimensionally in cocreating rhythmical patterns of relating while cotranscending with the possibles" (Parse, 1981, p. 67).

Middle-range theories are narrower in scope than grand theories, encompassing a limited number of concepts and a limited aspect of the real world. Middle-range theories are, therefore, made up of concepts and propositions that are empirically measurable. Examples of middle-range theories in nursing include Orlando's (1961) theory of the deliberative nursing process, Peplau's (1952, 1992) theory of interpersonal relations, and Watson's (1985) theory of human caring.

The specificity of middle-range theory concepts and propositions is illustrated by Orlando's theory, which predicts the effects of using a particular nursing process on patients' behavior. The relatively specific and concrete concepts of Orlando's theory are patient's behavior, with the dimensions of need for help and improvement; nurse's reaction, with the dimensions of perception, thought, and feeling; and nurse's activity, with the dimensions of automatic nursing process and deliberative nursing process. The theory contains nonrelational propositions that define each concept and its dimensions and relational propositions that specify the linkages between the concepts and their dimensions.

The definitional propositions of Orlando's theory, like those of other middle-range theories, include relatively precise theoretical definitions for each concept and operational definitions that specify how the concepts are measured. For example, the concept of nurse's activity is defined theoretically as "observable behavior, i.e., what the [nurse] says verbally and/or manifests nonverbally" (Orlando, 1961, p. 60). That concept can be operationally defined as the instructions, suggestions, directions, explanations, information, requests, and questions directed toward the patient that are identified in transcripts of tape recordings of nurse-patient contacts (Orlando, 1961, 1972).

The relational propositions of Orlando's theory, like those of all middle-range theories, specify empirically testable linkages between concepts. The link between nurse's activity and patient's behavior is specified in the following relational proposition: "An observation shared and explored with the nurse is immediately useful in ascertaining and meeting [the patient's] need [for help] or finding out that [the patient] is not in need at that time" (Orlando, 1961, p. 36).

Unique, Borrowed, and Shared Nursing Theories

Inasmuch as each theory deals only with a limited aspect of reality, many theories are needed to deal with all of the phenomena of interest to a discipline. Consequently, each conceptual model is more fully specified by several grand and/or middle-range theories, as indicated in Figure 1–1 by the subscript notation, 1 . . . n. Some of those theories are unique to nursing, and others are borrowed from adjunctive disciplines.

The theories developed by Leininger, Newman, Orlando, Parse, Peplau, and Watson are among a growing list of unique nursing theories. Other unique nursing theories, including King's (1990) theory of goal attainment and Orem's (1991) theories of self-care deficit, self-care, and nursing systems, are discussed in later chapters of this book.

Many other theories used by nurses have been borrowed from other disciplines. Theories of stress, coping, locus of control, and self-efficacy are just a few examples of borrowed theories. Unfortunately, these theories sometimes are used with no consideration given to their empirical adequacy in nursing situations. There is, however, increasing awareness of the need to test borrowed theories to determine if they are empirically adequate in nursing situations. The theory testing work by Lowery and associates (1987) is an outstanding example of what can happen when a theory, borrowed in this case from psychology, is tested in the real world of acute and chronic illness. The investigators determined that a basic proposition of attribution theory, stating that people search for causes to make sense of their lives, has not been fully supported in their research with patients with arthritis, diabetes, hypertension, or myocardial infarction. That result means that attribution theory cannot be considered a shared theory, that is, a theory that is borrowed from another discipline but found to be empirically adequate in situations that are relevant to nursing.

Further research should determine whether a modification of attribution theory is empirically adequate in nursing situations or if an entirely new theory is required. An example of a borrowed theory that appears to be developing into a shared theory is self-efficacy. That theory was developed initially in the discipline of social psychology and is beginning to receive support in nursing situations (e.g., Froman & Owen, 1990; Hickey, Owen, & Froman, 1992).

Some nurses continue to claim that there are few, if any, unique or shared nursing theories. It is likely, however, that the apparent paucity of recognizable nursing theories is due to some investigators' failure to be explicit about the theoretical components of their studies and to label their work as theories. Thus, the ideas presented by nurses in books, monographs, and journal articles should be closely examined for evidence of the concepts and propositions that make up theories. Identification of the components of a theory is accomplished by the technique of theory formalization, also called theoretical substruction. Discussion of that technique is beyond the scope of this book. Readers who are interested in theory formalization are, therefore, referred to Hinshaw's (1979) pioneering work and Fawcett and Downs' (1992) more recent work.

Distinctions Between Conceptual Models and Theories

Throughout this book, emphasis is placed on the point that a conceptual model is not a theory, and a theory is not a conceptual model. This point requires further discussion because there is still considerable confusion about these two components of the structural hierarchy of nursing knowledge in the minds of some students and scholars. The distinctions between conceptual models and theories described here and the meaning ascribed to conceptual models are in keeping with earlier works by Rogers (1970), Johnson (1974), and Reilly (1975) in nursing; Reese and Overton (1970) in developmental psychology; and Nye and Berardo (1966) in sociology.

Although some writers consider distinctions between conceptual models and theories a semantic point (e.g., Flaskerud & Halloran, 1980; Meleis, 1991), the issue should not be dismissed so easily. The distinction should be made because of the differences in the way that conceptual models and theories are used. Indeed, if one is to know what to do next, then one must know whether the starting point is a conceptual model or a theory. As can be seen in Figure 1–1, conceptual models and theories differ in their level of abstraction.

A conceptual model is an abstract and general system of concepts and propositions. A theory, in contrast, deals with one or more relatively specific and concrete concepts and propositions. Conceptual models are general guides that must be specified further by relevant and logically congruent theories before action can occur.

Distinguishing between conceptual models and theories on the basis of level of abstraction raises the question of how abstract is abstract enough for a work to be considered a conceptual model. Although the decision in a few cases may be somewhat arbitrary, the following rule serves as one guideline for distinguishing between conceptual models and theories. The rule requires determination of the purpose of the work.

If the purpose of the work was to articulate a body of distinctive knowledge for the whole of the discipline of nursing, the work most likely is a conceptual model. Given that that was the explicitly stated purpose of such authors as Johnson (1980), King (1971), Levine (1969), Neuman (Neuman & Young, 1972), Orem (1971), Rogers (1970), and Roy (1976), their works are classified as conceptual models.

If, however, the purpose of the work was to further develop one aspect of a conceptual model, the work most likely is a grand theory. For example, both Newman (1986) and Parse (1981, 1992) elected to further develop the concept of health from the perspective of Rogers' (1970) conceptual model. As can be discerned from these examples, nurse scholars who consider conceptual models and grand theories to be synonymous (e.g., Barnum, 1994; Kim, 1983; Marriner-Tomey, 1994) mislead their readers.

If the purpose was to describe, explain, or predict specific and concrete phenomena, the work most likely is a middle-range theory. For example, Peplau's (1952, 1992) theory of interpersonal relations is a description and classification of the stages of the nurse-patient relationship. Peplau neither did, nor did she intend to, address the entire domain of nursing. Consequently, her theory is classified as a middle-range theory.

In summary, if a given work is an abstract, general, and comprehensive perspective of the metaparadigm of nursing, it is a conceptual model. If the work is more specific, concrete, and restricted to a more limited range of phenomena than that identified by the conceptual model, it is a grand or middle-range theory.

Another rule for distinguishing between conceptual models and theories requires determination of how many levels of knowledge are needed before the work may be applied in particular nursing situations. If, for example, the work identifies physiological needs as an assessment parameter but does not explain the differences between normal and pathological functions of body systems in concrete terms, it most likely is a conceptual model. As such, the work is not directly applicable in clinical practice. A theory of normal and pathological functions must be linked with the conceptual model so that judgments about the physiological functions of body systems may be made. Conversely, if the work includes a detailed description of behavior, or an explanation of how particular factors influence particular behaviors, it most likely is a middle-range theory. In that case, the work may be directly applied in clinical practice.

The rule is also exemplified by the number of steps required before empirical testing can occur (Reilly, 1975). A conceptual model cannot be tested directly, because its concepts and propositions are not empirically measurable. More specific and concrete concepts and propositions have to be derived from the conceptual model; that is, a middle-range theory must be formulated. These more concrete concepts then must be defined in measurable ways, and hypotheses stating specific, observable relationships must be derived from the propositions of the theory. Four steps are, therefore, required before a conceptual model can be tested, albeit indirectly. First, the conceptual model must be formulated; second, a theory must be derived from the conceptual model; third, instruments or procedures that can measure the theory concepts must be identified; and fourth, empirically testable hypotheses must be specified. In contrast, only three steps are required for empirical testing of a middle-range theory. First, the theory must be stated; second, instruments or procedures that can measure the theory concepts must be identified; and third, empirically testable hypotheses must be specified.

Failure to distinguish between a conceptual model and a theory leads to considerable misunderstanding and inappropriate expectations about the work. When a conceptual model is labeled a theory, expectations regarding empirical testing and clinical applicability immediately arise. When such expectations cannot be met, the work is frequently regarded as inadequate. Similarly, when a theory is labeled a conceptual model, expectations regarding comprehensiveness arise. When those expectations cannot be met, that work also may be regarded as inadequate.

The meaning given to conceptual models in this book should not be confused with the meaning of model found in the philosophy of science literature and some nursing literature. The latter refers to representations of testable theories. Rudner (1966), for example, defined a model for a theory as "an alternative interpretation of the same calculus of which the theory itself is an interpretation" (p. 24). That kind of a model is made up of ideas or diagrams that are more familiar to the novice than are the concepts and propositions of the theory. Thus, the model is a heuristic device that facilitates understanding of the theory. Rudner illustrated this by the analogy of the flow of water through pipes as a model for a theory of electric current wires. So-called models that are actually diagrams of theories are found with increasing frequency in reports of nursing research. For example, Hawkes and Holm (1993) labeled their diagram of the relationships between the concepts of a middle-range theory of leisure-time physical activity as a model.

EMPIRICAL INDICATORS

The generation and testing of middle-range theories is accomplished through the use of **empirical indicators,** which are the fifth and final component in the structural hierarchy of contemporary nursing knowledge (see Figure 1–1). Empirical indicators are the very specific and concrete real world proxies for middle-range theory concepts. More specifically, they are the actual instruments, experimental conditions, and procedures that are used to observe or measure the concepts of a middle-range theory. For example, the Relationship Form (Forchuk & Brown, 1989) is the instrument that serves as the empirical indicator for the concept of the nurse-patient relationship in Peplau's (1952) theory of interpersonal relations in nursing. In particular, the instrument measures the progress of the nurse-patient relationship through the four phases delineated by Peplau: orientation, identification, exploitation, and resolution.

Conceptual Models, Empirical Indicators, Theories, Philosophies, and the Metaparadigm

Empirical indicators are directly connected to theories by means of the operational definition for each middle-range theory concept. As can be seen in Figure 1–1, there is no direct connection between empirical indicators and conceptual models, philosophies, or the metaparadigm. Consequently, these components of the structural hierarchy cannot be subjected to empirical testing. Rather, the credibility of a conceptual model is determined indirectly through empirical testing of middle-range theories that are derived from or linked with the model. Furthermore, philosophies cannot be empirically tested either directly or indirectly because they are statements of beliefs and values. Philosophies should, however, be defendable on the basis of logic or through dialogue (Salsberry, 1991). Similarly, the metaparadigm cannot be empirically tested but should be defendable on the basis of dialogue and debate about the phenomena of interest to the discipline as a whole.

CONCEPTUAL-THEORETICAL-EMPIRICAL SYSTEMS OF NURSING KNOWLEDGE

In nursing, conceptual models now are used as general guides for the design of research projects, educational curricula, administrative systems, and clinical protocols. Conceptual models can act as guides for those endeavors because they contain a set of statements about what sorts of entities and processes make up the domain of inquiry and a set of epistemic and methodological norms about how that domain can be applied in real world situations (Laudan, 1981).

The application of a domain of inquiry in the real world of research, education, administration, and practice occurs when a conceptual model is linked with relevant middle-range theories and empirical indicators to create a **conceptual-theoretical-empirical system of nursing knowledge.** Currently, many of the theories used to amplify the concepts and propositions of a nursing model are borrowed from adjunctive disciplines, including psychology, sociology, biology, physics, and chemistry. When borrowed theories are linked with conceptual models, care must be taken to ensure logical congruence. Whall (1980) presented the first substantial discussion in the nursing literature of elements to consider when assessing congruence between conceptual models of nursing and borrowed theories. She proposed that conceptual models and theories must be examined for their stands on holism and linearity. Holism is a major characteristic of both the reciprocal interaction and simultaneous action world views, whereas linearity is a central characteristic of the reaction world view. These three world views were discussed earlier in this chapter. Whall's discussion suggested that if the conceptual model and the theory are not congruent with regard to world view, the theory should be discarded and another more congruent one chosen; otherwise the theory should be reformulated so that it is congruent with the model. Inasmuch as the conceptual model is the more abstract starting point, the theory — not the model — is reformulated to ensure congruence.

Examples of construction of logically congruent conceptual-theoretical systems of nursing knowledge using reformulated borrowed theories are given in Fitzpatrick and associates (1982), Whall (1986), and McFarlane (1988). The same care to ensure logical congruence must be taken if a borrowed theory is to be linked with a conceptual model of nursing, or if a unique nursing theory not directly derived from the conceptual model of interest is to be linked with that model.

The instruments and procedures selected to measure theory concepts must not only be valid empirical indicators of those concepts but also they must be logically congruent with the conceptual model that is guiding the practical activity. Inasmuch as most instruments currently used by nurses are borrowed from other disciplines, extreme care must be taken to ensure that the instruments represent the intent of the conceptual model. Instruments that have been directly derived from conceptual models of nursing are discussed in later chapters.

The following discussion focuses on general considerations in constructing conceptual-theoretical-empirical systems of nursing knowledge in the areas of research, education, administration, and clinical practice. Later chapters document the use of conceptual models of nursing and related theories and empirical indicators in various situations.

Nursing Research

The function of nursing research is to generate or test nursing theories. Every theory development effort is guided by a conceptual model, which acts as a research tradition. Laudan (1981) explained the relationships between conceptual models as research traditions, theories, and empirical testing. He stated,

> Research traditions are not directly testable, both because their ontologies are too general to yield specific predictions and because their methodological components, being rules or norms, are not straightforwardly testable assertions about matters of fact. Associated with any active research tradition is a family of theories. . . . The theories . . . share the ontology of the parent research tradition and can be tested and evaluated using its methodological norms. (p. 151)

When a conceptual model is used to guide research, the metaparadigm concept *person* becomes the study subject. *Environment* becomes the relevant surroundings of the subject, as well as the research infrastructure available to the investigator. *Health* refers to the subject's state of wellness or illness, and *nursing* refers to the research processes. A fully developed conceptual model reflects a particular research tradition that includes the following six rules that guide theory generation and testing through all phases of a study:

- The first rule identifies the phenomena that are to be studied.

- The second rule identifies the distinctive nature of the problems to be studied and the purposes to be fulfilled by the research.

- The third rule identifies the subjects who are to provide the data and the settings in which data are to be gathered.

- The fourth rule identifies the research designs, instruments, and procedures that are to be employed.

- The fifth rule identifies the methods to be employed in reducing and analyzing the data.

- The sixth rule identifies the nature of contributions that the research will make to the advancement of knowledge. (Laudan, 1981; Schlotfeldt, 1975)

Thus, a conceptual model contains the concepts from which specific variables are derived for the research and the general propositions from which testable hypotheses eventually are derived. In addition, the conceptual model guides the selection of appropriate empirical indicators. The subject matter of the study might be one concept or the relations between two or more concepts. Theories borrowed from other disciplines may be linked with the conceptual model in order to test the empirical adequacy of the theory in nursing situations. Also, a study may involve generation or testing of a unique nursing theory.

The findings of research based on explicit conceptual-theoretical-empirical systems of nursing knowledge are, of course, used to evaluate the empirical adequacy of the theory. These findings also constitute indirect evidence regarding the conceptual model and are used to evaluate its credibility. Thus, the credibility of the conceptual model should be considered in addition to the empirical adequacy of the theory whenever research is conducted. Further discussion of credibility determination is presented in Chapter 2.

Nursing Education

In nursing education, the conceptual model, or conceptual framework as it usually is called, provides the general outline for curriculum content and teaching-learning activities. *Person* becomes the student, and *environment* becomes the educational setting. *Health* refers to the student's state of wellness or illness, and *nursing* refers to the educational goals, outcomes, and processes. Consequently, a fully developed conceptual model represents a particular view of and approach to nursing education. The curricular structure and educational processes are specified in the following four rules inherent in each conceptual model:

- The first rule identifies the distinctive focus of the curriculum and the purposes to be fulfilled by nursing education.

- The second rule identifies the general nature and sequence of the content to be presented.

- The third rule identifies the settings in which nursing education occurs and the characteristics of the students.

- The fourth rule identifies the teaching-learning strategies to be employed.

When a conceptual model is used for curriculum construction, it must be linked with theories about education and the teaching-learning process, as well as with substantive theoretical content from nursing and adjunctive disciplines (Fawcett, 1985). In addition, appropriate empirical indicators, in the form of the actual classroom content, clinical experiences, and student assignments, must be identified. The resulting conceptual-theoretical-empirical system then applies to the patient, the student, and the educator.

Nursing Administration

When a conceptual model is used in nursing administration, it provides a systematic structure for thinking about administrative structures, for observations of the administrative situation, and for interpreting what is seen in administrative settings (Fawcett et al., 1989). *Person* may refer to the staff of a clinical agency, the department of nursing as a whole, or even to the entire agency. *Environment* becomes the relevant clinical milieu for the staff and the surroundings of the department of nursing and the clinical agency. *Health* refers to the wellness or illness of the staff or the functional state of the department or agency. *Nursing* encompasses the management strategies and administrative policies used by the nurse administrator on behalf of or in conjunction with the staff, the department of nursing, and the agency.

Each fully developed conceptual model, then, represents a particular view of and approach to administration of nursing services. The administrative structure and management practices are specified in the following three rules that are inherent in each conceptual model:

- The first rule identifies the distinctive focus of nursing in the clinical agency and the purpose to be fulfilled by nursing services.

- The second rule identifies the characteristics of nursing personnel and the settings in which nursing services are delivered.

- The third rule identifies the management strategies and administrative policies to be employed.

When a conceptual model is used to guide administrative practices, it must be linked with theories of organization and management developed in nursing and adjunctive disciplines. Moreover, empirical indicators in the form of specific management strategies must be identified, and administrative policies must be formulated. The resulting conceptual-theoretical-empirical structure is then applicable to the patient, the nursing staff, and the nurse administrator.

Clinical Nursing Practice

Conceptual models of nursing also provide general guidelines for nursing practice. More specifically, a fully developed conceptual model represents a particular view of and approach to nursing practice. The original meaning ascribed to each metaparadigm concept (p. 7) is used when a conceptual model guides nursing practice. The domain of nursing practice and nursing processes are specified in the following four rules that are inherent in the conceptual model:

- The first rule identifies the purposes to be fulfilled by nursing practice and the general nature of the clinical problems to be considered.

- The second rule identifies the settings in which nursing practice occurs and the characteristics of legitimate recipients of nursing care.

- The third rule identifies the nursing process to be employed and the technologies to be used, including parameters for assessment, labels for patient problems, a strategy for planning, a typology of interventions, and criteria for evaluation of outcomes.

- The fourth rule identifies the nature of contributions that nursing practice makes to the well-being of recipients of nursing care.

Thus, a conceptual model guides all aspects of clinical practice and all steps of the nursing process. The specifics of nursing assessment, diagnosis, intervention, and evaluation, must, however, come from theories. Although the conceptual model may, for example, direct the clinician to look for certain categories of problems in adaptation, theories of adaptation are needed to describe, to explain, and to predict manifestations of actual or potential patient problems in particular situations. Similarly, theories are needed to direct the particular nursing interventions required in such situations. The conceptual-theoretical-empirical structure is completed when relevant empirical indicators are identified, including standards for nursing practice, a patient classification system, a quality assurance program, a method of nursing care delivery, and a clinical information system.

CONCLUSION

This chapter presented the definition and function of each component of the structural hierarchy of nursing knowledge. In addition, the distinctions between conceptual models and theories were discussed, and the formation of conceptual-theoretical-empirical systems of nursing knowledge was described. The distinctions between conceptual models and theories mandate separate analysis and evaluation schemes. Chapter 2 will present a framework expressly designed for the analysis and evaluation of conceptual models of nursing. A framework for analysis and evaluation of nursing theories is given in the companion to this book, *Analysis and Evaluation of Nursing Theories* (Fawcett, 1993).

REFERENCES

Ackoff, R.L. (1974). *Redesigning the future: A systems approach to societal problems.* New York: John Wiley & Sons.

Akinsanya, J.A. (1989). Introduction. *Recent Advances in Nursing, 24,* i–ii.

Altman, I., & Rogoff, B. (1987). World views in psychology: Trait, interactional, organismic, and transactional perspectives. In D. Stokols & I. Altman (Eds.), *Handbook of environmental psychology* (pp. 7–40). New York: John Wiley & Sons.

Barnum, B.J.S. (1994). *Nursing theory: Analysis, application, evaluation* (4th ed.). Philadelphia: JB Lippincott.

Benoliel, J.Q. (1977). The interaction between theory and research. *Nursing Outlook, 25,* 108–113.

Ben-Sira, Z. (1987). Social work in health care: Needs, challenges and implications for structuring practice. *Social Work in Health Care, 13,* 79–100.

Bertalanffy, L. (1968). *General system theory.* New York: George Braziller.

Biley, F. (1990). Wordly wise. *Nursing (London), 4*(24), 37.

Chin, R. (1980). The utility of systems models and developmental models for practitioners. In J.P. Riehl & C. Roy, *Conceptual models for nursing practice* (2nd ed., pp. 21–37). New York: Appleton-Century-Crofts.

Christensen, P.J., & Kenney, J.W. (Eds.), (1990). *Nursing process: Application of conceptual models* (3rd ed.). St. Louis: CV Mosby.

Conway, M.E. (1985). Toward greater specificity in defining nursing's metaparadigm. *Advances in Nursing Science, 7*(4), 73–81.

Conway, M.E. (1989, April). Nursing's metaparadigm: Current perspectives. Paper presented at the Spring Doctoral Forum, Medical College of Georgia School of Nursing, Augusta.

Donaldson, S.K. & Crowley, D.M. (1978). The discipline of nursing. *Nursing Outlook, 26,* 113–120.

Eckberg, D.L., & Hill, L., Jr. (1979). The paradigm concept and sociology: A critical review. *American Sociological Review, 44,* 925–937.

Eriksson, K. (1989). Caring paradigms. A study of the origins and the development of caring paradigms among nursing students. *Scandinavian Journal of Caring Sciences, 3,* 169–176.

Fawcett, J. (1978). The "what" of theory development. In *Theory development: What, why, how?* (pp. 17–33). New York: National League for Nursing.

Fawcett, J. (1984a). *Analysis and evaluation of conceptual models of nursing.* Philadelphia: FA Davis.

Fawcett, J. (1984b). The metaparadigm of nursing. Current status and future refinements. *Image: The Journal of Nursing Scholarship, 16,* 84–87.

Fawcett, J. (1985). Theory: Basis for the study and practice of nursing education. *Journal of Nursing Education, 24,* 226–229.

Fawcett, J. (1989). Analysis and evaluation of conceptual models of nursing (2nd ed.). Philadelphia: FA Davis.

Fawcett, J. (1992). The metaparadigm of nursing: International in scope and substance. In K. Krause & P. Åstedt-Kurki (Eds.), International perspectives on nursing: A joint effort to explore nursing internationally (Serie A 3/92, pp. 13–21). Tampere, Finland: Tampere University Department of Nursing.

Fawcett, J. (1993). Analysis and evaluation of nursing theories. Philadelphia: FA Davis.

Fawcett, J., Botter, M.L., Burritt, J., Crossley, J.D., & Frink, B.B. (1989). Conceptual models of nursing and organization theories. In B. Henry, C. Arndt, M. Di Vincenti, & A. Marriner-Tomey (Eds.), Dimensions of nursing administration: Theory, research, education, practice (pp. 143–154). Boston: Blackwell Scientific Publications.

Fawcett, J., & Downs, F.S. (1992). The relationship of theory and research (2nd ed.). Philadelphia: FA Davis.

Fitzpatrick, J.J., Whall, A.L., Johnston, R.L., & Floyd, J.A. (1982). Nursing models and their psychiatric mental health applications. Bowie, MD: Brady.

Flaskerud, J.H., & Halloran, E.J. (1980). Areas of agreement in nursing theory development. Advances in Nursing Science, 3(1), 1–7.

Forchuk, C., & Brown, B. (1989). Establishing a nurse-client relationship. Journal of Psychosocial Nursing and Mental Health Services, 27(2), 30–34.

Frank, L.K. (1968). Science as a communication process. Main Currents in Modern Thought, 25, 45–50.

Froman, R.D., & Owen, S.V. (1990). Mothers' and nurses' perceptions of infant care skills. Research in Nursing and Health, 13, 247–253.

Fry, S. (1981). Accountability in research: The relationship of scientific and humanistic values. Advances in Nursing Science, 4(1), 1–13.

Gortner, S.R. (1980). Nursing science in transition. Nursing Research, 29, 180–183.

Gortner, S.R. (1990). Nursing values and science: Toward a science philosophy. Image: Journal of Nursing Scholarship, 22, 101–105.

Hall, B.A. (1981). The change paradigm in nursing: Growth versus persistence. Advances in Nursing Science, 3(4), 1–6.

Hall, B.A. (1983). Toward an understanding of stability in nursing phenomena. Advances in Nursing Science, 5(3), 15–20.

Hall, K.V. (1979). Current trends in the use of conceptual frameworks in nursing education. Journal of Nursing Education, 18(4), 26–29.

Hall, A.D., & Fagen, R.E. (1968). Definition of system. In W. Buckley (Ed.), Modern systems research for the behavioral scientist (pp. 81–92). Chicago: Aldine.

Hardy, M.E. (1978). Perspectives on nursing theory. Advances in Nursing Science, 1(1): 37–48.

Hawkes, J.M., & Holm, K. (1993). Gender differences in exercise determinants. Nursing Research, 42, 166–172.

Heiss, J. (1976). Family roles and interaction (2nd ed.). Chicago: Rand McNally.

Heiss, J. (1981). The social psychology of interaction. Englewood Cliffs, NJ: Prentice-Hall.

Hickey, M.L., Owen, S.V., & Froman, R.D. (1992). Instrument development: Cardiac diet and exercise self-efficacy. Nursing Research, 41, 347–351.

Hinshaw, A.S. (1979). Theoretical substruction: An assessment process. Western Journal of Nursing Research, 1, 319–324.

Hinshaw, A.S. (1987). Response to "Structuring the nursing knowledge system: A typology of four domains." Scholarly Inquiry for Nursing Practice, 1, 111–114.

Jennings, B.M. (1987). Nursing theory development: Successes and challenges. Journal of Advanced Nursing, 12, 63–69.

Johnson, D.E. (1974). Development of theory: A requisite for nursing as a primary health profession. Nursing Research, 23, 372–377.

Johnson, D.E. (1980). The behavioral system model for nursing. In J.P. Riehl & C. Roy, Conceptual models for nursing practice (2nd ed., pp. 207–216). New York: Appleton-Century-Crofts.

Johnson, D.E. (1987). Evaluating conceptual models for use in critical care nursing practice. [Guest editorial]. Dimensions of Critical Care Nursing, 6, 195–197.

Johnson, D.E. (1990). The behavioral system model for nursing. In M.E. Parker (Ed.), Nursing theories in practice (pp. 23–32). New York: National League for Nursing.

Kershaw, B. (1990). Nursing models as philosophies of care. Nursing Practice, 4(1), 25–27.

Kim, H.S. (1983). The nature of theoretical thinking in nursing. Norwalk, CT: Appleton-Century-Crofts.

Kim, H.S. (1987). Structuring the nursing knowledge system: A typology of four domains. Scholarly Inquiry for Nursing Practice, 1, 99–110.

Kim, H.S. (1989). Theoretical thinking in

nursing: Problems and prospects. *Recent Advances in Nursing, 24,* 106–122.

King, I.M. (1971). *Toward a theory for nursing: General concepts of human behavior.* New York: John Wiley & Sons.

King, I.M. (1981). *A theory for nursing: Systems, concepts, process.* New York: John Wiley & Sons.

King, I.M. (1984). Philosophy of nursing education: A national survey. *Western Journal of Nursing Research, 6,* 387–406.

King, I.M. (1990). King's conceptual framework and theory of goal attainment. In M.E. Parker (Ed.), *Nursing theories in practice* (pp. 73–84). New York: National League for Nursing.

Kolcaba, K.Y., & Kolcaba, R.J. (1991). *In defense of the metaparadigm for nursing.* Unpublished manuscript.

Kuhn, T.S. (1970). *The structure of scientific revolutions* (2nd ed.). Chicago: University of Chicago Press.

Kuhn, T.S. (1977). Second thoughts on paradigms. In F. Suppe (Ed.), *The structure of scientific theories* (2nd ed., pp. 459–517). Chicago: University of Illinois Press.

Lachman, V.D. (1993, June). *Communication skills for effective interpersonal relations.* Concurrent session presented at the American Nephrology Nurses Association 24th National Symposium, Orlando, FL.

Laudan, L. (1981). A problem-solving approach to scientific progress. In I. Hacking (Ed.), *Scientific revolutions* (pp. 144–155). Fair Lawn, NJ: Oxford University Press.

Leininger, M.M. (1988). Leininger's theory of nursing: Cultural care diversity and universality. *Nursing Science Quarterly, 1,* 152–160.

Leininger, M.M. (1990). Historic and epistemologic dimensions of care and caring with future directions. In J.S. Stevenson & T. Tripp-Reimer (Eds.), *Knowledge about care and caring: State of the art and future developments* (pp. 19–31). Kansas City, MO: American Academy of Nursing.

Leininger, M.M. (1991a). The theory of culture care diversity and universality. In M.M. Leininger (Ed.), *Culture care diversity and universality: A theory of nursing* (pp. 5–65). New York: National League for Nursing.

Leininger, M.M. (1991b). Looking to the future of nursing and the relevancy of culture care theory. In M.M. Leininger (Ed.), *Culture care diversity and universality: A theory of nursing* (pp. 391–418). New York: National League for Nursing.

Leininger, M.M. (1991c). Letter to the editor: Reflections on an international theory of nursing. *International Nursing Review, 38,* 152.

Levine, M.E. (1969). *Introduction to clinical nursing.* Philadelphia: FA Davis.

Levine, M.E. (1991). The conservation principles: A model for health. In K.M. Schaefer & J.B. Pond (Eds.), *Levine's conservation model: A framework for nursing practice* (pp. 1–11). Philadelphia: FA Davis.

Lippitt, G.L. (1973). *Visualizing change: Model building and the change process.* Fairfax, VA: NTL Learning Resources.

Lowery, B.J., Jacobsen, B.S., & McCauley, K. (1987). On the prevalence of causal search in illness situations. *Nursing Research, 36,* 88–93.

Malloch, K., Martinez, R., Nelson, L., Predeger, B., Speakman, L., Steinbinder, A., & Tracy, J. (1992). To the editor [Letter]. *Advances in Nursing Science, 15(2),* vi–vii.

Mandelbaum, J. (1991). Why there cannot be an international theory of nursing. *International Nursing Review, 38,* 48, 53–55.

Marriner-Tomey, A. (1994). *Nursing theorists and their work* (3rd ed.). St. Louis: Mosby-Year Book.

McFarlane, A.J. (1988). A nursing reformulation of Bowen's family systems theory. *Archives of Psychiatric Nursing, 2,* 319–324.

Meleis, A.I. (1991). *Theoretical nursing: Development and progress* (2nd ed.). Philadelphia: JB Lippincott.

Moore, S. (1990). Thoughts on the discipline of nursing as we approach the year 2000. *Journal of Advanced Nursing, 15,* 825–828.

Morse, J.M., Solberg, S.M., Neander, W.L., Bottorff, J.L., & Johnson, J.L. (1990). Concepts of caring and caring as a concept. *Advances in Nursing Science, 13(1),* 1–14.

Nagle, L.M., & Mitchell, G.J. (1991). Theoretic diversity: Evolving paradigmatic issues in research and practice. *Advances in Nursing Science, 14(1),* 17–25.

Neuman, B. (1989). *The Neuman systems model* (2nd ed.). Norwalk, CT: Appleton & Lange.

Neuman, B., & Young, R.J. (1972). A model for teaching total person approach to patient problems. *Nursing Research, 21,* 264–269.

Newman, M.A. (1983). The continuing revolution: A history of nursing science. In N.L. Chaska (Ed.), *The nursing profession: A time to speak* (pp. 385–393). New York: McGraw-Hill.

Newman, M.A. (1986). *Health as expanding consciousness.* St. Louis: CV Mosby.

Newman, M.A. (1992). Prevailing paradigms

in nursing. *Nursing Outlook, 40,* 10–13, 32.

Newman. M.A., Sime, A.M., & Corcoran-Perry, S.A. (1991). The focus of the discipline of nursing. *Advances in Nursing Science, 14*(1), 1–6.

Newman, M.A., Sime, A.M., & Corcoran-Perry, S.A. (1992). Authors' reply [letter to the editor]. *Advances in Nursing Science, 14*(3), vi–vii.

Nightingale, F. (1859). *Notes on nursing: What it is, and what it is not.* London: Harrison. Reprinted 1946. Philadelphia: JB Lippincott.

Nursing Development Conference Group. (1973). *Concept formalization in nursing: Process and product.* Boston: Little, Brown.

Nursing Development Conference Group. (1979). *Concept formalization in nursing: Process and product* (2nd ed.). Boston: Little, Brown.

Nye, F.I., & Berardo, F.N. (Eds.). (1966). *Emerging conceptual frameworks in family analysis.* New York: Macmillan.

Nye, F.I., & Berardo, F.N. (Eds.). (1981). *Emerging conceptual frameworks in family analysis.* New York: Praeger.

Orem, D.E. (1971). *Nursing: Concepts of practice.* New York: McGraw-Hill.

Orem, D.E. (1991). *Nursing: Concepts of practice* (4th ed.). St. Louis: Mosby-Year Book.

Orem, D.E., & Taylor, S.G. (1986). Orem's general theory of nursing. In P. Winstead-Fry (Ed.), *Case studies in nursing theory* (pp. 37–71). New York: National League for Nursing.

Orlando, I.J. (1961). *The dynamic nurse-patient relationship.* New York: GP Putnam's Sons.

Orlando, I.J. (1972). *The discipline and teaching of nursing process (an evaluation study).* New York: GP Putnam's Sons.

Parse, R.R. (1981). *Man-living-health: A theory of nursing.* New York: John Wiley & Sons.

Parse, R.R. (1987). *Nursing science: Major paradigms, theories, and critiques.* Philadelphia: WB Saunders.

Parse, R.R. (1992). Human becoming: Parse's theory of nursing. *Nursing Science Quarterly, 5,* 35–42.

Peplau, H.E. (1952). *Interpersonal relations in nursing.* New York: GP Putnam's Sons.

Peplau, H.E. (1992). Interpersonal relations: A theoretical framework for application in nursing practice. *Nursing Science Quarterly, 5,* 13–18.

Peterson, C.J. (1977). Questions frequently asked about the development of a conceptual framework. *Journal of Nursing Education, 16*(4), 22–32.

Reese, H.W., & Overton, W.F. (1970). Models of development and theories of development. In L.R. Goulet & P.B. Baltes (Eds.), *Life span developmental psychology: Research and theory* (pp. 115–145). New York: Academic Press.

Reilly, D.E. (1975). Why a conceptual framework? *Nursing Outlook, 23,* 566–569.

Riehl, J.P., & Roy, C. (1974). *Conceptual models for nursing practice.* New York: Appleton-Century-Crofts.

Riehl, J.P., & Roy, C. (1980). *Conceptual models for nursing practice* (2nd ed.). New York: Appleton-Century-Crofts.

Rogers, M.E. (1970). *An introduction to the theoretical basis of nursing.* Philadelphia: FA Davis.

Rogers, M.E. (1990). Nursing: Science of unitary, irreducible, human beings: Update 1990. In E.A.M. Barrett (Ed.), *Visions of Rogers' science-based nursing* (pp. 5–11). New York: National League for Nursing.

Rogers, M.E. (1992). Nursing science and the space age. *Nursing Science Quarterly, 5,* 27–34.

Roy, C. (1976). *Introduction to nursing: An adaptation model.* Englewood Cliffs, NJ: Prentice-Hall.

Roy, C. (1988). An explication of the philosophical assumptions of the Roy Adaptation Model. *Nursing Science Quarterly, 1,* 26–34.

Roy, C., & Andrews, H.A. (1991). *The Roy adaptation model: The definitive statement.* Norwalk, CT: Appleton & Lange.

Rudner, R.S. (1966). *Philosophy of social science.* Englewood Cliffs, NJ: Prentice-Hall.

Salsberry, P. (1991, May). *A philosophy of nursing: What is it? What is it not?* Paper presented at the Philosophy in the Nurse's World Conference, Banff, Alberta, Canada.

Schlotfeldt, R.M. (1975). The need for a conceptual framework. In P.J. Verhonick (Ed.), *Nursing research I* (pp. 3–24). Boston: Little, Brown.

Seaver, J.W., & Cartwright, C.A. (1977). A pluralistic foundation for training early childhood professionals. *Curriculum Inquiry, 7,* 305–329.

Swanson, K.M. (1991). Empirical development of a middle range theory of caring. *Nursing Research, 40,* 161–165.

Thomae, H. (1979). The concept of development and life-span developmental psychology. In P.B. Baltes & O.G. Brim, Jr.

(Eds.), *Life-span development and behavior* (Vol. 2, pp. 281–312). New York: Academic Press.

Wagner, J.D. (1986). Nurse scholars' perceptions of nursing's metaparadigm. *Dissertation Abstracts International, 47*, 1932B.

Watson, J. (1985). *Nursing: Human science and human care: A theory of nursing.* Norwalk, CT: Appleton-Century-Crofts.

Watson, J. (1990). Caring knowledge and informed moral passion. *Advances in Nursing Science, 13*(1), 15–24.

Wells, L.E., & Stryker, S. (1988). Stability and change in self over the life course. In P.B. Baltes, D.L. Featherman, & R.M. Lerner (Eds.), *Life-span development and*

behavior (pp. 191–229). Hillsdale, NJ: Lawrence Erlbaum Associates.

Whall, A.L. (1980). Congruence between existing theories of family functioning and nursing theories. *Advances in Nursing Science, 3*(1), 59–67.

Whall, A.L. (1986). *Family therapy theory for nursing: Four approaches.* Norwalk, CT: Appleton-Century-Crofts.

Yura, H., & Torres, G. (1975). Today's conceptual framework within baccalaureate nursing programs. In *Faculty-curriculum development, Part III: Conceptual framework—Its meaning and function* (pp. 17–25). New York: National League for Nursing.

BIBLIOGRAPHY

STRUCTURAL HIERARCHY OF NURSING KNOWLEDGE

Commentary

Adam, E. (1983). Frontiers of nursing in the 21st century: Development of models and theories on the concept of nursing. *Journal of Advanced Nursing, 8*, 41–45.

Adam, E. (1983). Modèles conceptuels (French). *Nursing Papers, 15*(2), 10.

  Winkler, J. (1983). Conceptual models [Response to Adam]. *Nursing Papers, 15*(4), 69–71.

  Adam, E. (1983). (Reply to Winkler). *Nursing Papers, 15*(4), 71.

Adam, E. (1985). Toward more clarity in terminology: Frameworks, theories and models. *Journal of Nursing Education, 24*, 151–155.

Adam, E. (1987). Nursing theory: What it is and what it is not. *Nursing Papers, 19*(1), 5–14.

  Hardy, L.K. (1987). A response to "Nursing theory: What it is and what it is not" (Letter). *Nursing Papers, 19*(3), 5–7.

Aggleton, P., & Chalmers, H. (1985). Critical examination. *Nursing Times, 81*(14), 38–39.

Aggleton, P., & Chalmers, H. (1986). Nursing research, nursing theory, and the nursing process. *Journal of Advanced Nursing, 11*, 197–202.

Aggleton, P., & Chalmers, H. (1989). Next year's models. *Nursing Times, 85*(51), 24–27.

Aggleton, P., & Chalmers, H. (1987). Models of nursing, nursing practice and nursing

education. *Journal of Advanced Nursing, 12*, 573–581.

Akinsanya, J.A. (1989). Introduction. *Recent Advances in Nursing, 24*, i–ii.

Algase, D.L., & Whall, A.F. (1993). Rosemary Ellis's views on the substantive structure of nursing. *Image: Journal of Nursing Scholarship, 25*, 69–72.

Antrobus, S. (1993). Nursing's nature and boundaries. *Senior Nurse, 13*(2), 46–50.

Barnum, B.J.S. (1994). *Nursing theory: Analysis, application, evaluation* (4th ed.). Philadelphia: JB Lippincott.

Betz, C.L. (1990). Where's the nursing? (Editorial). *Journal of Pediatric Nursing, 5*, 245.

Biley, F. (1990). Wordly wise. *Nursing (London), 4*(24), 37.

Botha, M.E. (1989). Theory development in perspective: The role of conceptual frameworks and models in theory development. *Journal of Advanced Nursing, 14*, 49–55.

Bridges, J. (1991). Distinct from medicine. *Nursing Times, 87*(27), 42–43.

Brink, H. (1992). The science of nursing: Current issues and dilemmas. *Curationis, 15*(2), 12–18.

Brower, H.T. (1985). Gerontological nursing: Movement towards a paradigm state. *Journal of Professional Nursing, 1*, 328–335.

Bunting, S.M. (1988). The concept of perception in selected nursing theories. *Nursing Science Quarterly, 1*, 168–174.

Burnard, P. (1991). Towards enlightenment. *Nursing Standard, 5*(45), 48–49.

Carryer, J. (1992). A critical reconceptualisation of the environment in nursing: Developing a new model. *Nursing Praxis in New Zealand, 7*(2), 9–14.

Cash, K. (1990). Nursing models and the idea of nursing. *International Journal of Nursing Studies, 27,* 249–256.

Cowling, W.R. III. (1987). Metatheoretical issues: Development of new theory. *Journal of Gerontological Nursing, 13*(9), 10–13.

Cruickshank, C.N. (1992). Creating your own conceptual framework. *The Canadian Nurse, 88*(2), 31–32.

Davis, M. (1992). Models for care: Part (i): Medical, social and nursing models. *Nursing Times, 88*(48), i–viii.

Davis, M. (1993a). Models for care: Part (ii): Two contrasting nursing models. *Nursing Times, 89*(4), i–viii.

Davis, M. (1993b). Models for care: Part (iii): Your own nursing model. *Nursing Times, 89*(5), i–viii.

Dickoff, J., & James, P. (1988). Theoretical pluralism for nursing diagnosis. In R.M. Carroll-Johnston (Ed.), *Classification of nursing diagnoses: Proceedings of the eighth conference: North American Nursing Diagnosis Association* (pp. 98–125). Philadelphia: JB Lippincott.

Draper, P. (1990). The development of theory in British nursing: Current position and future prospects. *Journal of Advanced Nursing, 15,*12–15.

Draper, P. (1991). The ideal and the real: Some thoughts on theoretical developments in British nursing. *Nurse Education Today, 11,* 292–294.

Dylak, P. (1986). The state of the art? *Nursing Times, 82*(42), 72.

Emden, C., & Young, W. (1987). Theory development in nursing: Australian nurses advance global debate. *Australian Journal of Advanced Nursing, 4*(3), 22–40.

Engstrom, J.L. (1984). Problems in the development, use and testing of nursing theory. *Journal of Nursing Education, 23,* 245–251.

Ellis, R. (1982). Conceptual issues in nursing. *Nursing Outlook, 32,* 406–410.

Falco, S.M. (1989). Major concepts in the development of nursing theory. *Recent Advances in Nursing, 24,* 1–17.

Fawcett, J. (1986). Conceptual models of nursing, nursing diagnosis, and nursing theory development. [Guest editorial]. *Western Journal of Nursing Research, 8,* 397–399.

Fawcett, J. (1988). Conceptual models and theory development. *Journal of Obstetric, Gynecologic, and Neonatal Nursing, 17,* 400–403.

Fawcett, J. (1991). Approaches to knowledge development in nursing. *Canadian Journal of Nursing Research, 23*(4), 23–34.

Dzurec, L.C. (1991). Prefacing knowledge development in nursing. Telling stories. *Canadian Journal of Nursing Research, 23*(4), 35–42.

Fitzpatrick, J.J., & Whall, A.L. (1989). *Conceptual models of nursing: Analysis and application* (2nd ed.). Norwalk, CT: Appleton & Lange.

Friedemann, M.L. (1989a). Closing the gap between grand theory and mental health practice with families. Part 1: The framework of systemic organization for nursing of families and family members. *Archives of Psychiatric Nursing, 3,* 10–19.

Friedemann, M.L. (1989b). Closing the gap between grand theory and mental health practice with families. Part 2: The control-congruence model for mental health nursing of families. *Archives of Psychiatric Nursing, 3,* 20–28.

Frost, S., & Nunkoosing, K. (1989). Building a strong foundation. *Nursing Times, 85*(1), 59–60.

George, J.B. (Ed.). (1989). *Nursing theories: The base for professional nursing practice* (3rd ed.). Norwalk, CT: Appleton & Lange.

Grahame, C. (1987). Frontline revolt. *Nursing Times, 83*(16), 60.

Grinnell, F. (1992). Theories without thought? *Nursing Times, 88*(22), 57.

Hardy, L.K. (1986). Identifying the place of theoretical frameworks in an evolving discipline. *Journal of Advanced Nursing, 11,* 103–107.

Hardy, L.K. (1988). Excellence in nursing through debate—the case of nursing theory. *Recent Advances in Nursing, 21,* 1–13.

Hardy, L.K. (1990). The path to knowledge-personal reflections. *Nurse Education Today, 10,* 325–332.

Hardy, M.E. (1978). Perspectives on nursing theory. *Advances in Nursing Science, 1*(1), 37–48.

Hawkett, S. (1989). A model marriage? *Nursing Times, 85*(1), 61–62.

Herbert, M. (1988). The value of nursing models. *The Canadian Nurse, 84*(11), 32–34.

Ho, P. (1990, March). Nursing theories and nursing diagnosis. *Hong Kong Nursing Journal,* 15–16.

Hodgson, R. (1992). A nursing muse. *British Journal of Nursing, 1,* 330–333.

Holden, R.J. (1990). Models, muddles and medicine. *International Journal of Nursing Studies, 27,* 223–234.

Holmes, C.A. (1990). Alternatives to natural science foundations for nursing. *International Journal of Nursing Studies, 27*, 187–198.

Huckabay, L.M.D. (1991). The role of conceptual frameworks in nursing practice, administration, education, and research. *Nursing Administration Quarterly, 15*(3), 17–28.

Ingram, R. (1991). Why does nursing need theory? *Journal of Advanced Nursing, 16*, 350–353.

Jackson, M. (1986). On maps and models. *Senior Nurse, 5*(4), 24–26.

Jacobs, M.K. (1986). Can nursing theory be tested? In P.L. Chinn (Ed.), *Nursing research methodology: Issues and implementation* (pp. 39–53). Rockville, MD: Aspen.

Johnson, D.E. (1987). Evaluating conceptual models for use in critical care nursing practice. [Guest editorial]. *Dimensions of Critical Care Nursing, 6*, 195–197.

Johnson, D.E. (1989). Some thoughts on nursing [Editorial]. *Clinical Nurse Specialist, 3*, 1–4.

Jones, S. (1989). Is unity possible? *Nursing Standard, 3*(1), 22–23.

King, I.M. (1991). Nursing theory 25 years later. *Nursing Science Quarterly, 4*, 94–95.

Koziol-McLain, J., & Maeve, M.K. (1993). Nursing theory in perspective. *Nursing Outlook, 41*, 79–81.

Levine, M.E. (1988). Antecedents from adjunctive disciplines: Creation of nursing theory. *Nursing Science Quarterly, 1*, 16–21.

Lippitt, G.L. (1973). *Visualizing change: Model building and the change process.* Fairfax, VA: NTL Learning Resources.

Lister, P. (1987). The misunderstood model. *Nursing Times, 83*(41), 40–42.

Lister, P. (1991). Approaching models of nursing from a postmodernist perspective. *Journal of Advanced Nursing, 16*, 206–212.

Lundh, U., Soder, M., & Waerness, K. (1988). Nursing theories: A critical view. *Image: Journal of Nursing Scholarship, 20*, 36–40.

Madden, B.P. (1990). The hybrid model for concept development: Its value for the study of therapeutic alliance. *Advances in Nursing Science, 12*(3), 75–87.

Maher, A.B. (1986). Putting nursing in your article on nursing care. *Orthopedic Nursing, 5*(2), 42–43. (Reprinted in *Dermatology Nursing, 2*(2), 88–89, 1990.)

Marriner-Tomey, A. (1994). *Nursing theorists and their work* (3rd ed.). St. Louis: Mosby-Year Book.

Martin, P.A., & Frank, B. (1988). NANDA nursing diagnostic categories and their relationship to specific nursing theories. In R.M. Carroll-Johnston (Ed.), *Classification of nursing diagnoses: Proceedings of the eighth conference: North American Nursing Diagnosis Association* (pp. 411–413). Philadelphia: JB Lippincott.

McGee, P. (1992). Developing a model for theatre nursing. *British Journal of Nursing, 2*, 262–264, 266.

McMahon, S. (1991). The quest for synthesis: Human-companion animal relationships and nursing theories. *Holistic Nursing Practice, 5*(2), 1–5.

Meleis, A.I. (1991). *Theoretical nursing. Development and progress* (2nd ed.). Philadelphia: JB Lippincott.

Murphey, C.J. (1987). The nurse's liberation: An evolutionary epistemological paradigm for nursing. *Dissertation Abstracts International, 48*, 1303B.

O'Berle, K., & Davies, B. (1992). Support and caring: Exploring the concepts. *Oncology Nursing Forum, 19*, 763–767.

Orr, J. (1991). Knowledge is power. *Health Visitor, 64*(7), 218.

Parker, M.E. (Ed.). (1990). *Nursing theories in practice.* New York: National League for Nursing.

Pearson, A., & Vaughan, B. (1986). *Nursing models for practice.* Rockville, MD: Aspen.

Randell, B.P. (1992). Nursing theory: The 21st century. *Nursing Science Quarterly, 5*, 176–184.

Rasch, R.F.R. (1988). The development of a taxonomy for the nursing process: A deductive approach based on an analysis of the discipline of nursing and set theory. *Dissertation Abstracts International, 49*, 2132B.

Reed, P.G. (1989). Nursing theorizing as an ethical endeavor. *Advances in Nursing Science, 11*(3), 1–9.

Riehl-Sisca, J.P. (1989). *Conceptual models for nursing practice* (3rd ed.). Norwalk, CT: Appleton & Lange.

Ramprogus, V. (1992). Developing nursing theory. *Senior Nurse, 12*(1), 46–51.

Reilly, D.E., & Oermann, M.H. (1992). *Clinical teaching in nursing education* (2nd ed.). New York: National League for Nursing.

Searle, C. (1988). Nursing theories. What is our commitment? *Nursing RSA Verpleging, 3*(2), 15–21.

Smith, M.C. (1992). The distinctiveness of

nursing knowledge. *Nursing Science Quarterly, 5,* 148–149.

Theory development. What, why, how? (1978). New York: National League for Nursing.

Thompson, J.E., Oakley, D., Burke, M., Jay, S., & Conklin, M. (1989). Theory building in nurse-midwifery. The care process. *Journal of Nurse-Midwifery, 34,* 120–130.

Thibodeau, J.A. (1983). *Nursing models: Analysis and evaluation.* Monterey, CA: Wadsworth.

Thompson, J.E., Oakley, D., Burke, M., Jay, S., & Conklin, M. (1989). Theory building in nurse-midwifery: The care process. *Journal of Nurse-Midwifery, 34,* 120–130.

Torres, G. (1986). *Theoretical foundations of nursing.* Norwalk, CT: Appleton-Century-Crofts.

Walker, L.O., & Avant, K.C. (1988). *Strategies for theory construction in nursing* (2nd ed.). Norwalk, CT: Appleton & Lange.

Walker, L., & Phillips, J.R. (1989). The future of theory development: Commentary and response. *Nursing Science Quarterly, 2,* 118–119.

Whall, A.L. (1987). Conceptual model directions [Guest editorial]. *Journal of Gerontological Nursing, 13*(9), 6–7.

Wheeler, K. (1989). Self-psychology's contributions to understanding stress and implications for nursing. *Journal of Advanced Medical-Surgical Nursing, 1*(4), 1–10.

Wilford, S.L. (1990). Knowledge development in nursing: Emergence of a paradigm. *Dissertation Abstracts International, 50,* 3408B.

Winstead-Fry, P. (Ed.). (1986). *Case studies in nursing theory.* New York: National League for Nursing.

Yeo, M. (1989). Integration of nursing theory and nursing ethics. *Advances in Nursing Science, 11*(3), 33–42.

Conceptual Models

Christensen, P.J., & Kenney, J.W. (Eds.). (1990). *Nursing process: Application of conceptual models.* St. Louis: CV Mosby.

Eckberg, D.L., & Hill, L., Jr. (1979). The paradigm concept and sociology: A critical review. *American Sociological Review, 44,* 925–937.

Erickson, H.C., Tomlin, E.M., & Swain, M.A.P. (1983). *Modeling and role-modeling: A theory and paradigm for nursing.* Englewood Cliffs, NJ: Prentice-Hall.

Johnson, D.E. (1974). Development of theory: A requisite for nursing as a primary health profession. *Nursing Research, 23,* 372–377.

Johnson, D.E. (1980). The behavioral system model for nursing. In J.P. Riehl & C. Roy, (Eds.),*Conceptual models for nursing practice* (2nd ed., pp. 207–216). New York: Appleton-Century-Crofts.

Johnson, D.E. (1990). The behavioral system model for nursing. In M.E. Parker (Ed.), *Nursing theories in practice* (pp. 23–32). New York: National League for Nursing.

King, I.M. (1981). *A theory for nursing: Systems, concepts, process.* New York: John Wiley & Sons.

King, I.M. (1990). King's conceptual framework and theory of goal attainment. In M.E. Parker (Ed.), *Nursing theories in practice* (pp. 73–84). New York: National League for Nursing.

Levine, M.E. (1973). *Introduction to nursing* (2nd ed.). Philadelphia: FA Davis.

Levine, M.E. (1991). The conservation principles: A model for health. In K.M. Schaefer & J.B. Pond (Eds.), *Levine's conservation model: A framework for nursing practice* (pp. 1–11). Philadelphia: FA Davis.

Neuman, B. (1989). *The Neuman systems model* (2nd ed.). Norwalk, CT: Appleton & Lange.

Nightingale, F. (1992). *Notes on nursing: What it is, and what it is not* (Commemorative ed.). Philadelphia: JB Lippincott (Originally published in 1859).

Nye, F.I. & Berardo, F.N. (Eds.). (1981). *Emerging conceptual frameworks in family analysis.* New York: Praeger.

Orem, D.E. (1991). *Nursing: Concepts of practice* (4th ed.). St. Louis: Mosby-Year Book.

Peterson, C.J. (1977). Questions frequently asked about the development of a conceptual framework. *Journal of Nursing Education, 16*(4), 22–32.

Reilly, D.E. (1975). Why a conceptual framework? *Nursing Outlook, 23,* 566–569.

Rogers, M.E. (1970). *An introduction to the theoretical basis of nursing.* Philadelphia: FA Davis.

Rogers, M.E. (1990). Nursing: Science of unitary, irreducible, human beings: Update 1990. In E.A.M. Barrett (Ed.), *Visions of Rogers' science-based nursing* (pp. 5–11). New York: National League for Nursing.

Roy, C., & Andrews, H.A. (1991). *The Roy Adaptation Model: The definitive statement.* Norwalk, CT: Appleton & Lange.

Webb, C. (1986). Nursing models: A personal view. *Nursing Practice, 1,* 208–212.

Williams, C.A. (1979). The nature and development of conceptual frameworks. In F.S. Downs & J.W. Fleming, (Eds.), *Issues in* nursing research (pp. 89–106). New York: Appleton-Century-Crofts.

Wright, S.C. (1986). *Building and using a model of nursing*. Baltimore: Edward Arnold.

The Metaparadigm

Conway, M.E. (1985). Toward greater specificity in defining nursing's metaparadigm. *Advances in Nursing Science, 7*(4), 73–81.

Donaldson, S.K. & Crowley, D.M. (1978). The discipline of nursing. *Nursing Outlook, 26*, 113–120.

Eriksson, K. (1989). Caring paradigms: A study of the origins and the development of caring paradigms among nursing students. *Scandinavian Journal of Caring Science, 3*, 169–176.

Fawcett, J. (1984). The metaparadigm of nursing: Current status and future refinements. *Image: The Journal of Nursing Scholarship, 16*, 84–87.

Brodie, J.M. (1984). A response to Dr. J. Fawcett's paper: "The metaparadigm of nursing: Present status and future refinements." *Image: The Journal of Nursing Scholarship, 16*, 87–89.

Fawcett, J. (1992). The metaparadigm of nursing: International in scope and substance. In K. Krause & P. Åstedt-Kurki (Eds.), *International perspectives on nursing: A joint effort to explore nursing internationally* (Serie A 3/92, pp. 13–21). Tampere, Finland: Tampere University Department of Nursing.

Flaskerud, J.H., & Halloran, E.J. (1980). Areas of agreement in nursing theory development. *Advances in Nursing Science, 3*(1), 1–7.

Forchuk, C. (1991). Reconceptualizing the environment of the individual with a chronic mental illness. *Issues in Mental Health Nursing, 12*, 159–170.

Gortner, S.R. (1980). Nursing science in transition. *Nursing Research, 29*, 180–183.

Hanna, K.M. (1989). The meaning of health for graduate nursing students. *Journal of Nursing Education, 28*, 372–376.

Janhonen, S. (1992). Swedish nursing instructors' views of nursing. *Nurse Education Today, 12*, 329–339.

Janhonen, S. (1993). Finish nurse instructors' view of the core of nursing. *International Journal of Nursing Studies, 30*, 157–169.

Jennings, B.M. (1987). Nursing theory development: Successes and challenges. *Journal of Advanced Nursing, 12*, 63–69.

Kleffel, D. (1991). An ecofeminist analysis of nursing knowledge. *Nursing Forum, 26*(4), 5–18.

Kleffel, D. (1991). Rethinking the environment as a domain of nursing knowledge. *Advances in Nursing Science, 14*(1), 40–51.

Kim, H.S. (1983). *The nature of theoretical thinking in nursing*. Norwalk, CT: Appleton-Century-Crofts.

Kim, H.S. (1987). Structuring the nursing knowledge system: A typology of four domains. *Scholarly Inquiry for Nursing Practice, 1*, 99–110.

Hinshaw, A.S. (1987). Response to "Structuring the nursing knowledge system: A typology of four domains." *Scholarly Inquiry for Nursing Practice, 1*, 111–114.

Kim, H.S. (1989). Theoretical thinking in nursing: Problems and prospects. *Recent Advances in Nursing, 24*, 106–122.

King, I.M. (1984). Philosophy of nursing education: A national survey. *Western Journal of Nursing Research, 6*, 387–406.

Kuhn, T.S. (1970). *The structure of scientific revolutions* (2nd ed.). Chicago: University of Chicago Press.

Kuhn, T.S. (1977). Second thoughts on paradigms. In F. Suppe (Ed.), *The structure of scientific theories* (2nd ed., pp. 459–517). Chicago: University of Illinois Press.

Mandelbaum, J. (1991). Why there cannot be an international theory of nursing. *International Nursing Review, 38*, 53–55, 48.

McKenna, G. (1993). Caring is the essence of nursing practice. *British Journal of Nursing, 2*, 72–76.

Newman, M.A. (1983). The continuing revolution: A history of nursing science. In N.L. Chaska (Ed.), *The nursing profession: A time to speak* (pp. 385–393). New York: McGraw-Hill.

Newman, M.A. (1991). Health conceptualizations. In J.J. Fitzpatrick, R.L. Taunton, & A.K. Jacox, (Eds.), *Annual review of nursing research* (Vol. 9, pp. 221–243). New York: Springer.

Newman, M.A., Sime, A.M., & Corcoran-Perry, S.A. (1991). The focus of the discipline of nursing. *Advances in Nursing Science, 14*(1), 1–6.

Fawcett, J. (1992). Letter to the editor. *Advances in Nursing Science, 14*(3), vi.

Newman, M.A., Sime, A.M., & Corcoran-Perry, S.A. (1992). Authors' reply (Letter). *Advances in Nursing Science, 14*(3), vi–vii.

Malloch, K., Martinez, R., Nelson, L., Predeger, B., Speakman, L., Steinbinder,

A., & Tracy, J. (1992). (Letter). *Advances in Nursing Science, 15*(2), vi–vii.

Olson, T.C. (1993). Laying claim to caring: Nursing and the language of training, 1915–1937. *Nursing Outlook, 41,* 68–72.

Stevens, P.E. (1989). A critical social reconceptualization of environment in nursing: Implications for methodology. *Advances in Nursing Science, 11*(3), 56–68.

Taylor, B.J. (1992). From helper to human: A reconceptualization of the nurse as person. *Journal of Advanced Nursing, 17,* 1042–1049.

Wagner, J.D. (1986). Nurse scholars' perceptions of nursing's metaparadigm. *Dissertation Abstracts International, 47,* 1932B.

Webb, C. (1992). What is nursing? *British Journal of Nursing, 1,* 567–568.

Woods, N.F., Laffrey, S., Duffy, M., Lentz, M.J., Mitchell, E.S., Taylor, D., & Cowan, K.A. (1988). Being healthy: Women's images. *Advances in Nursing Science, 11*(1), 36–46.

World Views

Allen, C.E. (1991). An analysis of the pragmatic consequences of holism for nursing. *Western Journal of Nursing Research, 13,* 256–272.

Altman, I., & Rogoff, B. (1987). World views in psychology: Trait, interactional, organismic, and transactional perspectives. In D. Stokols & I. Altman (Eds.), *Handbook of environmental psychology* (pp. 7–40). New York: John Wiley & Sons.

Barnum, B.J. (1987). Holistic nursing and nursing process. *Holistic Nursing Practice, 1*(3), 27–35.

Battista, J.R. (1977). The holistic paradigm and general system theory. *General Systems, 22,* 65–71.

Brouse, S.H. (1992). Analysis of nurse theorists' definition of health for congruence with holism. *Journal of Holistic Nursing, 10,* 324–336.

Cull-Wilby, B.L., & Pepin, J.I. (1987). Towards a coexistence of paradigms in nursing knowledge development. *Journal of Advanced Nursing, 12,* 515–521.

Fawcett, J. (1993). From a plethora of paradigms to parsimony in worldviews. *Nursing Science Quarterly, 6,* 56–58.

Gortner, S.R. (1990). Nursing values and science: Toward a science philosophy. *Image: Journal of Nursing Scholarship, 22,* 101–105.

Hall, B.A. (1981). The change paradigm in nursing: Growth versus persistence. *Advances in Nursing Science, 3*(4), 1–6.

Hall, B.A. (1983). Toward an understanding of stability in nursing phenomena. *Advances in Nursing Science, 5*(3), 15–20.

Johns, C. (1989). Developing a philosophy. *Nursing Standard, 3*(1 Suppl), 2–4.

Johnson, M.B. (1990). The holistic paradigm in nursing: The diffusion of an innovation. *Research in Nursing and Health, 13,* 129–139.

Kershaw, B. (1990). Nursing models as philosophies of care. *Nursing Practice, 4*(1), 25–27.

Kim, H.S. (1993). Identifying alternative linkages among philosophy, theory and method in nursing science. *Journal of Advanced Nursing, 18,* 793–800.

Kobert, L., & Folan, M. (1990). Coming of age in nursing: Rethinking the philosophies behind holism and nursing process. *Nursing and Health Care, 11,* 308–312.

Looft, W.R. (1973). Socialization and personality throughout the life span: An examination of contemporary psychological approaches. In P.B. Baltes & K.W. Schaie (Eds.), *Life span developmental psychology: Personality and socialization* (pp. 25–52). New York: Academic Press.

Muller-Smith, P.A. (1992). When paradigms shift. *Journal of Post-Anesthesia Nursing, 7,* 278–280.

Murphy, C.J. (1987). The nurse's liberation: An evolutionary epistemological paradigm for nursing. *Dissertation Abstracts International, 48*(05), 1303B.

Nagle, L.M., & Mitchell, G.J. (1991). Theoretic diversity: Evolving paradigmatic issues in research and practice. *Advances in Nursing Science, 14*(1), 17–25.

Newman, M.A. (1992). Prevailing paradigms in nursing. *Nursing Outlook, 40,* 10–13, 32.

Parse, R.R. (1987). *Nursing science: Major paradigms, theories, and critiques.* Philadelphia: WB Saunders.

Polifroni, E.C., & Packard, S. (1993). Psychological determinism and the evolving nursing paradigm. *Nursing Science Quarterly, 6,* 63–68.

Reese, H.W., & Overton, W.F. (1970). Models of development and theories of development. In L.R. Goulet & P.B. Baltes (Eds.), *Life span developmental psychology: Research and theory* (pp. 115–145). New York: Academic Press.

Sarkis, J.M., & Skoner, M.M. (1987). An analysis of the concept of holism in nursing literature. *Holistic Nursing Practice, 2*(1), 61–69.

Sarter, B. (1988). Philosophical sources of nursing theory. *Nursing Science Quarterly, 1,* 52–59.

Seaver, J.W., & Cartwright, C.A. (1977). A pluralistic foundation for training early childhood professionals. *Curriculum Inquiry, 7,* 305–329.

Sellers, S.C. (1991). A philosophical analysis of conceptual models of nursing. *Dissertation Abstracts International, 52,* 1937B.

Smith, M.J. (1988a). Perspectives on nursing science. *Nursing Science Quarterly, 1,* 80–85.

Smith, M.J. (1988b). Perspectives of wholeness: The lens makes a difference. *Nursing Science Quarterly, 1,* 94–95.

Smith, M.J. (1988c). Wallowing while waiting. *Nursing Science Quarterly, 1,* 3.

Smith, M.J. (1989). Knowledge development: Pushing from within or pulling from without. *Nursing Science Quarterly, 2,* 156.

Upvall, M.J. (1993). Therapeutic syncretism: A conceptual framework of persistence and change for international nursing. *Journal of Professional Nursing, 9,* 56–62.

Williams, K. (1988). World view and the facilitation of wholeness. *Holistic Nursing Practice, 2*(3), 1–8.

Categories of Knowledge

Ackoff, R.L. (1974). *Redesigning the future: A systems approach to societal problems.* New York: John Wiley & Sons.

Barnum, B.J.S. (1990). *Nursing theory: Analysis, application, evaluation* (3rd ed.). Glenview, IL: Scott, Foresman/Little, Brown Higher Education.

Benoliel, J.Q. (1977). The interaction between theory and research. *Nursing outlook, 25,* 108–113.

Bertalanffy, L. (1968). *General system theory.* New York: George Braziller.

Chin, R. (1980). The utility of systems models and developmental models for practitioners. In J.P. Riehl & C. Roy (Eds.), *Conceptual models for nursing practice* (2nd ed., pp. 21–37). New York: Appleton-Century-Crofts.

Hall, A.D., & Fagen, R.E. (1968). Definition of system. In W. Buckley (Ed.), *Modern systems research for the behavioral scientist* (pp. 81–92). Chicago: Aldine.

Heiss, J. (1981). *The social psychology of interaction.* Englewood Cliffs, NJ: Prentice-Hall.

Marriner-Tomey, A. (1989). *Nursing theorists and their work* (2nd ed.). St. Louis: CV Mosby.

Meleis, A.I. (1991). *Theoretical nursing: Development and progress* (2nd ed.). Philadelphia: JB Lippincott.

Thomae, H. (1979). The concept of development and life-span developmental psychology. In P.B. Baltes & O.G. Brim, Jr. (Eds.), *Life-span development and behavior* (Vol. 2, pp. 281–312). New York: Academic Press.

Theories

Chinn, P.L., & Kramer, M.K. (1991). *Theory and nursing: A systematic approach* (3rd ed.). St. Louis: Mosby-Year Book.

Duldt, B.W., & Giffin, K. (1985). *Theoretical perspectives for nursing.* Boston: Little, Brown.

Fawcett, J. (1993). *Analysis and evaluation of nursing theories.* Philadelphia: FA Davis.

Henderson, V. (1966). *The nature of nursing: A definition and its implications for practice, research, and education.* New York: Macmillan.

Leininger, M.M. (Ed.). (1991). *Culture care diversity and universality: A theory of nursing.* New York: National League for Nursing.

McKenna, G. (1993). Unique theory—Is it essential in the development of a science of nursing? *Nurse Education Today, 13,* 121–127.

Newman, M.A. (1986). *Health as expanding consciousness.* St. Louis: CV Mosby.

Orlando, I.J. (1961). *The dynamic nurse-patient relationship.* New York: GP Putnam's Sons.

Orlando, I.J. (1972). *The discipline and teaching of nursing process (An evaluation study).* New York: GP Putnam's Sons.

Parse, R.R. (1981). *Man-living-health: A theory of nursing.* New York: John Wiley & Sons.

Parse, R.R. (1992). Human becoming: Parse's theory of nursing. *Nursing Science Quarterly, 5,* 35–42.

Paterson, J.G., & Zderad, L.T. (1988). *Humanistic nursing.* New York: National League for Nursing (Originally published in 1976).

Peplau, H.E. (1952). *Interpersonal relations in nursing.* New York: GP Putnam's Sons.

Peplau, H.E. (1992). Interpersonal relations: A theoretical framework for application in nursing practice. *Nursing Science Quarterly, 5,* 13–18.

Rubin, R. (1984). *Maternal identity and the maternal experience.* New York: Springer.

Travelbee, J. (1966). *Interpersonal aspects of nursing.* Philadelphia: FA Davis.

Watson, J. (1985). *Nursing: Human science and human care: A theory of nursing.* Norwalk, CT: Appleton-Century-Crofts.

Theory Reformulation

Engle, V.F. (1988). Reformulating middle-range nursing theory. *Journal of Gerontological Nursing*, 14(9), 8–10.

Fitzpatrick, J.J., Whall, A.L., Johnston, R.L., & Floyd, J.A. (1982). *Nursing models and their psychiatric mental health applications*. Bowie, MD: Brady.

McFarlane, A.J. (1988). A nursing reformulation of Bowen's family systems theory. *Archives of Psychiatric Nursing*, 2, 319–324.

Reed, P.G. (1991). Toward a nursing theory of self-transcendence: Deductive reformulation using developmental theories. *Advances in Nursing Science*, 13(4), 64–77.

Whall, A.L. (1980). Congruence between existing theories of family functioning and nursing theories. *Advances in Nursing Science*, 3(1), 59–67.

Whall, A.L. (1986). *Family therapy theory for nursing: Four approaches*. Norwalk, CT: Appleton-Century-Crofts.

Empirical Indicators

Creasia, J.L. (1991). Nursing theories, measurement resources, and methods for data collection in nursing. In C.F. Waltz, O.L. Strickland, & E.R. Lenz, *Measurement in nursing research* (2nd ed., pp. 461–511). Philadelphia: FA Davis.

Quayhagen, M.P., & Roth, P.A. (1989). From models to measures in assessment of mature families. *Journal of Professional Nursing*, 5, 144–151.

Conceptual Models and Nursing Research

Allen, M.N. & Hayes, P. (1989). Models of nursing: Implications for research in nursing. *Recent Advances in Nursing*, 24, 77–92.

Beck, C.T. (1985). Theoretical frameworks cited in Nursing Research from January 1974–June 1985. *Nurse Educator*, 10(6), 36–38.

Brallier, M.F. (1991). Research: Concept and theory identification in nursing administration. *Nursing Administration Quarterly*, 15(3), 79–80.

Fawcett, J., & Downs, F.S. (1992). *The relationship of theory and research* (2nd ed). Philadelphia: FA Davis.

Flaskerud, J.H. (1984). Nursing models as conceptual frameworks for research. *Western Journal of Nursing Research*, 6, 153–155, 197–199.

Grant, J.S., Kinney, M.R., & Davis, L.L. (1993). Using conceptual frameworks of models to guide nursing research. *Journal of Neuroscience Nursing*, 25, 52–56.

Haller, K.B. (1988). Theoretically speaking. *American Journal of Maternal Child Nursing*, 13, 238.

Hardy, L.K. (1982). Nursing models and research—a restricting view? *Journal of Advanced Nursing*, 7, 447–451.

Hinshaw, A.S. (1979). Theoretical substruction: An assessment process. *Western Journal of Nursing Research*, 1, 319–324.

Hymovich, D.P. (1993). Designing a conceptual or theoretical framework for research. *Journal of Pediatric Oncology Nursing*, 10, 75–78.

Jaarsma, T., & Dassen, T. (1993). The relationship of nursing theory and research: The state of the art. *Journal of Advanced Nursing*, 18, 783–787.

Laschinger, H.K., Docherty, S., & Dennis, C. (1992). Helping students use nursing models to guide research. *Nurse Educator*, 17(2), 36–38.

Laudan, L. (1977). *Progress and its problems*. Berkeley: University of California Press.

Laudan, L. (1981). A problem-solving approach to scientific progress. In I. Hacking (Ed.), *Scientific revolutions* (pp. 144–155). Fair Lawn, NJ: Oxford University Press.

McSkimming, S., Johnson, K., & Harrison, C. (1991). Proposed role of a clinical conceptual framework in the development of a research program. *Western Journal of Nursing Research*, 13, 539–542.

Moody, L.E., & Hutchinson, S.A. (1989). Relating your study to a theoretical context. In H.S. Wilson, *Research in nursing* (2nd ed., pp. 275–332). Redwood City, CA: Addison-Wesley.

Penticuff, J.H. (1991). Conceptual issues in nursing ethics research. *Journal of Medicine and Philosophy*, 16, 235–258.

Schlotfeldt, R.M. (1975). The need for a conceptual framework. In P.J. Verhonick (Ed.), *Nursing research I* (pp. 3–24). Boston: Little, Brown.

Schoenhofer, S.O. (1993). What constitutes nursing research? *Nursing Science Quarterly*, 6, 509–560.

Silva, M.C. (1986). Research testing nursing theory: State of the art. *Advances in Nursing Science*, 9(1), 1–11.

Silva, M.C. (1987). Conceptual models of nursing. In J.J. Fitzpatrick & R.L. Taunton (Eds.), *Annual review of nursing research* (Vol. 5, pp. 229–246). New York: Springer.

VanCott, M.L., Tittle, M.B., Moody, L.E., & Wilson, M.E. (1991). Analysis of a decade of critical care nursing practice research: 1979 to 1988. *Heart and Lung*, 20, 394–397.

Wells, T.J. (1987). Nursing model and research compatibility: Concerns and possibilities. *Journal of Gerontological Nursing*, *13*(9), 20–23.

Conceptual Models and Nursing Education

Batra, C. (1987). Nursing theory for undergraduates. *Nursing Outlook, 35*, 189–192.

Bramadat, I.J., & Chalmers, K.I. (1989). Nursing education in Canada: Historical "progress"—contemporary issues. *Journal of Advanced Nursing, 14*, 719–726.

Clifford, C. (1989). An experience of transition from a medical model to a nursing model in nurse education. *Nurse Education Today, 9*, 413–418.

Curriculum innovation through framework application. (1975). Loma Linda, CA: Loma Linda University School of Nursing.

DeBeck, V. (1981). The relationship between senior nursing students' ability to formulate nursing diagnoses and the curriculum model. *Advances in Nursing Science, 3*(3), 51–66.

Derdiarian, A.K. (1970). Education: A way to theory construction in nursing. *Journal of Nursing Education, 18*(2), 35–47.

Dowie, S., & Park, C. (1988). Relating nursing theory to students' life experiences. *Nurse Education Today, 8*, 191–196.

Faculty-curriculum development. Part III: Conceptual framework — its meaning and function. (1975). New York: National League for Nursing.

Fawcett, J. (1985). Theory: Basis for the study and practice of nursing education. *Journal of Nursing Education, 24*, 226–229.

Flaskerud, J.H. (1983). Utilizing a nursing conceptual model in basic level curriculum development. *Journal of Nursing Education, 22*, 224–227.

Gould, D. (1989). Teaching theories and models of nursing: Implications for a common foundation programme for nurses. *Recent Advances in Nursing, 24*, 93–105.

Green, C. (1985). An overview of the value of nursing models in relation to education. *Nurse Education Today, 5*(2), 67–71.

Hall, K.V. (1979). Current trends in the use of conceptual frameworks in nursing education. *Journal of Nursing Education, 18*(4), 26–29.

Jacobs-Kramer, M.K., & Huether, S.E. (1988). Curricular considerations for teaching nursing theory. *Journal of Professional Nursing, 4*, 373–380.

Jopp, M.C. (1989). Nursing conceptual frameworks: Content analysis of themes related to humans, environment, health, and nursing used in nursing education. In J.P. Riehl-Sisca, *Conceptual models for*

nursing practice (3rd ed., pp. 35–46). Norwalk, CT: Appleton & Lange.

Kermode, S. (1988). How nurses use curriculum concepts. *Australian Journal of Advanced Nursing, 6*, 21–26.

Kuhn, R.C., Alspach, J.A.G., & Roberts, W.L. (1985). Educational standards for critical care nursing: Conceptual framework. *Heart and Lung, 14*, 187–190.

Laschinger, H.K., & Boss, M.K. (1989). Learning styles of baccalaureate nursing students toward theory-based nursing. *Journal of Professional Nursing, 5*, 215–223.

Lutjens, L.R.J., & Horan, M.L. (1992). Nursing theory in nursing education: An educational imperative. *Journal of Professional Nursing, 8*, 276–281.

MacNeil, M. (1987). Models and the curriculum. *Senior Nurse, 6*(6), 22.

Masters, M. (1988). Nursing theory: An eclectic approach in baccalaureate education. *The Kansas Nurse, 63*(12), 1–2.

McCaugherty, D. (1991). The theory-practice gap in nurse education: Its causes and possible solutions. Findings from an action research study. *Journal of Advanced Nursing, 16*, 1055–1061.

Murphy, R.M. (1991). Creatively teaching the interrelationships of a nursing model. *Nurse Educator, 16*(4), 24–29.

Orb, A., & Reilly, D.E. (1991). Changing to a conceptual base curriculum. *International Nursing Review, 38*, 56–60.

Radke, K.J., Adams, B.N., Anderson, J., Bouman, C., Rideout, K., & Zigrossi, S. (1991). Curriculum blueprints for the future: The process of blending beliefs. *Nursing Educator, 16*(2), 9–13.

Rambur, B. (1991). Human environments, phenomena, crises, and lifestyles: Unifying concepts of a nursing curriculum. *Nursing and Health Care, 12*, 464–468.

Smith, L. (1987). Application of nursing models to a curriculum: Some considerations. *Nurse Education Today, 7*, 109–115.

Greenwood, J. (1988). More considerations concerning the application of nursing models to curricula: A reply to Lorraine Smith. *Nurse Education Today, 8*, 187–190.

Sohn, K.S. (1991). Conceptual frameworks and patterns of nursing curriculum. *Journal of Advanced Nursing, 16*, 858–866.

Toney, S.P. (1989). Relationship between conceptual frameworks, selected program, faculty, and student variables and faculty's perceived competency of graduates in associate degree nursing programs. *Dissertation Abstracts International, 50*, 2344B.

Webb, C. (1990). Nursing models in the curriculum: The nursing degree course at Bristol Polytechnic. *Nurse Education Today, 10*, 299–306.

White, M.B. (Ed.). (1983). *Curriculum development from a nursing model: The crisis theory framework.* New York: Springer.

Conceptual Models and Nursing Administration

Anderson, R.A. (1988). Development of a strategy for testing borrowed theory: An analysis using a conceptual model of nursing administration and contingency theory. *Dissertation Abstracts International, 48,* 3530B.

Anderson, R.A., & Scalzi, C. (1989). A theory development role for nurse administrators. *Journal of Nursing Administration, 19*(5), 23–29.

Davis, D.L., & Salmen, K.M. (1991). Nursing, planning, and marketing: From theory to practice. *Nursing Administration Quarterly, 15*(3), 66–71.

Fawcett, J., Botter, M.L., Burritt, J., Crossley, J.D., & Frink, B.B. (1989). Conceptual models of nursing and organization theories. In B. Henry, C. Arndt, M. Di Vincenti, & A. Marriner-Tomey (Eds.), *Dimensions of nursing administration: Theory, research, education, practice* (pp. 143–154). Boston: Blackwell Scientific Publications.

Flarey, D.L. (1991). Nursing practice in an osteopathic community. *Nursing Administration Quarterly, 15*(3), 29–36.

Haddon, R. (1991). The implications of shifting paradigms. *Aspen's Advisor for Nurse Executives, 6*(22), 1, 3–6.

Marriner-Tomey, A. (1989). Survey of theory in nursing administration textbooks. *Nursing Administration Quarterly, 13*(4), 69–70.

Mayberry, A. (1991). Merging nursing theories, models, and nursing practice: More than an administrative challenge. *Nursing Administration Quarterly, 15*(3), 44–53.

Pagana, K.D. (1986). Consider this. *Journal of Nursing Administration, 16*(2), 4.

Silver, J.I. (1991). Nursing theory (Management readings). *Journal of Nursing Administration, 21*(2), 11.

Smith, M.C. (1993). The contribution of nursing theory to nursing administration practice. *Image: Journal of Nursing Scholarship, 25,* 63–67.

Sorrentino, E.A. (1991). Making theories work for you. *Nursing Administration Quarterly, 15*(3), 54–59.

Conceptual Models and Nursing Practice

Akinsanya, J.A. (1984). The uses of theories in nursing. *Nursing Times, 80*(28), 59–60.

Ali, L. (1990). Clinical nursing assessment: Models in accident and emergency. *Nursing Standard, 5*(3), 33–35.

Bélanger, P. (1991). Nursing models—a major step towards professional autonomy. *AARN Newsletter, 48*(8), 13 (Alberta Association of Registered Nurses [Canada]).

Biley, F. (1991). The divide between theory and practice. *Nursing (London), 4*(29), 30–33.

Biley, F. (1992). Nursing models redundant in practice. *British Journal of Nursing, 1,* 219.

Carveth, J.A. (1987). Conceptual models in nurse-midwifery. *Journal of Nurse-Midwifery, 32,* 20–25.

Chalmers, H.A. (1989). Theories and models of nursing and the nursing process. *Recent Advances in Nursing, 24,* 32–46.

Chalmers, H., Kershaw, B., Melia, K., & Kendrich, M. (1990). Nursing models: Enhancing or inhibiting practice? *Nursing Standard, 5*(11), 34–40.

Christmyer, C.S., Catanzariti, P.M., Langford, A.M., & Reitz, J.A. (1988). Bridging the gap: Theory to practice—Part I, Clinical applications. *Nursing Management, 19*(8), 42–50.

Curtin, L.L. (1988). Thought-full nursing practice (Editorial). *Nursing Management, 19*(10), 7–8.

Davis, B., & Simms, C.L. (1992). Are we providing safe care? *The Canadian Nurse, 88*(1), 45–47.

Derstine, J.B. (1989). The development of theory-based practice by graduate students in rehabilitation nursing. *Rehabilitation Nursing, 14,* 88–89.

Derstine, J.B. (1992). Theory-based advanced rehabilitation nursing: Is it a reality? *Holistic Nursing Practice, 6*(2), 1–6.

Dyer, S. (1990). Team work for personal patient care. *Nursing the Elderly, 3*(7), 28–30.

Fawcett, J. (1990). Conceptual models and rules for nursing practice. In N.L. Chaska (Ed.), *The nursing profession: Turning points* (pp. 255–262). St. Louis: CV Mosby.

Fawcett, J., Archer, C.L., Becker, D., Brown, K.K., Gann, S., Wong, M.J., & Wurster, A.B. (1992). Guidelines for selecting a conceptual model of nursing: Focus on the individual patient. *Dimensions of Critical Care Nursing, 11,* 268–277.

Field, P.A. (1987). The impact of nursing

theory on the clinical decision making process. *Journal of Advanced Nursing, 12,* 563–571.

Field, P.A. (1989). Brenda, Beth, and Susan. Three approaches to health promotion. *The Canadian Nurse, 85*(5), 20–24.

Fitzpatrick, J.J. (1987). Use of existing nursing models. *Journal of Gerontological Nursing, 13*(9), 8–9.

Fitzpatrick, J.J. (1988). How can we enhance nursing knowledge and practice? *Nursing and Health Care, 9,* 517–521.

Freda, M.C. (1991). Home care for preterm birth prevention: Is nursing monitoring the interventions? *American Journal of Maternal-Child Nursing, 16,* 9–14.

Gilbert, E.S., & Harmon, J.S. (1986). *High-risk pregnancy and delivery: Nursing perspectives.* St. Louis: CV Mosby.

Godin, M.E. (1991). Using conceptual models (Letter). *Focus on Critical Care, 18,* 108.

Rodgers, B.L. (1991). Reply. (Letter). *Focus on Critical Care, 18,* 108.

Gordon, M. (1990). Toward theory-based diagnostic categories. *Nursing Diagnosis, 1*(1), 5–11.

Hanchett, E.S. (1988). *Nursing frameworks and community as client: Bridging the gap.* Norwalk, CT: Appleton & Lange.

Hanchett, E.S., & Clarke, P.N. (1988). Nursing theory and public health science: Is synthesis possible? *Public Health Nursing, 5*(1), 2–6.

Hawkett, S. (1991). A gap which must be bridged: Nurses' attitudes to theory and practice. *Professional Nurse, 6,* 166, 168–170.

Huch, M.H. (1988). Theory-based practice: Structuring nursing care. *Nursing Science Quarterly, 1,* 6–7.

Hughes, D.J.F., & Goldstone, L.A. (1989). Frameworks for midwifery care in Great Britain: An exploration of quality assurance. *Midwifery, 5,* 163–171.

Kappeli, S. (1987). The influence of nursing models on clinical decision making I. In K.J. Hannah, M. Reimer, W.C. Mills, & Letourneau, S. (Eds.), *Clinical judgment and decision making: The future with nursing diagnosis* (pp. 33–41). New York: John Wiley & Sons.

Kennedy, A. (1989). How relevant are nursing models? *Occupational Health, 41,* 352–354.

Lansberry, C.R., & Richards, E. (1992). Family nursing practice paradigm perspectives and diagnostic approaches. *Advances in Nursing Science, 15*(2), 66–75.

Laschinger, H.S. (1991). Nurses' attitudes about nursing models in practice. *Journal of Nursing Administration, 21*(10), 12, 15, 18.

Laschinger, H.K., & Duff, V. (1991). Attitudes of practicing nurses towards theory-based nursing practice. *Canadian Journal of Nursing Administration, 4*(1), 6–10.

Lindsay, B. (1990). The gap between theory and practice. *Nursing Standard, 5*(4), 34–35.

Loughlin, M. (1988). Modelled, muddled and befuddled. *Nursing Times, 84*(5), 30–31.

Luker, K. (1988). Do models work? *Nursing Times, 84*(5), 26–29.

MacVicar, B., & Swan, J. (1992). Mental health: Theory into practice. *Nursing Times, 88*(12), 38–40.

McCaugherty, D. (1992). The concepts of theory and practice. *Senior Nurse, 12*(2), 29–33.

McCaugherty, D. (1992). The gap between nursing theory and practice. *Senior Nurse, 12*(6), 44–48.

McCaugherty, D. (1992). Integrating theory and practice. *Senior Nurse, 12*(1), 36–39.

McKenna, H.P. (1990). The perception of psychiatric-hospital ward sisters/charge nurses towards nursing models. *Journal of Advanced Nursing, 15,* 1319–1325.

Mitchell, G.J. (1992). Specifying the knowledge base of theory in practice. *Nursing Science Quarterly, 5,* 6–7.

Norberg, A., & Wickstrom, E. (1990). The perception of Swedish nurses and nurse teachers of the integration of theory with nursing practice: An explorative qualitative study. *Nurse Education Today, 10,* 38–43.

Northrup, D.T., & Barrett, E.A.M. (1992). Disciplinary perspective: Unified or diverse? Commentary and response. *Nursing Science Quarterly, 5,* 154–157.

Oliver, N.R. (1991). True believers: A case for model-based nursing practice. *Nursing Administration Quarterly, 15*(3), 37–43.

Parse, R.R. (1990). Nursing theory-based practice: A challenge for the 90s (Editorial). *Nursing Science Quarterly, 3,* 53.

Savage, P. (1991). Patient assessment in psychiatric nursing. *Journal of Advanced Nursing, 16,* 311–316.

Schneider, P. (1991). Is an educational paradigm fundamental to clinical nursing practice? *The Lamp, 48*(2), 23–27.

Selanders, L., & Dietz-Omar, M. (1991). Making nursing models relevant for the practicing nurse. *Nursing Practice, 4*(2), 23–25.

Sirra, E. (1986). Using nursing models for nursing practice. *Nursing Journal of India, 77,* 301–304.

Smith, M.C. (1991). Evaluating nursing theory-based practice. *Nursing Science Quarterly, 4,* 98–99.

Speedy, S. Theory-practice debate: Setting the scene. *Australian Journal of Advanced Nursing, 6*(3), 12–20.

Story, E.L., & DuGas, B.W. (1988). A teaching strategy to facilitate conceptual model implementation in practice. *Journal of Continuing Education in Nursing, 19,* 244–247.

Villeneuve, M.J., & Ozolins, P.H. (1991). Sexual counseling in the neuroscience setting: Theory and practical tips for nurses. *AXON, 12*(3), 63–67.

Wardle, M.G., & Mandle, C.L. (1989). Conceptual models used in clinical practice. *Western Journal of Nursing Research, 11,* 108–114.

2

Analysis and Evaluation of Conceptual Models of Nursing

This chapter presents a framework for analysis and evaluation of conceptual models of nursing that highlights their most important features and is appropriate to their level of abstraction. The framework was first published several years ago (Fawcett, 1980) and has undergone revisions for each edition of this book. The initial and continued development of the framework has been motivated by dissatisfaction with other frameworks primarily because of their failure to distinguish between conceptual models and theories (e.g., Barnum, 1994; Fitzpatrick & Whall, 1989; George, 1990; Marriner-Tomey, 1994; Meleis, 1991). The current version of the framework reflects increased understanding of the relationship of conceptual models to the other components of the structural hierarchy of contemporary nursing knowledge, that is, the metaparadigm, philosophies, theories, and empirical indicators.

The major components of analysis and evaluation of conceptual models of nursing are identified in the following key terms. Each component is discussed in detail in this chapter.

KEY TERMS

ANALYSIS	Generation of Theory
Origins	Credibility
Unique Focus and Content	*Social Utility*
EVALUATION	*Social Congruence*
Explication of Origins	*Social Significance*
Comprehensiveness of Content	Contributions to Nursing
Logical Congruence	

A FRAMEWORK FOR ANALYSIS AND EVALUATION OF NURSING MODELS

The framework that is used in this book for analysis and evaluation of conceptual models of nursing separates questions dealing with analysis from those more appropriate to evaluation (Table 2–1). The questions for analysis follow directly from the discussion of the structural hierarchy of contemporary nursing knowledge that was presented in Chapter 1. The intent of the analysis is to present an objective and nonjudgmental description of the origins and content of the conceptual model. The evaluation, in contrast, requires judgments to be made about the conceptual model with regard to the extent to which it satisfies specific external criteria.

ANALYSIS OF CONCEPTUAL MODELS OF NURSING

Analysis of a conceptual model of nursing, using the framework presented in this chapter, requires a systematic, detailed review of all available publications and presentations by the author of the model to determine exactly what has been said, rather than relying on inferences about what might have been meant or by referring to other authors' interpretations of the conceptual model. When the author of the conceptual model has not been clear about a point or has not presented certain information, it may be necessary to make inferences or to turn to other reviews of the model. That, however, must be noted explicitly, so the distinction between the words of the conceptual model author and those of others is clear. The analysis targets the *origins* of the conceptual model, as well as its *unique focus* and *content*.

Origins of the Conceptual Model

The first step in the analysis of a conceptual model of nursing is examination of four aspects of its *origins*. First, the historical evolution of the conceptual model is described, and the author's motivation for developing the conceptual model is explicated. Second, the author's philosophical claims about nursing and the knowledge development strategies used to formulate the conceptual model are examined. Third, the influences on the author's thinking from nurse scholars and scholars of adjunctive disciplines are identified. Fourth, the world view reflected by the conceptual model is specified.

A conceptual model is derived from an author's philosophical claims about the phenomena of interest to nursing and the development of knowledge. The development of a conceptual model is a more intellectual than empirical endeavor, although empirical observations certainly may influence the work. Because it is not unusual to find that the content of a

TABLE 2–1. **A FRAMEWORK FOR ANALYSIS AND EVALUATION OF CONCEPTUAL MODELS OF NURSING**

Questions for Analysis

- What are the origins of the conceptual model?
  What is the historical evolution of the conceptual model?
  What motivated the development of the conceptual model?
  On what philosophical beliefs and values about nursing is the conceptual model based?
  What strategies for knowledge development were used to formulate the conceptual model?
  What scholars influenced the model author's thinking?
  What world view is reflected in the conceptual model?
- What is the unique focus of the conceptual model?
- How are nursing's four metaparadigm concepts explicated in the model?
  How is person defined and described?
  How is environment defined and described?
  How is health defined?
  How are wellness and illness differentiated?
  How is nursing defined?
  What is the goal of nursing?
  How is the nursing process described?
- What statements are made about the relationships among the four metaparadigm concepts?

Questions for Evaluation

- Are the philosophical claims on which the conceptual model is based explicit?
- Are the scholars who influenced the model author's thinking acknowledged, and are bibliographical citations given?
- Does the conceptual model provide adequate descriptions of all four concepts of nursing's metaparadigm?
- Do the relational propositions of the conceptual model completely link the four metaparadigm concepts?
- Is the researcher given sufficient direction about what questions to ask and what methodology to use?
- Does the educator have sufficient guidelines to construct a curriculum?
- Does the administrator have sufficient guidelines to organize and deliver nursing services?
- Is the clinician given sufficient direction to be able to make pertinent observations, decide that a nursing problem exists, and prescribe and execute a course of action that achieves the goal specified in a variety of clinical situations?
- Is the internal structure of the conceptual model logically congruent?
  Does the model reflect more than one contrasting world view?
  Does the model reflect characteristics of more than one category of nursing knowledge?
  Do the components of the model reflect logical translation/reformulation of diverse perspectives?
- What theories have been generated from the conceptual model?
- Are education and skill training required prior to application of the conceptual model in nursing practice?
- Is it feasible to implement clinical protocols derived from the conceptual model and related theories?
- To what extent is the conceptual model actually used to guide nursing research, education, administration, and practice?
- Does the conceptual model lead to nursing activities that meet the expectations of nursing care recipients and health care team members of various cultures and in diverse geographic regions?
- Does application of the conceptual model, when linked with relevant theories and appropriate empirical indicators, make important differences in the person's health status?
- What is the overall contribution of the conceptual model to the discipline of nursing?

conceptual model has undergone revisions as the author refines concepts and propositions and formulates new ideas about nursing, it is important to trace the evolution of the model from its initial version to the present one. The content of the conceptual model evolves as the author engages in inductive and/or deductive reasoning. The extensive review of the model author's publications and presentations will provide clues or explicit descriptions of the underlying beliefs and values and the factors that motivated model development, as well as the inductive and/or deductive strategies used to transform an implicit private image of nursing into an explicit conceptual model.

The author's use of either or both inductive and deductive reasoning reflects a certain philosophical orientation to the development of knowledge and to the relationship between the person and the environment. This orientation often can be traced to the author's educational experiences as well as to exposure to the thinking of other nursing scholars and scholars of adjunctive disciplines. Accordingly, analysis of the origins of the conceptual model should include identification of the author's references to the works of earlier scholars in nursing and other disciplines. In addition, the analysis of origins should include identification of the world view reflected by the conceptual model. The contrasting world views of reaction, reciprocal interaction, and simultaneous action, discussed in Chapter 1, are appropriate here. The questions to ask are:

- What are the origins of the conceptual model?

  What is the historical evolution of the conceptual model?

  What motivated the development of the conceptual model?

  On what philosophical beliefs and values about nursing is the conceptual model based?

  What strategies for knowledge development were used to formulate the conceptual model?

  What scholars influenced the model author's thinking?

  What world view is reflected in the conceptual model?

Unique Focus and Content of the Conceptual Model

The second step in the analysis of a conceptual model of nursing is examination of its *unique focus* and its *content*. The need to identify the unique focus of the conceptual model stems from the fact that although most authors start with the same view of the general purpose of nursing, in final form the nursing models present distinctive views of the metaparadigm concepts (Johnson, 1974). Indeed, different models are concerned with different problems in nurse-patient situations or different problems in person-environment interactions (Christensen & Kenney,

1990; Duffey & Muhlenkamp, 1974). They also may be concerned with different actual and potential deviations from desired health states and with different modes of nursing intervention (Johnson, 1987).

The factors that are thought to influence the development of problems or deviations and to direct types of nursing interventions also may vary from model to model. The unique focus of a conceptual model is specified by its classification regarding one or more categories of nursing knowledge. As explained in Chapter 1, the relevant categories are developmental, systems, or interaction; needs or outcomes; client-focused, person-environment interaction focused, or nursing therapeutics-focused; humanistic or energy field; and intervention, substitution, conservation, sustenance, or enhancement. The question is:

- What is the unique focus of the conceptual model?

The content of a conceptual model is presented in the form of abstract and general concepts and propositions. Most authors of nursing models have not presented their ideas in the form of explicit statements about each of the metaparadigm concepts. Therefore, this part of the analysis is most readily accomplished first by categorizing the content of the model into definitions and descriptions of person, environment, health, and nursing. Then, in the language of the conceptual model, statements reflecting the linkage of the metaparadigm concepts can be extracted. The questions are:

- How are nursing's four metaparadigm concepts explicated in the model?

How is person defined and described?

How is environment defined and described?

How is health defined? How are wellness and illness differentiated?

How is nursing defined? What is the goal of nursing?

How is the nursing process described?

- What statements are made about the relationships among the four metaparadigm concepts?

QUESTIONS FOR EVALUATION

Evaluation of a conceptual model of nursing is accomplished by comparing its content with criteria that address *explication of origins, comprehensiveness of focus and content, logical congruence, theory generating capabilities, credibility, and contributions to nursing knowledge.* The evaluation is based on the results of the analysis, as well as on a review of previously published critiques, research reports, and reports of the application of the conceptual model in nursing education, administration, and practice.

Explication of Origins

The first step of evaluation concerns the *origins* of the conceptual model. Identification of the author's beliefs and values yields information about the philosophical foundations of the model and helps to identify special points of emphasis in the view of nursing put forth by the conceptual model. The expectation is that those philosophical claims have been made explicit by the author. Indeed, "a statement of one's value system is an essential accompaniment to a model" (Johnson, 1987, p. 197). Furthermore, because the content of most conceptual models of nursing draws from existing knowledge in nursing and adjunctive disciplines (Levine, 1988, 1992), it is expected that the works of other scholars were cited. The questions to ask when evaluating the origins of the conceptual model are:

- Are the philosophical claims on which the conceptual model is based explicit?

- Are the scholars who influenced the model author's thinking acknowledged, and are bibliographical citations given?

Comprehensiveness of Content

The second step of evaluation deals with the *comprehensiveness of the content* of the model, with emphasis placed on the depth and breadth of content. No well-established criterion for the depth of the content of a conceptual model has been established. It seems reasonable to expect, however, that the content should encompass the four metaparadigm concepts and that that content is relatively unambiguous. Consequently, the expectation is that the conceptual model presents a description of the person, an identification of the person's environment, a discussion of the author's meaning of health, a definition of nursing, a statement of nursing goals or outcomes, and an outline of the nursing process. In addition, the nursing process should be grounded in a base of scientific knowledge, permit dynamic movement between each step, and be compatible with ethical standards for nursing practice (Walker & Nicholson, 1980).

Furthermore, it seems reasonable to expect the relational propositions of the conceptual model to link all four metaparadigm concepts. This may be done in a series of statements linking two or more concepts, or it may be accomplished by one summary statement encompassing all four concepts. These statements will, of course, use the vocabulary of the particular conceptual model. The questions to ask when evaluating the depth of the content of a conceptual model are:

- Does the conceptual model provide adequate descriptions of all four concepts of nursing's metaparadigm?

- Do the relational propositions of the conceptual model completely link the four metaparadigm concepts?

The criterion for the breadth of the content of a conceptual model requires that it is sufficiently broad in scope to provide guidance in clinical situations of normalcy, risk, crisis, and morbidity (Magee, 1991) and to also serve as a basis for research, education, and administration. Although the expectation is that the conceptual model is a useful frame of reference for many nursing activities, it is recognized that any one conceptual model may not be appropriate for *all* clinical situations. In fact, it is entirely possible that the content of the model precludes certain situations. In such a case, we must decide if the limitations are sufficient to warrant elimination of the model as a viable one for nursing. The questions to ask when evaluating the breadth of the content of the conceptual model are based on suggestions from Johnson (1987) and reflect the rules for nursing research, education, administration, and practice that were described in Chapter 1. The questions are:

- Is the researcher given sufficient direction about what questions to ask and what methodology to use?

- Does the educator have sufficient guidelines to construct a curriculum?

- Does the administrator have sufficient guidelines to organize and deliver nursing services?

- Is the clinician given sufficient direction to be able to make pertinent observations, decide that a nursing problem exists, and prescribe and execute a course of action that achieves the goal specified in a variety of clinical situations?

Logical Congruence

The third step of evaluation of a conceptual model considers the logic of its internal structure. Logical congruence is evaluated through the intellectual process of critical reasoning, which "highlights strengths and explores problems inherent in a line of reasoning" (Silva & Sorrell, 1992, p. 17). The process involves judging the congruence of the model author's espoused philosophical claims with the content of the model. Critical reasoning also involves judgments regarding the world view(s) and category(ies) of nursing knowledge reflected by the model. Evaluation of logical congruence is especially important if the conceptual model incorporates more than one contrasting world view or category of nursing knowledge. This is because different schools of thought cannot be combined easily, if at all. However, viewpoints sometimes may be merged or translated by redefining all concepts in a consistent manner. More specifically, conceptual models of nursing that strive to combine concepts and propositions derived from different world views and/or different categories of nursing knowledge must first reformulate or translate the concepts and propositions to ensure just one congruent frame of reference.

Reformulation or translation is accomplished by redefining concepts and restating propositions that do not reflect the preferred world view or category of nursing knowledge, so that all ideas presented in the conceptual model are consistent (Reese & Overton, 1970; Whall, 1980). The expectation is that all elements of the conceptual model are logically congruent. The questions to be asked when evaluating logical congruence are:

- Is the internal structure of the conceptual model logically congruent?

- Does the model reflect more than one contrasting world view?

- Does the model reflect characteristics of more than one category of nursing knowledge?

- Do the components of the model reflect logical reformulation/ translation of diverse perspectives?

Generation of Theory

The fourth step of the evaluation of a conceptual model of nursing reflects the relationship between models and theories. As explained in Chapter 1, grand and middle-range theories can be derived from conceptual models of nursing. Thus, *the theory-generating contributions* of the model should be judged.

The need for logically congruent conceptual-theoretical systems of nursing knowledge for nursing activities mandates that at least some theories be derived from each conceptual model. The expectation is, therefore, that the concepts and propositions of the model be sufficiently clear so that the relatively specific and concrete concepts and propositions of grand and middle-range theories can be deduced, and testable hypotheses can be formulated. The question is:

- What theories have been generated from the conceptual model?

Credibility of Conceptual Models

The fifth step of evaluation focuses attention on the *credibility* of the conceptual model. Credibility determination is necessary to avoid the danger of uncritical acceptance and adoption of conceptual models, which could easily lead to their use as ideologies. Indeed, critical reviews of the evidence regarding the credibility of each conceptual model must be encouraged, and acceptance of work that is "fashionable, well-trodden or simply available in the nursing library" (Grinnell, 1992, p. 57) must be avoided.

The ultimate aim of credibility determination is to ascertain which conceptual models are appropriate for use in which clinical settings and with which patients. It is likely that determination of credibility will either support or refute the impression that any conceptual model "can explain or guide any nursing intervention in any setting, and that all [models] are equally relevant for guiding the practice of nursing" (See, 1986, p. 355). Confirmation or refutation of that impression through a thorough evaluation of the credibility of each conceptual model is crucial if nursing is to continue to advance as a respected discipline characterized by excellence in scientific and clinical scholarship.

The credibility of a conceptual model cannot be determined directly. Rather, the abstract and general concepts and propositions of the conceptual model must be linked with the more specific and concrete concepts and propositions of a middle-range theory and appropriate empirical indicators to determine credibility. The resulting conceptual-theoretical-empirical system of nursing knowledge then is used to guide nursing activities, and the results of use are examined. Thus, credibility of conceptual models is determined through tests of conceptual-theoretical-empirical systems of nursing knowledge. Credibility determination is examined by means of the criteria of <u>social utility</u>, <u>social congruence</u>, and <u>social significance</u> of the conceptual model. Judgments regarding the extent to which the conceptual model meets those criteria require a review of all publications and presentations by the author of the conceptual model, as well as those by other nurses who have used the model.

Social Utility

Social utility addresses the special education required to apply the conceptual model; the feasibility of implementing the conceptual model in nursing practice; and the extent to which the conceptual model is actually used to guide nursing research, education, administration, and practice. Although model authors should strive to write and discuss their work clearly and concisely (Cormack & Reynolds, 1992), the abstract and general nature of conceptual models and the special vocabulary of each one typically require collegiate or continuing education for mastery. In addition, special training in interpersonal and psychomotor skills may be necessary to apply the model in clinical situations (Magee, 1991). The expectation is that the nurse has a full understanding of the conceptual model content as well as the interpersonal and psychomotor skills necessary to apply it. Thus, the first question to be asked when evaluating the social utility of a conceptual model is:

■ Are education and skill training required prior to application of the conceptual model in nursing practice?

The evaluation of social utility also considers the feasibility of implementing clinical protocols derived from the conceptual model and related theories in nursing practice. The expectation is, of course, that the implemention of such protocols is feasible. Feasibility is determined by evaluating the human and material resources needed to establish the model-based nursing actions as customary practice (Magee, 1991). Requisite resources include the time required to learn and implement the protocols; the number, type, and expertise of personnel required for their application; and the funds for continuing education, salaries, equipment, and protocol-testing procedures. The question is:

- Is it feasible to implement clinical protocols derived from the conceptual model and related theories?

Evaluation of social utility also requires consideration of the extent to which the conceptual model is actually used to guide nursing research, education, administration, and practice. Although a completely accurate appraisal of actual use is impossible, a rapidly growing body of literature documents the application of conceptual models to the design of nursing studies, the construction of educational programs and administrative structures, and the care of people who require nursing. The question is:

- To what extent is the conceptual model actually used to guide nursing research, education, administration, and practice?

Social Congruence

Social congruence refers to the compatibility of conceptual model-based nursing activities with the expectations of the patient, the community, and the health care system for nursing practice (Magee, 1991). In particular, the patient's and the community's culturally determined expectations, as well as various health care team members' discipline-oriented expectations, with regard to appropriate areas of assessment, relevant goals and outcomes, and appropriate nursing interventions must be taken into account (Aggleton & Chalmers, 1985; Jones, 1989; McLane, 1983). Furthermore, expectations based on the system of health care delivery in various countries should be considered (Cormack & Reynolds, 1992). If others' expectations for nursing are not congruent with the practice that is derived from the conceptual model, then they must be helped to expect a different kind of nursing. This is especially important, for without the expected affirmative answer to the question of social congruence, "nursing will not continue to be sanctioned as a profession or an occupation, and in a nursing shortage situation [or in the current era of health care reform], . . . the nurse may be replaced with other health professionals" (Johnson, 1987, p. 197). The question is:

- Does the conceptual model lead to nursing activities that meet the expectations of nursing care recipients and health care team members of various cultures and in diverse geographic regions?

Social Significance

The criterion of social significance requires a judgment to be made with regard to the social value of a conceptual model, with emphasis placed on the effect of use of a conceptual model on patients' health status (Magee, 1991). "This criterion," according to Johnson (1974), "recognizes that a professional service is a highly valued one because it is critical to people in some way" (p. 376). The social significance of a conceptual model can be determined by informal and formal methods.

The informal method of determining social significance is accomplished in three phases. First, prototype conceptual-theoretical systems of nursing knowledge are developed for each clinical specialty area or each nursing department and for various patient populations. Next, an individualized system of knowledge is developed by each nurse for each patient. Nursing care then is carried out in accordance with the nursing process of the selected conceptual model, which is amplified by logically congruent middle-range theories. Finally, the results of the evaluation of the process provide data that may be used to determine credibility of the knowledge system. The conceptual-theoretical system of knowledge is considered credible if patient outcomes are in accordance with expectations. If, however, patient outcomes are not in accordance with expectations, the credibility of the knowledge system, and hence the conceptual model, must be questioned.

The formal method of determining social significance is accomplished by examining the findings of research guided by conceptual-theoretical-empirical systems of nursing knowledge. First, the influence of the conceptual model on the research process is evaluated in relation to the following criteria, which were adapted from work by Silva (1986):

1. The conceptual model of nursing is explicitly identified as the underlying guide for the research.

2. The conceptual model of nursing is discussed in sufficient breadth and depth so that the relationship between the model and the study purpose and research question(s) is clear.

3. The linkages between conceptual model concepts and propositions and middle-range theory concepts and propositions are stated explicitly.

4. The study methodology reflects the conceptual model.
 (a). The study subjects are drawn from a population that is appropriate for the unique focus of the conceptual model.
 (b). The instruments are appropriate empirical indicators of conceptual model concepts.
 (c). The study design clearly reflects the unique focus of the conceptual model.
 (d). The data analysis techniques are in keeping with the unique focus of the conceptual model.

5. The data are interpreted in terms of evidence regarding the middle-range theory that was derived from or linked with the conceptual model.

6. Discussion of study results includes conclusions regarding the empirical adequacy of the middle-range theory and the credibility of the conceptual model.

The systematic application of those criteria is especially important because some researchers do little more than cite a particular conceptual model in the study report (Silva, 1987). If a research report satisfies the criteria, determination of credibility may proceed to a comparison of the research findings with the propositions of the conceptual-theoretical system of nursing knowledge that was used to guide the research. If the research findings support the empirical adequacy of the theory, then it is likely that the conceptual model is credible. If, however, the research findings do not support hypothesized expectations, both the empirical adequacy of the theory and the credibility of the conceptual model must be questioned.

The expectation for the criterion of social significance is that the use of the conceptual model has a significant, positive impact on the person's well-being. The question is:

- Does application of the conceptual model, when linked with relevant theories and appropriate empirical indicators, make important differences in the person's health status?

Contributions to the Discipline of Nursing

The sixth and final step of evaluation of nursing models, which is as general as the models themselves, requires a judgment to be made with regard to the *contribution of the model to the discipline of* nursing. The judgment is made following a thorough review of all of the literature dealing with the conceptual model. Judgments should not be made on the basis of the comparison of one conceptual model with another. Rather, each conceptual model should be judged on its own merits and in accord with its own philosophical claims. Thus, one should not, for example, criticize a conceptual model for failing to consider problems in patients' self-care abilities when the model emphasizes the nurse's management of stimuli to promote the patient's adaptation. The expectation is that the conceptual model enhances understanding of the phenomena of interest to nursing. The question is:

- What is the overall contribution of the conceptual model to the discipline of nursing?

CONCLUSION

In this chapter, a framework for analysis and evaluation of conceptual models was presented. The framework will be applied in the next seven chapters, each of which will present a comprehensive examination of one conceptual model of nursing.

The framework for analysis and evaluation of conceptual models of nursing presented in this chapter is not appropriate for examination of nursing theories. Readers who are interested in that component of nursing knowledge are referred to the text *Analysis and Evaluation of Nursing Theories* (Fawcett, 1993).

REFERENCES

Aggleton, P., & Chalmers, H. (1985). Critical examination. Nursing Times, 81(14), 38–39.

Barnum, B.J.S. (1994). Nursing theory: Analysis, application, evaluation (4th ed.). Philadelphia: JB Lippincott.

Christensen, P.J., & Kenney, J.W. (Eds.). (1990). Nursing process: Application of conceptual models. St. Louis: CV Mosby.

Cormack, D.F., & Reynolds, W. (1992). Criteria for evaluating the clinical and practical utility of models used by nurses. Journal of Advanced Nursing, 17, 1472–1428.

Duffey, M., & Muhlenkamp, A.F. (1974). A framework for theory analysis. Nursing Outlook, 22, 570–574.

Fawcett, J. (1980). A framework for analysis and evaluation of conceptual models of nursing. Nurse Educator, 5(6), 10–14.

Fawcett, J. (1993). Analysis and evaluation of nursing theories. Philadelphia: FA Davis.

Fitzpatrick, J.J., & Whall, A.L. (1989). Conceptual models of nursing: Analysis and application (2nd ed.). Norwalk, CT: Appleton & Lange.

George, J.B. (Ed.). (1990). Nursing theories: The base for professional nursing practice (3rd ed.). Norwalk, CT: Appleton & Lange.

Grinnell, F. (1992). Theories without thought? Nursing Times, 88(22), 57.

Johnson, D.E. (1974). Development of theory: A requisite for nursing as a primary health profession. Nursing Research, 23, 372–377.

Johnson, D.E. (1987). Evaluating conceptual models for use in critical care nursing practice. [Guest editorial]. Dimensions of Critical Care Nursing, 6, 195–197.

Jones, S. (1989). Is unity possible? Nursing Standard, 3(1), 22–23.

Levine, M.E. (1988). Antecedents from adjunctive disciplines: Creation of nursing theory. Nursing Science Quarterly, 1, 16–21.

Levine, M.E. (1992, February). Nursing knowledge: Improving education and practice through theory. Paper presented at the Sigma Theta Tau International Conference, "Improving Education and Practice through Theory," Chicago.

Magee, M. (1991, May). Eclecticism in nursing philosophy: Problem or solution? Paper presented at the Philosophy in the Nurse's World Conference, Banff, Alberta, Canada.

Marriner-Tomey, A. (1994). Nursing theorists and their work (3rd ed.). St. Louis: Mosby-Year Book.

McLane, A. (1983). Book review of Fawcett, J. Analysis and evaluation of conceptual models of nursing. The Leading Edge (Newsletter of Delta Gamma Chapter of Sigma Theta Tau), 3(2), 15–16.

Meleis, A.I. (1991). Theoretical nursing: Development and progress (2nd ed.). Philadelphia: JB Lippincott.

Reese, H.W., & Overton, W.F. (1970). Models of development and theories of development. In L.R. Goulet & P.B. Baltes (Eds.), Life span development psychology: Research and theory (pp. 116–145). New York: Academic Press.

See, E.M. (1986). Book review of George, J. (Ed.). Nursing theories: The base for nursing practice (2nd ed.). Research in Nursing and Health, 9, 355–356.

Silva, M.C. (1986). Research testing nursing theory: State of the art. Advances in Nursing Science, 9(1), 1–11.

Silva, M.C. (1987). Conceptual models of nursing. In J.J. Fitzpatrick & R.L. Taunton (Eds.), Annual review of nursing research (Vol. 5, pp. 229–246). New York: Springer.

Silva, M.C., & Sorrell, J.M. (1992). Testing of nursing theory: Critique and philosophical expansion. Advances in Nursing Science, 14(4), 12–23.

Walker, L.O., & Nicholson, R. (1980). Criteria for evaluating nursing process models. Nurse Educator, 5(5), 8–9.

Whall, A.L. (1980). Congruence between existing theories of family functioning and nursing theories. Advances in Nursing Science, 3(1), 59–67.

BIBLIOGRAPHY

Aggleton, P., & Chalmers, H. (1985). Critical examination. *Nursing Times, 81*(14), 38–39.

Aggleton, P., & Chalmers, H. (1986). Model choice. *Senior Nurse, 5*(5/6), 18–20.

Barnum, B.J.S. (1994). *Nursing theory: Analysis, application, evaluation* (4th ed.). Philadelphia: JB Lippincott.

Biley, F. (1990). How to analyse nursing models. *Nursing (London), 4*(12), 8–10.

Buchanan, B.F. (1987). Conceptual models: An assessment framework. *Journal of Nursing Administration, 17*(10), 22–26.

Chinn, P.L., & Kramer, M.K. (1991). *Theory and nursing: A systematic approach* (3rd ed.). St. Louis: Mosby-Year Book.

Chalmers, H.A. (1989). Theories and models of nursing and the nursing process. *Recent Advances in Nursing, 24*, 32–46.

Cormack, D.F., & Reynolds, W. (1992). Criteria for evaluating the clinical and practical utility of models used by nurses. *Journal of Advanced Nursing, 17*, 1472–1478.

Duffey, M., & Muhlenkamp, A.F. (1974). A framework for theory analysis. *Nursing Outlook, 22*, 570–574.

Engstrom, J.L. (1984). Problems in the development, use and testing of nursing theory. *Journal of Nursing Education, 23*, 245–251.

Fitzpatrick, J.J., & Whall, A.L. (1989). *Conceptual models of nursing: Analysis and application* (2nd ed.). Norwalk, CT: Appleton & Lange.

George, J.B. (Ed.). (1990). *Nursing theories: The base for professional nursing practice* (3rd ed.). Norwalk, CT: Appleton & Lange.

Hoon, E. (1986). Game playing: A way to look at nursing models. *Journal of Advanced Nursing, 11*, 421–427.

Jacobson, S.F. (1984). A semantic differential for external comparison of conceptual nursing models. *Advances in Nursing Science, 6*(2), 58–70.

Johnson, D.E. (1974). Development of theory: A requisite for nursing as a primary health profession. *Nursing Research, 23*, 372–377.

Johnson, D.E. (1987). Evaluating conceptual models for use in critical care nursing practice. [Guest editorial]. *Dimensions of Critical Care Nursing, 6*, 195–197.

Jones, S. (1989). Is unity possible? *Nursing Standard, 3*(1), 22–23.

Levine, M.E. (1988). Antecedents from adjunctive disciplines: Creation of nursing theory. *Nursing Science Quarterly, 1*, 16–21.

Marriner-Tomey, A. (1994). *Nursing theorists and their work* (3rd ed.). St. Louis: Mosby-Year Book.

Meleis, A.I. (1991). *Theoretical nursing: Development and progress* (2nd ed.). Philadelphia: JB Lippincott.

Mooney, M.M. (1960). The ethical component of nursing theory: An analysis of ethical components of four nursing theories. *Image: The Journal of Nursing Scholarship, 12*, 7–9.

Nicoll, L., Myer, P., & Abraham, I. (1985). Critique: External comparison of conceptual nursing models. *Advances in Nursing Science, 7*(4), 1–9.

O'Toole, M. (Ed.). (1992). *Miller-Keane encyclopedia and dictionary of medicine, nursing, and allied health* (5th ed.). Philadelphia: WB Saunders.

Peterson, C.J. (1977). Questions frequently asked about the development of a conceptual framework. *Journal of Nursing Education, 16*(4), 22–32.

Reese, H.W., & Overton, W.F. (1970). Models of development and theories of development. In L.R. Goulet & P.B. Baltes (Eds.), *Life span development psychology: Research and theory* (pp. 116–145). New York: Academic Press.

Riehl-Sisca, J.P. (1989). *Conceptual models for nursing practice* (3rd ed.). Norwalk, CT: Appleton & Lange.

Silva, M.C. (1986). Research testing nursing theory: State of the art. *Advances in Nursing Science, 9*(1), 1–11.

Silva, M.C. (1987). Conceptual models of nursing. In J.J. Fitzpatrick & R.L. Taunton (Eds.), *Annual review of nursing research* (Vol. 5, pp. 229–246). New York: Springer.

Sohn, K.S. (1991). One method for comparing different nursing models. *Nursing and Health Care, 12*, 410–413.

Thibodeau, J.A. (1983). *Nursing models: Analysis and evaluation.* Monterey, CA: Wadsworth.

Thomas, C.L. (Ed.). (1993). *Taber's cyclopedic medical dictionary* (17th ed.). Philadelphia: FA Davis.

Torres, G. (1986). *Theoretical foundations of nursing.* Norwalk, CT: Appleton-Century-Crofts.

Uys, L.R. (1987). Foundation studies in

nursing. *Journal of Advanced Nursing, 12,* 275–280.

Walker, L.O., & Nicholson, R. (1980). Criteria for evaluating nursing process models. *Nurse Educator, 5*(5), 8–9.

Winstead-Fry, P. (Ed.). (1986). *Case studies* in nursing theory. New York: National League for Nursing.

Winter, E.J.S., Bender, A.W., Hertz, J.E., & Reider, J.A. (1987). Analyzing and evaluating a baccalaureate nursing curriculum framework. *Nurse Educator, 12*(4), 10–13.

3

Johnson's Behavioral System Model

This chapter presents an analysis and evaluation of Dorothy Johnson's Behavioral System Model. Her work clearly fits the definition of conceptual model used in this book, and she has always classified it as such.

The concepts of Johnson's Behavioral System Model and their dimensions are listed below. Each concept and its dimensions are defined and described later in this chapter.

KEY CONCEPTS

BEHAVIORAL SYSTEM
SUBSYSTEMS
Attachment or Affiliative Behavior
Dependency Behavior
Ingestive Behavior
Eliminative Behavior
Sexual Behavior
Aggressive Behavior
Achievement Behavior
SUBSYSTEM FUNCTIONAL
   REQUIREMENTS
Protection
Nurturance
Stimulation
SUBSYSTEM STRUCTURAL
   COMPONENTS
Drive or Goal
Set
Choice
Action or Behavior
BEHAVIORAL SYSTEM BALANCE
   AND STABILITY

Purposeful, Orderly, and Predictable
   Behavior
GOAL OF NURSING
Restore, Maintain, or Attain
   Behavioral System Balance and
   Stability
NURSING DIAGNOSTIC AND
   TREATMENT PROCESS
Determination of the Existence of a
   Problem
Diagnostic Classification Schemes
   Internal Subsystem Problems
   Intersystem Problems
Management of Nursing Problems
   Fulfill Functional Requirements
   Impose External Regulatory or
     Control Mechanisms
   Change Structural Components
Evaluation of Behavioral System
   Balance and Stability

ANALYSIS OF JOHNSON'S BEHAVIORAL SYSTEM MODEL

This section presents an analysis of Johnson's Behavioral System Model. The analysis relies heavily on Johnson's 1980 and 1990a publications, "The Behavioral System Model for Nursing" and also draws from her 1992 publication, "The Origins of the Behavioral System Model."

Origins of the Model

Historical Evolution and Motivation

The rudimentary ideas of the Behavioral System Model were evident in Johnson's 1959 article, "A Philosophy of Nursing" and in her 1961 article, "The Significance of Nursing Care." However, Johnson did not present her entire conceptual model in the literature until she prepared a chapter for the second edition of Riehl and Roy's (1980) book, *Conceptual Models for Nursing Practice*. Prior to that publication, the only public records of the model were a widely cited paper that Johnson presented at Vanderbilt University in 1968 and an audiotape of her 1978a presentation at the Second Annual Nurse Educator Conference. Versions of the model had, however, been available to interested nurses since Grubbs published her interpretation of the Behavioral System Model in 1974 and Auger published her interpretation in 1976.

Johnson has not presented any major revisions in her conceptual model since the 1980 publication, although she continued to discuss and provide more detail about various aspects of the model in her 1990a publication and presented a very informative discussion of the origins of the model in her 1992 publication.

Johnson (1990a) noted that the Behavioral System Model "has been in the process of development for nearly the entire course of my professional life" (p. 23). The unique focus and content of the model evolved over a period of 20 years, beginning in the early 1940s when she began to teach nursing. As she developed baccalaureate nursing courses, she was motivated to ask several questions, including:

> What content is properly included in a course in nursing because it constitutes nursing knowledge?
> Knowledge for what purpose, to what end?
> What is the explicit, ideal goal of nursing? (Johnson, 1990a, p. 23)

In answering those questions, the task as Johnson saw it was to clarify nursing's social mission from the perspective of a theoretically sound view of the person served by nursing and to identify the nature of the body of knowledge needed to attain the goal of nursing. Johnson (1990a) stated that she approached that task historically, empirically, and analytically. The historical approach led her to accept from Nightingale nursing's traditional concern with the person who is ill, rather than with the person's disease, per se, as well as "a focus on the basic human needs of the person and a concern for the relationship between the person and the environment" (Johnson, 1992, p. 24). The empirical approach led to a review of studies of nursing tasks. Johnson noted that that approach, which defines nursing as what nurses do, was not fruitful. However, it kept the focus on people who are ill or who might be prevented from becoming ill. Finally, the analytical approach led Johnson to consider what reason suggests. That turned out to be the most useful approach.

"The work began," as Johnson (1992) explained, "with the effort to develop course content in the basic curriculum by focusing on common human needs, moving on to 'care and comfort' as organizing principles, and then to stress and tension reduction as the major principles" (p. 24). Through reasoning, Johnson (1980, 1990a) explained that she finally came to conceive of nursing's specific contribution to patient welfare as "the fostering of efficient and effective behavioral functioning in the patient to prevent illness and during and following illness" (1980, p. 207). That perspective led Johnson to accept "a theoretical view of the client, the person, as a behavioral system in much the same way that physicians have accepted a theoretical view of the person as a biological system" (1990a, p. 24).

Elaborating, Johnson (1992) explained that the behavioral system orientation leads nursing to fulfill its social mission through the special responsibility of promoting "the most effective and efficient behavioral system possible, as well as to prevent specific problems from occurring in the system. Meeting this responsibility would also contribute to healthier biologic and social systems" (pp. 26–27).

Philosophical Claims

Johnson has presented the philosophical claims undergirding the Behavioral System Model in the form of beliefs, assumptions, premises, and a value system. She noted that her student nursing experiences instilled certain beliefs about nursing. She commented,

> My own educational experience had led me to believe that nursing was a profession, or at least an emerging one, and that as a profession nursing makes a unique and significant contribution to patients—a contribution that differs from but is complementary to those made by medicine and other health professions. (Johnson, 1992, p. 24)

Johnson's beliefs about the nature and operation of the behavioral system are stated in the following 12 assumptions:

1. A system is a whole which functions as a whole.
2. Parts or elements of a system are organized, interactive, interdependent, and integrated.

3. The system tends to achieve a balance among various forces acting within and upon it.

4. Man strives continually to maintain behavioral system balance and a steady state by more or less automatic adjustments and adaptations to the natural forces impinging upon him.

5. Man actively seeks new experiences that may disturb balance and may require small or large behavioral system modification to reestablish balance.

6. Observed regularities and constancies in human behavior that result from behavioral system balance and stability are functionally significant for the individual and for social life.

7. When behavioral regularities are disturbed, integrity of the person is threatened and functions served by such order are less than adequately fulfilled.

8. Behavioral system balance represents adjustments and adaptations that are successful to some degree and in some way, even though observed behavior may not match cultural or biologic norms for acceptable or healthy behavior.

9. Living systems can and do operate at varying levels of efficiency and effectiveness, but in order for a system to operate at all, it must maintain a certain level of balance and stability internally and in its environmental interactions.

10. Behavioral systems have sufficient flexibility to take account of the usual fluctuations in the impinging forces and enough stress tolerance for adjustment to many common, but extreme, fluctuations.

11. During their lives, most individuals probably experience a psychologic or social crisis or physical illness grave enough to disturb system balance and require external assistance.

12. Nursing is, or could be, the force that supplies assistance both when disturbances in system balance occur and at other times to prevent such disturbances. (Johnson, 1980, pp. 208–209)

Additional beliefs about the behavioral system are specified in the following three premises, which undergird Johnson's view of the goal of nursing:

1. If extraordinarily strong impinging forces, or a lowered resistance to or capacity to adjust to more moderate forces, disturb behavioral system balance, the integrity of the person is threatened.

2. The attempt by man to preserve or re-establish behavioral system balance in the face of continuing excessive forces making for imbalance requires an extraordinary expenditure of energy.

3. Insofar as behavioral system balance requires a minimum (for the moment at least and in reference to a particular individual) expenditure of energy, a larger supply of energy is available in the service of biologic processes and recovery. (Johnson, 1968, p. 4).

Johnson's value system, which is capsulized in the following quotation, sets forth her beliefs about behavior:

There is a wide range of behavior which is tolerated in this society or any other, and only the middle section of the continuum can be said to represent the cultural norms. So long as behavior does not threaten the survival of society, either directly through the death or lack of productivity of individuals or indirectly through the creation of massive disorder or deviance from established social values, it appears to be acceptable. The outer limits of acceptable, and therefore tolerated, behavior are thus set for the professions by society, but in fact, the limits of acceptable behavior set by the health professions, including nursing, probably tend to be narrower in some areas and in some respects than those set by the larger society.

Since the professions have an obligation which goes beyond accepting the current state of affairs to shaping the reality of the future, an additional facet of this problem of values is that of determining what is desirable, rather than simply acceptable behavior. At least two closely related facts must be remembered in this connection. In the first place, forced change in behavior in one area of life may and often does require other behavioral modifications. The consequences may be unforeseen, unintended, and undesirable. Secondly, the current status of knowledge about man and his universe does not allow us to predict, with reasonable certainty, a configuration of behavioral responses which measured against some established standards could be said to be of a "better" or "higher" level in an absolute way.

Applying these considerations to the establishment of a value system for the use of this model leads us to certain conclusions. First of all nursing must not, in our opinion, purposefully support, certainly over a prolonged period or in the absence of other counteractive measures, behavioral responses which are so deviant that they are intolerant to society or constitute a threat to the survival of the individual, either socially or biologically, and thus ultimately are a threat to society. We believe further that while nursing has an obligation to [help the person] seek the highest possible level of behavioral functioning, and to contribute, through research, to the specification of what that level might be, we cannot afford to go very far beyond what is known. Quite specifically, we do not think that nursing can presume to transform the values, beliefs, and norms of the individuals we serve to those in accordance with the culture of middle-class, urban, American society which we generally represent. We cannot, and must not, substitute our judgments at any given point in time for those of the individual or of the larger society. (Johnson, 1968, pp. 4–5)

In her 1978a presentation, Johnson added to her value system by stating that the final judgment of the desired level of functioning is the right of the individual, given that that level is within survival limits and that the individual has been provided with adequate understanding of the potential for and the means to obtain a more optimal level of behavioral functioning than is evident at the present time.

Strategies for Knowledge Development

Johnson's conception of the person as a behavioral system reflects a synthesis of knowledge from the literature of many disciplines, as well as from nursing's historical past. Her description of the development of the Behavioral System Model suggests that she used both inductive and deductive reasoning. She explained, "Over a period of some twenty years and in the light of my clinical experiences, thinking, reading, and conversations with colleagues, I evolved the notion that one potentially useful way of viewing man is as a behavioral system" (Johnson, 1978b, pp. 7–8).

Influences from Other Scholars

Starting with Nightingale, Johnson acknowledged the influences of many scholars on the development of the Behavioral System Model. She explained that she received a facsimile edition of Nightingale's *Notes on Nursing* in 1946. The book "came just at the right time to have a profound influence on the course of my professional experience" (Johnson, 1992, p. 23). Johnson went on to explain that Nightingale's work "provided direction to my thinking" (p. 24). Two points in particular influenced the beginning of the development of the Behavioral System Model: "A focus on the basic human needs of the person and a concern for the relationship between the person and the environment" (p. 24).

Johnson (1988) commented that her teacher and subsequent colleague, Lulu Wolfe Hassenplug, convinced her that nursing is a profession. Moreover, she acknowledged the contributions made by her colleagues at the University of California, Los Angeles, to the continuing development of the Behavioral System Model.

The influence of nursing, behavioral, and biological scientists, as well as animal and human ethologists, on the development of the Behavioral System Model is evident in Johnson's many citations to an interdisciplinary literature that focuses on the observable features and actions that make up social behavior and on behavior that has major adaptive significance. The acceptance of the idea of the person as a behavioral system is, according to Johnson (1980), "made possible by the relatively recent development and rapid expansion of . . . an interdisciplinary literature . . . focused on the behavior of the individual as a whole — on what he does, why, and on the consequences of that behavior — not on why or how he has changed over time in an intraorganismic sense" (p. 207). Scholars whose writings influenced the identification and content of seven behavioral subsystems include Ainsworth (1964; 1972); Atkinson and Feather (1966); Crandal (1963); Fesbach (1970); Gewirtz (1972); Heathers (1955); Kagan (1964); Lorenz (1966); Mead (1953); Resnik (1972); Robson (1967); Rosenthal (1967); Sears, Maccoby, and Levin (1954); and Walike, Jordan, and Stellar (1969).

Johnson (1980, 1990a, 1992) also acknowledged the influence of general system theory, as set forth by Buckley (1968), Chin (1961), and Rapoport (1968), on her thinking. She explained,

Although general system theory was in its infancy, it did seem valid enough to support the notion of humans as behavioral systems, developing and changing, reacting and adapting to their respective environments, including other behavioral systems in that environment. (1992, p. 25)

World View

The Behavioral System Model reflects the *reciprocal interaction* world view. The focus on the behavioral system as a whole and emphasis on behavior, per se, indicate a holistic view of the person. Subsystems are explicitly identified as parts of the whole behavioral system, rather than as discrete entities.

The reciprocal interaction world view also is reflected in Johnson's (1980) description of the person as actively seeking new experiences. The active organism perspective is underscored by the ideas that each subsystem strives to achieve a particular goal and that each person makes certain behavioral choices. This perspective is further documented by Johnson's (1990a) statement that the behavioral system "determines and limits the interactions between the person and his or her environment, and establishes the relationship of the person to the objects, events, and situations in the environment" (p. 25). In fact, Johnson (personal communication cited in Conner, Magers, & Watt, 1994) views the behavioral system as active, not reactive. Furthermore, she believes that individuals are active beings who adjust environments to ensure better functioning for themselves.

Consistent with the reciprocal interaction world view, the Behavioral System Model incorporates elements of both persistence and change. As Johnson (1980) noted, the behavioral system "both requires and results in some degree of regularity and constancy in behavior. . . . Behavioral system balance reflects adjustments and adaptations that are successful in some way and to some degree" (p. 208).

Persistence is reflected in Johnson's emphasis on behavioral system balance and stability. Hall (1981) explained,

Interestingly, one of the first of the current nursing theorists, Dorothy Johnson, tried to head the profession in the direction of persistence. She takes equilibrium as a starting point in her original conception. The goal of nursing care, in her model, emphasizes balance, order, stability, and maintenance of the integrity of the patient. (p. 5)

Change is postulated to occur only when necessary for survival. More specifically, behavior changes when it no longer is "functionally efficient and effective . . . in managing the individual's relationship to the environment . . . or when some more optimal level of functioning is perceived as desirable by the individual" (Johnson, 1990a, p. 25).

Unique Focus of the Model

The unique focus of the Behavioral System Model is the person as a behavioral system. Indeed, "the acceptance of the behavioral system as the client is the primary component of this nursing model" (Johnson, 1990a, p. 24). Johnson (1980) maintained that "The conception of man as a behavioral system, or the idea that man's specific response patterns form an organized and integrated whole is original with me, so far as I know" (p. 208). She further noted that the literature indicates that others support her idea. Indeed, Ackoff used the term behavioral system in 1960.

The Behavioral System Model focuses on social behavior, that is, "the observable features and actions of the person that take into account the actual or implied presence of other social beings. In particular, the focus is on those forms of behavior that have been shown to have major adaptive significance" (Johnson, 1990a, p. 25). Particular attention is given to actual or potential structural or functional problems in the behavioral system as a whole and in the various subsystems and to behavioral functioning that is at a less than desired or optimal level. Two types of behavioral system disorders are considered relevant:

> 1. Those that are related tangentially or peripherally to disorder in the biological system; that is, they are precipitated simply by the fact of illness or the situational context of treatment.
>
> 2. Those that are an integral part of a biological system disorder in that they are either directly associated with or a direct consequence of a particular kind of biological system disorder or its treatment. (Johnson, 1968, pp. 6–7)

Factors that contribute to the development of those problems include inadequate or inappropriate formation of the system and its parts, a breakdown in internal regulatory and control mechanisms of the system, the system's exposure to noxious influences, its failure to be adequately stimulated, or lack of adequate environmental input (Johnson, 1980).

The Behavioral System Model was classified as a systems model by Barnum (1994), Marriner-Tomey (1989), and Riehl and Roy (1980). The appropriateness of this categorization is evident in the following comparison of the concepts and propositions of the Behavioral System Model with the characteristics of the systems category of knowledge.

The Behavioral System Model addresses system in the definition of the person as a behavioral system. The integration of the parts, called subsystems, is evident in the comment that they are "linked and open, as is true in all systems, and a disturbance in one subsystem is likely to have an effect on others" (Johnson, 1980, p. 210).

Environment is addressed throughout the presentation of the model, although its parameters are never identified beyond the comment that it is both internal and external. Boundary is not addressed explicitly in the

Behavioral System Model, although boundary permeability is alluded to in this statement: "There appears to be built into the system sufficient flexibility to take account of the usual fluctuations in the impinging forces and enough stress tolerance for the system to adjust to many common, but extreme, fluctuations" (Johnson, 1980, p. 209).

The systems model characteristic of tension, stress, strain, and conflict is addressed through the discussion of the "natural" forces impinging upon the behavioral system. Those forces lead to "more or less automatic adjustments and adaptations" required for continuing behavioral system balance and stability (Johnson, 1980, p. 208).

Johnson (1980) used the term steady state in conjunction with behavioral system balance. Although the concept of behavioral system balance and stability implies that the system is at a fixed point or achieves an equilibrium when stable, Johnson apparently regarded stability as a dynamic equilibrium. That aspect of the conceptual model requires clarification.

The characteristic of feedback is addressed only briefly in the Behavioral System Model, when Johnson (1978a) commented that it is necessary to understand input, output, feedback, and regulatory control mechanisms to analyze behavioral system functioning. However, the nature of those system operations was not described.

Meleis (1991) regarded the Behavioral System Model as a prominent example of the outcome category of models and also classified the model as client-focused. Although Barnum (1994) classified the Behavioral System Model as a systems model, she also placed it within the intervention category of her classification scheme.

Content of the Model: Concepts

Person

The person of interest in the Behavioral System Model is the individual **behavioral system**. The model focuses on the whole individual, defined as a behavioral system. "All patterned, repetitive, and purposeful ways of behaving that characterize each man's life are considered to comprise his behavioral system" (Johnson, 1980, p. 209). The parts of the behavioral system are called **subsystems**. They carry out specialized tasks or functions needed to maintain the integrity of the whole behavioral system and manage its relationship to the environment.

Johnson (1980, 1990a) identified seven behavioral subsystems. Those subsystems and their specialized functions are listed below.

1. *Attachment or affiliative subsystem:* Functions are attainment of the security needed for survival as well as social inclusion, intimacy, and the formation and maintenance of social bonds.

2. *Dependency subsystem:* Functions are succoring behavior that calls for a response of nurturance as well as approval, attention or recognition, and physical assistance.

3. *Ingestive subsystem:* Function is appetite satisfaction, with regard to when, how, what, how much, and under what conditions the individual eats, which is governed by social and psychological considerations as well as biological requirements for food and fluids.

4. *Eliminative subsystem:* Function is elimination, with regard to when, how, and under what conditions the individual eliminates wastes.

5. *Sexual subsystem:* Functions are procreation and gratification, with regard to behaviors dependent upon the individual's biological sex and gender role identity, including but not limited to courting and mating.

6. *Aggressive subsystem:* Function is protection and preservation of self and society.

7. *Achievement subsystem:* Function is mastery or control of some aspect of self or environment, with regard to intellectual, physical, creative, mechanical, social, and care-taking (of children, spouse, home) skills, and as measured against some standard of excellence.

Johnson (1990a) explained that each behavioral subsystem evolves "to carry out its own specialized tasks for the system as a whole. . . . [The] responses are differentiated, developed, and modified through maturation, experience, and learning. They are determined and are continuously governed by a multitude of physical, biological, psychological, and social factors operating in a complex and interlocking fashion" (p. 26).

Johnson (1990a) regards the attachment subsystem as "one of the first response systems to emerge developmentally . . . [and as] probably the most critical subsystem for it forms the basis for all social organization" (p. 27). Dependency behavior, according to Johnson (1990a) "in the socially optimum case evolves [developmentally] from almost total dependence on others to a greater degree of dependence on self, with a certain amount of interdependence essential to the survival of social groups" (p. 28).

The ingestive and eliminative subsystems extend beyond the biological functions of ingestion of substances and elimination of waste products. "Ingestive behavior," in Johnson's (1990a) view, "serve[s] the broad function of appetitive satisfaction in its own right, [which] may be and all too often is at odds with biological requirements for [f]oods and fluids" (p. 28). The function of the eliminative subsystem, Johnson (1990a) admitted, "is more difficult to differentiate from that of the biological system" (p. 28) but she went on to explain that "clearly all humans . . . must learn expected modes of behavior in the excretion of wastes, and these behaviors often take precedence over or strongly influence otherwise purely biological acts" (p. 28). The sexual subsystem, which as Johnson (1990a) pointed out "also has strong biological underpinnings . . . probably originates with the development of a gender role identity and covers the broad range of those behaviors dependent upon that identity" (p. 28).

Johnson's (1990a) view of the aggressive subsystem "follows the thinking of animal behaviorists [and is in sharp contrast to] that of the behavioral reinforcement school, which maintains that aggressive behavior is not only learned, but has as its primary intent the injury of others" (p. 29). The achievement subsystem, according to Johnson (1990a), probably develops through "exploratory behavior and attempts to manipulate the environment" (p. 29).

Johnson (1980, 1990a) maintained that the subsystems are found cross-culturally and across a broad range of the phylogenetic scale, suggesting that they are genetically programmed. She also noted the significance of social and cultural factors involved in the development of the subsystems. The seven subsystems are not, however, to be regarded as a complete set, because "the ultimate group of response systems to be identified in the behavioral system will undoubtedly change as research reveals new systems or indicates changes in the structure, functions, or behavior pattern groupings in the original set" (1980, p. 212).

Johnson (1980) explained that the subsystems "are linked and open, . . . and a disturbance in one subsystem is likely to have an effect on others" (p. 210). She further explained that "although each subsystem has a specialized task or function, the system as a whole depends on an integrated performance" (p. 210).

The ability of the subsystems to fulfill their functions depends upon certain requirements "that must be met through the individual's own efforts, or through outside assistance" (Johnson, 1980, p. 212). The **functional requirements** are:

1. *Protection* from noxious influences with which the system cannot cope

2. *Nurturance* through the input of appropriate supplies from the environment

3. *Stimulation* to enhance growth and prevent stagnation

In addition to function, each subsystem has structure. The four **structural components** of each are *drive or goal, set, choice,* and *action or behavior.* The *drive or goal* of a subsystem refers to motivation for behavior and is regarded by Johnson (1990a) as "perhaps the most significant" (p. 27) structural component. The drive is "that which is a stimulant to action [whereas] the goal is that which is sought" (Johnson, 1990a, p. 27). In general, the drive of each subsystem is the same for all people, "but there are variations among individuals in the specific objects or events that are drive-fulfilling, in the value placed on goal attainment, and in drive strength" (Johnson, 1980, p. 210). The specific drive of each subsystem cannot be observed directly but must be inferred from the individual's actual behavior and from the consequences of that behavior.

Set, which is also inferred from observed behavior, refers to the individual's predisposition to act in certain ways, rather than in other ways, to fulfill the function of each subsystem. Johnson (1980) explained that "through maturation, experience, and learning, the individual comes to develop and use preferred ways of behaving under particular circumstances and with selected individuals" (p. 211).

Choice refers to the individual's total behavior repertoire for fulfilling subsystem functions and achieving particular goals. The behavioral repertoire encompasses the scope of action alternatives from which the person can choose. Johnson (1980) pointed out that the individual rarely uses all those alternatives but, rather, chooses certain preferred behaviors. However, the other behaviors are available if the preferred ones do not work in a certain situation. She also noted that people continuously acquire new choices and modify old ones, and that the most adaptable individuals are those with the largest repertoires of choices.

Action refers to the actual organized and patterned behavior in a situation and is the only structural component that can be directly observed. Johnson (1980) commented that behavior is instigated, inhibited, shaped, continued, or terminated by the complex biological, psychological, sociological, and physical factors that constitute the other structural components. She described behavior as "a set of behavioral responses, responsive tendencies, or actions systems" (p. 209). She went on to say, "These responses are developed and modified over time through maturation, experience, and learning. They are determined developmentally and are continuously governed by a multitude of physical, biologic, psychologic, and social factors operating in a complex and interlocking fashion. These responses are reasonably stable, though modifiable, and regularly recurrent, and their action pattern is observable" (p. 209).

Environment

Johnson (1980) referred to the internal and external environment of the system, as well as to "the interaction between the person and his environment and . . . to the objects, events and situations in his environment" (p. 209). She also referred to forces that impinge on the person and to which the person adjusts and adapts. However, Johnson gave no specific definition for environment. Moreover, although she noted that the internal environment includes "the composition, quantity, temperature, and distribution of body fluids" (Johnson, 1961, p. 64), she neither identified other components of the internal environment nor identified any components of the external environment. Her discussion suggests that objects, events, situations, and forces are part of the environment. This was not, however, made explicit.

Health

Johnson (1978b) commented that health in its most global sense is a concern of the members of all health professions, political scientists, agronomists, and others. Her particular focus, however, and one that she considered appropriate for nursing, is the behavioral system. This focus is reflected in Johnson's (1968) statement, "One or more of [the behavioral system] subsystems is likely to be involved in any episode of illness, whether in an antecedent or a consequence way, or simply in association, directly or indirectly, with the disorder or its treatment" (p. 3). In various presentations and publications, Johnson has mentioned behavioral system balance and stability, efficient and effective behavioral functioning, behavioral system imbalance and instability, and the person who is ill.

Johnson (1978a) stated that **behavioral system balance and stability** is demonstrated by *observed behavior* that is *purposeful, orderly, and predictable. Purposeful behavior* is goal directed; that is, actions reveal a plan and cease at an identifiable point. Orderly behavior is methodical and systematic, as opposed to diffuse and erratic. Furthermore, *orderly behavior* encompasses actions that build sequentially toward a goal and form a recognizable pattern. *Predictable behavior* is that which is repetitive under particular circumstances.

Purposeful, orderly, and predictable behavior is maintained when it is efficient and effective in managing the person's relationship to the environment. Individuals are said to achieve efficient and effective behavioral functioning when their behavior is commensurate with social demands, when they are able to modify their behavior in ways that support biological imperatives, when they are able to benefit to the fullest extent during illness from the physician's knowledge and skill, and when their behavior does not reveal unnecessary trauma as a consequence of illness (Johnson, 1978a, 1980). Behavior changes when efficiency and effectiveness are no longer evident or when a more optimal level of functioning is perceived as desirable (Johnson, 1978a, 1990).

Behavioral system imbalance and instability is not described explicitly but can be inferred to be a malfunction of the behavioral system from the following statement:

> The subsystems and the system as a whole tend to be self-maintaining and self-perpetuating so long as conditions in the internal and external environment of the system remain orderly and predictable, the conditions and resources necessary to their functional requirements are met, and the interrelationships among the subsystems are harmonious. If those conditions are not met, malfunction becomes apparent in behavior that is in part disorganized, erratic, and dysfunctional. Illness or other sudden internal or external environmental change is most frequently responsible for such malfunctions. (Johnson, 1980, p. 212)

Johnson did not define illness. She mentioned psychological and social crisis and physical illness (Johnson, 1978a, 1980), but did not describe manifestations of those conditions. Although it may be inferred that behavioral system imbalance and instability are equated with illness, the previous quotation suggests that Johnson may view illness as separate from behavioral system functioning.

Furthermore, although Johnson (1980) referred to physical and social health, she did not explicitly define wellness. Just as an inference about illness may be made, it may be inferred that wellness is behavioral system balance and stability, in the form of purposeful, orderly, and predictable behavior that supports efficient and effective behavioral functioning. These inferences suggest that Johnson views health as a dichotomy, rather than a continuum. Caution must be observed, however, when assessing the validity of those inferences. In fact, Johnson (1990b) commented that health is neither a continuum nor a dichotomy, but she did not explain the meaning of her comment or identify her view of health.

Nursing

Johnson (1980, 1990a) clearly distinguished nursing from medicine by stating that nursing views the patient as a behavioral system, and medicine views the patient as a biological system. She views nursing as "a service that is complementary to that of medicine and other health professions, but which makes its own distinctive contribution to the health and well-being of people" (1980, p. 207). More specifically, she described nursing "as an external regulatory force that acts to preserve the organization and integration of the patient's behavior at the highest possible level under those conditions in which the behavior constitutes a threat to physical or social health, or in which illness is found" (1990a, p. 29).

The **goal of nursing** action is "*to restore, maintain, or attain behavioral system balance and dynamic stability* [italics mine] at the highest possible level for the individual" (Johnson, 1980, p. 214; 1990a, p. 29). This goal may be expanded to include helping the person to achieve a more optimum level of balance and functioning when that is possible and desired (Johnson, 1978a). "The need for nursing," according to Johnson (1990a), "arises when there are disturbances in the structure or function of the system as a whole or in one or more subsystems, or when behavioral functioning is at a less than desired level for the individual" (p. 29).

Johnson (1992) also indicated that there is a need for nursing when prevention is the goal. Indeed, she has stated that nursing should concentrate on "developing preventive nursing to fulfill its social obligations" (p. 26) and that "Clarifying nursing's social mission through an explicit goal in patient care and using a specific body of knowledge relevant to that goal therefore enables the discipline to work toward completing its special tasks in prevention, thus contributing to a high level of wellness in society" (p. 27).

Johnson (1990a) referred to the nursing process, which is summarized in Table 3–1, as the **nursing diagnostic and treatment process**. The first step of the process focuses on *determination of the existence of a problem*. Problems are identified by means of interviews to obtain past and present family and individual behavioral system histories, structured and unstructured observations, and objective methodologies. Emphasis is placed on the nature of behavioral system functioning in terms of the efficiency and effectiveness with which the individual's goals are obtained, with special attention directed toward the amount of energy required to achieve desired goals, the compatibility of the individual's behavior with survival imperatives and its congruence with the social situation, and the individual's degree of satisfaction with the behavior. Emphasis is also placed on the degree to which the behavior is purposeful, orderly, and predictable.

Problem determination continues with specification of the condition of the structural components for each subsystem. The patient is interviewed so that inferences can be made with regard to "the drive strength, direction, and value to the individual; the solidity and specificity of the set; the range of behavior patterns available to the individual; and the usual behavior of the individual under given conditions and its effectiveness in goal attainment" (Johnson, 1990a, p. 30). In addition, "information is required about the organization, interaction, and integration of the sybsystems" (p. 30), including any hierarchical structure or conflicts between subsystems.

Problem determination concludes with a comparison of the observed behavior with several indices of behavioral system balance and stability. Emphasis is placed on determination of the efficiency and effectiveness of the behavior in goal attainment. Johnson (1968, 1978a, 1980, 1990a) has identified several characteristics of behavior that can be considered indices of behavioral system stability and balance. They include successful achievement of the sought-after consequences; adequate motor, expressive, and social skills; purposeful, orderly, and predictable actions; expenditure of an acceptable amount of energy; compatibility of actions with biological survival imperatives; congruence of actions with the particular social situation; and the individual's satisfaction with the behavior.

The second step of the nursing process is the labeling of the nurse's impressions about the nature of the problem(s). Johnson (1990a) offered two types of *diagnostic classification schemes*. One scheme deals with internal subsystem problems. One class of problems "are those that arise because the functional requirements of the subsystems are not being met" (p. 30). Another class of problems are those "that result from some inconsistency or disharmony among the structural components of the subsystems" (p. 30). Still another class of problems "occur when the behavior is disapproved or punished by the ambient culture; that is, [when] behavior appropriate in one setting becomes culturally unacceptable in another"

TABLE 3–1. **THE BEHAVIORAL SYSTEM MODEL: NURSING DIAGNOSTIC AND TREATMENT PROCESS**

I. Determination of the existence of a problem
   A. Obtain past and present family and individual behavioral system histories
   B. Specify condition of the subsystem structural components
      1. Determine drive strength, direction, and value
      2. Determine the solidity and specificity of the set
      3. Identify the range of behavior patterns available to the individual
      4. Identify the usual behavior in a given situation
      5. Assess and compare behavior with indices of behavioral system balance and stability
         a. Determine whether the behavior is succeeding or failing to achieve the consequences sought
         b. Determine whether more effective motor, expressive, or social skills are needed
         c. Determine whether the behavior is purposeful, that is, whether actions are goal directed, reveal a plan and cease at an identifiable point, and are economical in sequence
         d. Determine whether the behavior is orderly, that is, whether actions are methodical, systematic, build sequentially toward a goal, and form a recognizable pattern
         e. Determine whether the behavior is predictable, that is, whether actions are repetitive under particular circumstances
         f. Determine whether the amount of energy expended to achieve desired goals is acceptable
         g. Determine whether behavior reflects appropriate choices
            (1) Determine whether actions are compatible with survival imperatives
            (2) Determine whether actions are congruent with the social situation
         h. Determine whether the individual is sufficiently satisfied with the behavior
      6. Determine the organization, interaction, and integration of the subsystems
II. Diagnostic classification of problems
   A. Internal subsystem problems
      1. Functional requirements not met
      2. Inconsistency of disharmony among structural components of subsystems
      3. Behavior inappropriate in the ambient culture
   B. Intersystem problems
      1. Domination of entire system by one or two subsystems
      2. Conflict between two or more subsystems
III. Management of nursing problems
   A. General goal of action
      1. Restore, maintain, or attain the patient's behavioral system balance and stability
      2. Help the patient achieve a more optimum level of balance and functioning when this is possible and desired
   B. Determine what nursing is to accomplish on behalf of the behavioral system
      1. Determine what level of behavioral system balance and stability is acceptable
      2. Determine who makes the judgment regarding acceptable level of behavioral system balance and stability
         a. Identify value system of nursing profession
         b. Identify own explicit value system
   C. Select a type of treatment
      1. Fulfill functional requirements of the subsystems
         a. Protect patient from overwhelming noxious influences
         b. Supply adequate nurturance through an appropriate input of essential supplies
         c. Provide stimulation to enhance growth and to inhibit stagnation
      2. Temporarily impose external regulatory or control measures
         a. Set limits for behavior by either permissive or inhibitory means
         b. Inhibit ineffective behavioral responses
         c. Assist patient to acquire new responses
         d. Reinforce appropriate behaviors

TABLE 3–1. **THE BEHAVIORAL SYSTEM MODEL: NURSING DIAGNOSTIC AND TREATMENT PROCESS** (Continued)

---

    3. Repair damaged structural units in desirable direction
      a. Reduce drive strength by changing attitudes
      b. Redirect goal by changing attitudes
      c. Alter set by instruction or counseling
      d. Add choices by teaching new skills
  D. Negotiate treatment modality with patient
    1. Establish a contract with the patient
    2. Help patient understand meaning of nursing diagnosis and proposed treatment
    3. If diagnosis and/or proposed treatment are rejected, continue to negotiate with the patient until agreement is reached
IV. Compare behavior after treatment to indices of behavioral system balance and stability (c.f. I.B.5.a–h)

Constructed from Johnson, D.E. (1968, April). *One conceptual model of nursing.* Paper presented at Vanderbilt University, Nashville, TN; Johnson, D.E. (1978, December). *Behavioral system model for nursing.* Paper presented at Second Annual Nurse Educator Conference, New York. (Cassette recording); Johnson, D.E. (1980). The behavioral system model for nursing. In J.P. Riehl & C. Roy, *Conceptual models for nursing practice* (2nd ed., pp. 207–216). New York: Appleton-Century-Crofts; and Johnson, D.E. (1990). The behavioral system model for nursing. In M.E. Parker (Ed.), *Nursing theories in practice* (pp. 23–32). New York: National League for Nursing.

(p. 30). The second scheme deals with <u>intersystem problems</u>. In this scheme, one class of problems "arise because one (or perhaps two) subsystems dominate the entire system" (p. 30). Another class of problems arise "as a result of a conflict between two or more subsystems" (p. 30).

The third step of the nursing process focuses on the *management of nursing problems.* Johnson (1980, 1990a) identified three types of treatments that constitute the external regulatory force that is nursing. The types of treatments are nursing actions that: (1) <u>fulfill the functional requirements of the subsystems</u>, (2) <u>impose external regulatory or control mechanisms</u>, or (3) <u>change the structural components</u> in desirable directions.

Johnson (1990a) indicated that the functional requirements of protection, nurturance, and stimulation can be fulfilled by nursing actions that "provide the [essential] conditions and resources [such as] information giving, role modeling, attention to the food being offered or the way in which it is being served, and seeing that infants or young children have access to their parents or elderly people to their pets" (p. 31). She explained that external regulatory or control mechanisms are imposed temporarily and are directed toward inhibition, stimulation, or reinforcement of certain behaviors. Repairing disordered structural components, Johnson (1990a) contends, "is the most difficult approach since it involves changes in the drive (goal), the set, the choices, and the behavior itself and requires such things as attitudinal changes, redirection of goals, and sometimes reduction in drive strength" (p. 31).

Johnson (1968) indicated that she expects the nurse to base judgments about behavioral system balance and stability on an explicit value system. Her own value system was previously discussed in the section on philosophical claims. Furthermore, Johnson (1978a) maintained that continuous negotiation between nurse and patient is necessary, especially if the initial diagnosis or proposed treatment is rejected by the patient. In fact, she maintained that the nurse should establish a contract with the patient and help the patient to understand the diagnosis and proposed treatment.

The final step of the nursing process is *evaluation*. The efficacy of nursing action is determined by means of a comparison of the individual's behavior after the treatment with the indices of behavioral system balance and stability used at the conclusion of the problem determination step of the process (Johnson, 1978a).

Content of the Model: Propositions

The linkage of the metaparadigm concepts, person and environment is reflected in the following statements:

> All the patterned, repetitive, and purposeful ways of behaving that characterize each man's life are considered to comprise his behavioral system. These ways of behaving form an organized and integrated functional unit that determines and limits the interaction between the person and his environment and establishes the relationship of the person to the objects, events, and situations in his environment. (Johnson, 1980, p. 209)
>
> The behavioral system has many tasks or missions to perform in maintaining its own integrity and in managing the system's relationship to its environment. (Johnson, 1980, p. 209)

The concepts, person, environment, and health, are linked in the following statement:

> The subsystems and the system as a whole tend to be self-maintaining and self-perpetuating so long as conditions in the internal and external environment of the system remain orderly and predictable, the conditions and resources necessary to their functional requirements are met, and the interrelationships among the subsystems are harmonious. If these conditions are not met, malfunction becomes apparent in behavior that is in part disorganized, erratic, and dysfunctional. Illness or other sudden internal or external environmental change is most frequently responsible for such malfunctions. (Johnson, 1980, p. 212)

The linkages among the metaparadigm concepts, person, health, and nursing, are evident in these statements:

> Most individuals probably experience at one or more times during their lives a psychologic crisis or a physical illness grave enough to disturb the system balance and to require external assistance. Nursing is

(or could be) the force that supplies assistance both at the time of occurrence and at other times to prevent such occurrences. (Johnson, 1980, p. 209)

Nursing is thus seen as an external regulatory force which acts to preserve the organization and integration of the patient's behavior at an optimal level under those conditions in which the behavior constitutes a threat to physical or social health, or in which illness is found. (Johnson 1980, p. 214)

EVALUATION OF JOHNSON'S BEHAVIORAL SYSTEM MODEL

This section presents an evaluation of the Behavioral System Model. The evaluation is based on the results of the analysis of the model as well as on publications and presentations by others who have used or commented on Johnson's work.

Explication of Origins

Johnson explicated the origins of the Behavioral System Model clearly and concisely. She chronicled the development of the model over time and indicated what motivated her to formulate a conceptual model of nursing. Furthermore, she explicitly stated her philosophical claims in the form of beliefs about the profession of nursing, assumptions and premises about the nature and operation of the behavioral system, and a comprehensive value system regarding what should be considered acceptable behavior.

Johnson stated that the use of the Behavioral System Model is based on values of the nursing profession, as well as those of the individual nurse. She values a focus on the person's behavior and views this behavior as a manifestation of the momentary condition of the whole behavioral system as well as the subsystems. Johnson also values nursing intervention before, during, and following illness. Moreover, she values the patient's contributions to his or her care, as indicated by her recommendation that a contract for nursing intervention be established between the nurse and the patient.

Johnson explicitly acknowledged other scholars and cited the knowledge she drew on from nursing and adjunctive disciplines. She was especially informative with regard to the influence of Nightingale's work and general system theory on the development of the Behavioral System Model.

Comprehensiveness of Content

The Behavioral System Model is sufficiently comprehensive with regard to depth of content, although clarity could be enhanced in some instances. Johnson addressed all four concepts of nursing's metaparadigm —person, environment, health, and nursing. Person is clearly defined and described. Although environment is mentioned repeatedly in Johnson's publications, the term is not defined explicitly. Furthermore, the parameters of the relevant environment are not clearly specified beyond a reference to the internal environment and the external environment. Randell (1991) presented work that has expanded the concept of environment through the specification of internal and external environmental regulators. "Regulators," Randell (1991) explained, "represent specific units of the environment that simultaneously influence and are influenced by behavior" (p. 157). The internal environment is made up of the biophysical regulator, the psychological regulator, and the developmental regulator. The external environment is made up of the sociocultural, the family, and the physical environmental regulators.

Health also is not defined explicitly. As a consequence, inferences must be made about what Johnson meant by wellness and illness, as well as how one is distinguished from the other. In particular, the relation of health to behavioral system balance and stability versus imbalance and instability needs to be articulated. Furthermore, although behavioral system balance and stability is clearly and comprehensively described, the description of behavioral system imbalance and instability is not explicit. It must be inferred that this is the converse of behavioral system balance and stability.

Other aspects of Johnson's discussion of health also require clarification. Although the model clearly focuses on behavior, Johnson uses the terms psychological and social crises and physical illness. The meaning of these terms in relation to the various subsystems of the behavioral system is not clear. One interpretation of Johnson's statements about illness is that the condition is separate from behavioral system functioning. Thus, it is not clear if illness (physical, psychological, or social) is an external condition that affects certain subsystems, or if it is manifested when those subsystems are not functioning efficiently and effectively. Similarly, the meaning of the terms physical and social health and their relation to the condition of the behavioral system require specification.

It must be pointed out, however, that Johnson (1978b) regarded health as "an extremely elusive state" (p. 6). It is not surprising, then, that her conceptual model does not include an explicit definition of health and that there is some lack of clarity about aspects of this concept.

Nursing is defined and described adequately, as are the goal of nursing and the nursing process. Johnson (1980) emphasized that judgments regarding behavioral system functioning are to be based on theoretical and empirical knowledge of systems, as well as on the scientific knowledge dealing with each subsystem. The nursing process of the Behavioral System Model is not presented as a particularly dynamic activity, although some dynamism is evident in the negotiation of proposed treatment between patient and nurse. Johnson's explication of her own value system, her statement that the use of the model should be based on the values of the nursing profession as well as those of the individual nurse, and the inclusion of negotiation of treatment between patient and nurse all attest to her concern for ethical standards for nursing practice.

The propositions of the Behavioral System Model link the person and the environment; the person, the environment, and health; and the person, health, and nursing. No one statement links all four metaparadigm concepts, and there is no direct link between environment and nursing. That linkage was implied, however, when Johnson (1980) stated that nursing is "an external regulatory force . . . that operates through the imposition of external regulatory or control mechanisms" (p. 214). It may be inferred that nursing is part of the environment.

Some limitations of the Behavioral System Model, especially those related to the lack of comprehensive descriptions of some metaparadigm concepts, have been overcome by others who have extended the model. Auger (1976) provided an interpretation of the model that focused on the person as a personality system (Johnson, personal communication, October 17, 1977), thus extending the model further into the psychological realm. Grubbs (1974, 1980) presented an interpretation of the model that expanded each of the metaparadigm concepts.

The Behavioral System Model is also sufficiently comprehensive in breadth of content. Johnson has specified a broad goal for nursing that focuses attention on correction of existing behavioral system problems as well as the prevention of problems. Sensitive to a criticism that the Behavioral System Model does not permit preventive nursing actions, Johnson (1990a) pointed out, "that is not true" (p. 31). Elaborating, she stated, "The fact is, however, that like medicine where problems in the biological system cannot be prevented until the nature of the problem is fully explained, preventive nursing is not possible until problems in the behavioral system are explicated. To the extent that any problem that might arise can be anticipated, and appropriate methodologies are available, preventive action is in order" (p. 31).

Moreover, Johnson (1990a) continues to maintain that the seven subsystems encompass all relevant behavior, despite others' attempts to add an eighth subsystem dealing with restorative behavior (e.g., Grubbs, 1974) and to interpret the functions of some of the subsystems in other ways (e.g., Auger, 1976). She stated that her discussion of the seven subsystems and their functions "is my original conception and the one to which I still subscribe. This point needs to be emphasized, since major changes to the model have been made over the years by those using it, and these changes have appeared in the literature. The changes are such that they alter the fundamental nature of the behavioral system as originally proposed, and I do not agree with them" (p. 27).

The comprehensiveness of the breadth of the Behavioral System

Model is further supported by the direction it provides for research, education, administration, and practice. Although rules for each area are not explicit in Johnson's writings, many can be extracted from the focus and content of the model.

The developing rules for research indicate that the research task "is to identify and explain the behavioral system disorders which arise in connection with illness, and to develop the rationale for and the means of management" (Johnson, 1968, p. 6). The phenomena to be studied are the behavioral system as a whole, as well as the structural components and the functional requirements of the behavioral subsystems. The problems to be studied are those that represent actual or potential imbalances and instability in the behavioral system and subsystems.

The ultimate purpose of research is to determine the effects of nursing actions, in the form of fulfillment of functional requirements, temporary imposition of external regulatory or control mechanisms, and changes in structural components on behavioral system balance and stability. It may be inferred that subjects may be individuals of all ages in various clinical settings. Definitive rules regarding methodological issues, including research designs, instruments, procedures, and data analysis techniques, remain to be developed. Lovejoy (1986) suggested that data may be collected via interview; observation, including participant observation, filming, and photographing; and projective techniques. It is clear that Behavioral System Model–based research findings will enhance understanding of factors that affect human behavioral system functioning.

The rules for nursing education that can be extracted from the Behavioral System Model stipulate that the focus of the curriculum is the behavioral system and subsystems. Johnson (1980) implied a sequence of content when she discussed levels of basic instruction. The first level is "a thorough grounding in the underlying natural and social sciences" (p. 214). The second level is "nursing's basic science — the study of man as a behavioral system" (p. 214). That level also should include "the study of pathophysiology of the biologic system, of medicine's clinical science, and of the health system as a whole" (p. 214). The third level emphasizes "nursing's clinical science, the study of behavioral system problems in man, which would include the relevant diagnostic and treatment rationales and methodologies" (p. 214). Johnson (1989) maintains that basic education for professional nursing practice should be at the postbaccalaureate level. She stated, "The entry level for the practice of professional nursing [should] be through graduate education. Even now the 4 or 5 years of college required is not a great enough time span to permit the acquisition of the knowledge and skill needed or the maturity and wisdom required for professional practice" p. 4). She went on to say that the entry level for technical nursing practice probably should be at the associate degree level, with the proviso that associate degree programs be redesigned and "deprofessionalized" so that the focus of the curriculum is appropriately on "the knowledge and skill needed to follow prescriptions for nursing and medical care and document outcomes and to allow perceptive and intelligent observation" (p. 4).

Accordingly, students interested in professional practice would have to meet the requirements for graduate school, and those interested in technical practice would have to meet the requirements of associate degree programs. Rules regarding teaching-learning strategies remain to be developed.

The rules for nursing service administration that can be extracted from the content of the Behavioral System Model suggest that the distinctive focus of nursing in the clinical agency is the individual behavioral system. The purpose of nursing services is to facilitate the delivery of nursing care that will promote behavioral system balance and stability. Johnson's focus on preventive nursing as well as the nursing care of ill people implies that nursing services could be delivered in diverse settings, ranging from people's homes to clinicians' private offices to ambulatory clinics to the critical care units of tertiary medical centers. Nursing personnel include both professional and technical nurses. Johnson (1989) dreams of the time when professional nurses, "whether salaried or in solo or group practice, will be independent practitioners, licensed to practice nursing and solely responsible for professional decisions and actions" (p. 3). These nurses would have a caseload of patients on both an inpatient and an outpatient basis. Technical nurses, Johnson continued, would be "employed by hospitals or other institutions or by professionals including nurses, in private practice" (p. 3). The rules regarding management strategies and administrative policies remain to be developed.

The rules for nursing practice indicate that nursing care is directed toward restoration, maintenance, or attainment of behavioral system balance and stability, and that clinical problems encompass conditions in which behavior is a threat to health or in which illness is found. As noted previously, nursing practice apparently can occur in many different clinical settings. Legitimate recipients of Behavioral System Model-based nursing care are those who are experiencing actual or potential threats to behavioral system balance and stability. The nursing process associated with the Behavioral System Model involves determination of the existence of a problem, diagnosis, treatment, and evaluation (Johnson, 1990a). Behavioral System Model–based nursing practice contributes to the well-being of individuals by promoting behavioral system balance and stability.

Logical Congruence

The Behavioral System Model is logically congruent. The content of the model clearly flows from Johnson's philosophical claims, and it reflects the reciprocal interaction world view. Although elements of the reaction world view are suggested by references to forces that operate on the system and the characterization of nursing as an external regulatory force, Johnson (1980) has reconciled the two world views in a satisfactory manner. She explained, "Man strives continually to maintain a behavioral system balance and steady states by more or less automatic adjustments and adaptations to the 'natural' forces impinging upon him. At the same time, . . . man also actively seeks new experiences that may disturb his balance" (p. 208). Furthermore, although nursing is defined as an external regulatory force, negotiation between the nurse and the patient is a key feature of the diagnostic and treatment process.

The Behavioral System Model clearly reflects a systems approach. Although Johnson discusses some subsystem behavior in a developmental context, the systems approach is the dominant and overriding perspective.

Generation of Theory

The formation of conceptual-theoretical-empirical systems of nursing knowledge is evident in many of the applications of the Behavioral System Model listed in the bibliography at the end of this chapter. In several instances, selected concepts of the model were linked with theories and empirical indicators borrowed from other disciplines. For example, Wilkie, Lovejoy, Dodd, and Tesler (1988) linked the aggressive subsystem with the gate control theory of pain in their study of the relationship of cancer pain control behaviors and pain intensity. The empirical indictors for this study were a Demographic Pain Data Form, which was adapted from existing pain assessment questionnaires, a Behavioral Observation-Validation Form, and a visual analog scale.

Lachicotte and Alexander (1990) linked the Behavioral System Model with the Nadler-Tushman Congruence Model to guide their study of the relationship between nurse administrators' attitudes toward nurse impairment and their method of dealing with the impairment. The empirical indicators were the Attitudes Toward Nurse Impairment Inventory and the Methods for Dealing with Nurse Impairment Questionnaire.

Holaday (personal communication, August 26, 1987) has begun to develop an original middle-range theory dealing with the structural components and functional requirements (sustenal imperatives) of the Behavioral System Model. This theory development work was part of a study of what chronically ill 10- to 12-year-old children do with their out-of-school time. The conceptual-theoretical framework for that study linked the Behavioral System Model with Bronfenbrenner's model of the ecology of human development. Holaday commented that she and a colleague "are interested in identifying the important sustenal imperatives for each subsystem and how they influence choice and action. We will attempt to see if there is a hierarchy of sustenal imperatives for each subsystem."

Although reports of the study have been published, (Bossert, Holaday, Harkins, & Turner-Henson, 1990; Holady & Turner-Henson, 1987; Turner-Henson, 1993), the theory has not yet been formalized.

Although some theory development work has been done, no theories of the behavioral system as a whole have been formulated yet. Commenting on that, Johnson (1990a) stated,

> An empirical literature supporting the conception of a behavioral system composed of *all* of the person's patterned and purposeful behavior is largely to be developed. There has been considerable research and theoretical attention, however, directed toward specific response systems within what I consider to be the total complex of the whole behavioral system. This is not unlike the case of knowledge about the biological system where knowledge of parts, the subsystems, preceded knowledge of the whole. Fortunately, we can tentatively rely on a developing body of knowledge about systems in general and the laws that govern the operation of all systems until further knowledge of the behavioral system as a whole is developed. (p. 25)

Credibility

Social Utility

Johnson (1980) claimed that the Behavioral System Model "has already proved its utility in providing clear direction for practice, education, and research" (p. 215). Articles by proponents of the Behavioral System Model indicate that it also has provided useful guidelines for administration.

Johnson's Behavioral System Model is especially attractive to those nurses who are familiar with system theory and the attendant vocabulary. Although Rawls (1980) regarded the complex and unique terminology used to explain the model as a disadvantage, this limitation is readily overcome by studying the model's vocabulary. Indeed, Johnson (1988) maintained that an understanding of the vocabulatory of any science or framework is a prerequisite to description of relevant phenomena. In addition, study is required to fully understand the unique focus and content of the Behavioral System Model. Johnson (1980) explained:

> Adoption of this model for practice carries with it direct responsibilities in education. The user will need a thorough grounding in the underlying natural and social sciences. Emphasis should be placed in particular on the genetic, neurologic, and endocrine bases of behavior; psychologic and social mechanisms for the regulation and control of behavior; social learning theories; and motivational structures and processes. (p. 214)

Furthermore, Johnson (1990a) pointed out that the effective use of the Behavioral System Model in practice requires "intensive study of the rich literature available on the seven response [sub]systems" (p. 32). She went on to explain:

The nurse must know, for example, how these [sub]systems develop over time, the many factors that influence that development, the
cultural variations in the basic response [sub]systems to be expected,
and much more. The nurse must also acquire an understanding of how
living systems operate. Only with such knowledge and understanding is
it possible for the practitioner to be aware of the kinds of data needed
about the individual. Only with such knowledge can the practitioner
analyze [those] data and intervene effectively. (p. 32)

Johnson (1980) also stated that the user of the model must study the
behavioral system as a whole and as a composite of subsystems, pathophysiology, medicine's and nursing's clinical sciences, and the health
care system. In addition, the potential user of the Behavioral System
Model must understand Johnson's value system and accept as appropriate
a wide range of behavior. In addition, the user of the model must be
willing to negotiate nursing treatment options with the patient.

The implementation of Behavioral System Model–based nursing
practice is feasible. Herbert (1989) commented that "considerable changes
in education and resources would be necessary to allow general implementation" (p. 34). She did not, however, identify the specific changes
that would be required. Dee (1990) maintained, "The challenge to nurse
executives is to create environments that promote optimal professional
practice so that the quality of patient care can be sustained and further
enhanced" (p. 41). Her description of the implementation of Behavioral
System Model–based nursing practice at the University of California, Los
Angeles (UCLA) Neuropsychiatric Institute and Hospital indicated that
administrators at that agency committed the time and human and material resources required to revise existing nursing assessment forms; develop teaching materials; conduct ongoing inservice education programs
to orient staff to the model and provide a forum for ongoing dialogue on
the refinement of the model; conduct orientation classes for new employees and supervise those employees in the application of the model;
develop strategies to overcome resistance to change; develop a patient
classification instrument that includes parameters to determine staffing
needs; and develop standardized nursing care plans, model-based nursing
diagnoses, and criteria to evaluate patient outcomes.

NURSING RESEARCH. The utility of the Behavioral System Model for
nursing research is documented by several studies that have been guided
by the model. Doctoral dissertations that could be located in *Dissertation
Abstracts International* are listed in the bibliography at the end of this
chapter. Holaday (personal communication, August 26, 1987) reported
that master's theses based on the Behavioral System Model were conducted by Broering (1985), Dawson (1984), Kizpolski (1985), Miller (1987),
Moran (1986), and Wilkie (1985). A computer-assisted literature search
was unable to retrieve published abstracts of those theses but did yield
the one citation that is listed in the chapter bibliography.

Instruments that measure Behavioral System Model concepts have been developed by Auger and Dee (1983; Dee, 1986; Dee & Auger, 1983); Bruce, Hinds, Hudak, Mucha, and Taylor (1980); Derdiarian (1983, 1988); Derdiarian and Forsyth (1983); Hadley (1990); Lovejoy (1982, 1983); and Majesky, Brester, and Nishio (1978). Auger and Dee developed and Dee validated the comprehensive Patient Classification Instrument (PCI) based on the Behavioral System Model. Bruce and associates developed a Behavioral System Model-based tool to measure outcome criteria for fluid and electrolyte balance in patients with end-stage renal disease.

Derdiarian developed the Derdiarian Behavioral System Model (DBSM) instrument, which was designed to measure cancer patients' perceived behavioral changes in all behavioral subsystems. Two forms of that instrument are now available — the DBSM Self-Report instrument for patients and the DBSM-O, which is the observational counterpart used by nurses (Derdiarian, 1990a). Hadley, along with colleagues J. Wood, A. McCracken, and G. Warshaw, developed the Behavioral Capabilities Scale for Older Adults, which measures stability and change in the behavioral capabilities of older adults in nursing homes. Lovejoy developed the Johnson Model First-Level Family Assessment Tool (JFFA — J), which is a projective instrument that measures the needs of families with a chronically ill child. Majesky et al. (1978) developed the Patient Indicators of Nursing Care instrument, a quality assurance tool that measures the quality of nursing care in terms of the prevention of nursing care complications.

Descriptive and correlational studies also have been derived from the Behavioral System Model. One of the earliest published full reports of research based on the model was Stamler and Palmer's (1971) investigation of dependency behaviors in children who made repetitive visits to an elementary school nurse. Damus (1980) also used the model to guide her study of patients who had post-transfusion hepatitis. She investigated "the relationship between selected physiologic disequilibria and behavioral disequilibria as well as the correlation of particular nursing diagnoses with effective nursing interventions" (p. 275). Damus used the behavioral subsystems as the classification scheme for nursing diagnoses and the functional requirements to classify nursing interventions.

Furthermore, Small (1980) discussed the findings of her comparison of the perceived body image and spatial awareness of visually handicapped preschool children with that of normally sighted preschoolers in the context of the Behavioral System Model. Moreover, Lachicotte and Alexander (1990) used the Behavioral System Model to study the relationship between nurse administrators' attitudes toward nurse impairment and their method of dealing with nurses who were impaired by alcoholism or other drug dependency.

Lovejoy (1985) conducted a Behavioral System Model–based study of the needs of visitors of patients in cancer research units. She compared the needs of visitors who maintained vigils at the patient's bedside with the needs of visitors who did not maintain vigils. Lovejoy and Moran (1988) studied the AIDS beliefs, behaviors, and informational needs of patients with AIDS or AIDS-related complex. The sexual and aggressive behavioral subsystems provided the focus for the study. Moreover, reasoning that "aggressive subsystem behaviors are developed and modified over time to protect the individual from pain" (p. 724), Wilkie et al. (1988) studied the relationship between pain control behaviors and pain intensity in a sample of 17 adult patients with solid tumor malignancies.

Although much of the Behavioral System Model-based research is limited to a single study on a single topic, some programmatic research is evident. Derdiarian has used the DBSM instrument in a series of studies to determine the quality of nursing care (1991); cancer patients' and nurses' satisfaction with Behavioral System Model-based nursing care (1990a); AIDS patients' perceived changes in the direction, quality, and relative importance of subsystem behaviors (Derdiarian & Schobel, 1990); and the relationship between the aggressive subsystem and the other subsystems of the Behavioral System Model (1990b). The latter study findings are especially salient in that they provide empirical support for Johnson's (1980) contention that the subsystems are "linked and open, . . . and a disturbance in one subsystem is likely to have an effect on others" (p. 210).

In addition, Holaday has conducted several Behavioral System Model–based studies dealing with children. For one investigation, Holaday (1974) used the concepts of the achievement subsystem, behavioral system balance, drive, and set to study the differences in achievement behavior between chronically ill and well children. In another study, Holaday (1981) used the concept of behavioral set to guide her investigation of the effects of degree of illness, infant's sex, and ordinal position on maternal response to infants' crying. In two other studies, Holaday (1982, 1987) again used the concept of behavioral set to continue her examination of mothers' responses to the crying behaviors of their chronically ill infants. Holaday (personal communication, August 26, 1987) explained that her 1987 study was "a 'second check' on the structural component of conceptual set" and that the data from that study led to identification of "the general characteristics of the stages of conceptual set." Holaday and associates have extended the research to studies of chronically ill children's use of out-of-school time (Bossert et al., 1990; Holaday & Turner-Henson, 1987).

NURSING EDUCATION. The utility of the Behavioral System Model for nursing education is documented by its use as a guide for curriculum construction in nursing education programs. Hadley (1970) described the use of the model at the University of Colorado in Denver. Harris (1986) explained how a modified version of the Behavioral System Model guided curriculum design at the University of California in Los Angeles. Fleming (1990) described the use of the Behavioral System Model by the Department of Nursing at California State University in Bakersfield. Carino (personal communication, January 24, 1990) explained how the Behavioral System Model was operationalized in the curriculum at the University of Hawaii in Honolulu in the 1960s. The utility of the Behavioral System Model for nursing education is also documented by Derdiarian (1981), who discussed the application of the model to cancer nursing education.

NURSING ADMINISTRATION. The utility of the Behavioral System Model for nursing administration is documented by its use as a guide for the nursing administrative structures of clinical agencies. Hackley (1987) reported the work she did to redesign nursing care processes within the context of the Behavioral System Model for the psychiatric unit at the U.S. Naval Hospital in Philadelphia, Pennsylvania. She noted that the model guided the practice of all health care team members, from orderlies to nurses to the staff psychiatrist.

Dee (1990) presented a detailed description of the use of the model at the UCLA Neuropsychiatric Institute and Hospital in Los Angeles, California. She explained that the Behavioral System Model is implemented in the child and adult psychiatric inpatient services with patients ranging from 2 to more than 90 years of age. Clinical settings include a child and an adolescent psychiatric unit, a child and an adolescent developmental disabilities unit, general adult psychiatric units, and a geropsychiatry unit.

Dee and Auger (1983) described the application of their Patient Classification Instrument (PCI) at the Neuropsychiatric Institute. The PCI operationalizes each behavioral subsystem as critical behaviors. Overall level of behavior for each patient is categorized as adaptive, in the process of being learned and/or minimally maladaptive, or maladaptive. Nursing interventions are linked to behaviors and also categorized according to the level of nursing care required. The authors maintained that although the patient classification system was developed for use in psychiatric settings, it can be extended to other clinical settings by identifying the relevant patient behaviors and nursing interventions in each setting. It is noteworthy that the patient classification system encompasses all subsystems and the entire nursing process. Indeed, Dee and Auger (1983) commented that use of the system led to many practical benefits and had a major impact on all phases of the nursing process. They explained,

> The assessment of patient behaviors . . . [is] now systematically and comprehensively reviewed within the framework of the behavioral subsystems. . . . The correlated nursing care actions with patient behaviors has assisted in both the planning and the intervention phases of the process by identifying a broad range of general areas of potential nursing activity. . . . The use of a model also provides an objective means for evaluating the quality of nursing care. . . . Instead of evaluating patient outcome for groups based on medical diagnoses, it becomes feasible to evaluate outcomes for groups of patients based on common behavioral problems or nursing treatment approaches. (p. 23)

A Behavioral System Model–based nursing diagnostic system also was developed for use at the UCLA Neuropsychiatric Institute and Hospital. Randell (1991) and Lewis and Randell (1991) described the development of the diagnostic system and documented its advantages over the North American Nursing Diagnosis Association (NANDA) system. Randell (1991) explained that the Behavioral System Model–based nursing diagnoses "reflect the nature of the ineffective behavior and its relationship to the regulators in the environment" (p. 154). She went on to point out that the Behavioral System Model "helps distinguish what counts as a problem and what counts as etiology, calling into question existing [NANDA] labels" (p. 159).

Chance (1982) claimed that nursing models provide guidelines for professional accountability and quality of nursing care. Although she reviewed the major concepts of the Behavioral System Model, she did not demonstrate their application to quality assurance programs. Application of the Behavioral System Model to quality assurance programs was, however, demonstrated by Majesky et al. (1978), who explained how their Patient Indicators of Nursing Care instrument can be used to assess the "degree to which nursing intervention contributes to the deterioration or improvement of a patient's condition, based on selected physiological measures, over a seven- to nine-day (hospital or nursing home) stay" (p. 366).

Bruce et al. (1980) also used the Behavioral System Model for a quality assurance program for patients with end-stage renal disease. The tool they designed to measure outcome criteria for fluid and electrolyte balance includes items that reflect the ingestive, eliminative, and achievement subsystems.

Glennin (1980) developed Behavioral System Model–based standards of nursing practice for hospitalized patients receiving acute care from professional registered nurses. Emphasis was placed on psychosocial, rather than physiological, management. Glennin classified the standards according to the nursing process areas of data-gathering, assessment, diagnosis, prescription, implementation, and evaluation. In each area, specific standards were formulated for relevant concepts and propositions of the model.

Rogers (1973) proposed that the behavioral subsystems represent areas for clinical specialization in nursing. One could, for example, be a clinical specialist in the aggressive subsystem or the attachment subsystem. There is no evidence to indicate that her innovative proposal has ever been implemented.

Initial empirical evidence supporting the utility of the Behavioral System Model for nursing administration is provided by the findings of Derdiarian's (1991) study of the effects of using two Derdiarian Behavioral System Model assessment instruments on the quality of nursing care. She found that when compared with routine nursing assessment, the use of the model-based instruments resulted in a statistically significant increase in the completeness of objective and subjective data gathered; the quality of the nursing diagnosis; the compatibility and specificity of nursing interventions with the nursing diagnoses; and the appropriateness and recording of follow-ups, evaluation of outcomes, and discharge plans.

NURSING PRACTICE. Evidence supporting the utility of the Behavioral System Model in various clinical settings is accumulating. The publications cited here, along with others listed in the bibliography at the end of this chapter, indicate that the Behavioral System Model can be used in many different clinical practice situations with patients of all ages.

Holaday (1980) used the model to assess health status and to derive nursing interventions for a 6-year-old child scheduled for surgery, for a 12-year-old child with meningomyelocele and multiple urinary tract problems, and for a 15-year-old retarded child with a discrepancy of the eliminative subsystem. Skolny and Riehl (1974) used the model to guide their actions to promote development of hope for the mother of a dying brain-injured 22-year-old man. Rawls (1980) used the model to guide nursing care of an adult amputee with a problem in body image. McCauley et al. (1984) used the model to guide assessment and nursing intervention for family-centered nursing care of the patient with ventricular tachycardia. Wilkie (1990) conceptualized cancer pain management within the Behavioral System Model and identified interdependent and independent nursing functions for management of cancer patients' pain. Herbert (1989) described the intellectual challenges posed by using the Behavioral System Model to guide the care of a 75-year-old woman who suffered flaccid hemiplegia due to a cerebrovascular accident. Furthermore, B. Sanchez, J. de Uriza, and M. Orjuela (personal communication, March 18, 1986) reported the progress they had made in using the Behavioral System Model to guide the nursing care of elderly patients in Colombia, South America.

The Behavioral System Model emphasizes and focuses explicitly on the individual behavioral system. Johnson (1978a) suggested the use of Chin's (1961) intersystem model for nurses who are interested in the care of families and other groups. This approach permits consideration of each individual behavioral system and the interaction of those systems. Furthermore, Conner, Harbour, Magers, and Watt (1994) briefly explained how the model could be used in community health nursing. Fruehwirth (1989) reported the results of using the Behavioral System Model for a support group for the caregivers of patients with Alzheimer's Disease.

Social Congruence

The Behavioral System Model is generally congruent with contemporary social expectations regarding nursing practice. Commenting on that criterion, Johnson (1980) stated, "Insofar as it has been tried in practice, the resulting nursing decisions and actions have generally been judged acceptable and satisfactory by patients, families, nursing staff, and physicians" (p. 215). Furthermore, Grubbs (1980) maintained that the role of the nurse, as described in this model, "is congruent with society's expectations of nursing and that nursing's contribution to health care is a socially valued service" (p. 218). In a recent publication, Johnson (1990a) noted that the Behavioral System Model "is commensurate with what nurses and the public perceive as nursing's function" (p. 31). Dee (1990) added, "The Johnson Model has provided nurses with a framework not only to describe phenomena, but also to explain, predict, and control clinical phenomena for the purpose of achieving desired patient outcomes. Levels of nursing care provided for the patient are, therefore, purposeful and nursing practice is more meaningful for the practitioner" (p. 41).

Empirical evidence supporting the claims made by Johnson, Grubbs, and Dee comes from Derdiarian (1990a), who reported a statistically significant increase in both cancer patients' and nurses' satisfaction with the nursing process, including the comprehensiveness of assessment, the appropriateness and priority rank of diagnoses, the interventions, and the effectiveness of outcomes, when nursing assessments were structured according to the Behavioral System Model compared with routine clinical assessment.

Johnson (1968) deliberately attempted to structure nursing practice so that it would be congruent with societal expectations. She maintained, "The value of the model does not lie so much in the fact that it leads to very different forms of action — if it did depart markedly from currently accepted practice, it would perhaps be open to greater question than it otherwise might be" (p. 6).

In contrast with her 1968 comment, 10 years later Johnson (1978a) indicated that in some situations, the nurse and/or the patient may accept a wider range of behavior than prescribed by cultural norms. In such cases, society would have to be helped to accept variances from the average. Additionally, society may have to be helped to accept the role of nursing in assisting people to maintain efficient and effective behavioral functioning when the threat of illness exists. This is because even though there is increased worldwide attention on primary health care with its emphasis on health promotion and illness prevention, some people still do not expect nursing care prior to the onset of illness. Indeed, Johnson (personal communication cited in Conner et al., 1994) maintained that preventive nursing — whether aimed at prevention of behavioral system disorder or some other goal — needs to be developed.

Social Significance

Johnson (1980) claimed that the Behavioral System Model leads to nursing actions that are socially significant, stating that "resulting [nursing] actions have been thought to make a significant difference in the lives of the persons involved" (p. 215). Grubbs (1980) agreed with Johnson, noting that the model "provides the framework for categorizing all aspects of the nursing process so that the science of nursing, the personal satisfaction of the nurse, and ultimately the welfare of the patient will improve" (p. 249). Neither Johnson nor Grubbs, however, supported her claim with empirical evidence.

Rawls (1980) provided anecdotal evidence of the social significance of the Behavioral System Model. She stated:

> Use of the Model allowed me to systematically assess the patient and facilitated identification of specific factors which influenced the effectiveness of nursing care. The assessment data allowed identification of interventions which had the desired effect and resulted in effective care for the patient. (p. 16)

Poster (1989) provided initial empirical evidence of the social significance of the Behavioral System Model. Using the Patient Classification Instrument developed by Auger and Dee (1983), she found that 90 percent of the 38 adolescent psychiatric inpatients studied had an adaptive change in at least one behavioral category after 1 week of Behavioral System Model–based nursing care.

Contributions to the Discipline of Nursing

Johnson certainly may be considered a pioneer in the development of distinctive nursing knowledge, despite the fact that she did not publish her model until relatively recently. The Behavioral System Model makes a substantial contribution to nursing knowledge by focusing attention on the person's behavior, rather than on his or her health state or disease condition. Johnson used this distinction to clarify the different foci of nursing and medicine, a clarification that is especially important for continued development of nursing as a distinct discipline. However, she recognized the boundary overlaps that are inevitable in all disciplines. That point is elaborated in the following quotation:

> This model attempts to specify [the goal of nursing] in keeping with our historical concerns, and to reclarify nursing's mission and area of responsibility. In doing so, no denial of nursing's old relationship with medicine is intended. Nursing has, and undoubtedly always will play an important role in assisting medicine to fulfill its mission. We do this directly by taking on activities delegated by medicine, but also, and perhaps more importantly, we may contribute to the achievement of medicine's goals by fulfilling our own mission. (Johnson, 1968, p. 9)

Johnson (1968) identified the advantages she saw in the Behavioral System Model. The list adequately summarizes the many contributions her conceptual model makes to the discipline of nursing.

1. The assumptions and values of the model are made explicit. This allows their examination and offers the possibility that those assumptions which have not been adequately verified can be logically and perhaps empirically tested.

2. The model offers a reasonably precise and limited ideal goal for nursing by stating the end product desired. Specification of this ideal state or condition is the first step in its operational definition in the concrete case. It thus offers promise for the establishment of standards against which to measure the effectiveness and significance of nursing actions.

3. The model directs our attention to those aspects of the patient, in all his complex reality, with which nursing is concerned, and provides a systematic way to approach the identification of nursing problems.

4. It provides us with clues as to the source of difficulty (i.e., either functional or structural stress).

5. It offers a focus for intervention and suggests the major modes of intervention which will be required.

6. It opens the door to focused research programs in nursing and the possibility that the findings of individual investigators will become cumulative and of theoretical as well as of practical significance. (pp. 7–8)

Commenting on the contributions of the Behavioral System Model in a recent paper, Johnson (1992) stated:

Admittedly even now knowledge about the behavioral patterns in the response or action systems is greater than knowledge of the underlying structures, and knowledge about the parts or subsystems is greater than knowledge of the system as a whole. Nonetheless, the body of knowledge about the behavioral system and its subsystems is sufficiently substantial to allow pertinent observations and useful interpretations in practice. It also points to many possibilities for intervention as well as avenues for research. In this way a body of knowledge about disorders in the behavioral system and their prevention and treatment will be developed and expanded over time and will be known as nursing science. (p. 26)

In conclusion, the Behavioral System Model has been enthusiastically adopted by many nurses interested in a systematic approach to nursing. It has documented utility in nursing practice, administration, and research, and it provides direction for curriculum development. The credibility of the Behavioral System Model is beginning to be established by means of studies directly derived from several of its components and linked with relevant theories and appropriate empirical indicators. This empirical work needs to be expanded, and more systematic evaluations of the use of the model in various clinical situations and educational settings are needed.

REFERENCES

Ackoff, R.L. (1960). Systems, organizations, and interdisciplinary research. *General Systems, 5,* 1–8.

Ainsworth, M. (1964). Patterns of attachment behavior shown by the infant in interaction with mother. *Merrill-Palmer Quarterly, 10*(1), 51–58.

Ainsworth, M. (1972). Attachment and dependency: A comparison. In J. Gewirtz (Ed.), *Attachment and dependency* (pp. 97–137). Englewood Cliffs, NJ: Prentice-Hall.

Atkinson, J.W., & Feather, N.T. (1966). *A theory of achievement maturation.* New York: John Wiley & Sons.

Auger, J.R. (1976). *Behavioral systems and nursing.* Englewood Cliffs, NJ: Prentice-Hall.

Auger, J.R., & Dee, V. (1983). A patient classification system based on the behavioral system model of nursing: Part I. *Journal of Nursing Administration, 13*(4), 38–43.

Barnum, B.J.S. (1994). *Nursing theory: Analysis, application, evaluation* (4th ed.). Philadelphia: JB Lippincott.

Bossert, E., Holaday, B., Harkins, A., & Turner-Henson, A. (1990). Strategies of normalization used by parents of chronically ill school age children. *Journal of Child and Adolescent Psychiatric and Mental Health Nursing, 3,* 57–61.

Broering, J. (1985). *Adolescent juvenile status offenders' perceptions of stressful life events and self-perception of health status.* Unpublished master's thesis, University of California, San Francisco.

Bruce, G.L., Hinds, P., Hudak, J., Mucha, A., Taylor, M.C., & Thompson, C.R. (1980). Implementation of ANA's quality assurance program for clients with end-stage renal disease. *Advances in Nursing Science, 2*(2), 79–95.

Buckley, W. (Ed.). (1968). *Modern systems research for the behavioral scientist.* Chicago: Aldine.

Carino, C. (1976). Behavioral responses of disoriented patients compared to oriented patients in intensive care units. *Dissertation Abstracts International, 37,* 162B.

Chance, K.S. (1982). Nursing models: A requisite for professional accountability. *Advances in Nursing Science, 4*(2), 57–65.

Chin, R. (1961). The utility of system models and developmental models for practitioners. In W.G. Bennis, K.D. Beene, & R. Chin (Eds.), *The planning of change* (pp. 201–214). New York: Holt, Rinehart & Winston.

Conner, S.S., Harbour, LS, Magers, J.A., & Watt, J.K., (1994). Dorothy E. Johnson: Behavioral system model. In A. Marriner-Tomey, *Nursing theorists and their work* (3rd ed., pp. 231–245). St. Louis: Mosby-Year Book.

Crandal, V. (1963). Achievement. In H.W. Stevenson (Ed.), *Child psychology* (pp. 416–459). Chicago: University of Chicago Press.

Damus, K. (1980). An application of the Johnson behavioral system model for nursing practice. In J.P. Riehl & C. Roy, *Conceptual models for nursing practice* (2nd ed., pp. 274–289). New York: Appleton-Century-Crofts.

Dawson, D.L. (1984). *Parenting behaviors of mothers with hospitalized children under two years of age.* Unpublished master's thesis, University of California, San Francisco.

Dee, V. (1986). Validation of a patient classification instrument for psychiatric patients based on the Johnson model for nursing. *Dissertation Abstracts International, 47,* 4822B.

Dee, V. (1990). Implementation of the Johnson model: One hospital's experience. In M.E. Parker (Ed.), *Nursing theories in practice* (pp. 33–44). New York: National League for Nursing.

Dee, V., & Auger, J.A. (1983). A patient classification system based on the behavioral system model of nursing: Part 2. *Journal of Nursing Administration, 13*(5), 18–23.

Derdiarian, A.K. (1981). Nursing conceptual frameworks: Implicataions for education, practice, and research. In D.L. Vredevoe, A.K. Derdiarian, L.P. Sarna, M. Eriel, & J.C. Shipacoff, *Concepts of oncology nursing* (pp. 369–385). Englewood Cliffs, NJ: Prentice-Hall.

Derdiarian, A.K. (1983). An instrument for theory and research using the behavioral systems model for nursing: The cancer patient (Part I). *Nursing Research, 32,* 196–201.

Derdiarian, A.K. (1988). Sensitivity of the Derdiarian behavioral system model instrument to age, site, and stage of cancer: A preliminary validation study. *Scholarly Inquiry for Nursing Practice, 2,* 103–121.

Derdiarian, A.K. (1990a). Effects of using systematic assessment instruments on patient and nurse satisfaction with nursing care. *Oncology Nursing Forum, 17,* 95–101.

Derdiarian, A.K. (1990b). The relationships

among the subsystems of Johnson's behavioral system model. *Image: Journal of Nursing Scholarship, 22,* 219–225.

Derdiarian, A.K. (1991). Effects of using a nursing model-based assessment instrument on quality of nursing care. *Nursing Administration Quarterly, 15*(3), 1–16.

Derdiarian, A.K., & Forsythe, A.B. (1983). An instrument for theory and research using the behavioral systems model for nursing: The cancer patient (Part II). *Nursing Research, 32,* 260–266.

Derdiarian, A.K., & Schobel, D. (1990). Comprehensive assessment of AIDS patients using the behavioural systems model for nursing practice instrument. *Journal of Advanced Nursing, 15,* 436–446.

Feshbach, S. (1970). Aggression. In P. Mussen (Ed.), *Carmichael's manual of child psychology* (Vol. 2, 3rd ed., pp. 159–259). New York: John Wiley & Sons.

Fruehwirth, S.E.S. (1989). An application of Johnson's behavioral model: A case study. *Journal of Community Health Nursing, 6*(2), 61–71.

Fleming, B.H. (1990, September). *Use of the Johnson model in nursing education.* Paper presented at the National Nursing Theory Conference, UCLA Neuropsychiatric Institute and Hospital Nursing Department, Los Angeles, CA.

Gewirtz, J. (Ed.). (1972). *Attachment and dependency.* Englewood Cliffs, NJ: Prentice-Hall.

Glennin, C.G. (1980). Formulation of standards for nursing practice using a nursing model. In J.P. Riehl & C. Roy, *Conceptual models for nursing practice* (2nd ed., pp. 290–301). New York: Appleton-Century-Crofts.

Grubbs, J. (1974). An interpretation of the Johnson Behavioral System Model. In J.P. Riehl & C. Roy, *Conceptual models for nursing practice* (pp. 160–197). New York: Appleton-Century-Crofts.

Grubbs, J. (1980). An interpretation of the Johnson Behavioral System Model. In J.P. Riehl & C. Roy, *Conceptual models for nursing practice* (2nd ed., pp. 217–254). New York: Appleton-Century-Crofts.

Hackley, S. (1987, February). *Application of Johnson's behavioral system model.* Paper presented at the University of Pennsylvania School of Nursing, Philadelphia.

Hadley, B.J. (1970, March). *The utility of theoretical frameworks for curriculum development in nursing: The happening at Colorado.* Paper presented at WICHEN General Session, Honolulu, Hawaii.

Hadley, B.J. (1990, September). *The Dorothy*

Johnson behavioral systems model in clinical nursing research—A tale of two studies. Paper presented at the National Nursing Theory Conference, UCLA Neuropsychiatric Institute and Hospital Nursing Department, Los Angeles, CA.

Hall, B.A. (1981). The change paradigm in nursing: Growth versus persistence. *Advances in Nursing Science, 3*(4), 1–6.

Harris, R.B. (1986). Introduction of a conceptual nursing model into a fundamental baccalaureate course. *Journal of Nursing Education, 25,* 66–69.

Heathers, G. (1955). Acquiring dependence and independence: A theoretical orientation. *Journal of Genetic Psychology, 87,* 277–291.

Herbert, J. (1989). A model for Anna. *Nursing, 3*(42), 30–34.

Holaday, B. (1974). Achievement behavior in chronically ill children. *Nursing Research, 23,* 25–30.

Holaday, B. (1980). Implementing the Johnson model for nursing practice. In J.P. Riehl & C. Roy, *Conceptual models for nursing practice* (2nd ed., pp. 255–263). New York: Appleton-Century-Crofts.

Holaday, B. (1981). Maternal response to their chronically ill infants' attachment behavior of crying. *Nursing Research, 30,* 343–348.

Holaday, B. (1982). Maternal conceptual set development: Identifying patterns of maternal response to chronically ill infant crying. *Maternal-Child Nursing Journal, 11,* 47–59.

Holaday, B. (1987). Patterns of interaction between mothers and their chronically ill infants. *Maternal-Child Nursing Journal, 16,* 29–45.

Holaday, B., & Turner-Henson, A. (1987). Chronically ill school-age children's use of time. *Pediatric Nursing, 13,* 410–414.

Johnson, D.E. (1959). A philosophy of nursing. *Nursing Outlook, 7,* 198–200.

Johnson, D.E. (1961). The significance of nursing care. *American Journal of Nursing, 61*(11), 63–66.

Johnson, D.E. (1968, April). *One conceptual model of nursing.* Paper presented at Vanderbilt University, Nashville, TN.

Johnson, D.E. (1978a, December). *Behavioral system model for nursing.* Paper presented at the Second Annual Nurse Educator Conference, New York. (Cassette recording).

Johnson, D.E. (1978b). State of the art of theory development in nursing. In *Theory development: What, why, how?* (pp. 1–10). New York: National League for Nursing.

Johnson, D.E. (1980). The behavioral system model for nursing. In J.P. Riehl & C. Roy, *Conceptual models for nursing practice* (2nd ed., pp. 207–216). New York: Appleton-Century-Crofts.

Johnson, D.E. (1988). *The nurse theorists: Portraits of excellence—Dorothy Johnson.* Oakland, CA: Studio Three. (Videotape).

Johnson, D.E. (1989). Some thoughts on nursing (Editorial). *Clinical Nurse Specialist, 3,* 1–4.

Johnson, D.E. (1990a). The behavioral system model for nursing. In M.E. Parker (Ed.), *Nursing theories in practice* (pp. 23–32). New York: National League for Nursing.

Johnson, D.E. (1990b, September). Response to V. Dee & B.P. Randell, *The Johnson behavioral systems model: Conceptual issues and dilemmas.* Paper presented at the National Nursing Theory Conference, UCLA Neuropsychiatric Institute and Hospital Nursing Department, Los Angeles, CA.

Johnson, D.E. (1992). The origins of the behavioral system model. In F.N. Nightingale, *Notes on nursing: What it is, and what it is not* (Commemorative edition, pp. 23–27). Philadelphia: JB Lippincott.

Kagan, J. (1964). Acquisition and significance of sex typing and sex role identity. In M. Hoffman & L. Hoffman (Eds.), *Review of child development research* (Vol. 1, pp. 137–167). New York: Russell Sage Foundation.

Kizpolski, P.A. (1985). *Family adaptation during the midstage of cancer.* Unpublished master's thesis, University of California, San Francisco.

Lachicotte, J.L., & Alexander, J.W. (1990). Management attitudes and nurse impairment. *Nursing Management, 21,* 102–104, 106, 108, 110.

Lewis, C., & Randell, B.P. (1991). Alteration in self-care: An instance of ineffective coping in the geriatric patient. In R.M. Carroll-Johnson (Ed.), *Classification of nursing diagnoses: Proceedings of the ninth conference: North American Nursing Diagnosis Association* (pp. 264–265). Philadelphia: JB Lippincott.

Lorenz, K. (1966). *On aggression.* New York: Harcourt.

Lovejoy, N.C. (1982). An empirical verification of the Johnson behavioral system model for nursing. *Dissertation Abstracts International, 42,* 2781B.

Lovejoy, N.C. (1983). The leukemic child's perceptions of family behaviors. *Oncology Nursing Forum, 10*(4), 20–25.

Lovejoy, N.C. (1985). Needs of vigil and non-vigil visitors in cancer research units. In *Fourth Cancer Nursing Research Conference Proceedings* (pp. 142–164). Honolulu: American Cancer Society.

Lovejoy, N.C. (1986, March). *Johnson's behavioral system model.* Paper presented at the Sigma Theta Tau conference—Nursing Knowledge: Improving Research Through Theory, San Francisco, CA.

Lovejoy, N.C., & Moran, T.A. (1988). Selected AIDS beliefs, behaviors and informational needs of homosexual/bisexual men with AIDS or ARC. *International Journal of Nursing Studies, 25,* 207–216.

Majesky, S.J., Brester, M.H., & Nishio, K.T. (1978). Development of a research tool: Patient indicators of nursing care. *Nursing Research, 27,* 365–371.

Marriner-Tomey, A. (1989). *Nursing theorists and their work* (2nd ed). St. Louis: CV Mosby.

McCauley, K., Choromanski, J.D., Wallinger, C., & Liu, K. (1984). Current management of ventricular tachycardia: Symposium from the Hospital of the University of Pennsylvania. Learning to live with controlled ventricular tachycardia: Utilizing the Johnson model. *Heart and Lung, 13,* 633–638.

Mead, M. (1953). *Cultural patterns and technical change.* World Federation for Mental Health: UNESCO.

Meleis, A.I. (1991). *Theoretical nursing: Development and progress* (2nd ed.). Philadelphia: JB Lippincott(MDNM).

Miller, M. (1987). *Uncertainty, coping, social support and family functioning in parents of children with myelomeningocele.* Unpublished master's thesis. University of California, San Francisco.

Moran, T.A. (1986). *The effect of an AIDS diagnosis on the sexual practices of homosexual men.* Unpublished master's thesis, University of California, San Francisco.

Nightingale, F.N. (1946). *Notes on nursing: What it is, and what it is not* (Facsimile ed.). Philadelphia: JB Lippincott. (Originally published in 1859).

Poster, E.C. (1989). Behavioral category ratings of adolescents on an inpatient psychiatric unit: The use of the Johnson behavioral system model (Abstract). In A. Brackston, L. Cooper-Pagé, S. Edwards, M., Light, S. Cardinal, B. Du Gas, C. Hinds, & M. McNamara (Eds.), *Proceedings: Putting it all together* (p. 99). Ottawa, Ontario, Canada: University of Ottawa.

Randell, B.P. (1991). NANDA versus the Johnson behavioral systems model: Is there a diagnostic difference? In R.M.

Carroll-Johnson (Ed.), *Classification of nursing diagnoses: Proceedings of the ninth conference: North American Nursing Diagnosis Association* (pp. 154–160). Philadelphia: JB Lippincott.

Rapoport, A. (1968). Forward. In W. Buckley (Ed.), *Modern systems research for the behavioral scientist* (pp. xiii–xxii). Chicago: Aldine.

Rawls, A.C. (1980). Evaluation of the Johnson Behavioral Model in clinical practice. *Image: Journal of Nursing Scholarship, 12,* 13–16.

Resnik, H.L.P. (1972). *Sexual behaviors.* Boston: Little, Brown.

Riehl, J.P., & Roy, C. (1980). *Conceptual models for nursing practice* (2nd ed.). New York: Appleton-Century-Crofts.

Robson, K.K. (1967). Patterns and determinants of maternal attachment. *Journal of Pediatrics, 77,* 976–985.

Rogers, C.G. (1973). Conceptual models as guides to clinical nursing specialization. *Journal of Nursing Education, 12*(4), 2–6.

Rosenthal, M. (1967). The generalization of dependency from mother to a stranger. Journal of Child Psychology and Psychiatry, 8, 177–183.

Sears, R., Maccoby, E., & Levin, H. (1954). *Patterns of child rearing.* White Plains, NY: Row, Peterson.

Skolny, M.S., & Riehl, J.P. (1974). Hope:

Solving patient and family problems by using a theoretical framework. In J.P. Riehl & C. Roy, *Conceptual models for nursing practice* (pp. 206–218). New York: Appleton-Century-Crofts.

Small, B. (1980). Nursing visually impaired children with Johnson's model as a conceptual framework. In J.P. Riehl & C. Roy, *Conceptual models for nursing practice* (2nd ed., pp. 264–273). New York: Appleton-Century-Crofts.

Stamler, C., & Palmer, J.O. (1971). Dependency and repetitive visits to the nurse's office in elementary school children. *Nursing Research, 20,* 254–255.

Walike, B., Jordan, H.A., & Stellar, E. (1969). Studies of eating behavior. *Nursing Research, 18,* 108–113.

Wilkie, D. (1985). *Pain intensity and observed behaviors of adult cancer patients experiencing pain.* Unpublished master's thesis, University of California, San Francisco.

Wilkie, D. (1990). Cancer pain management: State-of-the-art care. *Nursing Clinics of North America, 25,* 331–343.

Wilkie, D., Lovejoy, N., Dodd, M., & Tesler, M. (1988). Cancer pain control behaviors: Description and correlation with pain intensity. *Oncology Nursing Forum, 15,* 723–731.

BIBLIOGRAPHY

Primary Sources

Johnson, D.E. (1959). A philosophy of nursing. *Nursing Outlook, 7,* 198–200.

Johnson, D.E. (1961). The significance of nursing care. *American Journal of Nursing, 61*(11), 63–66.

Johnson, D.E. (1980). The behavioral system model for nursing. In J.P. Riehl & C. Roy, *Conceptual models for nursing practice* (2nd ed., pp. 207–216). New York: Appleton-Century-Crofts.

Johnson, D.E. (1990). The behavioral system model for nursing. In M.E. Parker (Ed.), *Nursing theories in practice* (pp. 23–32). New York: National League for Nursing.

Johnson, D.E. (1992). The origins of the behavioral system model. In F.N. Nightingale, *Notes on nursing: What it is, and what it is not* (Commemorative edition, pp. 23–27). Philadelphia: JB Lippincott.

Commentary

Aggleton, P., & Chalmers, H. (1984). Defining the terms. *Nursing Times, 80*(36), 24–28.

Auger, J.R. (1976). *Behavioral systems and nursing.* Englewood Cliffs, NJ: Prentice-Hall.

Barnum, B.J.S (1994). *Nursing theory: Analysis, application, evaluation* (4th ed.). Philadelphia: JB Lippincott.

Conner, S.S., Harbour, L.S., Magers, J.A., & Watt, J.K. (1994). Dorothy E. Johnson: Behavioral system model. In A. Marriner-Tomey, *Nursing theorists and their work* (3rd ed., pp. 231–245). St. Louis: Mosby-Year Book.

Conner, S.S., Magers, J.A., & Watt, J.K. (1989). Dorothy E. Johnson: Behavioral system model. In A. Marriner-Tomey, *Nursing theorists and their work* (2nd ed., pp. 309–324). St. Louis: CV Mosby.

Connor, S.S., & Watt, J.K. (1986). Dorothy E. Johnson: Behavioral system model. In A. Marriner, *Nursing theorists and their work* (pp. 283–296). St. Louis: CV Mosby.

Crawford, G. (1982). The concept of pattern in nursing: Conceptual development and measurement. *Advances in Nursing Science, 5* (1), 1–6.

Derdiarian, A.K. (1981). Nursing conceptual frameworks: Implications for education, practice, and research. In D.L. Vredevoe, A.K. Derdiarian, L.P. Sarna, M. Eriel, & J.C. Shipacoff, Concepts of oncology nursing (pp. 369–385). Englewood Cliffs, NJ: Prentice-Hall.

Grubbs, J. (1974). An interpretation of the Johnson Behavioral system model. In J.P. Riehl & C. Roy, Conceptual models for nursing practice (pp. 160–197). New York: Appleton-Century-Crofts. Reprinted in J.P. Riehl & C. Roy (1980). Conceptual models for nursing practice (2nd ed., pp. 217–254). New York: Appleton-Century-Crofts.

Holaday, B.J. (1981). The Johnson Behavioral system model for nursing and the pursuit of quality health care. In G.E. Lasker (Ed.), Applied systems and cybernetics. Vol. 4. Systems research in health care, biocybernetics and ecology (pp. 1723–1728). New York: Pergamon.

Johnson, D.E. (1967). Powerlessness: A significant determinant in patient behavior? Journal of Nursing Education, 6(2), 39–44.

Johnson, D.E. (1974). Development of theory: A requisite for nursing as a primary health profession. Nursing Research, 23, 372–377.

Johnson, D.E. (1959). The nature of a science of nursing. Nursing Outlook, 7, 291–294.

Johnson, D.E. (1978). State of the art of theory development in nursing. In Theory development: What, why, how? (pp. 1–10). New York: National League for Nursing.

Johnson, D.E. (1987). Evaluating conceptual models for use in critical care nursing practice. [Guest editorial]. Dimensions of Critical Care Nursing, 6, 195–197.

Johnson, D.E. (1989). Some thoughts on nursing (Editorial). Clinical Nurse Specialist, 3, 1–4.

Lobo, M.L. (1985). Dorothy E. Johnson. In Nursing Theories Conference Group, Nursing theories: The base for professional practice (2nd ed., pp. 195–213). Englewood Cliffs, NJ: Prentice-Hall.

Lobo, M.L. (1990). Dorothy E. Johnson. In J.B. George (Ed.), Nursing theories: The base for professional nursing practice (3rd ed., pp. 113–128). Norwalk, CT: Appleton & Lange.

Loveland-Cherry C., & Wilkerson, S.A. (1983). Dorothy Johnson's behavioral system model. In J.J. Fitzpatrick & A.L. Whall, Conceptual models of nursing: Analysis and application (pp. 117–135). Bowie, MD: Brady.

Loveland-Cherry C., & Wilkerson, S.A. (1989). Dorothy Johnson's behavioral system model. In J.J. Fitzpatrick & A.L. Whall, Conceptual models of nursing: Analysis and application (2nd ed., pp. 147–163). Norwalk, CT: Appleton & Lange.

Meleis, A.I. (1991). Theoretical nursing: Development and progress (2nd ed.). Philadelphia: JB Lippincott.

Reynolds, W., & Cormack, D.F.S. (1991). An evaluation of the Johnson behavioural system model of nursing. Journal of Advanced Nursing, 16, 1122–1130.

Riegel, B. (1989). Social support and psychological adjustment to chronic coronary heart disease: Operationalization of Johnson's behavioral system model. Advances in Nursing Science, 11(2), 74–84.

Silva, M.C. (1987). Conceptual models of nursing. In J.J. Fitzpatrick & R.L. Taunton (Eds.), Annual review of nursing research (Vol. 5, pp. 229–246). New York: Springer.

Wu, R. (1973). Behavior and illness. Englewood Cliffs, NJ: Prentice-Hall.

Research

Auger, J.A., & Dee, V. (1983). A patient classification system based on the behavioral system model of nursing: Part 1. Journal of Nursing Administration, 13(4), 38–43.

Bossert, E., Holaday, B., Harkins, A., & Turner-Henson, A. (1990). Strategies of normalization used by parents of chronically ill school age children. Journal of Child and Adolescent Psychiatric and Mental Health Nursing, 3, 57–61.

Bruce, G.L., Hinds, P., Hudak, J., Mucha, A., Taylor, M.C., & Thompson, C. R. (1980). Implementation of ANA's quality assurance program for clients with end-stage renal disease. Advances in Nursing Science 2(2), 79–95.

Dee V., & Auger, J.A. (1983). A patient classification system based on the behavioral system model of nursing: Part 2. Journal of Nursing Administration, 13(5), 18–23.

Derdiarian, A.K. (1983). An instrument for theory and research using the behavioral systems model for nursing: The cancer patient (Part I). Nursing Research, 32, 196–201.

Derdiarian, A.K. (1984). An investigation of the variables and boundaries of cancer nursing: A pioneering approach using Johnson's behavioral systems model for nursing. In Proceedings of the 3rd International Conference on Cancer Nursing (pp. 96–102). Melbourne, Australia: The Cancer Institute/Peter MacCallum Hospital and the Royal Melbourne Hospital.

Derdiarian, A.K. (1988). Sensitivity of the Derdiarian behavioral system model instrument to age, site, and stage of cancer: A preliminary validation study. *Scholarly Inquiry for Nursing Practice, 2*, 103–121.

Holaday, B. (1989). Response to "Sensitivity of the Derdiarian behavioral system model instrument to age, site, and stage of cancer: A preliminary validation study." *Scholarly Inquiry for Nursing Practice, 2*, 123–125.

Derdiarian, A.K. (1990). Effects of using systematic assessment instruments on patient and nurse satisfaction with nursing care. *Oncology Nursing Forum, 17*, 95–101.

Derdiarian, A.K. (1990). The relationships among the subsystems of Johnson's behavioral system model. *Image: Journal of Nursing Scholarship, 22*, 219–225.

Derdiarian, A.K. (1991). Effects of using a nursing model-based assessment instrument on quality of nursing care. *Nursing Administration Quarterly, 15*(3), 1–16.

Derdiarian, A.K., & Forsythe, A.B. (1983). An instrument for theory and research using the behavioral systems model for nursing: The cancer patient (Part II). *Nursing Research, 32*, 260–266.

Derdiarian, A.K., & Schobel, D. (1990). Comprehensive assessment of AIDS patients using the behavioural systems model for nursing practice instrument. *Journal of Advanced Nursing, 15*, 436–446.

Dimino, E. (1988). Needed: Nursing research questions which test and expand our conceptual models of nursing. *Virginia Nurse, 56*(3), 43–46.

Hadley, B.J. (1990). Response to "Hardiness, self-perceived health, and activity among independently functioning older adults." *Scholarly Inquiry for Nursing Practice, 4*, 185–188.

Holaday, B.J. (1974). Achievement behavior in chronically ill children. *Nursing Research, 23*, 25–30.

Holaday, B.J. (1981). Maternal response to their chronically ill infants' attachment behavior of crying. *Nursing Research, 30*, 343–348.

Holaday, B. (1982). Maternal conceptual set development: Identifying patterns of maternal response to chronically ill infant crying. *Maternal-Child Nursing Journal, 11*, 47–69.

Holaday, B. (1987). Patterns of interaction between mothers and their chronically ill infants. *Maternal-Child Nursing Journal, 16*, 29–45.

Holaday, B., & Turner-Henson, A. (1987).

Chronically ill school-age children's use of time. *Pediatric Nursing, 13*, 410–414.

Lachicotte, J.L., & Alexander, J.W. (1990). Management attitudes and nurse impairment. *Nursing Management, 21*, 102–104, 106, 108, 110.

Lovejoy, N. (1983). The leukemic child's perception of family behaviors. *Oncology Nursing Forum, 10*(4), 20–25.

Lovejoy, N. (1985). Needs of vigil and nonvigil visitors in cancer research units. In *Fourth Cancer Nursing Research Conference Proceedings* (pp. 142–164). Honolulu, HI, American Cancer Society.

Lovejoy, N.C., & Moran, T.A. (1988). Selected AIDS beliefs, behaviors and informational needs of homosexual/bisexual men with AIDS or ARC. *International Journal of Nursing Studies, 25*, 207–216.

Majesky, S.J., Brester, M.H., & Nishio, K.T. (1978). Development of a research tool: Patient indicators of nursing care. *Nursing Research, 27*, 365–371.

Randell, B.P. (1991). NANDA versus the Johnson behavioral systems model: Is there a diagnostic difference? In R.M. Carroll-Johnson (Ed.), *Classification of nursing diagnoses: Diagnosis Association* (pp. 154–160). Philadelphia: JB Lippincott.

Small, B. (1980). Nursing visually impaired children with Johnson's model as a conceptual framework. In J.P. Riehl & C. Roy, *Conceptual models for nursing practice* (2nd ed., pp. 264–273). New York: Appleton-Century-Crofts.

Stamler, C., & Palmer, J.O. (1971). Dependency and repetitive visits to the nurse's office in elementary school children. *Nursing Research, 20*, 254–255.

Wilkie, D., Lovejoy, N., Dodd, M., & Tesler, M. (1988). Cancer pain control behaviors: Description and correlation with pain intensity. *Oncology Nursing Forum, 15*, 723–731.

Master's Thesis

Devlin, S.L. (1992). The relationship between nurse managers' and staff nurses' return to school. *Master's Abstracts International, 30*, 707.

Doctoral Dissertations

Carino, C. (1976). Behavioral responses of disoriented patients compared to oriented patients in intensive care units. *Dissertation Abstracts International, 37*, 162B.

Dee, V. (1986). Validation of a patient classification instrument for psychiatric patients based on the Johnson model for nursing. *Dissertation Abstracts International, 47,* 4822B.

Kosten, P.A. (1977). Professional nurses' assessment of practice in psychiatric settings. *Dissertation Abstracts International, 38,* 140B.

Lovejoy, N.C. (1982). An empirical verification of the Johnson behavioral system model for nursing. *Dissertation Abstracts International, 42,* 2781B.

Nishimoto, P.W. (1987). Perceived impact of prostate surgery on sexual stability. *Dissertation Abstracts International, 47,* 4114B.

Riegel, B.J. (1991). Social support and cardiac invalidism following acute myocardial infarction. *Dissertation Abstracts International, 52,* 1959B.

Turner-Henson, A. (1993). Chronically ill children's mothers' perceptions of environmental variables. *Dissertation Abstracts International, 53,* 3405B.

Education

Harris, R.B. (1986). Introduction of a conceptual nursing model into a fundamental baccalaureate course. *Journal of Nursing Education, 25,* 66–69.

Administration

Dee, V. (1990). Implementation of the Johnson model: One hospital's experience. In M.E. Parker (Ed.), *Nursing theories in practice* (pp. 33–44). New York: National League for Nursing.

Glennin, C.G. (1974). Formulation of standards of nursing practice using a nursing model. In J.P. Riehl & C. Roy, *Conceptual models for nursing practice* (pp. 234–246). New York: Appleton-Century-Crofts. Reprinted in J.P. Riehl & C. Roy (1980), *Conceptual models for nursing practice* (2nd ed., pp. 290–301). New York: Appleton-Century-Crofts.

Moreau, D., Poster, E.C., & Niemela, K. (1993). Implementing and evaluating an attending nurse model. *Nursing Management, 24*(6), 56–58, 60, 64.

Niemela, K., Poster, E.C., & Moreau, D. (1992). The attending nurse: A new role for the advanced clinician . . . adolescent inpatient unit. *Journal of Child and Adolescent Psychiatric and Mental Health Nursing, 5*(3), 5–12.

Rogers, C.G. (1973). Conceptual models as guides to clinical nursing specialization. *Journal of Nursing Education, 12*(4), 2–6.

Practice

Broncatello, K.F. (1980). Auger in action: Application of the model. *Advances in Nursing Science, 2*(2), 13–24.

Damus, K. (1974). An application of the Johnson behavioral system model for nursing practice. In J.P. Riehl & C. Roy, *Conceptual models for nursing practice* (pp. 218–233). New York: Appleton-Century-Crofts. Reprinted in J.P. Riehl & C. Roy (1980). *Conceptual models for nursing practice* (2nd ed., pp. 274–289). New York: Appleton-Century-Crofts.

Fruehwirth, S.E.S. (1989). An application of Johnson's behavioral model: A case study. *Journal of Community Health Nursing, 6*(2), 61–71.

Herbert, J. (1989). A model for Anna. *Nursing, 3*(42), 30–34.

Holaday, B.J. (1974). Implementing the Johnson model for nursing practice. In J.P. Riehl & C. Roy, *Conceptual models for nursing practice* (pp. 197–206). New York: Appleton-Century-Crofts. Reprinted in J.P. Riehl & C. Roy (1980). *Conceptual models for nursing practice* (2nd ed., pp. 255–263). New York: Appleton-Century-Crofts.

Iveson-Iveson, J. (1982). Standards of behaviour. *Nursing Mirror, 155*(20), 38.

Lewis, C., & Randell, B.P. (1991). Alteration in self-care: An instance of ineffective coping in the geriatric patient. In R.M. Carroll-Johnson (Ed.), *Classification of nursing diagnoses: Proceedings of the ninth conference: North American Nursing Diagnosis Association* (pp. 264–265). Philadelphia: JB Lippincott.

McCauley, K., Choromanski, J.D., Wallinger, C., & Liu, K. (1984). Current management of ventricular tachycardia: Symposium from the Hospital of the University of Pennsylvania. Learning to live with controlled ventricular tachycardia: Utilizing the Johnson model. *Heart and Lung, 13,* 633–638.

Rawls, A.C. (1980). Evaluation of the Johnson Behavioral Model in clinical practice. *Image, 12,* 13–16.

Skolny, M.A., & Riehl, J.P. (1974). Solving patient and family problems by using a theoretical framework. In J.P. Riehl & C. Roy, *Conceptual models for nursing practice* (pp. 206–218). New York: Appleton-Century-Crofts.

Spratlen, L.P. (1976). Introducing ethnic-cultural factors in models of nursing: Some mental health care applications. *Journal of Nursing Education, 15*(2), 23–29.

Wilkie, D. (1990). Cancer pain management: State-of-the-art care. *Nursing Clinics of North America, 25,* 331–343.

4

King's General Systems Framework

This chapter presents an analysis and evaluation of Imogene M. King's General Systems Framework and a discussion of her Theory of Goal Attainment, which she derived from the framework. King has always been very clear about the separation of her work into a conceptual framework and a theory, which fit the definition of a conceptual model and a middle-range theory, respectively, used in this book. In accordance with King's preference, the term conceptual framework, rather than conceptual model, is used throughout this chapter.

Until recently, King did not provide an explicit title for her conceptual framework. In previous editions of this book, it was referred to as the Open Systems Model (Fawcett, 1984) and the Interacting Systems Framework (Fawcett, 1989). Within the past few years, King (1989a, 1992b) has begun to title her work the General Systems Framework. Accordingly, this title is used in this edition.

The concepts of the General Systems Framework and the Theory of Goal Attainment and their dimensions are listed below. Each concept and its dimensions are defined and described later in this chapter.

KEY TERMS

PERSONAL SYSTEM	Transaction
Perception	Role
Self	Stress
Growth and Development	Coping
Body Image	SOCIAL SYSTEM
Time	Organization
Space	Authority
Learning	Power
INTERPERSONAL SYSTEM	Status
Interaction	Decision Making
Communication	Control

HEALTH
Dynamic Life Experiences
Ability to Function in Social Roles
GOAL OF NURSING
Help Individuals Maintain Their
  Health So They Can Function in
  Their Roles
INTERACTION-TRANSACTION
  PROCESS MODEL
Perception
Judgment
Action
Reaction
Disturbance
Mutual Goal Setting
Exploration of Means to Achieve Goal

Agreement on Means to Achieve
  Goal
Transaction
Attainment of Goal
THEORY OF GOAL ATTAINMENT
Perception
Communication
Interaction
Transaction
Self
Role
Growth and Development
Coping with Stress
Time
Personal Space

ANALYSIS OF KING'S GENERAL SYSTEMS FRAMEWORK

This section presents an analysis of King's General Systems Framework and her Theory of Goal Attainment. The analysis relies heavily on King's (1981) book, *A Theory for Nursing: Systems, Concepts, Process*; her book chapter (1990b), "King's conceptual framework and theory of goal attainment"; and her journal article (1992a), "King's theory of goal attainment" and draws from several other recent publications.

Origins of the Model

Historical Evolution and Motivation

King presented the foundation for the General Systems Framework in the 1964 publication, "Nursing theory—Problems and prospect." She then identified several concepts of the framework in her 1968 article, "A conceptual frame of reference for nursing." In 1971, the entire conceptual framework was presented in her book, *Toward a Theory for Nursing*. King then described refinements of the framework in her 1978 speech at the Second Annual Nurse Educator Conference. Further refinements in the General Systems Framework were presented in her 1981 book, *A Theory for Nursing: Systems, Concepts, Process*, and the Theory of Goal Attainment was introduced. Overviews of the framework and theory, with some refinements, were subsequently published in a book (King, 1986a), book chapters (King, 1986b, 1987b, 1989a, 1990b, in press a, in press b), and a journal article (King, 1992a). In 1987, King (personal communication, July 18, 1987) stated that her conceptual framework "will not change but will continue to generate theories."

King began to develop the General Systems Framework at a time when nursing was striving for status as a science and hence as a legitimate profession. She, along with other writers of the 1960s (e.g., Moore, 1968, 1969), maintained that the delineation of a theoretical body of knowledge was necessary for the advancement of nursing. Indeed, King (1964) voiced her concern that an existing "antitheoretical bias" in nursing had resulted in "nursing theory . . . based on practical techniques — the 'how' rather than the 'why'" (p. 395). She therefore deliberately set out to develop a conceptual frame of reference for nursing as a precursor to a theory that would explicate the "why" of nursing actions. King (1988b) stated that the specific motivation to develop her conceptual framework was the need to select essential content for a new master's degree program in nursing.

King (1971) explained that the particular concepts of her framework were formulated in response to several questions emanating from her "personal concern about the changes influencing nursing, a conscious awareness of the knowledge explosion, and a hunch that some of the essential components of nursing have persisted" (p. 19). The questions were:

1. What are some of the social and educational changes in the United States that have influenced changes in nursing?

2. What basic elements are continuous throughout these changes in nursing?

3. What is the scope of the practice of nursing, and in what kind of settings do nurses perform their functions?

4. Are the current goals of nursing similar to those of the past half century?

5. What are the dimensions of practice that have given the field of nursing unifying focus over time?

King (1971) then noted, "These questions established a framework for thinking about nursing today, for reading about nursing in society, for discussing ideas with nurses and other individuals" (p. 19). These activities led King to the literature of systems analysis and general system theory, and hence to another set of questions. The questions were:

1. What kind of decisions are nurses required to make in the course of their roles and responsibilities?

2. What kind of information is essential for them to make decisions?

3. What are the alternatives in nursing situations?

4. What alternative courses of action do nurses have in making critical decisions about another individual's care, recovery, and health?

5. What skills do nurses now perform and what knowledge is essential for nurses to make decisions about alternatives? (pp. 19–20)

King (1985a) later commented that her perspective of nursing evolved in response to the questions,

1. What is the essence of nursing?
2. What is the human act?

Still later, King (1992a) stated that the following questions served as "guides for a review and analysis of the [nursing] literature" (p. 19):

(a) Who are nurses and how are they educated?
(b) How and where is nursing practiced?
(c) Who needs nursing in society?
(d) What is the overall goal of nursing?
(e) What is the nursing act?
(f) What is the nursing process? (p. 19)

Elaborating on the origin of her conceptual framework, King (1971) explained, "Concepts that consistently appeared in nursing literature, in research findings, in speeches by nurses, and were observable in the world of nursing practice were identified and synthesized into a conceptual framework" (pp. 20–21). This synthesis resulted in selection of four universal ideas—social systems, health, perception, and interpersonal relations. King (1971) maintained that these ideas formed a conceptual framework that "suggests that the essential characteristics of nursing are those properties that have persisted in spite of environmental changes" (p. ix). The four universal ideas were then used as a general frame of reference for identification of the other concepts of the framework.

Furthermore, King (1992a) stated that the literature review revealed three major ideas about nursing. "One idea was that nursing is complex because of the human variables found in nursing situations. . . . A second idea . . . was that nurses play different roles in health care organizations of varying sizes and organizational structure. Nurses are expected to perform many functions in these organizations. A third idea was that changes in society, changes in the role of women, and advancement in knowledge from research and technology have influenced changes in nursing" (pp. 19–20).

In a recent recounting of the development of the General Systems Framework, King (1990b) acknowledged the influence of general system theory on her thinking. She stated, "After studying the research on General System Theory, I was able to synthesize my analysis of the nursing literature and my knowledge from other disciplines into a conceptual framework" (p. 74).

Philosophical Claims

King presented the philosophical claims undergirding the General Systems Framework and the Theory of Goal Attainment in the form of a philosophical orientation to science and a philosophical orientation to nursing.

Recently, King (1989a, 1990b) revealed that her philosophical orientation to science is general system theory. She requested that her work be read "from the perspective of General System Theory and a science of wholeness, which is my philosophical position" (1990b, p. 74).

King (1990b) pointed out that her philosophical orientation to science is congruent with her philosophical orientation to nursing, which is expressed in propositions, beliefs, and assumptions. Two major and several minor propositions express what King (1964) regarded "not as a theory of nursing but rather [as] another approach in thinking about fundamental concepts in nursing" (p. 401).

Major proposition: The nursing process is conducted within a social system. The dimensions include:

1. The nursing process
2. The individuals involved in the nursing process
3. The individuals involved in the environment within which the nursing process is activated
4. The social organization within which the process takes place
5. The community within which the social organization functions

Minor propositions:

> The nursing process will differ, dependent upon the individual nurse and each recipient of nursing service.
> The nursing process will differ relative to all individuals in the environment.
> The nursing process will differ relative to the social organization in which the nursing process takes place.
> The relationships among the dimensions have an effect upon the nursing process.

Major proposition: Nursing includes specific components.

1. Nursing judgment
2. Nurse action
3. Communication
4. Evaluation
5. Coordination

Minor propositions:

> The nursing judgment will vary relative to each nursing action.
> The effectiveness of nursing action will vary with the extent to which it is communicated to those responsible for its implementation.
> Nursing action is more effectively assured if the goals are communicated and standards of nursing performance have been established.
> Nursing action is based on facts, which may change; thus, nursing judgments and action are evaluated and revised as the situation changes.
> Nursing action is one component of health care; thus health care is effected by the coordination of nursing with health services. (pp. 401–402)

A fundamental belief undergirding the General Systems Framework and Theory of Goal Attainment is that the focus of nursing is the human being and human acts (King, 1985a). Other beliefs are:

> Nurses, in the performance of their roles and responsibilities, assist individuals and groups in society to attain, maintain, and restore health.
> In the process of functioning in social institutions, nurses assist individuals to meet their basic needs at some point in time in the life cycle when they cannot do this for themselves.
> An understanding of basic human needs in the physical, social, emotional, and intellectual realm of the life process from conception to old age, within the context of social systems of the culture in which nurses live and work, is essential and basic content for learning the practice of nursing. (King, 1971, p. 22)

King (1981) explained that the General Systems Framework and the Theory of Goal Attainment are based on the following overall assumption: "The focus of nursing is human beings interacting with their environment leading to a state of health for individuals, which is an ability to function in social roles" (p. 143).

King (1981) identified several specific assumptions about human beings:

> Individuals are social beings.
> Individuals are sentient beings.
> Individuals are rational beings.
> Individuals are reacting beings.
> Individuals are perceiving beings.
> Individuals are controlling beings.
> Individuals are purposeful beings.
> Individuals are action-oriented beings.
> Individuals are time-oriented beings. (p. 143)

Recently, King (1990b) added the following assumption about human beings:

> Individuals are spiritual beings. (p. 77)

In her latest overview of the Theory of Goal Attainment, King (in press b) explicated her philosophical assumptions as follows:

> My assumptions about human beings are that they are open systems in transaction with the environment. Transaction connotes that there is no separateness between human beings and environment. Characteristics that are common to human beings are that they are unique, holistic, individuals of intrinsic worth who are capable of rational thinking and decision making. Individuals are sentient and social, as observed by their interactions with persons and objects in the environment. They are perceived and reacting beings who are controlling, purposeful, action oriented, and time oriented in their behavior. Individuals have the capacity to think, to know, to make choices and select alternative courses of actions. Human beings have the ability through their language and other symbols to record their history and to preserve their culture. Individuals differ in their needs, wants, and goals. Since each

person is unique, the nature of values emanates from the nature of human beings. Values form the basis for each person's goals. Values are demonstrated in the standards of human conduct that have been handed down from one generation to another called social expectations. Values are linked to cultures and, therefore, vary from person to person, family to family, and society to society. When there is disagreement between two or more individuals, value conflict may occur. When one is pressured to make choices, intrapersonal conflicts in values may occur.

King (1981, 1992a) also identified several specific assumptions about nurse-client interactions. Those assumptions are:

Perceptions of nurse and of client influence the interaction process.
Goals, needs, and values of nurse and client influence the interaction process.
Individuals and families have a right to knowledge about their health.
Individuals and families have a right to participate in decisions that influence their life, their health, and community services.
Health professionals have a responsibility to share information that can help individuals make informed decisions about their health care.
Individuals and families have a right to accept or to reject health care.
The goals of health professionals and goals of recipients of health care may be incongruent.
Health professionals have a responsibility to gather relevant information about the perceptions of the client so that their goals and the goals of the client are congruent. (1981, pp. 143–144; 1992a, p. 21)

Still another assumption, which extends the scope of the General Systems Framework to family phenomena, is: "The assumption that individuals (nurse and client) are capable of interacting to set mutual goals and agree on means to achieve the goals has been extended to include mutual goal setting with family members in relation to clients and families" (King, 1986b, p. 200).

Strategies for Knowledge Development

King used both inductive and deductive thought processes to formulate the General Systems Framework and Theory of Goal Attainment. Explaining her approach, King (1975) commented:

My personal approach to synthesizing knowledge for nursing was to use data and information available from research in nursing and related fields and from my 25 years in active practice, teaching, and research. . . . A search of the literature in nursing and other behavioral science fields, discussion with colleagues, attendance at numerous conferences, inductive and deductive reasoning, and some critical thinking about the information gathered, led me to formulate my own framework. (pp. 36–37)

Elaborating on the process she used to review the literature, King (1992a) stated, "The process used . . . to identify relevant concepts began with a review of the literature. . . . From the literature review, a list of words were [sic] recorded using content analysis. A reconceptualization of this list provided the comprehensive concepts for the King conceptual system. . . . Subsequent to the review of literature and discussions with colleagues and with nurses giving direct care, and with critical thinking about the information gathered, the author was led to formulate the conceptual system" (pp. 19–20).

Influences from Other Scholars

King (1971, 1975, 1981, 1989a, 1992a) has repeatedly mentioned the influence of the literature of nursing and adjunctive disciplines on the development of the General Systems Framework and Theory of Goal Attainment. She recently explained,

> I know of no other discipline that deals with knowledge that is so vitally essential in the empirical world of application to practice as the knowledge we expect nurses to have for decision making for immediate action in many situations. If one analyzes the knowledge required for nurses to function in the complex world of practice, that knowledge is composed of concepts in every discipline in higher education. This is what motivated me to identify those concepts in other disciplines that give nurses specific knowledge that is applied in real world situations. (1989a, p. 150)

Furthermore, although King (1981) cited the influence of general system theory on the formulation of her conceptual framework in the past, she has underscored that influence in recent publications (King, 1989a, 1990b). Among the numerous authors from many disciplines whose works King cited are Benne and Bennis (1959), Bertalanffy (1956, 1968), Boulding (1956), Bross (1953), Bruner and Krech (1968), Cherry (1966), DiVincenti (1977), Erikson (1950), Etzioni (1975), Fisher and Cleveland (1968), Fraser (1972), Freud (1966), Gesell (1952), Gibson (1966), Griffiths (1959), Haas (1964), Hall (1959), Hall and Fagen (1956), Havighurst (1953), Ittleson and Cantril (1954), Janis (1958), Jersild (1952), Katz and Kahn (1966), Klein (1970), Linton (1963), Lyman and Scott (1967), Monat and Lazarus (1977), Orme (1969), Parsons (1951), Piaget (1969), Ruesch and Kees (1972), Schilder (1951), Selye (1956), Shontz (1969), H.A. Simon (1957), Y.R. Simon (1962), Sommer (1969), Wapner and Werner (1965), Watzlawick, Beavin, and Jackson (1967), and Zald (1970). Furthermore, King (1992a) commented that the term transaction came from a study of Dewey's theory of knowledge (Dewey & Bentley, 1949)" (p. 21).

King (1971, 1981) has also noted the influence of students, academic colleagues, nurse researchers, and clinicians on her thinking. During an interview conducted a few years ago, King (1988b) highlighted the contributions to her thinking made by Kaufmann (1958), Orlando (1961), and Peplau (1952). King (1988b) explained that Kaufmann's (1958) doctoral dissertation led her to explore the concepts of perception, time, and stress. She also noted that the research conducted at Yale University School of

Nursing to test Orlando's (1961) theory of the deliberative nursing process influenced her thinking. King and Peplau (cited in Takahashi, 1992) pointed out the connections between their works with regard to patient outcomes. Peplau commented, "When [King] talks about setting goals and I talk about beneficial outcomes for the patient in relation to the nurse's interventions in presenting phenomena, I think you have a very close connection" (p. 86). King responded by saying, "And I have to tell you all publicly that Dr. Peplau's [1952] work influenced my work" (p. 86).

Furthermore, King (1988b) noted that a review of her 1971 book by Rosemary Ellis (1971) encouraged her to continue her work by deriving a theory from the General Systems Framework. The result was the Theory of Goal Attainment.

World View

The General Systems Framework reflects a *reciprocal interaction* world view. The holistic element of that world view is indicated by the focus of the framework on three systems—the personal, interpersonal, and social—as wholes. The concepts associated with each system in no way represent parts or subsystems. Rather, they may be construed as global characteristics of the system. In fact, no parts or subsystems are ever mentioned. Holism is further indicated by King's (1989a) statement that her focus is holistic, "that is, the total human being's interactions with another total human being in a specific situation" (p. 155).

Moreover, the reciprocal interaction world view is reflected by King's view of human beings as active participants in interaction with one another and her philosophical allegiance to "a science of wholeness" (King, 1990b, p. 74).

In keeping with the reciprocal interaction world view, the General Systems Framework emphasizes change, as attested to by King's (1981) statement that health is a dynamic life experience implying continuous adjustment to environmental stressors. Change is viewed as continuous, natural, and desirable, as is documented by King's (1981) comment that normal changes in growth and development take place continuously.

Unique Focus of the Model

King (1989a) identified the unique focus of the General Systems Framework as "human beings interacting with their environment" (p. 150), and more specifically as "individuals whose interactions in groups within social systems influence behavior within the systems" (p. 152). Particular attention is given to the continuing ability of individuals to meet their basic needs so that they may function in their socially defined roles. Factors that contribute to problems in the individual's ability to function in social roles may be inferred to be stressors in the internal and external environment. This interpretation is supported by the following statement:

> Health is defined as dynamic life experiences of a human being, which implies continuous adjustment to stressors in the internal and external environment through optimum use of one's resources to achieve maximum potential for daily living. (King, 1981, p. 5)

King has maintained for many years that the General Systems Framework is a derivative of systems thinking. Recently, she explained, "When I was studying systems research in the late 1960s, this movement in general [system] theory provided information for me to think about the complexities and variability in the field of nursing" (King, 1989a, p. 150). King (personal communication, May 12, 1980) also acknowledged the contributions of social psychology to her thinking, although she stated that she "never followed the symbolic interactionist school." Close examination of the content of the framework, however, revealed that characteristics of both systems and interaction models are evident.

The General Systems Framework addresses most of the characteristics of systems models. System is addressed through the personal, interpersonal, and social systems, which King (1981) viewed as open, dynamic, and interacting.

The General Systems Framework addresses environment in terms of internal and external components. King (1981) repeatedly referred to the interaction between open systems and environment and indicated that matter, energy, and information are exchanged. The dynamic quality of that interaction is evident in the following quotation from Daubenmire and King (1973):

> The nursing process is defined as a dynamic, ongoing interpersonal process in which the nurse and the patient are viewed as a system with each affecting the behavior of the other and both being affected by factors within the situation. (p. 513)

Boundary was addressed in the General Systems Framework in the following statement: "Open systems, such as man interacting with the environment, exhibit permeable boundaries permitting an exchange of matter, energy, and information" (King, 1981, p. 69). In speaking of the characteristic of boundaries in the Theory of Goal Attainment, King (1989a) noted, "The structure of the theory indicates some semipermeable boundaries of two or more individuals interacting in a health care system for a purpose that leads to goal attainment" (p. 155). King (1981) also referred to the "artificial boundaries of nursing," which she identified as "individuals and groups interacting with the environment" (p. 1).

The systems model characteristic of tension, stress, strain, and conflict is addressed in King's (1981) discussion of stress and transaction as they relate to the interpersonal system. She commented, "When transactions are made, tension or stress is reduced in a situation" (p. 82).

The characteristic of equilibrium or steady state is not explicitly addressed in the General Systems Framework. King (1981) did, however, note that the dynamic life experience of health involves continuous adjustment to environmental stressors. That statement suggests that King would accept the idea of a steady state, rather than a fixed point equilibrium.

The characteristic of feedback is dealt with in a dynamic manner in King's (1971) discussion of nurse-patient interaction. She states: "Perception of the nurse leads to judgments and to action by the nurse. Simultaneously, the perception of the patient leads to judgments and then to actions by the patient. This is a continuous dynamic process rather than separate incidents in which the action of one person influences the perceptions of the other and vice versa" (p. 92).

The General Systems Framework also addresses each of the characteristics of interaction models. A major feature of the framework is the social act of human interaction that occurs in the relationship between nurse and patient. In fact, King (1981) indicated that a social psychological perspective is reflected in her description of human interaction.

The characteristic of perception is considered in detail as a major concept of the personal system. Moreover, perception is a central aspect of the process of human interaction described in the General Systems Framework.

Communication is a concept associated with the interpersonal system. According to King (1981), communication is used to establish and maintain relationships between human beings. Furthermore, nurses and patients communicate to establish mutual goals and decide on the means to achieve these goals.

Role is another concept related to the interpersonal system. The attention given to role is evident in King's (1981) definition of health as "an ability to function in social roles" (p. 143).

The interaction model characteristic of self-concept is addressed in the General Systems Framework through the concept of self, which is associated with the personal system. In fact, King's use of Jersild's (1952) definition of the self as "a composite of thoughts and feelings, which constitute a person's awareness of his individual existence, his conception of who and what he is" (p. 9), coincides with Heiss' (1981) definition of self-concept as "the individual's thoughts and feelings about himself" (p. 83), which is explicitly identified as a part of symbolic interactionism.

Meleis (1991) classified the General Systems Framework as interaction-focused, and Marriner-Tomey (1989) placed the framework in her interpersonal relationships category. Barnum (1994) did not place the General Systems Framework in any of the categories of her classification scheme. In a previous edition of her book, she commented that King's work cannot be "categorized according to the classification of intervention, conservation, substitution, sustenance, and enhancement [because it] seems to desire interaction for its own sake rather than for the sake of a determined change (intervention), for conservation, for substitution, for sustenance, or for enhancement" (Stevens, 1984, p. 259).

Content of the Model: Concepts

Person

King (1981) stated, "human beings are the focus for nursing" (p. 13). The primary concerns of nursing are human behavior, social interaction, and social movements (King, 1976). Thus, within the context of the meta-paradigm concept of person, King (1971) included three dynamic interacting open systems—**personal systems, interpersonal systems,** and **social systems**.

Each system is described through a major concept and a set of what King (1986a) called subconcepts. King (1989a) explained that the placement of particular concepts and subconcepts within each system required arbitrary decisions because they are "so interrelated in the interactions of human beings with their environment" (p. 151).

The major concepts and subconcepts can be considered the dimensions of the three systems. King (1989a) maintained that knowledge of those dimensions is necessary for the nurse's thorough understanding of the three systems. Indeed, although "the concepts in all three systems were interrelated when one observed any concrete nursing situation, the purpose for placing these concepts in [a particular] system was to facilitate learning about self as an individual and about interactions with other individuals" (King, 1992a, p. 20).

King (1981) characterized individuals, or **personal systems,** as social beings who are rational and sentient. She conceptualized the individual as a personal system who processes selective inputs from the environment through the senses. King (1990a) explained that "At a personal systems level, individuals generally wish to preserve life, avoid pain, procreate, gratify desires, and insure their security. In addition, individuals want to perform functions associated with activities of daily living" (p. 127). Moreover, King (1992b) noted that the personal system considers the individual "whether healthy or ill" (p. 604). The major concept associated with personal systems is perception, and the subconcepts are *self, growth and development, body image, time, space,* and *learning* (King, 1986a).

King (1989a) maintained that *perception* "is a comprehensive concept in personal systems" and that "knowledge of perception is essential for nurses to understand self and to understand other individuals" (pp. 152–153). She defined perception as "a process of organizing, interpreting, and transforming information from sense data and memory. It is a process of human transactions with the environment. It gives meaning to one's experience, represents one's image of reality, and influences one's behavior" (King, 1981, p. 24). King (1989a) noted that "perception varies from one individual to another because each human being has different backgrounds of knowledge, skills, abilities, needs, values, and goals" (p. 152). In formulating that definition of perception, King drew upon the work of Bruner and Krech (1968), Gibson (1966), and Klein (1970), among others. The incorporation of the notion of transactions in the definition is based on the work of Ittleson and Cantril (1954).

King (1981) described the personal system as "a unified, complex whole, self who perceives, thinks, desires, imagines, decides, identifies goals and selects means to achieve them" (p. 27). She accepted as her definition of the *self* that proposed by Jersild (1952):

> The self is a composite of thoughts and feelings which constitute a person's awareness of his individual existence, his conception of who and what he is. A person's self is the sum total of all he can call his. The self includes, among other things, a system of ideas, attitudes, values and commitments. The self is a person's total subjective environment. It is a distinctive center of experience and significance. The self constitutes a person's inner world as distinguished from the outer world consisting of all other people and things. The self is the individual as known to the individual. It is that to which we refer when we say "I." (pp. 9–10)

King's (1981) description of *growth and development* drew from the works of Erikson (1950), Freud (1966), Gesell (1952), Havighurst (1953), and Piaget (1969). She identified two characteristics of growth and development:

> 1. Growth and development include cellular, molecular, and behavioral changes in human beings.
> 2. Growth and development are a function of genetic endowment, meaningful and satisfying experiences, and an environment conducive to helping individuals move toward maturity. (pp. 30–31)

The concept of *body image* was defined by King (1981) as "a person's perceptions of his own body, others' reactions to his appearance, and is a result of others' reactions to self" (p. 33). That definition was derived from the writings of Fisher and Cleveland (1968), Schilder (1951), Shontz (1969), and Wapner and Werner (1965).

King (1981) defined *time* as "the duration between the occurrence of one event and the occurrence of another event" (p. 44). She noted that the term is used "to give order to events and to determine duration based on perceptions of each person's experiences" (p. 45). That definition was based on the writings of Fraser (1972) and Orme (1969), among others.

Space was defined by King (1981) as "existing in all directions and is the same everywhere. . . . as the physical area called territory and by the behavior of individuals occupying space" (pp. 37–38). She incorporated territory and the related idea of personal space into her discussion, citing the works of Hall (1959), Lyman and Scott (1967), and Sommer (1969).

King (1986a) added *learning* to the list of concepts related to the personal system in her discussion of use of the General Systems Framework as a guide for curriculum development. She did not, however, define or describe that concept.

King (1981) linked all concepts except learning related to the personal system in the following statement:

> An individual's perceptions of self, of body image, of time and space influence the way he or she responds to persons, objects, and events in his or her life. As individuals grow and develop through the life span, experiences with changes in structure and function of their bodies over time influence their perceptions of self. (p. 19)

The **interpersonal system** is composed of "two, three, or more individuals interacting in a given situation" (King, 1976, p. 54). King (1990a) explained that "At the interpersonal systems level, individuals increase consciousness and are open to interpersonal perceptions in the communications and interactions with persons and things in the environment. Individuals have the potential to make transactions that include goal setting, and choosing means to attain goals to maintain their health and function in roles" (p. 127). The interpersonal system moves the focus from the individual alone to individuals interacting in dyads, triads, small groups, and large groups (King, 1989a). The major concept of the interpersonal system is *interaction*; the subconcepts are *communication, transaction, role, stress,* and *coping* (King, 1986a, 1987a).

King (1989a) noted that "*interaction* is a comprehensive concept in interpersonal systems" and that "knowledge of interaction is essential for nurses to understand a fundamental process for gathering information about human beings" (p. 153). She defined interactions as:

> The acts of two or more persons in mutual presence. Interactions can reveal how one person thinks and feels about another person, how each perceives the other and what the other does to him, what his expectations are of the other, and how each reacts to the actions of the other. (King, 1981, p. 85)

According to King (1981), "The process of interactions between two or more individuals represents a sequence of verbal and nonverbal behaviors that are goal directed" (p. 60). Following a social psychological perspective, King (1971, 1981) explained that this process consists of each person's simultaneous perceptions and judgments about the other in the interaction, the taking of some mental actions based on the judgments, and reacting to the other's perceptions. Interaction follows those mental processes, and this is followed in turn by transaction. Moreover, "In the interactive process, two individuals mutually identify goals and the means to achieve them. When they agree to the means to implement the goals, they move toward transactions. Transactions are defined as goal attainment" (King, 1981, p. 61).

King (1981) pointed out that the perceptions, judgments, actions, and reactions of the individuals cannot be directly observed but must be inferred from the directly observable interaction. Elaborating, she stated, "First, the informational component of interactions can be observed as communication. Second, the valuational component of interactions can be observed as transaction because one obviously values a goal, identifies means to achieve it, and takes action to attain it" (p. 62).

King (1981) viewed *communication* as "the vehicle by which human relations are developed and maintained" (p. 79). She went on to say that "all behavior is communication" (p. 80). The General Systems Framework focuses on intrapersonal and interpersonal communication as well as verbal and nonverbal communication. In formulating her view of communication, King drew primarily from works by Cherry (1966), Ruesch and Kees (1972), and Watzlawick et al. (1967).

Communication is involved in *transactions*, which is defined as "a process of interaction in which human beings communicate with environment to achieve goals that are valued. Transactions are goal directed human behaviors" (King, 1981, p. 82).

In the General Systems Framework, the concept of *role* was derived from the work of Benne and Bennis (1959), Haas (1964), and Parsons (1951). Three elements of role are of interest:

(1) Role is a set of behaviors expected when occupying a position in a social system; (2) rules or procedures define rights and obligations in a position in an organization; (3) role is a relationship with one or more individuals interacting in specific situations for a purpose. (King, 1981, p. 93)

King (1981) developed her definition of *stress* from the writings of Janis (1958), Monat and Lazarus (1977), and Selye (1956). She stated:

Stress is a dynamic state whereby a human being interacts with the environment to maintain balance for growth, development, and performance, which involves an exchange of energy and information between the person and the environment for regulation and control of stressors. (p. 98)

Stress is viewed as negative and positive as well as constructive and destructive. King (1981) explained that stress is reduced when transactions are made.

Coping, King (1987) maintained, is an essential area of knowledge related to the interpersonal system. However, she did not give a definition or description of that concept. In a later paper, King (1992a) targeted the object of coping through use of the phrase "coping with stress" (p. 21).

King (1981) defined a **social system** as "an organized boundary system of social roles, behaviors, and practices developed to maintain values and the mechanisms to regulate the practices and rules" (p. 115). She also stated, "Social systems describe units of analysis in a society in which individuals form groups to carry on activities of daily living to maintain life and health and, hopefully, happiness" (King, 1976, p. 54). Social systems encompass the family, school, industry, social organizations, and health care delivery systems (King, 1989a). King (1992b) pointed out that the inclusion of social systems in the General Systems Framework "reminds us that a variety of [such] systems provided the background for each person's growth, and development, etc., and health professionals assess situations on that basis" (p. 604). The major concept of the social system is *organization*, and the subconcepts are *authority, power, status, decision making,* and *control* (King, 1986a).

King (1989a) pointed out that *organization* is "a comprehensive concept in social systems" and that "knowledge of organization is essential for nurses to understand the variety of social systems within which individuals grow and develop" (p. 153). Her definition of organization, which was based on the work of DiVincenti (1977) and Katz and Kahn (1966), is as follows: "An organization is composed of human beings with prescribed roles and positions who use resources to accomplish personal and organizational goals" (King, 1981, p. 119).

King (1981) drew from Katz and Kahn (1966) and Simon (1962), among others, for her definition of *authority*. She states:

> Authority is a transactional process characterized by active, reciprocal relations in which members' values, background, and perception play a role in defining, validating, and accepting the authority of individuals within an organization. One person influences another, and he recognizes, accepts, and complies with the authority of that person. (p. 124)

The concept of *power* was defined as "the process whereby one or more persons influence other persons in a situation. Power defines a situation in a way that people will accept what is being done while they may not agree with it" (King, 1981, p. 127). This definition was based on the work of Etzioni (1975), Griffiths (1959), Katz and Kahn (1966), and Zald (1970).

King (1981) defined *status* as "the position of an individual in a group or a group in relation to other groups in an organization" (p. 129). She drew from Linton's (1963) work to characterize status as ascribed or achieved.

The works of Bross (1953) and Simon (1957) were used to formulate the definition of *decision making* used in the General Systems Framework. The definition is as follows:

> Decision making in organizations is a dynamic and systematic process by which goal-directed choice of perceived alternatives is made and acted upon by individuals or groups to answer a question and attain a goal. (King, 1981, p. 132)

King (1986a) added *control* to the list of concepts related to the social system in her discussion of the use of the General Systems Framework as

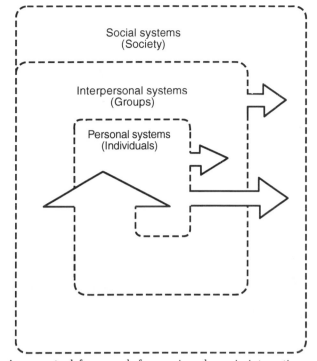

FIGURE 4–1. A conceptual framework for nursing: dynamic interacting systems. (From King, IM: A Theory for Nursing: Systems, Concepts, Process. John Wiley & Sons, New York, 1981, p 11, with permission.)

a guide for curriculum development. She did not, however, provide a definition or description of that concept.

The relationships among the personal, interpersonal, and social systems are illustrated in Figure 4–1. The figure depicts the three "open systems in a dynamic interacting framework" (King, 1981, p. 10).

Environment

King used the terms environment, health care environment, internal environment, and external environment. She linked the latter two terms in the following statement: "The internal environment of human beings transforms energy to enable them to adjust to continuous external environmental changes" (King, 1981, p. 5). She also noted that the person continuously adjusts to stressors in the internal and external environment. It appears, then, that those environments are the source of stressors.

In addition, King (1990a) noted that "environment is a function of balance between internal and external interactions" (p. 127). In particular, "the performance of activities of daily living . . . depends on one's external and internal environments working in some type of harmony and balance" (p. 125). She went on to say that "the social milieu is an environmental factor that influences health" (p. 125). She also has noted that the personal, interpersonal, and social systems "are elements in the total environment" (King, 1992a, p. 20). No other discussion of environment was provided, and no definitions of internal or external environment were given.

Health

King (1981) defined **health** as "*dynamic life experiences* of a human being, which implies continuous adjustment to stressors in the internal and external environment through optimum use of one's resources to achieve maximum potential for daily living" (p. 5). She also defined health as "an *ability to function in social roles*" (p. 143). King (1985b) maintained that the idea of health as functional ability is the predominant view of that concept in the General Systems Framework.

King (1990a) identified eight characteristics of health: "genetic, subjective, relative, dynamic, environmental, functional, cultural, and perceptual" (p. 127). She regards health as "a function of persons interacting with the environment," symbolized by the equation, $H = f (P \longleftrightarrow E)$ (p. 127).

King did not use the term wellness, and although she did mention illness, she "rejects a linear continuum of wellness-illness" (King, 1989a, p. 152). Elaborating on that point, King (1990a), speaking in the third person, recently explained that her concept of health "has been published since 1971. At that time she mentioned a continuum, and the definition indicated it was a dynamic process. The author has deleted the word continuum from her concept as it represents a linear concept" (p. 127). It seems that King would also regard a dichotomy of health and illness as a linear concept that is inconsistent with the general system orientation of her conceptual framework.

Instead, King (1989a) regards health as "a dynamic state of an individual in which change is a constant and an ongoing process" (p. 152). Disturbances in the dynamic state are regarded as illness or disability. King (1981) explicitly defined illness as "a deviation from normal, that is, an imbalance in a person's biological structure or in his psychological make-up, or a conflict in a person's social relationships" (p. 5). She went on to say that one kind of illness is disease. Other kinds of illnesses were not identified.

Nursing

King (1981) stated that nursing is

perceiving, thinking, relating, judging, and acting vis-a-vis the behavior of individuals who come to a nursing situation. A nursing situation is the immediate environment, spatial and temporal reality, in which nurse and client establish a relationship to cope with health states and adjust to changes in activities of daily living if the situation demands adjustment. (p. 2)

She went on to define nursing as "a process of action, reaction, and interaction whereby nurse and client share information about their perceptions in the nursing situation. Through purposeful communication they identify special goals, problems, or concerns. They explore means to achieve a goal and agree to [the] means to [achieve] the goal. When clients participate in goal setting with professionals, they interact with nurses to move toward goal attainment in most situations" (p. 2).

The domain of nursing "includes promotion of health, maintenance and restoration of health, care of the sick and injured, and care of the dying (King, 1981, p. 4). Furthermore, King (1976) viewed nursing as a helping profession that "provides a service to meet a social need" (p. 52). This service extends to the care of individuals and groups who are ill and hospitalized, those who have chronic diseases and require rehabilitation, and those who require guidance for the maintenance of health.

According to King (1976), nurses are key figures in health care delivery. She viewed nurses as "partners with physicians, social workers, and allied health professionals in promoting health, in preventing disease, and in managing patient care. They cooperate with physicians, families, and others to coordinate plans of health care" (p. 52).

The person seeks help from the nurse when he or she cannot perform usual daily activities (Daubenmire & King, 1973). Accordingly, the **goal of nursing** "is to help individuals maintain their health so they can function in their roles" (King, 1981, pp. 3–4). In particular,

> The goal of nursing is to help individuals and groups attain, maintain, and restore health. If this is not possible, nurses help individuals die with dignity. (King, 1981, p. 13)

Nursing is practiced through the nursing process. Daubenmire and King (1973) defined the nursing process as "a dynamic, ongoing interpersonal process in which the nurse and the patient are viewed as a system with each affecting the behavior of the other and both being affected by factors within the situation" (p. 513).

King (1976) likened the nursing process to all human processes. She commented:

> The nursing act [is] as all other human acts, that is, a sequence of behaviors of interacting persons that occur in the following three phases: recognition of presenting conditions, operations or activities related to the conditions or situations, and motivation to exert some control over the events to achieve goals. (p. 54)

The nursing process is elaborated through the Theory of Goal Attainment. King (1992b) explained that the theory "has identified an interaction process that leads to transactions and then to goal attainment"

(p. 604). Recently, King (1989a) began to refer to the nursing process described by the theory as an **"interaction-transaction process model"** (p. 153) and as a "transaction model" (p. 157). The components of the nursing process, or transaction model, were identified as *perception, judgment, action, reaction, disturbance, mutual goal setting, exploration of means to achieve the goal, agreement on means to achieve the goal, transaction,* and *attainment of the goal* (King, 1981, 1990b, 1992a).

The process, which is depicted in Figure 4–2, follows a sequence that encompasses two people—the nurse and the client—who meet in some situation. In the assessment phase of the process, the nurse and the client perceive each other, make mental judgments about the other, take some mental action, react to each one's perceptions of the other, communicate, and begin to interact (King, 1992a). King (1981, 1992a) pointed out that inferences must be made about each person's perceptions, mental judgments, and mental actions. "Accuracy of perception," King (1981) explained, "will depend upon verifying [the nurse's] inferences with the client" (p. 146). Action and reaction are "behaviors that are directly observable in concrete situations in nursing practice" (1992a, p. 22).

In the planning phase, interactions between the nurse and the client continue. Interactions can be observed directly, and data about those interactions can be recorded. The specific data of interaction are the concerns, problems, or disturbances identified by the client and the nurse, their mutual goal setting, their exploration of means to achieve the goal, and their agreement on the means required to achieve the goal. King (1992a) explained that goal setting "is based on the nurses' assessments of the clients' concerns, problems, and disturbances in health, their perceptions of problems, and their sharing of information with clients and families to move toward quality improvement in their health" (p. 22).

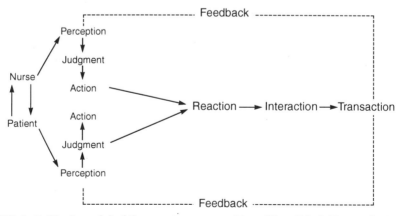

FIGURE 4–2. King's model of the nursing process. (From King, IM: A Theory for Nursing: Systems, Concepts, Process. John Wiley & Sons, New York, 1981, p 145, with permission of Delmar Publishers.)

The implementation phase of the process is when transactions are made. Transactions, which are "the valuational components of the interaction" (King, 1990a, p. 128), can be observed in the form of goal attainment measures (King, 1985b). The evaluation phase of the process requires a decision to be made with regard to whether the goal was attained and, if necessary, the determination of why the goal was not attained (King, 1992a).

King's version of the nursing process can be operationalized through two instruments, the Criterion-Referenced Measure of Goal Attainment Tool and the Goal-Oriented Nursing Record. The Criterion-Referenced Measure of Goal Attainment Tool (King, 1988a) can be used to assess and plan nursing care, as well as to evaluate outcomes. The Tool includes three scales: physical abilities, which addresses the functional, or physical ability of individuals to perform activities of daily living; behavioral response, which addresses the individual's response to the performance of activities of daily living; and goals to be attained, which addresses "the mutual goal setting by nurse and patient on the basis of data from the assessment of functional abilities and from the nurse-patient interactions in which they share information about the presenting conditions and/or problems to be solved" (p. 110). Each scale includes the following three subscales. The personal hygiene subscale addresses essential tasks in performing actions related to hygiene, including mouth care, bathing, eating, dressing, grooming, bladder, bowel, and continence. The movement subscale encompasses walking, wheelchair, in bed, exercises, range of motion, and sleep. The human interaction subscale encompasses consciousness; hearing; vision; smell; taste; touch; verbal communication, including speaking, listening, reading, and writing; nonverbal communication; and transactions in the form of decisions.

The Goal-Oriented Nursing Record (GONR) is a documentation system that can be used to record and evaluate the nurse's observations and actions and the client's responses to care. The major components of the GONR, which King (1981) adapted from Weed's (1969) Problem-Oriented Medical Record, are a data base, nursing diagnoses, goal list, nursing orders, flow sheets, progress notes, and discharge summary. King (1985a, 1987a) stated that nursing diagnoses taken from the North American Nursing Diagnosis Association (NANDA) list have replaced the problem list of Weed's format. Furthermore, although King included use of the SOAP format in her 1981 presentation of the GONR, she has since indicated that that format "is not logical" (King, 1985b). Nursing orders now identify the plan of nursing care (King, 1989b).

King (1981, 1985a, 1989b) explained that the GONR data base begins with a nursing history, which focuses on assessment of activities of daily living. A valid and reliable instrument, such as the Criterion-Referenced Measure of Goal Attainment Tool (King, 1988a), should be used to collect data. Additional data about roles, environmental stressors, the client's perceptions of what is happening, and the client's values, goals, and learning needs can be collected by means of an interview guide. King (1981) noted that all health care professionals contribute to the data base. Consequently, the medical history and physical examination, results of laboratory tests and x-ray examinations, and information from social workers and family members might also be included. The data base may also indicate the patient classification category, which could be based on the severity of the illness or the ability to perform activities of daily living.

Nursing diagnoses are made on the basis of the data collected. Goals are formulated from the nursing diagnoses and are written to reflect client outcome behaviors. Nursing orders, which are written only by professional nurses, should reflect a plan of care that is consistent with the goals. Flow sheets may be used to record such routine information as vital signs, routine daily care, cumulative data such as blood levels and special exercises, and specific information. Progress notes should be written in relation to the goals, as well as in relation to legal and ethical aspects of care. The discharge summary lists the nursing diagnoses and the extent to which each goal was attained, along with a list of future goals and a plan for continuity of care, if warranted. The components of the GONR are summarized in Table 4–1.

Content of the Model: Propositions

The propositions of the General Systems Framework encompass all four metaparadigm concepts. Person and environment are linked in the following statement:

> In open systems, such as human beings interacting with their environments, there is continuous and dynamic communication occurring. (King, 1981, p. 66)

The concepts of person, environment, and nursing are linked in the following quotation:

> The artificial boundaries of nursing are individuals and groups interacting with the environment. Nurses function in their roles in a variety of health care environments. (King, 1981, p. 1)

Person, health, and nursing are linked in this statement:

> As professionals, nurses deal with the behavior of individuals and groups in potentially stressful situations relative to health and illness and help people meet needs that are basic in performing activities of daily living. (King 1976, p. 51)

Finally, all four metaparadigm concepts are linked in the following quotation:

> The focus of nursing is human beings interacting with their environment leading to a state of health for individuals, which is an ability to function in social roles. (King, 1981, p. 143)

TABLE 4–1. **COMPONENTS OF THE GOAL-ORIENTED NURSING RECORD**

I.   Data base
   A. Nursing history
      1. Assessment of activities of daily living
      2. Additional data
         a. Client's roles
         b. Environmental stressors
         c. Client's perceptions
         d. Client's values, goals, learning needs
   B. Other information
      1. Medical history and physical examination
      2. Results of laboratory tests and x-ray examinations
      3. Information from sources such as social workers and family members
   C. Classification of client
      1. According to severity of illness
      2. According to ability to perform activities of daily living
II. Nursing diagnoses
III. Goal list
   A. Formulated from nursing diagnoses
   B. Written to reflect client outcome behaviors
IV. Nursing orders
   A. Plan is based on assessment, nursing diagnoses, and goal list
   B. Means agreed upon to resolve the problem reflected in each nursing diagnosis and goal
   C. May include client education as an integral component
V.   Flow sheets
   A. Routine information
   B. Daily routine care
   C. Cumulative data
   D. Specific information
VI. Progress notes
   A. Progress toward goal attainment
   B. Legal aspects of care
   C. Ethical aspects of care
VII. Discharge summary
   A. List of nursing diagnoses
   B. Statement of extent to which each goal was attained
   C. Future goals
   D. Plan for continuity of care

Constructed from King, I.M. (1981). *A theory for nursing: Systems, concepts, process* (pp. 164–176). New York: John Wiley & Sons; King, I.M. (1985, May). *Panel discussion with theorists.* Nurse Theorist Conference, Pittsburgh, PA. (Cassette recording); and King, I.M., (1989b). Theories and hypotheses for nursing administration. In B. Henry, M. DiVincenti, C. Arndt, & A. Marriner (Eds.), *Dimensions of nursing administration: Theory, research, education, and practice* (pp. 35–45). Boston: Blackwell Scientific Publications.

EVALUATION OF KING'S GENERAL SYSTEMS FRAMEWORK

This section presents an evaluation of the General Systems Framework. The evaluation is based on the results of the analysis of the framework as well as on publications and presentations by King and others who have used or commented on King's work.

Explication of Origins

King articulated the origins of the General Systems Framework and the Theory of Goal Attainment clearly and concisely. She outlined the development of the framework and theory over time and indicated her motivation for the work. Furthermore, she explicated the philosophical claims undergirding the framework and theory in the form of major and minor propositions about nursing, beliefs about nursing, and assumptions about human beings and nurse-client interactions.

The assumptions indicate that King values the client's participation in his or her nursing care. They also indicate that King values the client's right to accept or reject the care offered by nurses and other health care professionals.

King's discussions of interaction and the nursing process indicate that she values equally the nurse's and the client's perceptions of any given situation. In particular, her definition of nursing as a process indicates that both nurse and client participate in setting goals and determining the means to achieve the goals.

King explicitly acknowledged the influence of other scholars on her thinking and provided extensive bibliographic citations of relevant works. In her recent publications, she underscored the influence of general system theory on the development of her framework and theory.

Comprehensiveness of Content

The General Systems Framework is sufficiently comprehensive with regard to depth of content, although some inconsistencies are evident and some points require clarification. King provided a comprehensive discussion of the metaparadigm concept, person. In fact, her descriptions of the major concepts and subconcepts associated with personal systems, interpersonal systems, and social systems provide more specification of individuals, groups, and society than is usually found in a conceptual model. One inconsistency evident in King's discussion of the person is the designation of person as client in most of her writings and the designation of person as patient in others. Moreover, in some instances, she refers to the person as a client and as a patient in the same paper (e.g., King, 1990b). In addition, definitions of the subconcepts of learning in the personal system, coping in the interpersonal system, and control in the social system are needed to enhance the clarity of the General Systems Framework.

In contrast to the comprehensive consideration of the person, King's discussion of environment remains vague. She failed to define that concept and to identify the parameters of the internal and external components. Although King (personal communication to R. Martone, July 25, 1989) claimed that her concept of social systems "explains environments and internal [environment] is explained in [the] communication concept," further explication of the metaparadigm concept of environment would provide much needed clarification.

Health was clearly defined in the General Systems Framework. King recently revealed that she now rejects the idea of health as a continuum of wellness to illness because that is a linear notion. Using the same reasoning, it may be inferred that she also rejects the idea of health as a dichotomy of wellness and illness. That inference, however, requires explicit commentary by King. King defined illness and related that concept to her definition of health by indicating that disturbances in the dynamic state that is health are regarded as illness or disability.

King defined and described nursing in a comprehensive manner and clearly identified the goal of nursing as health. In recent publications and presentations, King has reinforced the fact that her version of the nursing process is part of the Theory of Goal Attainment.

A few points regarding the nursing process require clarification. First, although King has defined or described most of the terms making up the process, she never explained exactly what she means by the term reaction. Second, there is an inconsistency in her writings with regard to whether action and reaction are observable components of the process (King, 1981; 1992a). Third, it is unclear whether the process can be used not only with individuals but also with groups and social organizations, and if so, how this might be accomplished. King (1983a, 1983b, 1983c) has begun to extend the nursing process to families, although explicit use of the process of perception, judgment, action, reaction, interaction, and transaction was not evident in the examples given. In fact, King's extension of the nursing process to families contradicts her emphasis on the individual, as is evident in the following statement: "Although the primary point of interest in the [Theory of Goal Attainment] relates to interpersonal systems of an individual in the role of caregiver and an individual in the role of recipient of care, the goals to be attained relate to the individual receiving care" (King, 1989a, p. 155).

King deliberately related the concepts of the General Systems Framework to theoretical and empirical literature about human behavior. This is clearly evident in the strong scientific knowledge base used to describe each concept and subconcept of the personal, interpersonal, and social systems. Moreover, King has underscored the need for an extensive base of knowledge on which to base judgments regarding nursing diagnoses and goals. Indeed, King (1971) stated emphatically, "Judgments made by nurses will be influenced by their knowledge of the physical, psychological, and social components of man, by their system of values, and by their selected perceptions in the nursing situation" (p. 92). In particular, interaction is based on the perceptions, judgments, actions, and reactions of the nurse and the client engaged in a nursing situation. Furthermore, the data base requires collection of considerable information about the person for the identification of nursing diagnoses and goals.

King (1971) conceptualized human interaction as a dynamic process. She explained:

> Perception of the nurse leads to judgments and to action by the nurse. Simultaneously, the perception of the patient leads to judgments and then to action by the patient. This is a continuous dynamic process rather than separate incidents in which the action of one person influences the perceptions of the other and vice versa. (p. 92)

Furthermore, the GONR suggests a dynamic nursing process inasmuch as that nursing record involves continual monitoring of changes in the status of nursing diagnoses and recording of the client's current health status as well as frequent revisions in the nursing diagnoses and goal list on the basis of outcomes of nursing care.

King's concern for ethical standards for nursing practice is evident in her insistence on consideration of clients' perceptions of a situation. Her concern for ethical standards is also evident in her insistence that the client or a designée participate in goal setting and identification of the means to attain the goals.

The propositions of the General Systems Framework link all four metaparadigm concepts. In addition, the personal, interpersonal, and social systems are linked in the statement that "The focus [of the General Systems Framework] is on individuals whose interactions in groups within social systems influence behavior within the systems" (King, 1989a, p. 152).

The General Systems Framework is also sufficiently comprehensive in breadth of content. King has specified a relatively broad goal for nursing that focuses on the health of individuals, groups, and society. She has claimed that her concept of health "includes health promotion, health maintenance, and regaining health when there is some interference along the life cycle, such as an illness" (King, in press b). In addition, King (1981) maintained that

> Nurses play strategic roles in the process of human growth and development and in helping individuals cope with disturbances in their health. They have an essential role in community planning for the delivery of health services to the public. As professionals, nurses deal with behavior of individuals and groups in potentially stressful situations pertaining to health, illness, and crises [including death], and help people cope with changes in daily activities. (p. 13)

The General Systems Framework provides direction for research, education, administration, and practice. Many rules can be extracted from the focus and content of the framework.

The research rules are relatively well developed. The phenomena to be studied include transactions and health. King (1986b) identified transaction as "a critical dependent variable in nurse-client interactions that lead to goal attainment" (p. 202) and health, or the ability to function in social roles, as "an outcome variable" (p. 200) in the Theory of Goal

Attainment. King's (1968, 1971) typology of variables that could generate research hypotheses identifies more specific phenomena that could be studied within the context of the General Systems Framework.

One set of variables could serve as predictors of nurse behaviors. These include the nurse's education and experience, which could be used to predict effectiveness of nursing care. Another set of variables influences the whole complex of behaviors entering into the nursing process, such as patient perceptions and expectations as well as the structure of the clinical agency. Still another set focuses on situational behaviors related to nurse-patient interaction, including communication and interpersonal relationships, among others. A final set of variables encompasses criteria of effectiveness of nursing care, such as the patient's performance of activities of daily living and knowledge about health maintenance.

The problems to be studied are actual or potential disturbances in the ability to function in social roles. The ultimate purpose of research is to determine the effects of mutual goal setting and implementation of the nursing interventions related to goals on goal attainment. Study subjects may include individuals; dyads, triads, and other groups; and families, social organizations, and health care systems. Data may be gathered in health care systems within society, the home of the individual, a school, an industry or a business, or another social setting (King, 1989a).

Byers (1985) indicated that the Theory of Goal Attainment leads to both qualitative and quantitative research. She described experimental designs that are consistent with the theory and identified three approaches to measuring goal attainment. One approach is to view goal attainment as a dichotomy—the goal is attained or not attained. Another approach is to use King's (1988a) Criterion-Referenced Measure of Goal Attainment Tool, which yields ordinal scores. Still another approach is to adapt the technique of goal attainment scaling developed in psychology. Definitive rules regarding qualitative studies, instruments other than the Criterion-Referenced Measure of Goal Attainment Tool, procedures, and data analysis techniques remain to be developed. General Systems Framework-based research clearly will enhance understanding of factors that affect health in the form of the ability to function in social roles.

Some rules for nursing education can be extracted from the literature dealing with the General Systems Framework. King (1989a) pointed out that "the concepts in this framework provide a unique approach to curriculum development" (p. 154). Daubenmire (1989) stated that the General Systems Framework leads to a distinctive focus on the "dynamic interaction of the nurse-client dyad" (p. 168). Given that focus, emphasis is placed on nursing student behavior as well as client behavior. Speaking to the purposes of education, King (1986a) maintained that "Education provides for the intellectual, emotional, and social growth of human beings. Education demonstrates balance between freedom and individual responsibility. The ultimate goal of education is the pursuit and dissemination of truth" (p. 60). She also noted that the purpose of education is "to prepare individuals to be useful, productive, and relatively happy citizens" (p. 97). King (1986a) went on to say that the purposes of nursing education are to prepare people to become professional practitioners and to assist them "to acquire knowledge in the practice of nursing" (p. 63). The purposes of nursing education are, according to Daubenmire (1989), "to provide a curriculum, a climate for life-long learning, and resources whereby students acquire values, knowledge, and skills used in practicing theory-based nursing" (p. 167).

King (1986a) stated that the concepts related to the personal, interpersonal, and social systems serve as content for nursing courses. She explained:

> In my conceptual framework, the concepts [and subconcepts] are the specific content to be learned and this represents theoretical knowledge if one develops each concept. This theoretical knowledge is used by students when teachers plan learning experiences for them in concrete nursing situations. (p. 81)

King (1986a) pointed out that the concepts and subconcepts also identify the psychomotor skills that need to be taught.

The sequence of content, according to King (1986a) emphasizes "learning about individuals. . . . As students move from one course to another they expand their knowledge of each of [the concepts and subconcepts of the personal, interpersonal, and social systems] and add knowledge about family and health-care systems" (p. 81). King (1986a) noted that the curriculum should include related theory and practicum courses. She explained,

> A practicum course that accompanies a theory course provides selected experiences for students to use the knowledge beginning with experiences with relatively normal human beings, such as well child clinics, residents in nursing homes, children in the school system, and adults in industry and business. Then the knowledge can be used in experiences with individuals who have an interference in their ability to function in their usual roles and enter a health-care system for assistance. (p. 82)

Through her discussions of the use of the General Systems Framework in nursing education, King (1986a, 1989a) has implied that nursing education may occur in hospital-based diploma programs; in formal degree granting programs in community colleges, senior colleges, or universities; and in continuing education programs. Students would have to meet the requirements for admission to the program and have the ability to acquire "intellectual skills, interpersonal skills, and technical skills" (King, 1986a, p. 63). In addition, students must be able to be "active participants in the [educational] experiences and learn how to think, make decisions, and act consistently and reasonably as members of a profession and of a democratic society" (King, 1986a, p. 72).

Teaching-learning strategies should, according to King (1986a), be directed toward "providing a climate conducive to individual growth and freedom to inquire into the nature of the environment" (p. 72). She recommended an array of specific strategies, including lecture and discussion; group discussion; role playing; demonstrations of interviewing techniques, participant and nonparticipant observation techniques, and structured observations; and individual and group conferences between students and teacher.

The rules for nursing administration that can be extracted from the General Systems Framework indicate that the distinctive focus of nursing in health care organizations is the nurse and the client interacting for the purpose of mutual goal setting and goal attainment. Nursing personnel include both technical and professional nurses whose functions are clearly differentiated. Technical nurses are prepared in associate degree programs and "provide general nursing with supervision from professional nurses" (King, 1986a, p. 107). Professional nurses are prepared in baccalaureate degree programs and are able to supervise and manage care, observe behaviors "in the form of reactions [and] symptoms of disease and illness," record and report "facts about patients and clients and [evaluate] the total situation," implement nursing goals, direct "the nursing care of individuals and groups and [provide] for essential health education to help them maintain their health," supervise nursing personnel, and implement "physician's orders for treatments and medications based on [nursing] knowledge and understanding" (pp. 106–107).

King (1989b) identified some management strategies and administrative policies that could be used to direct the delivery of General Systems Framework and Theory of Goal Attainment-based nursing services. She suggested that nurse administrators should "restructure job descriptions to reflect differentiation in roles and functions of all nursing personnel . . . [and] change the organizational chart to clearly show the lines of communication and responsibility for each level of nursing personnel" (p. 43). She went on to point out that "knowledge of the [framework] concepts of power, authority, status, and role in planning for this change will prevent resistance" (p. 43), and recommended that the nursing personnel who will be affected should be encouraged to participate in the decision making about the changes in the job descriptions and the organizational chart. In addition, King (1989b) recommended the use of the GONR to document nursing care and to measure the effectiveness of that care.

The rules for nursing practice stemming from the General Systems Framework and Theory of Goal Attainment indicate that the purpose of nursing practice is to "help individuals attain and maintain their health, and if there is some disturbance such as illness or disability, nurses' actions are goal directed to help individuals regain health or live with a chronic illness or a disability" (King, 1989a, p. 152). Clinical problems to consider encompass activities of daily living related to the performance of social roles. Nursing extends to care of persons in acute and chronic care settings as well as in settings appropriate to delivery of care for the maintenance of health. Legitimate recipients of nursing care are people who can actively participate in decisions that influence their care as well as patients who have family members with whom nurses can make transactions until the patients can participate (King, 1986b).

The nursing process is clearly and explicitly identified as a process of perception, judgment, action, reaction, interaction, and transaction and is documented by use of the GONR. Behaviors required for transactions are specified clearly and precisely in the operational definition of that concept given below in the section on theory generation. Nursing practice based on the General Systems Framework and Theory of Goal Attainment contributes to the well-being of clients by enhancing their abilities to function in the activities of daily living associated with their social roles.

Logical Congruence

The General Systems Framework is generally logically congruent. The content of the framework follows logically from King's philosophical claims. Despite the use of terms such as action and reaction, the framework does not reflect the reaction world view. King (1981) effectively translated those terms to conform to the reciprocal interaction world view by describing the process of interaction as a dynamic "sequence of verbal and nonverbal behaviors that are goal-directed" in which both individuals participate (p. 60). Perhaps it was the terms action and reaction that led Magan (1987) to regard the framework as mechanistic and consistent with the totality paradigm. Parse's (1987) description of the totality paradigm suggests, however, that it actually is a bridge between the mechanistic elements of the reaction world view and the organismic, holistic elements of the reciprocal interaction world view. Furthermore, although King cited Freud's and Selye's essentially reactive views of the person, she provided definitions of growth and development and stress that depict the person as active.

The General Systems Framework reflects the characteristics of both the systems and interaction categories of nursing knowledge, but there is no evidence of logical incompatibility. The development of a conceptual framework combining all of those characteristics was accomplished by using an open systems approach along with a perspective of active participation of individuals in human interactions. In effect, the characteristics of the interaction approach represent the properties of the personal, interpersonal, and social systems.

Generation of Theory

Theories have been directly derived from the General Systems Framework by King (1981, 1989b, 1992a), Gonot (1986), Frey (1989), and Sieloff Evans (1991). King derived the **Theory of Goal Attainment** from the interpersonal system component of the General Systems Framework, as well as from certain concepts included in the personal system component. The theory encompasses the concepts of *perception, communication, interaction, transaction, self, role, growth and development, coping with stress, time,* and *personal space* (King, 1992a). The following constitutive definitions of those concepts were given by King (1986b), who cited pages in her 1981 book:

> Perception is each person's representation of a subjective world of experience (p. 146).
> Communication is a process whereby information is given from one person to another either directly in face-to-face meetings or indirectly through telephone, television, or the written word (p. 146).
> Interaction is a process of perception and communication between person and person and person and environment, represented by verbal and nonverbal behaviors that are goal-directed (p. 145).
> Transaction is defined as observable behavior of human beings interacting with their environment that leads to goal attainment (p. 147).
> Self is defined as a personal system synonymous with the terms I, me, and person. Self is a unified, complex whole [person] who perceives, thinks, desires, imagines, decides, identifies goals and selects means to achieve them (p. 27).
> Role is a set of behaviors expected of persons occupying a position in a social system; rules that define rights and obligations in a position; [and] a relationship with one or more individuals interacting in specific situations for a purpose (p. 147).
> Growth and development is defined as continuous changes in individuals at the cellular, molecular and behavioral levels of activities (p. 148).
> Stress is a dynamic state whereby a human being interacts with the environment to maintain balance for growth, development, and performance (p. 147).
> Time is a sequence of events moving onward to the future; a continuous flow of events in successive order that implies change; a past and a future (p. 148).
> Space is that element that exists in all directions and is the same everywhere. . . . a physical area called territory, and is defined by the behavior of individuals occupying space such as gestures, postures, and visible boundaries erected to mark off personal space (p. 148).

King (1992a) defined stress and space but she did not provide definitions for coping with stress or personal space.

Drawing from Dewey's (1963) theory of knowledge, King (1987a) commented that communication is the information component of the Theory of Goal Attainment, and transaction is the valuation component. Furthermore, King (1986b) considered transaction as "a critical dependent variable in nurse-client interactions that lead to goal attainment" (p. 202) and has developed an operational definition of the concept. The following operations, or behaviors, make up the operational definition of transaction.

> 1. One member of the nurse-client dyad initiates behavior: asks questions, makes statements, reaches out with arms, walks toward the other, looks at the other, gives something to the other.
>
> 2. The opposite member of the nurse-client dyad responds with behavior: answers questions, makes statements, reaches out with arms, walks toward the other, returns a look, gives or accepts something from the other.
>
> 3. Disturbance (or problem) is noted in the dyadic situation if a state or condition is identified.
>
> 4. Some goal is mutually agreed upon by both members of dyad; the goal may be implicit in behavior that is observed or verbalized, and each member shows or states agreement.
>
> 5. Exploration of means to achieve goals is initiated by one member of the dyad, or one member exhibits behavior that moves toward a goal.
>
> 6. The other member agrees to the means to achieve a goal, and both move toward the goal.
>
> 7. Transactions are made and the goal is attained. (King, 1981, pp. 150–151; 1986b, p. 202)

King (1989a) noted that health is the goal specified by the Theory of Goal Attainment. Consequently, health is regarded as an outcome variable. King (1986b) explained, "The outcome is a state of health for individuals. A state of health is an ability to function in social roles" (p. 200). Health is constitutively defined as "dynamic life experiences of a human being, which implies continuous adjustment to stressors in the internal and external environment through optimum use of one's resources to achieve maximum potential for daily living" (King, 1981, p. 5). King (1989a) regards the construct of health to be related to "individuals and their health, to groups and their health, and to society and health" (p. 155).

King's (1988a) Criterion-Referenced Measure of Goal Attainment Tool is an empirical indicator associated with the Theory of Goal Attainment. The instrument, which is previously described in the section on the nursing process, has predictive and content validity and is reliable.

With the exception of growth and development, all of the concepts of the Theory of Goal Attainment are linked in the following proposition. Note, however, that this proposition uses the terms stress and space, rather than the theory concepts coping with stress and personal space.

> Nurse and client interactions are characterized by verbal and nonverbal communication, in which information is exchanged and interpreted. This is accomplished through transactions in which the values, aspirations, and wants of each member of the dyad are shared through

the perceptions of the nurse, through the perceptions of the client and the situation, and through self in role of client and in role of nurse. Finally, interactions are characterized by stressors influencing each person and the situation in time and space. (King, 1992a, pp. 21–22)

King has continually refined the statements that link the various concepts of the Theory of Goal Attainment. The current list of specific propositions is as follows:

1. If perceptual accuracy is present in nurse-client interactions, transactions will occur.

2. If nurse and client make transactions, goals will be attained.

3. If goals are attained, effective nursing care will occur.

4. If transactions are made in nurse-client interactions, growth and development will be enhanced for both.

5. If nurses with special knowledge and skills communicate appropriate information to clients, mutual goal setting will occur.

6. When mutual goals have been identified, means have been explored, and nurse and client agree on means to achieve goals, transactions will be made and goals achieved.

7. If role expectations and role performance as perceived by nurse and client are congruent, transactions will occur.

8. If role conflict is experienced by nurse, client, or both, stress in nurse-client interactions will occur.

9. Accurate perception of time and space dimensions in nurse-client interactions leads to transactions.

10. Knowledge of one's concept of self will help bring about a helping relationship with clients. (King, 1986b, p. 203)

King (1986b, 1990b) derived the following hypotheses from the theory propositions:

1. Functional abilities will be greater in patients who participate in mutual goal setting than in those who do not participate.

2. Mutual goal setting will increase functional abilities in performance of activities of daily living.

3. Goal attainment will be greater in patients who participate in mutual goal setting than in patients who do not participate.

4. There is a positive relationship between functional abilities and goal attainment.

5. Perceptual congruence in nurse-patient interactions increases mutual goal setting.

6. Mutual goal setting will increase the morale of elderly patients.

7. Mutual goal setting decreases stress in planning and implementing decisions about goals to be attained.

8. Mutual goal setting increases transactions, which increases goal attainment, which leads to effective nursing care.

9. Goal attainment in nursing situations leads to growth and development in nurse and client.

10. Transactions increase nurses' and patients' self-awareness in goal attainment.

11. Congruence in role expectations and role performance increases transactions in nurse-patient interactions.

12. Accurate perceptions of time-space relations in nurse-client interactions increase transactions and goal attainment.

13. Goal attainment decreases stress and anxiety in nursing situations.

14. Goal attainment increases patients' learning and coping abilities in nursing situations. (1986b, p. 206; 1990b, pp. 81–82)

The Theory of Goal Attainment was developed to describe the nature of the interaction between nurses and clients. This middle-range theory is relatively broad in scope but does have certain boundaries. King (1981) delineated the interior and exterior boundaries of the theory as follows:

Interior Boundaries

1. Nurse and client do not know each other.

2. Nurse is licensed to practice professional nursing.

3. Client is in need of the services provided by the nurse.

4. Nurse and client are in a reciprocal relationship in that the nurse has special knowledge and skills to communicate appropriate information to help client set goals; client has information about self and perceptions of problems or concerns that when communicated to nurse will help in mutual goal setting.

5. Nurse and client are in mutual presence, purposefully interacting to achieve goals. (p. 150)

Exterior Boundaries

1. Interactions are in a two-person group.

2. Interactions [are] limited to licensed professional nurse and to client in need of nursing care.

3. Interactions [are] taking place in natural environments. (p. 150)

King (1987a) identified another boundary of the theory when she noted that the client's locus of control must be taken into account because it is difficult to set mutual goals with a client who has an external locus of control.

King (1989b) has also derived a middle-range theory of nursing administration from the General Systems Framework. This theory, which is still in rudimentary form, was derived from the social system component of the General Systems Framework, as well as from certain concepts included in the personal system and the interpersonal system components. The concepts of the theory are organization, power, authority, status, role, control, decision making, perception, communication, interaction, and transaction. King (1989b) explained that the theory, "when published in detail, will be useful in nursing service administration and in nursing education administration" (p. 42).

Another theory that could be useful in nursing administration is Sieloff's (in press; Sieloff Evans, 1991) middle-range theory of nursing departmental system power, which is being derived from the General Systems Framework. Frey (1989) derived her middle-range theory of social support and health from the General Systems Framework and theoretical and empirical literature from nursing and adjunctive disciplines. The concepts of the theory are child health, family health, and social support. The theory propositions, stated as hypotheses, are:

1. There is a positive and reciprocal relationship between family health and child health.

2. Parents' support has a direct and positive effect on family health.

3. Child's support has a direct and positive effect on child health.

4. There is a positive and reciprocal relationship between parents' support and child's support. (p. 141)

Gonot (1986) derived a theoretical and practice model of family therapy from King's General Systems Framework, her Theory of Goal Attainment, and her views of the family. Gonot explained that "The interpersonal system of the family is the focal system of the model. The personal systems of family members are the subsystems, and the environmental social systems comprise the familial suprasystem" (p. 46).

Credibility

Social Utility

The social utility of the General Systems Framework and Theory of Goal Attainment was highlighted by King's (1992a) statement that her framework and theory have been used "to generate hypotheses that have been tested, and some are being tested currently in research . . . Moreover, [the framework and theory have] been used as a guide to help nurses organize the delivery of nursing services in hospitals and in the community. The concepts [and subconcepts of the framework and theory] have served as the knowledge base for using the nursing process of assessing, planning, implementing, and evaluating nursing care. The [framework and theory have] helped teachers assist learners to organize a multitude of facts into meaningful wholes" (pp. 22–23). The social utility of the General Systems Framework and Theory of Goal Attainment are further documented by a book containing 20 chapters that present discussions of extensions or tests of King's work (Frey & Sieloff, in press).

King (cited in Takahashi, 1992) pointed out that the General Systems Framework and the Theory of Goal Attainment, per se, do not guide practical activities but that the knowledge of the content of the framework and theory is used. She stated, "What I am saying is that we often say that theory guides practice, or theory is applied to practice. Theory, as theory, is an abstraction. What we apply is the knowledge" (p. 89). That knowledge "is applied in nursing through the interaction-transaction process model in [the Theory of Goal Attainment]" (King, 1989a, p. 153).

The knowledge required for application of the General Systems Framework and Theory of Goal Attainment comes from extensive study of the major concepts and subconcepts of the personal, interpersonal, and social systems through course work in nursing and adjunctive disciplines. King (1986a) identified several courses in the adjunctive disciplines as prerequisite to the nursing major. Introductory courses in the behavioral sciences include sociology, psychology, anthropology, political science, and economics. Courses in the biophysical sciences include physics, biology, anatomy, physiology, biochemistry, microbiology, and immunology. Humanities courses include English, with an emphasis on communication, art and music appreciation, logic, philosophy, and history.

King (1986a) indicated that implementation of the framework and theory requires not only theoretical and empirical knowledge of the concepts and subconcepts of the personal, interpersonal, and social systems, but also the ability to use that knowledge to work with people of all ages with a focus on their activities of daily living. In addition, the application of the framework and theory require the perceptual and psychomotor skills necessary to assess individuals' health states and the interpersonal and communication skills necessary to engage in mutual goal setting.

Furthermore, the user of the framework and theory must learn to be sensitive to and accepting of the client's perception of what is happening. King (1992a) indicated that professional values must also be learned. Finally, King (1986a) identified four processes as essential nursing content that must be mastered in order to use the framework and theory: nursing process, teaching and learning processes, transaction process, and research process.

The many concepts that make up the General Systems Framework and Theory of Goal Attainment provide an extensive vocabulary. However, the concepts and their definitions were taken from well-known works. Thus, mastery of the vocabulary should not pose a major problem for potential users of the framework and theory.

Implementation of clinical protocols derived from the knowledge of the content of the General Systems Framework and Theory of Goal Attainment certainly is feasible but, as with the implementation of any conceptual model or theory, requires considerable time and effort. Byrne-Coker and Schreiber (1990a, 1990b) identified several strategies that facilitate General Systems Framework-based nursing practice in clinical agencies. One strategy is a 2-week orientation program that progresses from discussion of the personal system, with emphasis on comparison of the new employee's values with those of the hospital, to the social system, with emphasis on how the hospital defines the role of the nurse, to the interpersonal system, with emphasis on the nursing process. The orientation program concludes with a formal presentation of the framework. In addition, new nurses receive an exercise book "to help them practice applying the concepts in their clinical area" (Byrne-Coker & Schreiber, 1990b, p. 26).

Another strategy is 45-minute inservice education sessions offered on all shifts in all clinical areas to help continuing staff to learn the content and processes of the framework and theory. Still another strategy is ongoing inservice education in the form of a "concept of the month." Byrne-Coker and Schreiber (1990a) explained, "Each month, a concept [of the framework] was featured and information about the concept, taken from King's text, was posted. In addition, mini-discussions, 15 minutes each, highlighted the selected concept and encouraged nurses to begin thinking about it. Nurses thought about how the concept influenced their nursing care that particular month and were asked to write this on the perimeter of the poster" (p. 90).

Another strategy is to redesign existing nursing history and assessment forms, nursing diagnoses, patient teaching programs, and quality assurance programs so that they are consistent with the General Systems Framework. An additional strategy is to design computer software that is consistent with the framework and theory.

Finally, Byrne-Coker and Schreiber (1990a) drew attention to the need to employ morale-boosting strategies during periods of waning enthusiasm for framework and theory-based nursing. They cited the effectiveness of a visit to the clinical agency by King herself, as well as "Kingratulations" parties held at the completion of all the "concepts of the month" associated with each system (personal, interpersonal, and social).

Other strategies that make the implementation of the General Systems Framework and Theory of Goal Attainment feasible were described by Messmer (1992). She reported the effectiveness of case study presentations, a self-study module for staff nurses and newly employed nurses that carries 5 contact hours of continuing education credits, and "lunch and learn" inservice education sessions.

Even more strategies were described by West (1991). She commented on the effectiveness of a video and "resources nurses" for each unit who helped their peer staff nurses to "internalize theory (as they understood it) and accept it as an every day part of nursing" (p. 29). In addition, a coordinator supervised the overall implementation process on all nursing units.

Clearly, the administrators of the clinical agency must be willing to underwrite the cost of such strategies, in terms of the required personnel time and materials. In addition, the nurses must be willing to expend the time and energy required to revise forms and implement changes.

NURSING RESEARCH. The concepts and propositions of the General Systems Framework and Theory of Goal Attainment are guiding nursing research. A mark of the growing body of research focused on King's work is the research conference, held in February 1988 at the University of South Florida College of Nursing, which was devoted exclusively to presentation of studies that tested the Theory of Goal Attainment.

Several doctoral dissertations and master's theses have been guided by the General Systems Framework or the Theory of Goal Attainment. Those that were retrieved from a search of *Dissertation Abstracts International* and *Master's Abstracts International* are listed in the bibliography at the end of this chapter.

Published full reports of General Systems Framework or Theory of Goal Attainment-based research range from instrument development work to studies of the effects of nursing interventions on goal attainment. Instrument development studies include King's (1988a) work to develop and determine the psychometric properties of the Criterion-Referenced Measure of Goal Attainment Tool and Sieloff Evans' (1991) research, which focused on development and testing of a tool to measure nursing departmental power. In addition, Rawlins, Rawlins, and Horner (1990) based their Family Needs Assessment Tool, which was designed to evaluate the special needs of the families of chronically ill children, on the Theory of Goal Attainment.

Several other studies have been guided by the General Systems Framework and the Theory of Goal Attainment. King's (1981) descriptive study was designed to identify the elements of transactions. Rundell (1991) used a qualitative grounded approach to identify categories relating to interactions between nurses and patients on high dependency units, that is, units that are intermediate between surgical intensive care units and general surgical wards. Houfek (1992) studied nurses' perceptions of the dimensions of nursing care situations. Rooke and Norberg (1988) attempted to categorize nurses' descriptions of problematic and meaningful nursing situations within the context of King's framework. They reported that situations of an ethical, existential, educational, or technological nature did not fit into King's framework.

McGirr, Rukholm, Salmoni, O'Sullivan, and Koren (1990) examined the perceptions of cardiac rehabilitation program clients with regard to mood, severity of illness, and exercise. They found that the clients who exercised "felt healthy and merry, [and] those who did not exercise felt miserable" (p. 14). Kneeshaw (1990) studied nurses' perceptions of their coworkers' responses to the nurses' attempts to quit smoking. Levine, Wilson, and Guide (1988) surveyed 200 members of the American Association of Critical Care Nurses to determine their self-esteem, gender identify, and personality characteristics.

Spees (1991) based her investigation of the knowledge of common medical terms in a sample of 25 hospitalized clients and 25 family members on King's concept of communication. The results indicated that clients and family members may not understand medical terminology as well as nurses think they do. Davis and Dearman (1991) described the coping strategies used by infertile women. They discussed the results of their study in relation to King's personal system subconcept of time.

Rosendahl and Ross (1982) studied the effect of the investigator's attending behavior (making eye contact and making comments that reflected the topic introduced by the subject) on the mental status of older people. Brower (1981) found support for the hypothesis, derived from interaction theory and King's concept of social systems, that nurses' attitudes toward older persons are dependent on the type of institution in which they work. The findings indicated that nurses employed in visiting nurse home health agencies and nurses employed in hospitals had more favorable attitudes toward the aged than nurses employed in private home health agencies.

Frey's (1989) study findings provide some empirical support for her theory of the relationship of social support to child and family health. She claimed that the results provide "indirect validation of King's conceptual framework" (p. 144).

Martin (1990) found that a General Systems Framework–based nursing intervention improved awareness of prostate and testicular cancer in a sample of 448 men ranging in age from 18 to 64. Furthermore, Hanucharurnkul and Vinya-nguag (1991) found that patients undergoing pyelolithotomy or nephrolithotomy who received a nursing intervention based in part on the Theory of Goal Attainment had less pain sensation and distress, used fewer analgesics, ambulated more, had fewer complications, and had higher satisfaction with care than those who did not receive the intervention.

NURSING EDUCATION. The General Systems Framework and Theory of Goal Attainment have documented utility for nursing education. King (1989a) pointed out that the framework and theory have been used "in curriculum development, for teaching in higher education, and with undergraduate and graduate students to plan, implement, and evaluate nursing care" (p. 155). She noted that the framework and theory have guided curriculum development for programs "leading to a baccalaureate degree, a master's degree and an associate degree" as well as for a hospital-based diploma program in Canada (p. 154).

Gulitz and King (1988) described the process of curriculum development using the General Systems Framework. King (1986a) presented detailed descriptions of the nursing curriculum plans for a hypothetical associate degree program and a hypothetical baccalaureate program, including the philosophy of nursing education, curriculum conceptual framework, program objectives, prerequisite and concurrent courses in adjunctive disciplines, nursing courses, plan of study, and sample courses with course description, objectives, content, learning activities, teaching strategies, and strategies for formative and summative evaluation. She also outlined a curriculum to articulate associate degree and baccalaureate degree programs. In addition, King (1986a) shared her ideas, along with course titles and objectives, about undergraduate and graduate education in nursing for the future. Here, she emphasized professional education and learning about nursing as an academic discipline.

The Ohio State University College of Nursing in Columbus has used the General Systems Framework as a guide for the baccalaureate curriculum since 1970. Components of this curriculum were described by Daubenmire and King (1973) and Daubenmire (1989). Commenting on the success of the King-based curriculum, Daubenmire (1989) stated,

> Based on both internal and external evaluation, it is clear that King's framework continues to provide a viable curricular strategy for the education of baccalaureate nurses. Extensive curriculum revision is extremely costly in terms of faculty time and energy, which can be better used in conducting research, service, and other scholarly endeavors. A curriculum model which is conceptually based allows for updating content and skills without the necessity for major curriculum change." (p. 167)

The master's program at Loyola University of Chicago School of Nursing has also used King's conceptual framework (King, personal communication, February 23, 1982). Furthermore, Olivet Nazarene College in Kankakee, Illinois (Asay & Ossler, 1984) and a hospital-based school of nursing in Winnipeg, Manitoba, Canada, have used the conceptual framework as a curriculum guide (Fromen & Sanderson, 1985).

Brown and Lee (1980) proposed a model for continuing nursing education based on the General Systems Framework. They presented the following rationale for using King's framework as the foundation for their continuing education model:

> The concepts—social systems, health, perception, and interpersonal relationships—are relevant in every nursing situation; the interacting levels of operation—individuals, groups, and society—depict a reciprocal relationship between human behaviour and the environment; and the triad of elements—continuing nursing education, nursing practice, and nursing research are interrelated in the nursing profession (p. 473).

NURSING ADMINISTRATION. The utility of the General Systems Framework and Theory of Goal Attainment for nursing administration has begun to be documented. King (1989a) noted that the framework and theory have been used "as a guide to help individuals organize the delivery of nursing services in health care systems" (p. 155). Elberson (1989) linked the General Systems Framework and Arndt and Huckabay's (1980) theory of nursing administration to create a conceptual-theoretical structure for nursing administration. Elberson explained that "For King, the unit of analysis is the individual. The focus is the individual nurse managing care for patients and small groups of clients. For Arndt and Huckabay, the unit of analysis is also the individual, but in this case the focus is the individual nurse administrator managing the care provided by individual nurses and groups of nurses. Both perspectives are models of health-care management" (p. 49). Elberson continued her discussion by explaining how the content of the General Systems Framework can be adapted for nursing administration. For example, the interpersonal system can be adapted in the following manner:

> At the interpersonal level, nurse administrators organize information and communicate. The skills that effective nurse administrators possess include the ability to manage information. They determine the type of information that is needed, the best sources of information, optimal storage and retrieval methods, and how to analyze and disseminate the most useful information. (pp. 49–50)

The General Systems Framework and Theory of Goal Attainment are used to guide the delivery of nursing services at Tampa General Hospital (TGH) in Tampa, Florida (LaFontaine, 1989; Messmer, 1992). Messmer reported that the framework and theory guided the revision of a flow sheet and an assessment tool. She added that efforts are underway to integrate the framework and theory into the hospital's developing computerized information systems. She commented, "TGH's goal of fully automating the patient record requires that King's Theory of Goal Attainment become an integral part of the nursing documentation system" (p. 8).

Byrne-Coker and Schreiber (1989, 1990a, 1990b) described the strategies used to implement the General Systems Framework at Centenary Hospital in Scarborough, Ontario, Canada. Those strategies are outlined above at the beginning of the section on social utility. They found that the initial 23-page Nursing History and Assessment Record (NHAR) developed by members of the Nursing Quality Assurance Committee had to be revised to reflect the needs of each clinical unit and reported satisfactory progress with the revisions for the gerontology, rehabilitation, and psychiatric units (Byrne-Coker & Schreiber, 1989, 1990a). Schreiber (1991) explained the process of the revisions of the NHAR for the psychiatric unit. Byrne-Coker, Fradley, Harris, Tomarchio, Chan, and Caron (1990) described the Nursing Diagnosis Categorization Tool, which links the NANDA diagnoses with the systems, concepts, and subconcepts of the General Systems Framework.

West (1991) described the implementation of the General Systems Framework and Theory of Goal Attainment at Sunnybrook Health Science Centre in Toronto, Ontario, Canada. She noted that King's GONR is used to document nursing care.

King (personal communication, July 18, 1987) reported that the GONR system is being used in several nursing service areas. King (1981) claimed that use of the GONR would facilitate nursing audits. Such a measure of quality of nursing care would operationalize Chance's (1982) proposal concerning the use of nursing models for establishing standards of professional accountability. Given the focus of the Theory of Goal Attainment on process (action, reaction, interaction) and outcome (transaction or goal attainment regarding functional ability), quality assurance programs based on King's framework and theory certainly could be developed.

NURSING PRACTICE. King (1992a) stated that the General Systems Framework and the Theory of Goal Attainment provide a useful approach for nursing practice. She claims that although any one framework or theory "cannot cover every nursing situation [the nursing process of the Theory of Goal Attainment] can be used in most nursing situations" (p. 24). She went on to explain that "when clients cannot communicate with a nurse, they can nonverbally send and receive messages. In some situations, nurses use their judgment and set goals for the patients and families when they are unable to do this for themselves. . . . When working with patients who are comatose, nurses can verbally communicate and observe for nonverbal gestures such as muscle movement, the squeezing of the nurse's hand, or changes in facial expressions" (p. 24).

In a specific example, King (1986b) described the use of the Theory of Goal Attainment by a graduate student who was caring for a comatose patient. Because the patient could not communicate verbally, mutual goals were set with the patient's husband. The student, however, communicated verbally with the patient and observed and recorded her nonverbal responses. The student ascertained that goals set with the husband were attained after the patient regained consciousness and returned to her home.

The General Systems Framework and Theory of Goal Attainment have documented use for the care of individuals of various ages and with various medical conditions. Steele (1981) used the framework as the basis for her text on child health. Hughes (1983) gave a brief example of the application of the theory to the emergency department care of a 17-year-old high school student with an ankle injury. Davis (1987) described how the framework can be used to care for women who are infertile, whereas Smith (1988) applied the theory to the care of a 30-year-old woman who had had a cesarean birth, and Heggie and Gangar (1992) applied the framework to women experiencing menopause. King (1986b) described the use of the theory by a clinical specialist who was working with a 43-year-old man who had had coronary artery bypass surgery. She also described the use of the GONR for a 60-year-old man who had had a cerebral vascular accident (King, 1981).

Elderly individuals have also been the subject of publications describing the use of the General Systems Framework and Theory of Goal Attainment (Jonas, 1987; Kenny, 1990; Kohler, 1988; Miller, 1990). Filial caregivers of the elderly were the subject matter of Temple and Fawdry's 1992) application of the theory. King (1984a) adapted the GONR to the care of patients with end-stage renal disease. Messner and Smith (1986) explained the use of the theory with individuals who have neurofibromatosis. Husband (1988) applied the theory to the care of adults with diabetes. Gonot (1983) explained how the GONR could be used to care for individuals with psychiatric diagnoses. DeHowitt (1992) discussed individual psychotherapy from the perspective of the General Systems Framework and Theory of Goal Attainment. LaFontaine (1989) explained how the theory is used to alleviate the apprehensions and anxieties of individuals who require gastroendoscopic examinations, and Swindale (1989) explained the nurse's role in reducing preoperative anxiety by providing information.

The framework and theory also can be used to care for families and other groups. King (1983a, 1983b, 1983c) explained how the GONR can be applied to the family. Sirles and Selleck (1989) described the impact of cardiac disease on a family and identified family assessment techniques. Symanski (1991) focused on families with high-risk infants, and Norris and Hoyer (1993) focused on development of a King-based framework that promotes parenting while the infant is in a neonatal intensive care unit. Gonot (1986) described the use of her King-based model of family therapy for family assessment. Turning attention to groups other than families, Laben, Dodd, and Sneed (1991) focused on group therapy for offenders in the criminal justice system.

King (1984b) discussed the application of the framework and theory in community health nursing. Furthermore, Hanchett (1988, 1990) provided informative discussions of the use of King's work when the client is the community.

Social Congruence

The social congruence of the General Systems Framework and the Theory of Goal Attainment is based, in part, on the fact that King (1975) deliberately constructed the framework from "recurring ideas or . . . concepts that were undergoing verification through systematic investigation" (p. 37). Thus, the conceptual-theoretical system of knowledge emphasizes nursing care based on valid scientific findings and enduring traditions deemed acceptable by society.

Moreover, with its emphasis on mutual goal setting, the nursing process described by the Theory of Goal Attainment should be particularly appealing to health care consumers and nurses who believe that health care is a collaborative endeavor and to health care consumers who wish to participate actively in their nursing care. Indeed, King (1992b) noted that her formulation of the nursing process "is based on knowledge of human interactions in which a critical human variable (coping) should be of concern in helping those we serve to build collaborative relationships and participate as informed decision makers in their own health care" (p. 604).

Bramlett, Gueldner, and Sowell (1990) pointed out that King's assumptions about human beings and her emphasis on mutual goal setting "supports a need to redefine the concept of advocacy to accommodate a more active and less dependent client role in decision making" (p. 160). They also pointed out that "King's focus on the information giving role of the nurse is consistent with the concept of consumer-centric advocacy" (p. 160). Health care consumers and nurses who do not subscribe to such an approach to nursing care would have to be helped to see its value. This is especially so when caring for clients with external locus of control. In fact, the General Systems Framework and Theory of Goal Attainment may not be the appropriate perspective to guide the nursing care of such clients.

In addition, the client's cultural background should be considered prior to using the General Systems Framework and Theory of Goal Attainment. That is because, as Meleis (1985) pointed out, although the emphasis on mutual goal setting is congruent with values espoused by Western societies, including the United States, it may not be appropriate for people of other cultures. She commented,

> Many other societies that consider patients helpless, that espouse the sick role as abandonment of social roles and responsibilities, and that support the rights of patients to be sheltered from prognosis and health care goals (such as some middle-eastern cultures) would consider this theory culturally limited. Patients in these societies prefer to relinquish all decisions and goal setting to the expertise of the health care professionals. (p. 238)

King (cited in Takahashi, 1992), however, claimed that the General Systems Framework and Theory of Goal Attainment are applicable cross-culturally. She stated,

> My theory has been studied in Thailand, Sweden, Canada, the United States and Japan. My theory does help individuals coming from different cultures because it deals with human beings primarily and their interactions with other human beings. I am currently working with an investigator to design an intercultural study of the theory, and I have some Japanese nurses who said they would like to collect some data in Japan. We will be collecting data in Sweden and two other countries besides the United States. (p. 91)

The belief that King's work is appropriate cross-culturally is reflected in Spratlen's (1976) and Rooda's (1992) publications. Spratlen built on King's early work to develop "an approach to nursing education, research and practice which incorporates the cultural dimensions of attitudes and behavior in matters of health" (p. 23). Rooda described the conceptual model for multicultural nursing that she developed from the Theory of Goal Attainment. She noted that the model provides direction for nursing practice and research and prepares nurses to provide holistic nursing care in a global society.

West's (1991) experience with the implementation of the General Systems Framework and Theory of Goal Attainment provides empirical data regarding social congruence. She reported that a study of nurses' reactions to the implementation of General Systems Framework and Theory of Goal Attainment-based practice at Sunnybrook Health Science Centre in Toronto revealed mixed results. Interviews with nursing unit directors and discussions with staff nurses indicated a clear dichotomy — approximately equal numbers of nurses were "adamantly for theory or vehemently against it. There seemed to be little ambivalence" (p. 30). Chart audits of the GONR using a quality assurance tool to ensure non-biased, reliable, and valid assessments revealed "a wide range of comprehension and various levels of abilities to not only format a care plan reflecting the theory, but also to monitor the outcome of that theory and the patient's response to the plan" (p. 30). West concluded that greater attention needs to be paid to discussion of the value of conceptual model-based nursing practice prior to the selection and implementation of a particular model.

Additional empirical evidence of social congruence comes from a study by Hanucharurnkul and Vinya-nguag (1991). They found that patients who received a nursing intervention based in part on the Theory of Goal Attainment had higher satisfaction with care than those who did not receive the intervention. Furthermore, Jonas (1987) reported her own and the patient's satisfaction with nursing care based on the Theory of Goal Attainment.

Social Significance

King (1992b) claimed that the "use of my conceptual system and theory in nursing practice has shown cost containment, health care outcomes, and health team approach in using the same conceptual system" (p. 604). She did not, however, provide any empirical or anecdotal evidence to support that claim.

Anecdotal and empirical evidence supporting the contention that use of the General Systems Framework and Theory of Goal Attainment leads to improvements in individuals' health status is beginning to accrue. Smith's (1988) case presentation suggested that mutual goal setting resulted in attainment of goals and enhanced client health. Kohler (1988) indicated that mutual goal setting and agreement on means to achieve the goals increased compliance to the medication regimen. DeHowitt (1992) stated that individual psychotherapy guided by the Theory of Goal Attainment increased a patient's own goal setting and goal attainment, which in turn increased the patient's positive feelings about himself and his feelings of progress in therapy.

Martin's (1990) results supported the effectiveness of an intervention on men's awareness of prostate and testicular cancer. In addition, Hanucharurnkul and Vinya-nguag's (1991) results supported the effectiveness of an intervention based in part on the Theory of Goal Attainment on several measures of postoperative recovery.

Contributions to the Discipline of Nursing

King's General Systems Framework and her Theory of Goal Attainment represent substantial contributions to the discipline of nursing. The concepts and propositions of the framework, together with the content related to each concept of the personal, interpersonal, and social systems, form the beginning of conceptual-theoretical systems of nursing knowledge needed for various nursing activities. Furthermore, the Theory of Goal Attainment is a major contribution to the growing body of distinctive nursing theory. The fact that the theory has been tested empirically and has received initial support is especially significant. However, additional tests of the Theory of Goal Attainment are needed. Furthermore, the credibility of the General Systems Framework requires further investigation by means of systematic tests of conceptual-theoretical-empirical structures derived from the framework, the Theory of Goal Attainment or other relevant theories, and appropriate empirical indicators.

The emphasis on client participation in the General Systems Framework and Theory of Goal Attainment, including mutual goal setting and exploration of means to achieve goals, should be attractive to the many nurses who are consumer advocates. Some authors have maintained that this emphasis imposes a limitation on use of the conceptual framework and theory in situations in which clients cannot participate, such as infants or patients who are comatose or irrational (Austin & Champion, 1983; Barnum, 1994). In contrast, the evidence given in the section on social utility indicates that the framework and theory can be used with individuals who cannot interact verbally. However, as noted in the section on social congruence, the General Systems Framework may not be appropriate for use with clients who have external locus of control.

King, in a personal communication to Ackerman et al. (1994), summarized the contributions of her work by noting that her approach to nursing is the only one that "has provided a theory that deals with choices, alternatives, participation of all individuals in decision making and specifically deals with outcomes of nursing care" (p. 316).

REFERENCES

Ackerman, M.L., Brink, S.A., Clanton, J.A., Moody, S.L., Perlich, G.L., Price, D.L., & Prusinski, B.B. (1994). Imogene King: Theory of goal attainment. In A. Marriner-Tomey, Nursing theorists and their work, (3rd ed., pp. 305–322). St. Louis: Mosby-Year Book.

Arndt, C., & Huckabay, L.M.D. (1980). Nursing administration: Theory for practice with a systems approach (2nd ed). St. Louis: CV Mosby.

Asay, M.K., & Ossler, C.C. (Eds.) (1984). Conceptual models of nursing: Applications in community health nursing: Proceedings of the *Eighth Annual Community Health Nursing Conference*. Chapel Hill, NC: Department of Public Health Nursing, School of Public Health, University of North Carolina.

Austin, J.K., & Champion, V.L. (1983). King's theory for nursing: Explication and evaluation. In P.L. Chinn (Ed.), *Advances in nursing theory development* (pp. 47–61). Rockville, MD: Aspen.

Barnum, B.J.S. (1994). *Nursing theory: Analysis, application, evaluation* (3rd ed.). Glenview, IL: Scott, Foresman/Little, Brown Higher Education.

Benne, R.D., & Bennis, W.G. (1959). The role of the professional nurse. *American Journal of Nursing, 59*, 380–383.

Bertalanffy, L. (1956). General system theory. *Yearbook of the Society for the Advancement of General System Theory, 1*(1), 1–10.

Bertalanffy, L. (1968). *General system theory*. New York: George Braziller.

Boulding, K. (1956). General system theory —The skeleton of science. *Yearbook of the Society for the Advancement of General System Theory, 1*(1), 11–17.

Bramlett, M.H., Gueldner, S.H., & Sowell, R.L. (1990). Consumer-centric advocacy: Its connection to nursing frameworks. *Nursing Science Quarterly, 3*, 156–161.

Bross, I. (1953). *Design for decision*. New York: Macmillan.

Brower, H.T. (1981). Social organization and nurses' attitudes toward older persons. *Journal of Gerontological Nursing, 7*, 293–298.

Brown, S.T., & Lee, B.T. (1980). Imogene King's conceptual framework: A proposed model for continuing nursing education. *Journal of Advanced Nursing, 5*, 467–473.

Bruner, I.S., & Krech, W. (Eds.). (1968). *Perception and personality*. New York: Greenwood Press.

Byers, P. (1985, August). *Application of Imogene King's framework*. Paper presented at conference on Nursing Theory in Action, Edmonton, Alberta, Canada. (Cassette recording).

Byrne-Coker, E., Fradley, T., Harris, J., Tomarchio, D., Chan, V., & Caron, C. (1990). Implementing nursing diagnoses within the context of King's conceptual framework. *Nursing Diagnosis, 1*, 107–114.

Byrne-Coker, E., & Schreiber, R. (1989). Concept of the month: Implementing King's conceptual framework at the bedside. *Journal of Nursing Administration, 19*(2), 28–32.

Byrne-Coker, E., & Schreiber, R. (1990a). Implementing King's conceptual framework at the bedside. In M.E. Parker (Ed.), *Nursing theories in practice* (pp. 85–102. New York: National League for Nursing.

Byrne-Coker, E., & Schreiber, R. (1990b). King at the bedside. *The Canadian Nurse, 86*(1), 24–26.

Chance, K.S. (1982). Nursing models: A requisite for professional accountability. *Advances in Nursing Science, 4*(2), 57–65.

Cherry, C. (1966). *On human communication*. Cambridge, MA: MIT Press.

Daubenmire, M.J. (1989). A baccalaureate nursing curriculum based on King's conceptual framework. In J.P. Riehl-Sisca, *Conceptual models for nursing practice* (3rd ed., pp. 167–178). Norwalk, CT: Appleton & Lange.

Daubenmire, M.J., & King, I.M. (1973). Nursing process models: A systems approach. *Nursing Outlook, 21*, 512–517.

Davis, D.C. (1987). A conceptual framework for infertility. *Journal of Obstetric, Gynecologic, and Neonatal Nursing, 16*, 30–35.

Davis, D.C., & Dearman, C.N. (1991). Coping strategies of infertile women. *Journal of Obstetric, Gynecologic, and Neonatal Nursing, 20*, 221–228.

DeHowitt, M.C. (1992). King's conceptual model and individual psychotherapy. *Perspectives in Psychiatric Care, 28*(4), 11–14.

Dewey, J. (1963). *Experience and education*. New York: Collier Books.

Dewey, J., & Bentley, A. (1949). *Knowing and the known*. Boston: Beacon Press.

DiVincenti, M. (1977). *Administering nursing service* (2nd ed.). Boston: Little, Brown.

Elberson, K. (1989). Applying King's model to nursing administration. In B. Henry, M. DiVincenti, C. Arndt, & A. Marriner (Eds.). *Dimensions of nursing administration: Theory, research, education, and practice* (pp. 47–53). Boston: Blackwell Scientific Publications.

Ellis, R. (1971). Book review of King, I.M. (1971). Toward a theory for nursing: General concepts of human behavior. *Nursing Research, 20*, 462.

Erikson, E. (1950). *Childhood and society*. New York: Norton.

Etzioni, A.A. (1975). *Comparative analysis of complex organizations* (rev. ed.). New York: The Free Press.

Fawcett, J. (1984). *Analysis and evaluation of conceptual models of nursing*. Philadelphia: FA Davis.

Fawcett, J. (1989). *Analysis and evaluation*

of conceptual models of nursing (2nd ed.). Philadelphia: FA Davis.

Fisher, S., & Cleveland, S. (1968). Body image and personality. New York: Dover.

Fraser, J.T. (Ed.). (1972). The voices of time. New York: George Braziller.

Freud, S. (1966). Introductory lectures on psychoanalysis (J. Strachey, Ed. and trans.) New York: Norton.

Frey, M.A. (1989). Social support and health: A theoretical formulation derived from King's conceptual framework. Nursing Science Quarterly, 2, 138–148.

Frey, M.A., & Sieloff, C.L. (Eds.). (in press). King's conceptual framework and theory of goal attainment: Contributions to nursing science. Newbury Park: Sage.

Fromen, D., & Sanderson, H. (1985, August). Application of Imogene King's framework. Paper presented at conference on Nursing Theory in Action, Edmonton, Alberta, Canada. (Cassette recording.)

Gesell, A. (1952). Infant development. New York: Harper.

Gibson, J. (1966). The senses considered as perceptual systems. Boston: Houghton Mifflin.

Gonot, P.J. (1983). Imogene M. King: A theory for nursing. In J.J. Fitzpatrick & A.L. Whall, Conceptual models of nursing: Analysis and application (pp. 221–243). Bowie, MD: Brady.

Gonot, P.J. (1986). Family therapy as derived from King's conceptual model. In A.L. Whall, Family therapy theory for nursing: Four approaches (pp. 33–48). Norwalk, CT: Appleton-Century-Crofts.

Griffiths, D. (1959). Administrative theory. Englewood Cliffs, NJ: Prentice-Hall.

Gulitz, E.A., & King, I.M. (1988). King's general systems model: Application to curriculum development. Nursing Science Quarterly, 1, 128–132.

Haas, J.E. (1964). Role conception and group consensus: A study of disharmony in hospital work groups. Columbus, OH: Ohio State University College of Commerce and Administration, Bureau of Business Research, 1964.

Hall, E. (1959). The silent language. Greenwich, CT: Fawcett.

Hall, A.D., & Fagen, R.E. (1956). Definition of system. Yearbook of the Society for the Advancement of General System Theory, 1(1), 18–28.

Hanchett, E.S. (1988). Nursing frameworks and community as client: Bridging the gap. Norwalk, CT: Appleton & Lange.

Hanchett, E.S. (1990). Nursing models and community as client. Nursing Science Quarterly, 3, 67–72.

Hanucharurnkul, S., & Vinya-nguag, P. (1991). Effects of promoting patients' participation in self-care on postoperative recovery and satisfaction with care. Nursing Science Quarterly, 4, 14–20.

Havighurst, R. (1953). Human development and education. New York: McKay.

Heggie, M., & Gangar, E. (1992). A nursing model for menopause clinics. Nursing Standard, 6(21), 32–34.

Heiss, J. (1981). The social psychology of interaction. Englewood Cliffs, NJ: Prentice-Hall.

Houfek, J.F. (1992). Nurses' perceptions of the dimensions of nursing care episodes. Nursing Research, 41, 280–285.

Hughes, M.M. (1983). Nursing theories and emergency nursing. Journal of Emergency Nursing, 9, 95–97.

Husband, A. (1988). Application of King's theory of nursing to the care of the adult with diabetes. Journal of Advanced Nursing, 13, 484–488.

Ittleson, W., & Cantril, H. (1954). Perception: A transactional approach. Garden City, NY: Doubleday & Co.

Janis, I. (1958). Psychological stress. New York: John Wiley & Sons.

Jersild, A.T. (1952). In search of self. New York: Columbia University Teachers College Press.

Jonas, C.M. (1987). King's goal attainment theory: Use in gerontological nursing practice. Perspectives, 11(4), 9–12.

Katz, D., & Kahn, R.L. (1966). The social psychology of organizations. New York: John Wiley & Sons.

Kaufmann, M.A. (1958). Identification of theoretical bases for nursing practice. Unpublished doctoral dissertation, University of California, Los Angeles.

Kenny, T. (1990). Erosion of individuality in care of elderly people in hospital—an alternative approach. Journal of Advanced Nursing, 15, 571–576.

King, I.M. (1964). Nursing theory—problems and prospect. Nursing Science, 2, 394–403.

King, I.M. (1968). A conceptual frame of reference for nursing. Nursing Research, 17, 27–31.

King, I.M. (1971). Toward a theory for nursing: General concepts of human behavior. New York: John Wiley & Sons.

King, I.M. (1975). A process for developing concepts for nursing through research. In P.J. Verhonick (Ed.), Nursing research I (pp. 25–43). Boston, Little, Brown.

King, I.M. (1976). The health care system: Nursing intervention subsystem. In H. Werley, A. Zuzich, M. Zajkowski, & A.D.

Zagornik (Eds.), *Health research: The systems approach* (pp. 51–60). New York: Springer.

King, I.M. (1978, December). *King's conceptual model of nursing.* Paper presented at Second Annual Nurse Educator Conference, New York. (Cassette recording).

King, I.M. (1981). *A theory for nursing: Systems, concepts, process.* New York: John Wiley & Sons. Reissued 1990. Albany, NY: Delmar.

King, I.M. (1983a). King's theory of nursing. In I.W. Clements & F.B. Roberts, *Family health: A theoretical approach to nursing care* (pp. 177–188). New York: John Wiley & Sons.

King, I.M. (1983b). The family coping with a medical illness: Analysis and application of King's theory of goal attainment. In I.W. Clements & F.B. Roberts, *Family health: A theoretical approach to nursing care* (pp. 383–385). New York: John Wiley & Sons.

King, I.M. (1983c). The family with an elderly member: Analysis and application of King's theory of goal attainment. In I.W. Clements & F.B. Roberts, *Family health: A theoretical approach to nursing care* (pp. 341–345). New York: John Wiley & Sons.

King, I.M. (1984a). Effectiveness of nursing care: Use of a goal oriented nursing record in end stage renal disease. *American Association of Nephrology Nurses and Technicians Journal, 11*(2), 11–17, 60.

King, I.M. (1984b). A theory for nursing: King's conceptual model applied in community health nursing. In M.K. Asay & C.C. Ossler (Eds.), *Conceptual models of nursing. Applications in community health nursing: Proceedings of the Eighth Annual Community Health Nursing Conference* (pp. 13–34). Chapel Hill, NC: Department of Public Health Nursing, School of Public Health, University of North Carolina.

King, I.M. (1985a, May). *Panel discussion with theorists.* Nurse Theorist Conference, Pittsburgh, PA. (Cassette recording).

King, I.M. (1985b, August). *Imogene King.* Paper presented at conference on Nursing Theory in Action, Edmonton, Alberta, Canada. (Cassette recording).

King, I.M. (1986a). *Curriculum and instruction in nursing.* Norwalk, CT: Appleton-Century-Crofts.

King, I.M. (1986b). King's theory of goal attainment. In P. Winstead-Fry (Ed.), *Case studies in nursing theory* (pp. 197–213). New York: National League for Nursing.

King, I.M. (1987a, May). *King's theory.* Paper presented at Nurse Theorist Conference, Pittsburgh, PA. (Cassette recording).

King, I.M. (1987b). King's theory of goal attainment. In R.R. Parse, *Nursing science: Major paradigms, theories, and critiques* (pp. 107–113). Philadelphia: WB Saunders.

King, I.M. (1988a). Measuring health goal attainment in patients. In C.F. Waltz, & O.L. Strickland (Eds.), *Measurement of nursing outcomes. Vol. 1. Measuring client outcomes* (pp. 108–127). New York: Springer.

King, I.M. (1988b). *The nurse theorists: Portraits of excellence—Imogene King.* Oakland, CA: Studio Three. (Videotape).

King, I.M. (1989a). King's general systems framework and theory. In J.P. Riehl-Sisca, *Conceptual models for nursing practice* (3rd ed., pp. 149–158). Norwalk, CT: Appleton & Lange.

King, I.M. (1989b). Theories and hypotheses for nursing administration. In B. Henry, M. DiVincenti, C. Arndt, & A. Marriner (Eds.), *Dimensions of nursing administration: Theory, research, education, and practice* (pp. 35–45). Boston: Blackwell Scientific Publications.

King, I.M. (1990a). Health as the goal for nursing. *Nursing Science Quarterly, 3,* 123–128.

King, I.M. (1990b). King's conceptual framework and theory of goal attainment. In M.E. Parker (Ed.), *Nursing theories in practice* (pp. 73–84). New York: National League for Nursing.

King, I.M. (1992a). King's theory of goal attainment. *Nursing Science Quarterly, 5,* 19–26.

King, I.M. (1992b). Window on general systems framework and theory of goal attainment. In M. O'Toole (Ed.), *Miller-Keane encyclopedia and dictionary of medicine, nursing, and allied health* (p. 604). Philadelphia: WB Saunders.

King, I.M. (in press a). A systems framework for nursing. In M.A. Frey & C.L. Sieloff (Eds.), *King's conceptual framework and theory of goal attainment: Contributions to nursing science.* Newbury Park: Sage.

King, I.M. (in press b). The theory of goal attainment. In M.A. Frey & C.L. Sieloff (Eds.), *King's conceptual framework and theory of goal attainment: Contributions to nursing science.* Newbury Park: Sage.

Klein, G. (1970). *Perception, motivation and personality.* New York: Alfred A. Knopf.

Kneeshaw, M.F. (1990). Nurses' perceptions of co-worker responses to smoking cessation attempts. *Journal of the New York State Nurses' Association, 21*(9), 9–13.

Kohler, P. (1988). Model of shared control. *Journal of Gerontological Nursing, 14*(7), 21–25.

Laben, J.K., Dodd, D., & Sneed, L. (1991). King's theory of goal attainment applied in group therapy for inpatient juvenile sexual offenders, maximum security state offenders, and community parolees, using visual aids. *Issues in Mental Health Nursing, 12*(1), 51–64.

LaFontaine, P. (1989). Alleviating patient's apprehensions and anxieties. *Gastroenterology Nursing, 11*, 256–257.

Levine, C.D., Wilson, S.F., & Guido, G.W. (1988). Personality factors of critical care nurses. *Heart and Lung, 17*, 392–398.

Linton, R. (1963). *The study of man.* New York: Appleton-Century-Crofts.

Lyman, S., & Scott, M. (1967). Territoriality: A neglected sociological dimension. *Social Problems, 15*, 236–249.

Magan, S.J. (1987). A critique of King's theory. In R.R. Parse, *Nursing science: Major paradigms, theories, and critiques* (pp. 115–133). Philadelphia: WB Saunders.

Marriner-Tomey, A. (1989). *Nursing theorists and their work* (2nd ed). St. Louis: CV Mosby.

Martin, J.P. (1990). Male cancer awareness: Impact of an employee education program. *Oncology Nursing Forum, 17*, 59–64.

McGirr, M., Rukholm, E., Salmoni, A., O'Sullivan, P., & Koren, I. (1990). Perceived mood and exercise behaviors of cardiac rehabilitation program referrals. *Canadian Journal of Cardiovascular Nursing, 1*(4), 14–19.

Meleis, A.I. (1985). *Theoretical nursing: Development and progress.* Philadelphia: JB Lippincott.

Meleis, A.I. (1991). *Theoretical nursing: Development and progress* (2nd ed.). Philadelphia: JB Lippincott.

Messmer, P.R. (1992). Implementing theory based nursing practice. *Florida Nurse, 40*(3), 8.

Messner, R., & Smith, M.N. (1986). Neurofibromatosis: Relinquishing the masks: A quest for quality of life. *Journal of Advanced Nursing, 11*, 459–464.

Miller, C.A. (1990). *Nursing care of older adults.* Glenview, IL: Scott, Foresman/ Little, Brown Higher Education.

Monat, A., & Lazarus, R.S. (Eds.). (1977). *Stress and coping.* New York: Columbia University Press.

Moore, M.A. (1968). Nursing: A scientific discipline? *Nursing Forum, 7*, 340–348.

Moore, M.A. (1969). The professional practice of nursing: The knowledge and how it is used. *Nursing Forum, 8*, 361–373.

Norris, D.M., & Hoyer, P.J. (1993). Dynamism in practice: Parenting within King's framework. *Nursing Science Quarterly, 6*, 79–85.

Orlando, I.J. (1961). *The dynamic nurse-patient relationship.* New York: GP Putnam's Sons.

Orme, J.E. (1969). *Time, experience and behavior.* New York: American Elsevier.

Parse, R.R. (1987). *Nursing science: Major paradigms, theories, and critiques.* Philadelphia: WB Saunders.

Parsons, T. (1951). *The social system.* Glencoe, IL: The Free Press.

Peplau, H.E. (1952). *Interpersonal relations in nursing.* New York: GP Putnam's Sons. Reprinted 1991. New York: Springer.

Piaget, J. (1969). *The mechanisms of perception.* New York: Basic Books.

Rawlins, P.S., Rawlins, T.D., & Horner, M. (1990). Development of the family needs assessment tool. *Western Journal of Nursing Research, 12*, 201–214.

Rooda, L.A. (1992). The development of a conceptual model for multicultural nursing. *Journal of Holistic Nursing, 10*, 337–347.

Rooke, L., & Norberg, A. (1988). Problematic and meaningful situations in nursing interpreted by concepts from King's nursing theory and four additional concepts. *Scandinavian Journal of Caring Sciences, 2*, 80–87.

Rosendahl, P.B., & Ross, V. (1982). Does your behavior affect your patient's response? *Journal of Gerontological Nursing, 8*, 572–575.

Ruesch, J., & Kees, W. (1972). *Nonverbal communication.* Los Angeles: University of California Press.

Rundell, S. (1991). A study of nurse-patient interaction in a high dependency unit. *Intensive Care Nursing, 7*, 171–178.

Schilder, P. (1951). *The image and appearance of the human body.* New York: International Universities Press.

Schreiber, R. (1991). Psychiatric assessment —à la King. *Nursing Management, 22*(5), 90–94.

Selye, H. (1956). *The stress of life.* New York: McGraw-Hill.

Shontz, F. (1969). *Perceptual and cognitive aspects of body experience.* New York: Academic Press.

Sieloff, C.L. (in press). Development of a theory of departmental power. In M.A. Frey & C.L. Sieloff (Eds.), *King's conceptual framework and theory of goal attainment: Contributions to nursing science.* Newbury Park: Sage.

Sieloff Evans, C.L. (1991). *Imogene King: A conceptual framework for nursing.* Newbury Park, CA: Sage.

Simon, H.A. (1957). *Administrative behavior* (2nd ed.). New York: Macmillan.

Simon, Y.R. (1962). *A general theory of authority.* South Bend, IN: University of Notre Dame Press.

Sirles, A.T., & Selleck, C.S. (1989). Cardiac disease and the family: Impact, assessment, and implications. *Journal of Cardiovascular Nursing, 3*(2), 23–32.

Smith, M.C. (1988). King's theory in practice. *Nursing Science Quarterly, 1,* 145–146.

Sommer, R. (1969). *Personal space.* Englewood Cliffs, NJ: Prentice-Hall.

Spees, C.M. (1991). Knowledge of medical terminology among clients and families. *Image: Journal of Nursing Scholarship, 23,* 225–229.

Spratlen, L.P. (1976). Introducing ethnic-cultural factors in models of nursing: Some mental health care applications. *Journal of Nursing Education, 15*(2), 23–29.

Steele, S. (1981). *Child health and the family: Nursing concepts and management.* New York: Masson Publishing USA.

Stevens, B.J. (1984). *Nursing theory. Analysis, application, evaluation* (2nd ed.). Boston: Little, Brown.

Swindale, J.E. (1989). The nurse's role in giving pre-operative information to reduce anxiety in patients admitted to hospital for elective minor surgery. *Journal of Advanced Nursing, 14,* 899–905.

Symanski, M.E. (1991). Use of nursing theories in the care of families with high-risk infants: Challenges for the future. *Journal of Perinatal and Neonatal Nursing, 4*(4), 71–77.

Takahashi, T. (1992). Perspectives on nursing knowledge. *Nursing Science Quarterly, 5,* 86–91.

Temple, A., & Fawdry, K. (1992). King's theory of goal attainment: Resolving filial caregiver role strain. *Journal of Gerontological Nursing, 18*(3), 11–15.

Wapner, S., & Werner, H. (Eds.). (1965). *The body percept.* New York: Random House.

West, P. (1991). Theory implementation: A challenging journey. *Canadian Journal of Nursing Administration, 4*(1), 29–30.

Watzlawick, P., Beavin, J. H., & Jackson, D.D. (1967). *Pragmatics of human communication.* New York: Norton.

Weed, L.L. (1969). *Medical records, medical education, and patient care.* Cleveland: Case Western Reserve University Press.

Zald, M.N. (Ed.). (1970). *Power in organization.* Nashville, TN: Vanderbilt University Press.

BIBLIOGRAPHY

PRIMARY SOURCES

Frey, M.A., & Sieloff, C.L. (Eds.). (in press). *King's conceptual framework and theory of goal attainment: Contributions to nursing science.* Newbury Park: Sage.

King, I.M. (1964). Nursing theory—problems and prospect. *Nursing Science, 2,* 394–403.

King, I.M. (1968). A conceptual frame of reference for nursing. *Nursing Research, 17,* 27–31.

King, I.M. (1971). *Toward a theory for nursing: General concepts of human behavior.* New York: John Wiley & Sons.

King, I.M. (1976). The health care system: Nursing intervention subsystem. In H. Werley, A. Zuzich, M. Zajkowski, & A.D. Zagornik (Eds.), *Health research: The systems approach* (pp. 51–60). New York: Springer.

King, I.M. (1981). *A theory for nursing: Systems, concepts, process.* New York: John Wiley & Sons. Reissued 1990. Albany, NY: Delmar.

King, I.M. (1983). King's theory of nursing. In I.W. Clements & F.B. Roberts, *Family health: A theoretical approach to nursing care* (pp. 177–188). New York: John Wiley & Sons.

King, I.M. (1986). King's theory of goal attainment. In P. Winstead-Fry (Ed.), *Case studies in nursing theory* (pp. 197–213). New York: National League for Nursing.

King, I.M. (1987). King's theory of goal attainment. In R.R. Parse, *Nursing science. Major paradigms, theories, and critiques* (pp. 107–113). Philadelphia: WB Saunders.

King, I.M. (1988). Imogene M. King. In T.M. Schorr & A. Zimmerman, *Making choices.*

Taking chances: Nurse leaders tell their stories (pp. 146–153). St. Louis: CV Mosby.

King, I.M. (1989). King's general systems framework and theory. In J.P. Riehl-Sisca, *Conceptual models for nursing practice* (3rd ed., pp. 149–158). Norwalk, CT: Appleton & Lange.

King, I.M. (1990). Health as the goal for nursing. *Nursing Science Quarterly, 3,* 123–128.

King, I.M. (1990). King's conceptual framework and theory of goal attainment. In M.E. Parker (Ed.), *Nursing theories in practice* (pp. 73–84). New York: National League for Nursing.

King, I.M. (1992). King's theory of goal attainment. *Nursing Science Quarterly, 5,* 19–26.

King, I.M. (1992). Window on general systems framework and theory of goal attainment. In M. O'Toole (Ed.), *Miller-Keane encyclopedia and dictionary of medicine, nursing, and allied health* (p. 604). Philadelphia: WB Saunders.

Takahashi, T. (1992). Perspectives on nursing knowledge. *Nursing Science Quarterly, 5,* 86–91.

COMMENTARY

Ackerman, M.L., Brink, S.A., Clanton, J.A., et al. (1989). Imogene King: Theory of goal attainment. In A. Marriner-Tomey, *Nursing theorists and their work* (2nd ed., pp. 345–360). St. Louis: CV Mosby.

Ackerman, M.L., Brink, S.A., Clanton, J.A. et al. (1994). Imogene King. Theory of goal attainment. In A. Marriner-Tomey (Ed.), *Nursing theorists and their work* (3rd ed., pp. 305–322). St. Louis: Mosby-Year Book.

Ackerman, M.L., Brink, S.A., Jones, C.G., Moody, S.L., Perlich, G.L., & Prusinski, B.B. (1986). Imogene King. Theory of goal attainment. In A. Marriner, *Nursing theorists and their work* (pp. 231–245). St. Louis: CV Mosby.

Ackerman, M.L., Brink, S.A., Clanton, J.A., et al. (1989). Imogene King: Theory of goal attainment. In A. Marriner-Tomey, *Nursing theorists and their work* (2nd ed., pp. 345–360). St. Louis: CV Mosby.

Aggleton, P., & Chalmers, H. (1990). King's model. *Nursing Times, 86*(1), 38–39.

Austin, J. K., & Champion, V.L. (1983). King's theory for nursing: Explication and evaluation. In P.L. Chinn (Ed.), *Advances in nursing theory development* (pp. 49–61). Rockville, MD: Aspen.

Bramlett, M.H., Gueldner, S.H., & Sowell, R.L. (1990). Consumer-centric advocacy: Its connection to nursing frameworks. *Nursing Science Quarterly, 3,* 156–161.

Buchanan, B.F. (1987). Conceptual models: An assessment framework. *Journal of Nursing Administration, 17*(10), 22–26.

Burney, M.A. (1992). King and Newman: In search of the nursing paradigm. *Journal of Advanced Nursing, 17,* 601–603.

DeFeo, D.J. (1990). Change: A central concern of nursing. *Nursing Science Quarterly, 3,* 88–94.

DiNardo, P.B. (1989). Evaluation of the nursing theory of Imogene M. King. In J.P. Riehl-Sisca, *Conceptual models for nursing practice* (3rd ed., pp. 159–166). Norwalk, CT: Appleton & Lange.

Fitzpatrick, J.J., Whall, A.L., Johnston, R.L., & Floyd, J.A. (1982). *Nursing models and their psychiatric mental health applications.* Bowie, MD: Brady, 1982.

Frey, M.A. (1993). A theoretical perspective of family and child health derived from King's conceptual framework of nursing: A deductive approach to theory building. In S.L. Feetham, S.B. Meister, J.M. Bell, & C.L. Gillis (Eds.), *The nursing of families: Theory/research/education/practice* (pp. 30–37). Newbury Park, CA: Sage.

George, J.B. (1980). Imogene M. King. In Nursing Theories Conference Group, *Nursing theories: The base for professional nursing practice* (pp. 184–198). Englewood Cliffs, NJ: Prentice-Hall.

George, J.B. (1985). Imogene M. King. In Nursing Theories Conference Group, *Nursing theories: The base for professional nursing practice* (2nd ed., pp. 235–257). Englewood Cliffs, NJ: Prentice-Hall.

George, J.B. (1990). Imogene M. King. In J.B. George (Ed.), *Nursing theories: The base for professional nursing practice* (3rd ed., pp. 193–210). Norwalk, CT: Appleton & Lange.

Gonot, P.J. (1983). Imogene M. King: A theory for nursing. In J.J. Fitzpatrick & A.L. Whall, *Conceptual models of nursing: Analysis and application* (pp. 221–243). Bowie, MD: Brady.

Gonot, P.J. (1989). Imogene M. King: A theory for nursing. In J.J. Fitzpatrick & A.L. Whall, *Conceptual models of nursing: Analysis and application* (2nd ed., pp. 271–283). Norwalk, CT: Appleton & Lange.

Hanucharurnkul, S. (1989). Comparative analysis of Orem's and King's theories. *Journal of Advanced Nursing, 14,* 365–372.

Hawks, J.H. (1991). Power: A concept analysis. *Journal of Advanced Nursing, 16*, 754–762.

Huch, M.H. (1991). Perspectives on health. *Nursing Science Quarterly, 4*, 33–40.

King, I.M. (1978). The "why" of theory development. In *Theory development: What, why, how?* (pp. 11–16). New York: National League for Nursing.

King, I.M. (1988). Concepts: Essential elements of theories. *Nursing Science Quarterly, 1*, 22–25.

Magan, S.J. (1987). A critique of King's theory. In R.R. Parse, *Nursing science: Major paradigms, theories, and critiques* (pp. 115–133). Philadelphia: WB Saunders.

Meleis, A.I. (1991). *Theoretical nursing: Development and progress* (2nd ed.). Philadelphia: JB Lippincott.

Rooda, L.A. (1992). The development of a conceptual model for multicultural nursing. *Journal of Holistic Nursing, 10*, 337–347.

Sieloff Evans, C.L. (1991). *Imogene King: A conceptual framework for nursing.* Newbury Park, CA: Sage.

Spratlen, L.P. (1976). Introducing ethnic-cultural factors in models of nursing: Some mental health care applications. *Journal of Nursing Education, 15*(2), 23–29.

Uys, L.R. (1987). Foundational studies in nursing. *Journal of Advanced Nursing, 12*, 275–280.

RESEARCH

Brower, H.T. (1981). Social organization and nurses' attitudes toward older persons. *Journal of Gerontological Nursing, 7*, 293–298.

Davis, D.C., & Dearman, C.N. (1991). Coping strategies of infertile women. *Journal of Obstetric, Gynecologic, and Neonatal Nursing, 20*, 221–228.

Frey, M.A. (1989). Social support and health: A theoretical formulation derived from King's conceptual framework. *Nursing Science Quarterly, 2*, 138–148.

Hanucharurnkul, S., & Vinya-nguag, P. (1991). Effects of promoting patients' participation in self-care on postoperative recovery and satisfaction with care. *Nursing Science Quarterly, 4*, 14–20.

Houfek, J.F. (1992). Nurses's perceptions of the dimensions of nursing care episodes. *Nursing Research, 41*, 280–285.

King, I.M. (1975). A process for developing concepts for nursing through research. In P.J. Verhonick (Ed.), *Nursing research I* (pp. 25–43). Boston: Little, Brown.

King, I.M. (1988). Measuring health goal attainment in patients. In C.F. Waltz, & O.L. Strickland (Eds.), *Measurement of nursing outcomes. Vol. 1. Measuring client outcomes* (pp. 108–127). New York: Springer.

Kneeshaw, M.F. (1990). Nurses' perceptions of co-worker responses to smoking cessation attempts. *Journal of the New York State Nurses' Association, 21*(9), 9–13.

Levine, C.D., Wilson, S.F., & Guido, G.W. (1988). Personality factors of critical care nurses. *Heart and Lung, 17*, 392–398.

Martin, J.P. (1990). Male cancer awareness: Impact of an employee education program. *Oncology Nursing Forum, 17*, 59–64.

McGirr, M., Rukholm, E., Salmoni, A., O'Sullivan, P., & Koren, I. (1990). Perceived mood and exercise behaviors of cardiac rehabilitation program referrals. *Canadian Journal of Cardiovascular Nursing, 1*(4), 14–19.

Rawlins, P.S., Rawlins, T.D., & Horner, M. (1990). Development of the family needs assessment tool. *Western Journal of Nursing Research, 12*, 201–214.

Rooke, L., & Norberg, A. (1988). Problematic and meaningful situations in nursing interpreted by concepts from King's nursing theory and four additional concepts. *Scandinavian Journal of Caring Sciences, 2*, 80–87.

Rosendahl, P.B., & Ross, V. (1982). Does your behavior affect your patient's response? *Journal of Gerontological Nursing, 8*, 572–575.

Rundell, S. (1991). A study of nurse-patient interaction in a high dependency unit. *Intensive Care Nursing, 7*, 171–178.

Spees, C.M. (1991). Knowledge of medical terminology among clients and families. *Image: Journal of Nursing Scholarship, 23*, 225–229.

MASTER'S THESES

Dispenza, J.M. (1990). Relationship of husband and wife perceptions of the coping responses of the female spouse of males in high level stress. *Master's Abstracts International, 28*, 407.

Monti, A. (1992). Members' perceptions of the transactions within their psychosocial club. *Master's Abstracts International, 30*, 1296.

O'Shall, M.L. (1989). The relationship of

congruency of role conception between head nurse and staff nurse and staff nurse job satisfaction. *Master's Abstracts International, 27,* 379.

DOCTORAL DISSERTATIONS

Glenn, C.J. (1989). The development of autonomy in nurses. *Dissertation Abstracts International, 50,* 1852B.

Hanna, K.M. (1991). Effect of nurse-client transaction on female adolescents' contraceptive perceptions and adherence. *Dissertation Abstracts International, 51,* 3323B.

Hobdell, E.F. (in press). The relationship between chronic sorrow and accuracy of perception of cognitive development in parents of children with neural tube defect. *Dissertation Abstracts International.*

O'Connor, P. (1990). Service in nursing: Correlates of patient satisfaction. *Dissertation Abstracts International, 50,* 4985B.

Omar, M.A. (1990). Relationship of family processes to family life satisfaction in stepfamilies and biological families during pregnancy. *Dissertation Abstracts International, 51,* 1196B.

Rooke, L. (1990). Nursing and theoretical structures of nursing: A didactic attempt to develop the practice of nursing. *Dissertation Abstracts International, 51,* 239C.

Rubin, M. (in press). Perceived uncertainty, coping strategies, and adaptation in patients with human papilloma virus (HPV) on Papanicolaou smear. *Dissertation Abstracts International.*

Zurakowski, T.L. (1991). Interpersonal factors and nursing home resident health (anomia). *Dissertation Abstracts International, 51,* 4281B.

EDUCATION

Brown, S.T., & Lee, B.T. (1980). Imogene King's conceptual framework: A proposed model for continuing nursing education. *Journal of Advanced Nursing, 5,* 467–473.

Daubenmire, M.J. (1989). A baccalaureate nursing curriculum based on King's conceptual framework. In J.P. Riehl-Sisca, *Conceptual models for nursing practice* (3rd ed., pp. 167–178). Norwalk, CT: Appleton & Lange.

Daubenmire, M.J., & King, I.M. (1973). Nursing process models: A systems approach. *Nursing Outlook, 21,* 512–517.

Gulitz, E.A., & King, I.M. (1988). King's general systems model: Application to curriculum development. *Nursing Science Quarterly, 1,* 128–132.

King, I.M. (1978). JANFORUM: U.S.A.: Loyola University of Chicago School of Nursing. *Journal of Advanced Nursing, 3,* 390.

King, I.M. (1986). *Curriculum and instruction in nursing.* Norwalk, CT: Appleton-Century-Crofts.

ADMINISTRATION

Byrne-Coker, E., Fradley, T., Harris, J., Tomarchio, D., Chan, V., & Caron, C. (1990). Implementing nursing diagnoses within the context of King's conceptual framework. *Nursing Diagnosis, 1* 107–114.

Byrne-Coker, E., & Schreiber, R. (1989). Concept of the month: Implementing King's conceptual framework at the bedside. *Journal of Nursing Administration, 19*(2), 28–32.

Byrne-Coker, E., & Schreiber, R. (1990). Implementing King's conceptual framework at the bedside. In M.E. Parker (Ed.), *Nursing theories in practice* (pp. 85–102). New York: National League for Nursing.

Byrne-Coker, E., & Schreiber, R. (1990). King at the bedside. *Canadian Nurse, 86*(1), 24–26.

Elberson, K. (1989). Applying King's model to nursing administration. In B. Henry, M. DiVincenti, C. Arndt, & A. Marriner (Eds.), *Dimensions of nursing administration: Theory, research, education, and practice* (pp. 47–53). Boston: Blackwell Scientific Publications.

King, I.M. (1989). Theories and hypotheses for nursing administration. In B. Henry, M. DiVincenti, C. Arndt, & A. Marriner (Eds.), *Dimensions of nursing administration: Theory, research, education, and practice* (pp. 35–45). Boston: Blackwell Scientific Publications.

Messmer, P.R. (1992). Implementing theory based nursing practice. *Florida Nurse, 40*(3), 8.

Schreiber, R. (1991). Psychiatric assessment —à la King. *Nursing Management, 22*(5), 90–94.

West, P. (1991). Theory implementation: A challenging journey. *Canadian Journal of Nursing Administration, 4*(1), 29–30.

Practice

Bradley, J.C., & Edinberg, M.A. (1986). *Communication in the nursing context* (2nd ed.). Norwalk, CT: Appleton & Lange.

Davis, D.C. (1987). A conceptual framework for infertility. *Journal of Obstetric, Gynecologic, and Neonatal Nursing, 16,* 30–35.

DeHowitt, M.C. (1992). King's conceptual

model and individual psychotherapy. *Perspectives in Psychiatric Care, 28*(4), 11–14.

Gonot, P.W. (1986). Family therapy as derived from King's conceptual model. In A.L. Whall, *Family therapy theory for nursing: Four approaches* (pp. 33–48). Norwalk, CT: Appleton-Century-Crofts.

Hanchett, E.S. (1988). *Nursing frameworks and community as client: Bridging the gap.* Norwalk, CT: Appleton & Lange.

Hanchett, E.S. (1990). Nursing models and community as client. *Nursing Science Quarterly, 3,* 67–72.

Heggie, M., & Gangar, E. (1992). A nursing model for menopause clinics. *Nursing Standard, 6*(21), 32–34.

Hughes, M.M. (1983). Nursing theories and emergency nursing. *Journal of Emergency Nursing, 9,* 95–97.

Husband, A. (1988). Application of King's theory of nursing to the care of the adult with diabetes. *Journal of Advanced Nursing, 13,* 484–488.

Jonas, C.M. (1987). King's goal attainment theory: Use in gerontological nursing practice. *Perspectives, 11*(4), 9–12.

Kenny, T. (1990). Erosion of individuality in care of elderly people in hospital — an alternative approach. *Journal of Advanced Nursing, 15,* 571–576.

King, I.M. (1983). The family coping with a medical illness: Analysis and application of King's theory of goal attainment. In I.W. Clements & F.B. Roberts, *Family health: A theoretical approach to nursing care* (pp. 383–385). New York: John Wiley & Sons.

King, I.M. (1983). The family with an elderly member: Analysis and application of King's theory of goal attainment. In I.W. Clements & F.B. Roberts, *Family health: A theoretical approach to nursing care* (pp. 341–345. New York: John Wiley & Sons.

King, I.M. (1984). A theory for nursing: King's conceptual model applied in community health nursing. In M.K. Asay & C.C. Ossler (Eds.), *Conceptual models of nursing. Applications in community health nursing: Proceedings of the Eighth Annual Community Health Nursing Conference* (pp. 13–34). Chapel Hill, NC: Department of Public Health Nursing, School of Public Health, University of North Carolina.

King, I.M. (1984). Effectiveness of nursing care: Use of a goal-oriented nursing record in end stage renal disease. *American Association of Nephrology Nurses and Technicians Journal, 11*(2), 11–17, 60.

King, I.M. (1987). Keynote address: Translating research into practice. *Journal of Neuroscience Nursing, 19*(1), 44–48.

Kohler, P. (1988). Model of shared control. *Journal of Gerontological Nursing, 14*(7), 21–25.

Laben, J.K., Dodd, D., & Sneed, L. (1991). King's theory of goal attainment applied in group therapy for inpatient juvenile sexual offenders, maximum security state offenders, and community parolees, using visual aids. *Issues in Mental Health Nursing, 12*(1), 51–64.

LaFontaine, P. (1989). Alleviating patient's apprehensions and anxieties. *Gastroenterology Nursing, 11,* 256–257.

Messner, R., & Smith, M.N. (1986). Neurofibromatosis: Relinquishing the masks: A quest for quality of life. *Journal of Advanced Nursing, 11,* 459–464.

Miller, C.A. (1990). *Nursing care of older adults.* Glenview, IL: Scott, Foresman/Little, Brown Higher Education.

Norris, D.M., & Hoyer, P.J. (1993). Dynamism in practice: Parenting within King's framework. *Nursing Science Quarterly, 6,* 79–85.

Sirles, A.T., & Selleck, C.S. (1989). Cardiac disease and the family: Impact, assessment, and implications. *Journal of Cardiovascular Nursing, 3*(2), 23–32.

Smith, M.C. (1988). King's theory in practice. *Nursing Science Quarterly, 1,* 145–146.

Steele, S. (1981). *Child health and the family: Nursing concepts and management.* New York: Masson Publishing USA.

Swindale, J.E. (1989). The nurse's role in giving pre-operative information to reduce anxiety in patients admitted to hospital for elective minor surgery. *Journal of Advanced Nursing, 14,* 899–905.

Symanski, M.E. (1991). Use of nursing theories in the care of families with high-risk infants: Challenges for the future. *Journal of Perinatal and Neonatal Nursing, 4*(4), 71–77.

Temple, A., & Fawdry, K. (1992). King's theory of goal attainment: Resolving filial caregiver role strain. *Journal of Gerontological Nursing, 18*(3), 11–15.

Levine's Conservation Model

This chapter presents an analysis and evaluation of Myra E. Levine's Conservation Model. Levine's work clearly fits the definition of a conceptual model of nursing used in this book. In fact, Levine (1985, 1987) noted that her work is "a generalization" of nursing and agreed that it is indeed a conceptual model.

The concepts of the Conservation Model and their dimensions are listed below. Each concept and its dimensions are defined and described later in this chapter.

KEY CONCEPTS

HOLISM
WHOLENESS
CHANGE
ADAPTATION
INTERNAL ENVIRONMENT
Homeostasis
Homeorrhesis
EXTERNAL ENVIRONMENT
Perceptual
Operational
Conceptual
ORGANISMIC RESPONSES
Fight or Flight
Inflammatory-Immune
Stress
Perceptual Awareness
  Basic Orienting System
  Visual System
  Auditory System

Haptic System
Taste-Smell System
CONSERVATION
Health and Disease as Patterns of
  Adaptive Change
GOAL OF NURSING
Promotion of Wholeness for All
  People, Well or Sick
TROPHICOGNOSIS
Observation
Provocative Facts
Testable Hypothesis
INTERVENTION/ACTION
Therapeutic
Supportive
CONSERVATION PRINCIPLES
Conservation of Energy
Conservation of Structural Integrity
Conservation of Personal Integrity

Conservation of Social Integrity	THEORY OF THERAPEUTIC
EVALUATION OF NURSING	INTENTION
INTERVENTION/ACTION	THEORY OF REDUNDANCY

ANALYSIS OF LEVINE'S CONSERVATION MODEL

This section presents an analysis of Levine's Conservation Model. The analysis draws from several of Levine's publications, including three recent book chapters, "The conservation principles of nursing: Twenty years later" (Levine, 1989b), "Conservation and integrity" (Levine, 1990), and "The conservation principles: A model for health" (Levine, 1991).

Origins of the Model

Historical Evolution and Motivation

Levine (1966a) presented the rudiments of the Conservation Model in an article entitled "Adaptation and assessment: A rationale for nursing intervention." Additional elements of the model were presented in two other articles, "The four conservation principles of nursing" (Levine, 1967), and "The pursuit of wholeness" (Levine, 1969b). A comprehensive discussion of the model was presented in the book, *Introduction to Clinical Nursing* (1969a). The second edition of this book was published in 1973. Other features of the model were given in Levine's 1971 publication, "Holistic nursing," and her presentations at conferences (Levine, 1978a, 1984a, 1986), as well as her responses to a videotaped interview (Levine, 1987). The most recent explications of the Conservation Model are Levine's 1989b, 1990, and 1991 book chapters. Levine (personal communication, July 15, 1987) regarded the 1989b chapter as "a significant restatement of the model . . . a natural evolutionary statement of how the basic concepts are related to each other." Further refinements are evident in the 1990 and 1991 chapters.

Levine (1969a) commented that she was motivated to develop the Conservation Model as a starting point for the theory development needed to provide the "why's" of nursing activities. She stated, "The serious study of any discipline requires a theoretical baseline which gives it substance and meaning" (p. ix). Although Levine did not underestimate the importance of technical skills, she pointed out:

> Nursing . . . remain[s] characterized by a rigid dependence on procedures. The "why" is not entirely neglected, but it is often applied after the fact, as if such justification invested the procedure with a special scientific holiness. Nurses cherish "applied science principles" in an era when nursing is deeply involved in scientific research, but even the lessons learned from nurse researchers are too often ignored. (p. vii)

Levine's attention to the theoretical basis for nurses' actions came at a time when nursing was beginning to recognize the need for substantive knowledge (Newman, 1972). A major feature of her work is the explication of the scientific concepts underlying nursing processes. In fact, Levine (1969a) deliberately set out to provide "an intellectual framework for analysis and understanding of the scientific nature of nursing activity" (p. viii).

Levine (1988b) maintained that the universal importance of conservation made it essential knowledge about human life that must be included in the nursing curriculum. She went on to explain,

> The development of the four conservation principles grew naturally out of my desire to organize nursing knowledge so that the student would have a strong organizing basis for interpreting all kinds of nursing situations. It was easy to work with, and in its simplicity it seemed to open many channels of thinking that had not been obvious before. . . . I adopted it as the basis for a textbook in beginning nursing, *Introduction to Clinical Nursing*. I never dreamed that others would see in it a new [conceptual model of] nursing. I was certain it would educate good nurses. That is all I ever wanted to do. (p. 227)

Philosophical Claims

Levine has presented the philosophical claims undergirding the Conservation Model in the form of assumptions about nursing and about human beings, beliefs about nursing, and a value system.

Levine (1973) developed the Conservation Model from the basic assumption that nursing intervention is a conservation activity. Drawing from Tillich (1961), she assumed that the "multidimensional unity of life" must be conserved. She also assumed that "the human being responds to the forces in his environment in a singular yet integrated fashion" (p. 6). Elaborating, Levine explained:

> The holistic nature of the human response to the environment provides the rationale for substantive principles of nursing. A principle is a fundamental concept that forms the basis for a chain of reasoning. Formulated on a broad base, it establishes the relationships between apparently otherwise unrelated facts. Nursing principles are fundamental assumptions which provide a unifying structure for understanding a wide variety of nursing activities. Nursing principles are all "conservation" principles. (p. 13).

Levine's assumptions about human beings place the human being within the context of his or her surroundings. She stated:

> Living things of every kind share the earth, and the multitude of environmental habitats exist in a vital, changing harmony. To understand the individual, the place and time of his or her living must also be understood. (Levine, 1990, p. 196)

The individual cannot be understood outside of the context of a place and time. The individual cannot be separated from the influence of everything that is happening around him or her, nor indeed, from all those events—remembered and forgotten—which have created the individual as he or she is at this precise moment. Nursing can succeed only when it recognizes that the person is not summarized by the immediate present, but is burdened by a lifetime of experience—recorded not only on the tissues of the body, but on the spirit and mind as well. (Levine, 1990, p. 197)

Levine's belief's about nursing are summarized in the following quotations:

Emphasizing the integrity of the patient brings integrity to the nursing profession and the individual nurse. Bringing together the best science and the most devoted humanism is the ultimate aim of nursing. In finding, valuing, and cherishing the integrity of the patient, the nurse's integrity is acknowledged and rewarded. (Levine, 1990, p. 200)

All nursing actions are moral statements. . . . Expectations [regarding care] must be realistic. Goals that are impossible are more than merely frustrating; they are also unethical. Nurses cannot promise good health and long life to everyone, and it is cruel to place the onus of failure on the individual. Nurses have long been expert at celebrating small victories with patients. It may be, finally, that such moments most truly reflect the moral burden of nursing practice. Moral judgments must be reserved and patients must be accepted as they are—for what they are—with dignity and honesty. (Levine, 1989c, p. 6)

Levine has explicated a set of values about nursing and health care that is grounded in the two moral imperatives of Western democratic societies—the sanctity of life and the prevention or alleviation of suffering. "The fundamental belief of the sanctity of life," Levine (1989a) explained, "provides the structure upon which all moral systems are based" (p. 125). She went on to say,

All the efforts of the healing sciences are founded on the holiness and wholeness of the human being, and the special injunction this places on the caregiver to bring dignity and compassion to the tasks of caring for another person. . . . The sanctity of life . . . is the essence of the respectful relationship that one person must have for another. It is never more important than when a nurse-patient dyad is created whereby one individual enters dependency, willing or not, and places his trust in another person. . . . Every moment of a nurse-patient interaction requires recognition of the selfhood, the uniqueness of each individual: nurse and patient. . . . The nurse functions in the role of caregiver and assumes an additional moral burden to recognize, value, and defend the dependency of the patient. (p. 125)

Levine (1989a) maintained that the health care system is dedicated to the task of preventing or alleviating suffering. She stated:

It is the individual who enters "patienthood" who is the sufferer. It is the moral duty of the nurse to confront the suffering individual and bring all the skills of hand, heart, and mind to alleviate it. It is equally binding that once the conditions of patienthood have been successfully overcome, the individual is free of his dependent role. He ceases to be a patient. His privacy is restored. (p. 126)

In another paper, Levine (1989c) stated, "The fundamental moral responsibility of patient care is the limitation and relief of suffering" (pp. 4–5).

Levine (1989a) values the ultimate freedom of the individual to make decisions. She commented, "The patient's freedom must prohibit the imposition of the nurse's values into his decisions for his care" (p. 126). Indeed, "It is patients whose predicament of need sets the standards of ethical responsibility" (Levine, 1989c, p. 5). Consequently,

> It is the challenge of the nurse to provide the individual with appropriate care without losing sight of the individual's integrity, to honor the trust that the patient has placed in the nurse, and to encourage the participation of the individual in his or her own welfare. The patient comes in trust and dependence only for as long as the services of the nurse are needed. The nurse's goal is always to impart knowledge and strength so that the individual can resume a private life—no longer a patient, no longer dependent. (Levine, 1990, p. 199)

Levine (1989d) explicated guidelines that clearly reflect her values regarding the "personal responsibility that is the particular province of the caregivers, privileges of behavior that have been awarded by the community that licenses them to practice" (p. 88). The four guidelines are:

> 1. Persons who require [care] enter with a contract of trust. They place their well-being, and often their lives in the hand of caregivers. To respect that trust by the most vigorous effort is a moral responsibility.
>
> 2. It is not the task of the practitioner . . . to evaluate the social worth of the patient. Judgments as to the quality of life of individual patients are inappropriate and unsupportable and should never be used as a rationale for withholding or withdrawing essential care.
>
> 3. The decisions for introducing treatments should be based (as they have been historically) on the physician's evaluation of the patient's condition and the consequent appropriate interventions. The interference of third party payers in which therapeutic decisions are dictated by cost or any other extraneous factors is morally repugnant.
>
> 4. Life or death decisions are not properly those of caregivers and never should be left to those whose mission is to protect life and relieve suffering. Decisions to use extraordinary means of sustaining life processes should be made in advance of the actual events by the informed wisdom of the physician whenever possible. The caregivers— physicians and nurses—should bring all their skills to bear to alleviate suffering, but that does not include hastening the death of another human being. (pp. 88–89)

Levine's values extend to her choice of the term to describe the recipient of nursing care. She explained:

> The word "patient" has been deliberately used whenever the care recipient was discussed. The widespread use of the substitute term "client" was just as deliberately excluded even though many nurses use it habitually. Its original purpose, to add some professional elegance to nursing practice, does not justify the moral failure it reflects. The word client comes from the Latin root that means "follower." That idea is a pure derivative of the paternalistic-parentalistic relationship and ought to be forbidden in nursing on moral grounds. The word patient comes from the Latin word for "suffering." Job, for example, is often credited with patience, not because he was willing to wait without complaint until his ordeal was over, but because he was suffering. He was not a quiescent sufferer; he argued, complained, lamented, and despised his undeserved misfortune. (Levine, 1989a, p. 126)

In another publication, Levine (1990) commented, "The labeling of persons as clients reinforces . . . dependency because a client is a follower. The provenance of the word patient is sufferer. It is the condition of suffering that makes it possible to set independence aside and accept the services of another person" (p. 199).

Strategies for Knowledge Development

Levine's use of knowledge from a variety of adjunctive disciplines indicates that she used a deductive approach to develop the Conservation Model. That approach is further illustrated in the following comment:

> The essential science concepts develop the rationale [for nursing actions], using ideas from all areas of knowledge that contribute to the development of the nursing process in the specific area of the model. (Levine, 1969a, p. viii)

Influences from Other Scholars

Levine is known for her careful citations of the many scholars and scientists from nursing and adjunctive disciplines whose work has influenced her thinking. Levine (personal communication, February 2, 1982) stated that she "did not invent the notion of Conservation—I simply live in a natural world where it is a characteristic of experience." Indeed, Levine (1988b, 1991) pointed out that conservation is a natural law of science and cited Feynman (1965), who described conservation "as one of the 'great general principles [which] all detailed laws . . . seem to follow' (p. 59)," (1991, p. 3). She went on to explain that "No sophisticated theorizing can displace the fundamental importance of natural law" (1991, p. 3).

Levine (1990) commented that her use of concepts and theories from adjunctive disciplines "brings coherence to nursing problems, encouraging freedom of exploration in practice, research, and teaching without losing sight of the integrity of either the practitioner or the patient" (p. 196). She has explicitly acknowledged the contributions to her thinking made by the work of Bates (1967), Beland (1971), Cannon (1939), Dubos

(1961, 1965), Erikson (1964, 1968), Gibson (1966), Goldstein (1963), Hall (1959, 1966), Selye (1956), and Sherrington (1906), among others. She has disclaimed "even with some vigor," however, any dependence on Maslow and other more recent authors whose work focuses on holism (Levine, personal communication, February 2, 1982). Moreover, she has decried Maslow's influence on nursing education (Levine, 1991).

Furthermore, Levine (1992) identified parallels between the Conservation Model and Nightingale's (1859) ideas about observation, environment, and nursing. She explained, "I quoted [Nightingale's] words on 'observation' in my text (Levine, 1973), and emphasized, as I believe she did, that observation was a guardian activity" (p. 41). Nightingale's emphasis on environment influenced Levine in that "the Conservation Model insists that the person can only be understood in the context of environment" (p. 41).

Levine (1992) went on to discuss the link between Nightingale and the Conservation Model with regard to nursing:

> The nursing that Nightingale describes fits comfortably into the Conservation principles. She details the parameters of the conservation of energy. . . . Although her physiology is very limited, Nightingale recognizes the importance of conservation of structural integrity. . . . Those injunctions in Notes on Nursing that describe the experience of the patient seem very personal, even though her own invalidism had hardly begun. She lists many of the behaviors basic to the personal integrity of the patient and the nurse . . . Notes on Nursing was directed at the social integrity, health, and well-being of the English people. (pp. 41–42)

World View

The Conservation Model clearly reflects the *reciprocal interaction* world view. Levine regards the person as a holistic being who constantly strives to preserve wholeness and integrity. Furthermore, although Levine (1989b) discusses physiological and behavioral responses, she regards those responses as "one and the same—not merely parallel and not merely simultaneous—but essential portions of the same activity" (p. 330). Moreover, although she identified four principles of conservation, she views them as joined, not isolated or separate.

The characteristics of the reciprocal interaction world view are exemplified explicitly in the following quotations.

> Nursing intervention, traditionally directed by procedures or manifestations of disease symptoms, needs new directions if the holistic approach is to be utilized. The individual must be recognized in his wholeness, and the powerful influence of adaptation recognized as a dynamic and ever-present factor in evaluating his care. Instead of listing "needs" or "symptoms," it should be possible to identify for each individual the patterns of his adaptive response, and to tailor intervention to enhance their effectiveness. (Levine, 1971, pp. 257–258)

> All nursing care is focused on man and the complexity of his rela-
> tionships with his environment, both internal and external, and com-
> mon experience emphasizes that every response to every environmental
> stimulus results from the integrated and unified nature of the human
> organism. In other words, every response is an organismic one—no
> other kind is possible—and every adaptive change is accomplished by
> the entire individual. (Levine, 1967, p. 46)

The reciprocal interaction world view is also reflected in Levine's
characterization of the person as an active participant in interactions with
the environment. This is especially evident in her statement that "The
individual can . . . never be passive. He is an active participant in his
environment, not only altering it by his presence but also actively and
constantly seeking information from it" (Levine, 1969b, p. 96), and "The
person is an active participant, exploring, seeking, and testing understanding of the world he or she inhabits" (Levine, 1992, p. 41). The active
organism perspective is also reflected in Levine's discussion of the perceptual systems. For example, Levine (1973) commented, "The human being
is a sentient being, and the ability to interact with the environment seems
ineluctably tied to his sensory organs" (p. 446). She also noted, "The
perceptual systems provide information to the individual; usually this is
knowledge sought by the individual" (Levine, 1973, p. 450).

In keeping with the reciprocal interaction world view, the Conservation Model incorporates elements of both persistence and change. Persistence is reflected in the emphasis on homeostasis and conservation. Levine (1989b) regards homeostasis as "a state of energy-sparing" (p. 329); it
even "might be called the state of conservation" (p. 329). The essence of
conservation, in turn, is use of responses "that *cost the least* to the individual in expense of effort and demand on his or her well-being" (p. 329).

Change is evident in Levine's (1973) comments that "change is the
essence of life, and it is unceasing as long as life goes on" and that "change
is characteristic of life" (p. 10).

Despite the pervasiveness of change in the person's life, conservation,
and hence persistence, appears to be predominant. Apparently, Levine
regards the many changes that must occur as the person faces environmental challenges as necessary for survival. Conservation facilitates and
maintains the patterns and routines of human behavior, and adaptive
changes represent the invention of new routines to avoid extinction.

Unique Focus of the Model

The unique focus of the Conservation Model is the conservation of
the person's wholeness. More specifically, the focus is on adaptation as
the process by which individuals maintain their wholeness or integrity.
Thus, the model emphasizes the effectiveness of the person's adaptations.
Furthermore, the Conservation Model focuses the nurse's attention on the

person and the complexity of his or her relationships with the internal and external environments. The model also emphasizes the nurse's responsibility for conservation of the patient's energy, as well as his or her structural, personal, and social integrity.

The source of threats to the person's wholeness or integrity is environmental challenge. Apparently, challenges may come from the internal or external environment. This interpretation of Levine's ideas is supported by the following comment:

> The exquisite internal balance responds constantly to the external forces. . . . There is an intimate relationship between the internal and the external environments, much of it vividly understood in recent years by research in physiological periodicity and the circadian cycles. (Levine, 1973, p. 8)

This interpretation is supported further by Levine's (1973) reference to positive feedback in the internal environment, which is manifested when pathological processes occur and can be responsible for pathology.

Interestingly, Levine (cited in Riehl-Sisca, 1989) apparently regarded the Conservation Model as an interaction model, and Riehl-Sisca (1989) classified it as such. The content of the model does not, however, address any of the characteristics of the category as described in this book. Certainly the Conservation Model deals with the interaction between person and environment, but this is not the same as the symbolic interactionism emphasis of the interaction category. When asked about the interaction classification, Levine (personal communication, August 13, 1987) agreed that her conceptual model does not reflect symbolic interactionism. She went on to say that hers is "an adaptation model."

Close examination of the content of the Conservation Model indicates that the systems approach is the appropriate classification. The characteristic of integration of parts is reflected in the following quotations.

> The total life process of the entire organism is dependent upon the inter-relatedness of its component systems. In fact, the organism is a system of systems. (Levine, 1973, pp. 8–9)

> Human life must be described in the language of "wholes." . . . perceiving the "wholes" depends upon recognizing the organization and interdependence of observable phenomena. (Levine, 1971, p. 255)

Other than her comment regarding the organism as a system of systems, Levine does not explicitly address the characteristic of system. Environment, however, is addressed repeatedly and is viewed as both internal and external. The relationship of the person to the environment is expressed clearly in the following statement: "The person cannot be described apart from the specific environment in which he or she is found" (Levine, 1989b, p. 325). Levine (1973) related the idea of "wholeness" to that of the open system. Citing Erikson (1968), she stated that a whole is an open system and explained, "The unceasing interaction of the individual organism with its environments does represent an 'open and fluid' system" (p. 11).

The characteristic of boundary is explicitly addressed in the Conservation Model in the discussion of individual territoriality. Levine (1973) commented, "every individual requires space, and both the establishment of his personal boundaries and their defense are essential components of his behavior" (p. 459). Levine (1973) went on to cite Hall's (1966) work on human territorial behavior, with its identification of the intimate, personal distance, social distance, and public distance zones maintained between people.

The systems model characteristic of tension, stress, strain, and conflict is alluded to by Levine in her discussion of adaptation. She stated:

> Change is characteristic of life, and adaptation is the method of change. The organism retains its integrity in both the internal and external environment through its adaptive capability. Adaptation is the process of change whereby the individual retains his integrity within the realities of his environments. (Levine, 1973, pp. 10–11)

Levine's (1989b) use of the term environmental challenge suggests that this is what represents the factors or forces that are responsible for initiating change and adaptation.

Levine (1973) referred to the characteristic of steady state when she discussed homeorrhesis. This term denotes "a stabilized flow, rather than a static state" (p. 7). Levine (1973) commented, "The concept of stabilized flow more accurately reflects the reality of daily change as well as the alterations in physiological activity that characterize the processes of growth and development" (pp. 7–8). In her recent work, however, Levine (1989b, 1991) seemed to favor homeostasis as the best descriptor of internal environment, regarding it as a state that "provides the necessary baselines for a multitude of synchronized physiological and psychological factors," (1989b, p. 329) rather than a system of balance and quiescence. In fact, Levine (personal communication, August 13, 1987) indicated that homeostasis is the appropriate view of the internal environment because it captures the notion of the congruence of the person with the environment.

The characteristic of feedback is addressed in the Conservation Model in terms of physiological and pathological processes. In keeping with systems models, Levine (1973, 1989b) associated negative feedback with autoregulation of physiological systems and positive feedback with disruption of function seen in pathological processes.

Meleis (1991) regarded the Conservation Model as a prominent example of the outcome category of models. She also placed the Conservation Model in her nursing therapeutics category, noting that Levine's work focuses on nursing activities and actions designed to care for people. Marriner-Tomey (1989) placed the Conservation Model within her energy fields category. Barnum (1994) classified the Conservation Model in the conservation category.

Content of the Model: Concepts

Person

The Conservation Model focuses on the individual person, described as a **holistic being**. Citing Erikson's (1964) definition of **wholeness**, Levine (1969b) stated, "From the moment of birth until the instant of death, every individual cherishes and defends his 'wholeness' " (p. 93). In fact, "the experience of wholeness is the foundation of all human enterprise" (Levine, 1991, p. 3).

Levine (1973, 1989b) pointed out that Erikson's definition of wholeness emphasizes the mutuality between diversified functions and parts within an entirety. This definition also maintains that the boundaries between parts are open and fluid, such that the parts "have a yearning for each other" (Levine, 1978a).

Wholeness, according to Levine (1989b),

> can be used as a starting point of analysis only if it can be converted into manageable parts . . . but none of the isolated aspects of wholeness can have meaning outside of the context within which the individual experiences his or her life. . . . Only then are the "open and fluid" boundaries established. (pp. 325–326)

Wholeness is the equivalent of integrity. "Integrity," Levine (1990) explained, "is having the freedom to choose: to move without constraint, as slowly or as swiftly as desired, and to exercise decisions on all matters —trivial and otherwise—without apology, indebtedness, or guilt. Integrity is the experience of life, the sensations of the body and its limbs, the sensory recording of every place and time on the mind and in the spirit" (p. 193).

Levine (1973) further described the person as an organism that is a system of systems. She stated:

> The total life process of the entire organism is dependent upon the inter-relatedness of its component systems. In fact, the organism is a system of systems, and in its wholeness expresses the organization of all the contributing parts. (pp. 8–9)

Levine (1973) characterized the life process as unceasing **change** that has direction, purpose, and meaning. She explained:

> The organism represents a pattern of orderly, sequential change. Because it is both ordered and sequential, the pattern is a message. So long as the pattern is consistent, it is also understandable. . . . The change which supports the well-being of the organism can be predicted, measured, and observed, and therefore is a cogent message. (pp. 9–10)

According to Levine (1973), change occurs through **adaptation**. She explained, "The organism retains its integrity in both the internal and external environment through its adaptive capability" (p. 10). She went on to say:

> Adaptation is the process of change whereby the individual retains his integrity within the realities of his environments. Adaptation is basic to survival, and it is an expression of the integration of the entire organism. (pp. 10–11)

In fact, Levine (1989b) maintained that "the life process *is* the process of adaptation" (p. 326).

Further discussion of the person and adaptation within the context of the Conservation Model requires consideration of the relationship between the person and the environment. The next section focuses on Levine's view of environment. It is followed by consideration of the person-environment relationship and additional discussion of adaptation.

Environment

Levine referred to an **internal environment** and an **external environment**. She maintained that "the integrated response of the individual aris[es] from the internal environment" (Levine, 1973, p. 12). Drawing on the concept of the "milieu interne" that Claude Bernard discussed in the late nineteenth century, Levine (1973) explained:

> Bernard identified the primordial seas, captured within the integument of the human body and providing the organism with a tightly regulated solution of substances essential to its continuing well-being. . . . Man carried the essentials with him, safely packaged inside his skin. But it was apparent to Bernard, and to the army of investigators who followed him, that the internal environment was susceptible to constant change. (p. 7)

Levine (1973) traced the further development of the concept of internal environment to Cannon's (1939) formulation of *homeostasis* and finally to Waddington's (1968) idea of *homeorrhesis*. More specifically, Levine (1991) explained:

> Every successful living organism has the ability to select from the environment those elements that are essential to its welfare and to exclude those that are repetitive, harmful, or inconsequential. As Bernard (1957) and earlier Cannon (1939) emphasized, the organism must possess the ability to stabilize its internal environment in the face of the uncontrolled factors it may confront in its external environment. Such activity, resulting in the safety and well-being of the individual, was described as a stable state, or *homeostasis*. Waddington (1968) suggested, instead, the term *homeor[r]hesis* to emphasize the constant fluid and changing character of the *milieu interne*. (p. 5)

Homeostasis, maintained Levine (1989b), should not be viewed as a system of balance and quiescence but rather as "a state of energy-sparing that also provides the necessary baselines for a multitude of synchronized physiological and psychological factors" (p. 329). Levine (personal communication, August 13, 1987) explained that homeostatis reflects congruence of the person with the environment.

Homeorrhesis, as described by Levine (1973), is

> a stabilized flow rather than a static state. Such a concept emphasizes the fluidity of change within a space-time continuum and more nearly describes the remarkable patterns of adaptation which permit the individual's body to sustain its well-being within the vast changes which encroach upon it from the environment. (p. 7)

The internal environment is subject to continuous change from the challenges of the external environment, which always are a form of energy. The maintenance of the integration of bodily functions in the face of these changes depends on multiple negative feedback loops, which are control mechanisms that result in autoregulation of the internal environment (Levine, 1973). Collective synchronization of multiple negative feedback loops is accomplished through homeostasis and "creates the 'stable state' of the internal environment" (Levine, 1989b, p. 329).

Levine (1973) rejected the "simplistic view of the external environment [as] a kind of stage setting against which the individual plays out his life" (p. 12). In other words, the external environment "is not a drop on a stage where life events are acted" (Levine, 1990, p. 196). Rather, Levine adopted Bates' (1967) formulation of external environment as *perceptual, operational,* and *conceptual.*

The *perceptual environment* encompasses "that portion of the environment to which the individual responds with his sense organs" (Levine, 1973, p. 12). It includes "those factors which can be recorded on the sensory system—the energies of light, sound, touch, temperature, and chemical change that is smelled or tasted, as well as position sense and balance" (Levine, 1989b, p. 326). Levine (1971) pointed out that the person "is not a passive recipient of sensory input. [Rather], he seeks, selects, and tests information from the environment in the context of his definition of himself, and so constantly defends his safety, his identity, and in a larger sense, his purpose" (p. 262).

The *operational environment* is "that which interacts with living tissues even though the individual does not possess sensory organs that can record the presence of these external factors" (Levine, 1989b, p. 326). Thus, the operational environment is not directly perceived by the individual. It encompasses "every unseen and unheard aspect of the individual's life-space [including] all forms of radiation, microorganisms, [and] pollutants that are odorless and colorless" (Levine, 1989b, p. 326). Although that aspect of the environment cannot be apprehended by the senses or anticipated symbolically, it is of vital concern because of its potential danger to the well-being of the individual (Levine, 1971).

The *conceptual environment* is "the environment of language, ideas, symbols, concepts, and invention" (Levine, 1989b, p. 326). It encompasses "the exchange of language, the ability to think and to experience emotion . . . value systems, religious beliefs, ethnic and cultural traditions, and the individual psychological patterns that come from life experiences" (Levine, 1973, p. 12). That aspect of the environment takes into account the fact that "human beings are sentient, thinking, future-oriented and past-aware individuals" (Levine, 1989b, p. 326).

Levine (1973) mentioned the importance of both internal and external environments and noted that the interface between the two is involved in the person's adaptation. She explained:

> Separate consideration of either the internal or external environments can provide only a partial view of the complex interaction that is taking place between them. It is, in fact, at the interface where the exchange between internal and external environments occurs that the determinants for nursing interventions are found. In this broader sense, all adaptations represent the accommodation that is possible between the internal and external environments. (p. 12)

Person and Environment

The Conservation Model "emphasizes that the environment is not a passive stage setting, but rather that the person is an active participant, exploring, seeking, and testing understanding of the world he or she inhabits. The nurse cannot enter another person's environment without becoming an essential factor in it" (Levine, 1992, p. 41).

Moreover, Levine (1989b) maintained that the person is not separate from the environment. She stated, "The person cannot be described apart from the specific environment in which he or she is found. The precise environment necessarily completes the wholeness of the individual" (p. 325). Levine further stated:

> The interaction at the interface between individual and environment is an orderly, sometimes predictable, but always a limited process. The consequence of the interaction is invariably the product of the characteristics of the living individual *and* the external factors. . . . The *process* of the interaction is *adaptation*. (p. 326)

Levine (1989b) explained that adaptation can be thought of as a way in which the person and the environment become congruent over time or as the fit of the person with his or her "predicament of time and space" (p. 326). Indeed, "the ability of every individual not only to survive but to flourish is a consequence of the competence of the person's interactions with the environments in which he or she functions" (Levine, 1991, pp. 4–5).

Adaptation is characterized by history, specificity, and redundancy. The fundamental nature of adaptation is "a consequence of a historical progression: the evolution of the species through time, reflecting the sequence of change in the genetic patterns that have recorded the change in the historical environments" (Levine, 1989b, p. 327).

The specificity of adaptation is exemplified by the synchronized tasks of body systems. In particular, each body system has specific tasks involving biochemical changes in response to environmental challenges. Although the tasks are specific, they are synchronized with each other and serve the individual as a whole. Specificity in biochemistry is dependent upon sequential change that occurs in cascades. The cascade "is characterized by the intermingling of the steps with each other — the precursor is not entirely exhausted when the intermediate forms develop and the final stage is congruent with the steps that precede it" (Levine, 1989b, p. 328).

Levine (1989b) explained that the cascade of adaptations is characterized by redundancy, which refers to the series of wave-like adaptive responses that are available to the individual when environmental challenges arise. Examples of redundancy in adaptation include the "ubiquitous . . . 'fail-safe' options in the anatomy, physiology, and psychology of individuals" (Levine, 1991, p. 6). Some redundant systems respond instantly to threatened shifts in physiological parameters. Others are corrective and utilize the time interval provided by the instantaneous response to correct imbalances. Still other redundant systems function by reestablishing a previously failed response.

Redundancy is also seen in four levels of **organismic responses** to environmental challenges. These responses are considered to be "coexistent in a single individual, and in fact, often influence each other. They represent, however, an assembly of parts which have indeed entered into fruitful association and organization. Together they permit the person to protect and maintain his integrity as an individual" (Levine, 1969b, (p. 98).

Levine (1989b) pointed out that because the responses are redundant, "they do not follow one another in a prescribed sequence, but are integrated in individuals by their cognitive abilities, the wealth of their previous experience, their ability to define their relationships to the events and the strengths of their adaptive capabilities" (p. 330). She further noted that although some responses can be considered physiological and some, behavioral, "the integration of living processes argues that they are one and the same — not merely parallel and not merely simultaneous — but essential portions of the same activity" (p. 330).

The most primitive level of organismic response is the *fight or flight mechanism*. That adrenocortical-sympathetic reaction is an instantaneous response to a real or imagined threat. The fight or flight mechanism swiftly provides a condition of physiological and behavioral readiness for sudden and unexplained environmental challenges.

The second level is the *inflammatory-immune response*. This response to injury is important for maintenance of structural continuity and promotion of healing. It "assures restoration of physical wholeness and the expectation of complete healing" (Levine, 1989b, p. 330).

The third level is the *stress response*. Drawing from Selye's (1956) description of stress, Levine (1989b) stated that this response is "recorded over time and is influenced by the accumulated experience of the individual" (p. 330).

The fourth level of organismic response is *perceptual awareness*, as mediated through the sense organs. Perceptual awareness is concerned with gathering information from the environment and converting it to meaningful experience (Levine, 1969b, 1989b). "The human being," Levine (1973) explained, "is a sentient being, and the ability to interact with the environment seems ineluctably tied to his sensory organs" (p. 446). Drawing upon Gibson's (1966) formulation of perceptual systems to explain the mediation of behavior by sensory organs, Levine (1969b) commented, "Individual identity arises out of information received through these intact and functional perceptual systems" (p. 97).

Gibson (1966) proposed five perceptual systems. The basic orienting system provides a general orientation to the environment and is essential to the function of the other perceptual systems. The anatomical organ of that system is the balancing portion of the inner ear, which responds to changes in gravity, acceleration, and movement. The visual system permits the person to look, and the auditory system permits listening to sounds as well as identifying the direction from which they are coming. The haptic system responds to touch through reception of sensations by the skin, joints, and muscles. The taste-smell system provides information about chemical stimuli and facilitates safe nourishment (Levine, 1969b, 1973). Levine (1989b) pointed out that for Gibson, "individuals do not merely 'see'—they *look*; they do not merely 'hear'—they *listen*. Thus equipped with the ability to select information from the environment, the individual is an active, seeking participant in it—not merely reacting but influencing, changing, and creating the parameters of his or her life" (p. 330).

The product of adaptation, according to Levine (1989b), is **conservation**. She explained, "Survival depends on the adaptive ability to use responses that *cost the least* to the individual in expense of effort and demand on his or her well-being. That is, of course, the essence of *conservation*" (p. 329).

Levine (1990) regards conservation as "a universal concept" (p. 192). She explained:

> Conservation describes the way complex systems are able to continue to function even when severely challenged. They sustain them-

selves, not only in the face of immediate disruptive threats, but in such a way as to assure the vitality of future responses. This work is accomplished in the most economic way possible. . . . The . . . process of conservation is characteristic of the way that physiological functions are regulated in the body. Negative feedback is activated when something needs to be adjusted, but is quiescent otherwise. Conservation defends the wholeness of living systems by ensuring their ability to confront change appropriately and retain their unique identity. (p. 192)

Levine (1989b, 1991) has linked conservation to both homeostasis and homeorrhesis. With regard to homeostasis, she maintained, "Conservation is clearly the consequence of the multiple, interacting, and synchronized negative feedback systems that provide for the stability of the living organism. . . . [Indeed,] homeostasis might be called the state of conservation." (1989b, p. 329). Speaking of the link between homeorrhesis and conservation, she claimed, "Homeor[r]hesis . . . [is] a consequence of conservation: the frugal, economic, contained, and controlled use of environmental resources by the individual organism in his or her best interest. This is the achievement of adaptation" (1991, p. 5).

Levine (1991) pointed out that "every self-sustaining system monitors its own behavior by conserving the use of resources required to define its unique identity" (p. 4). The ultimate purpose of conservation is "to defend, sustain, maintain, and define the integrity of the system for which it functions" (p. 3). Indeed, conservation is the "guardian activity that defends and protects [wholeness, which is] the universal target of selfhood" (p. 4).

Health

"Inherent in the life experience," Levine (1991) maintained, "is a state of being described as 'health' . . . and . . . every individual defines health for himself or herself" (p. 4). Levine (1973, 1984a) characterized **health and disease as patterns of adaptive change**. She commented that adaptation is not an all or none process; rather, it is a matter of degree — some adaptations are successful and some are not; some work and some do not. There are, however, no maladaptations. Thus, adaptation has no value attached to it; it just is. Levine (1973) went on to explain:

The measure of effective adaptation is compatibility with life. A poor adaptation may threaten life itself, but at the same time the degree of adaptive potential available to the individual may be sufficient to maintain life at a different level of effectiveness. . . . All the processes of living are processes of adaptation. Survival itself depends upon the quality of the adaptation possible for the individual. (p. 11)

Levine (1989b) further explained, "The most successful adaptations are those that best fit the organism in its environment. A 'best fit' is accomplished with the least expenditure of effort, and with sufficient protective devices built in so that the goal is achieved in as economic and expeditious a manner as possible" (p. 330). In so saying, Levine clearly linked conservation to the health state of the person. In fact, "The goal of conservation is health" (Levine, 1990, p. 193). Levine (1991) went on to explain that "conservation of the integrity of the person is essential to assuring health, and providing the strength to confront disability. Indeed, the importance of conservation in the treatment of illness is precisely focused on the reclamation of wholeness, of health" (p. 3).

Levine (1990) underscored the importance of conservation to health in the following comment:

> The environment is not always "user-friendly." Successful engagement with the environment depends upon the individual's repertoire — that store of adaptations which is either built into the genes or achieved through life experience. While there are redundant or back-up systems that offer options when the initial response is insufficient, health and safety are products of a competent conservation. (p. 193)

Levine (1991) pointed out that health, whole, and healing all share the same root. She explained:

> Healing is the avenue of return to the daily activities compromised by ill health. It is not only the insult or injury that is repaired — but the person himself or herself as whole and healing. Indeed, the expectation that healing will restore the conditions that existed before the intrusion persists even in situations where the therapeutic outcome leaves a loss of function or effectiveness. It is not merely the healing of an afflicted part. It is, rather, a return to selfhood, where the encroachment of the disability can be set aside entirely, and the individual is free to pursue once more his or her own interests without constraint. (p. 4)

Levine (1984b) indicated that she does not like the term *wellness* and prefers the word *healthy*. It may be inferred from her description of health as "wholeness" (Levine, 1973, p. 11) and as "successful adaptation" (Levine, 1966a, p. 2452) that she used the term health to mean wellness.

It also may be inferred that wellness means social well-being. This inference is supported by the following statement: "One criterion of successful adaptation is the attainment of social well-being, but there is tremendous variation in the degree to which this is achieved" (Levine, 1966a, p. 2452). Indeed, Levine (1984b) has stated that health is socially defined in the sense of "Do I continue to function in a reasonably normal fashion?"

Levine used Wolf's (1961) concept of disease as adaptation to noxious environmental forces for her description of illness. She explained, "disease represents efforts of the individual to protect his integrity" (Levine, 1971, p. 257). In the same vein, Levine (1991) noted that inasmuch as "illness challenges the integrity of the person, defending his health — his unique wholeness — is a continuing endeavor" (p. 4).

Disease, for Levine, is undisciplined and unregulated change, a disruption in the orderly sequential pattern of change that is characteristic of life. This anarchy of pattern may not be successful in supporting life. Levine (1973) maintained that "Such anarchy, in fact, occurs in disease processes, and unless the pattern can be restored, the organism will die" (p. 9).

The anarchy of disease processes is a positive feedback mechanism. Levine (1973) noted that positive feedback "results in an increasing rate of function without the regulatory control that restores balance. Thus a 'vicious cycle' is instituted which produces more and more disruption of function" (p. 10).

Levine (1973) pointed out that individuals acknowledge illness through their perceptual systems. She stated:

> Physical well-being is dependent upon an experienced body which is communicating the "right" signals. The constancy of awareness of the internal feeling of the body is the baseline against which well-being is measured. . . . Individuals can acknowledge "illness" only in recognizing an alteration in their perception of internal feelings. (p. 456)

Levine's description of health indicates that she conceptualized that concept as a continuum. This interpretation is supported by the following comment:

> Adaptation . . . is susceptible to an infinite range within the limits of life compatibility. Within that range, there are numerous possible degrees of adaptation. Thus, the dynamic processes establishing balance along the continuum are adaptations. (Levine, 1973, p. 11)

Nursing

Levine (1973) described nursing as a human interaction. "It is a discipline rooted in the organic dependency of the individual human being on his relationships with other human beings" (p. 1). She further described nursing as "a subculture, possessing ideas and values which are unique to nurses, even though they mirror the social template which created them" (p. 3).

The **goal of nursing**, according to Levine (1984a), is the *promotion of wholeness for all people, well or sick.* She maintained:

> The goal of all nursing care should be to promote wholeness, realizing that for every individual that requires a unique and separate cluster of activities. The individual's integrity—his one-ness, his identity as an individual, his wholeness—is his abiding concern, and it is the nurse's responsibility to assist him to defend and to seek its realization. (Levine, 1971, p. 258)

The nursing process of the Conservation Model is conservation. Levine (1989b) defined conservation as "keeping together" and stated that conversation—the "keeping together" function—should be the major guideline for all nursing intervention (p. 331). Indeed, "every nursing act is dedicated to the conservation or the 'keeping together' of the wholeness of the individual" (Levine, 1991, p. 3).

Levine (1973) emphasized the roles of both nurse and patient in conservation, as illustrated in the following statement.

> "To keep together" means to maintain a proper balance between active nursing intervention coupled with patient participation on the one hand and the safe limits of the patient's ability to participate on the other. (p. 13)

In fact, Levine (1984b) stated that she regards patients as partners or participants in nursing care. As elaborated previously in the section on philosophical claims, Levine views the person who is a patient as being temporarily dependent on the nurse. The nurse's goal is to end the dependence, that is, the person's patient status, as quickly as possible. Levine (1989b) noted that as part of the patient's environment, the nurse brings to the nursing care situations his or her "own cascading repertoire of skill, knowledge, and compassion. It is a shared enterprise and each participant is rewarded" (p. 336).

Although Levine did not identify an explicit nursing process, it is possible to extract a format from several of her publications. The process, which Levine (1966b) regards as a "scientific approach in the determination of nursing care" (p. 57), consists of three major phases: **trophicognosis**, **intervention**, and **evaluation**.

Trophicognosis, which is defined as "a nursing care judgment arrived at by the scientific method" (Levine, 1966b, p. 57), is presented as an alternative to nursing diagnosis. Tracing the development of nursing diagnosis and its legal interpretation, Levine (1966b) pointed out that the term always referred to "diagnosis of disease made by a nurse" (p. 55). Then, citing the only dictionary definition of diagnosis, she maintained that it is "incorrect to use the term diagnosis as a synonym for observations, judgments, problems, needs or assessments" (pp. 56–57). In concluding her argument, Levine stated:

> Because the term, nursing diagnosis, is now susceptible of legal interpretation, and other usages of the term are semantically incorrect, it is proposed that a new nursing term be used to describe the scientific approach in the determination of nursing care. Such a method of ascribing nursing care needs may be called trophicognosis. (p. 57)

Citing Feiblemann's (1959) description of the scientific method, Levine (1966b) explained that the first step in trophicognosis is *observation*. Observations that are relevant to the formulation of a trophicognosis focus on data that will influence nursing care rather than medical care. Levine (1966b) noted:

> The development of a trophicognosis requires a reorientation in the selection of data because the information required to project nursing care needs differs somewhat from the kind of information required to

direct medical therapy. Although nurses are exhorted to observe from the first day of clinical practice, the focus of attention is almost invariably on collecting data for the physician's use. Too infrequently does the nurse observe with the primary purpose of illuminating her own role in the care of the patient. And yet the nurse does have responsibilities to the patient which she does not share with the physician. Thus her observations may be primarily useful to the physician, primarily useful to the nurse, or useful in some degree to both. In selecting observations to be used to construct the trophicognosis, emphasis should be placed on those which influence nursing care. (p. 58)

Levine (1966b) went on to say that "By its very nature, nursing responsibility involves gathering data which includes all the information available from every source involved in the care of the patient, including medical and paramedical information as well as that data which is specifically and uniquely the province of the nurse herself" (p. 58).

Observations result in the next step, which is the awareness of provocative facts, which in turn leads to the third step, construction of a testable hypothesis. The hypothesis represents the trophicognosis. Summarizing the trophicognosis phase of the nursing process, Levine (1966b) stated, "In developing the trophicognosis, the observations and assembled data provide the 'provocative facts.' The testable hypothesis formulated on the basis of strength of this information is the trophicognosis" (pp. 57–58).

The elements of trophicognosis are listed in Table 5–1. Levine (personal communication, August 13, 1987) stated that she and her colleagues are developing a taxonomy of trophicognoses. To date, no presentations or publications have given any details of the taxonomy, although Schaefer (1991b), citing a personal communication (September 21, 1989), reported that Levine "supports the development of [trophicognoses] from the clustering of provocative facts that recur in practice and become the focus of nursing intervention" (p. 221).

The trophicognosis forms the basis for the second phase of the nursing process, **intervention**, or **action**. Nursing intervention may be therapeutic or supportive. Levine (1973) explained:

> When nursing intervention influences adaptation favorably, or toward renewed social well-being, then the nurse is acting in a therapeutic sense. When nursing intervention cannot alter the course of the adaptation—when her best efforts can only maintain the status quo or fail to halt a downward course—then the nurse is acting in a supportive sense. (p. 13)

According to Levine (1973), "nursing intervention must be designed so that it fosters successful adaptation whenever possible" (p. 13). Thus, nursing must view individuals so that the best fit available to each person can be sustained (Levine, 1989b). Interestingly, however, adaptation is impossible to measure or quantify. Levine (1991) explained, "While certain, generalized adaptations can be described—the required oxygen

TABLE 5 - 1. **ELEMENTS OF TROPHICOGNOSIS**

I. Establishing an objective and scientific rationale for nursing care
    A. Basis for implementation of prescribed medical regime
        1. Knowledge and understanding of the medical diagnosis
        2. Evaluation of the medical history with specific reference to areas influencing the nursing care plan
        3. Knowledge of laboratory and x-ray reports emphasizing factors that influence nursing care
        4. Consultation with physician to share information and clarify nursing care decisions
        5. Knowledge of aspects of prescribed medical regime (expected and untoward effects) as contributing to the evaluation of the effectiveness of the therapy
    B. Basis for implementation of prescribed paramedical regime
        1. Knowledge of paramedical diagnoses and prescriptions for care
        2. Clear definition of nurse's role in paramedical prescriptions
    C. Determination of nursing processes demanded by medical treatment
        1. Observation of effects of prescribed medical aspects of patient's care on individual progress
        2. Adaptation of nursing techniques to the unique cluster of needs demonstrated in the individual patient
    D. Basis for implementation of the unique nursing needs of the individual patient
        1. Knowledge and understanding of the principles of nursing science
        2. Provision for gathering a nursing history with specific reference to aspects that will influence the nursing care plan
        3. Accurate recording and transmittal of observations and evaluation of patient's response to nursing processes
        4. Utilization of knowledge gained in consultation with family members or other individuals concerned with the patient including the religious counselor
II. Implementation of nursing care within the structure of administrative policy, availability of equipment, and established standards of nursing care

From Levine, M.E. (1966b). Trophicognosis: An alternative to nursing diagnosis. In *American Nurses' Association regional clinical conference* (Vol. 2, pp. 59–60). New York: American Nurses' Association, with permission.

tension, [the] temperature tolerance of living cells, the effect of atmospheric pressure on physiological function, as examples — precise identification of the adaptive condition is not [yet] possible" (pp. 6–7). Inasmuch as adaptation cannot be directly observed, the goal of nursing intervention, Levine (1991) maintained, "must be on the consequences of care rather than on algorithms designed to display the adaptive patterns. . . . The research necessary to describe adaptation patterns and the therapeutic interventions that will support them has yet to be done" (p. 7).

Nursing intervention is structured according to four **conservation principles**: *conservation of energy, conservation of structural integrity, conservation of personal integrity,* and *conservation of social integrity.*

Conservation of energy, according to Levine (1988b), "refers to balancing energy output and energy input to avoid excessive fatigue, that is, adequate rest, nutrition, and exercise" (p. 227). Levine (1989b) explained that the conservation of energy is a natural law "found to hold everywhere in the universe for all animate and inanimate entities" (p. 331). Energy, according to Levine (1991), is not directly observable, although "the consequences of its exchange are predictable, manageable, and quantifiable. Instruments can monitor, measure, produce or capture energy" (p. 7). Examples of energy parameters of concern to nurses include body temperature; pulse, respiratory, and metabolic rates; blood gases; and blood pressure. There are, Levine (1991) maintained, finite sources of energy available to the person. Conservation of energy assures that "energy is spent carefully with essential priorities served first" (p. 7). Although individuals conserve their energy, the energy from life-sustaining activities, such as biochemical changes, is expended even at perfect rest. Levine (1989b) commented, "The conservation of energy is clearly evident in the very sick, whose lethargy, withdrawal, and self-concern are manifested while, in its wisdom, the body is spending its energy resource on the processes of healing" (p. 332).

Conservation of structural integrity focuses on the person's ability to move and choose activities freely. More specifically, this principle of conservation "refers to maintaining or restoring the structure of the body, that is, preventing physical breakdown and promoting healing" (Levine, 1988b, p. 227). Levine pointed out that we expect and have confidence in the ability of our bodies to heal. Healing, according to Levine (1989b), "is the defense of wholeness . . . [and] a consequence of an effective immune system" (p. 333). Conservation of structural integrity "emphasizes that the individual's defense[s] against the hazards of the environment are achieved with the most economical expense of effort" (Levine, 1991, p. 8). It results in repair and healing to sustain the wholeness of structure and function" (Levine, 1991, p. 7).

Conservation of personal integrity underscores the fact that "every individual defends his unique personhood, the individual within known as the 'self.' Wholeness is summarized in that knowledge [of self]" (Levine, 1991, p. 8). This conservation principle, then, focuses on "the maintenance or restoration of the patient's sense of identity, self-worth, and acknowledgement of uniqueness" (Levine, 1988b, p. 227). The self, according to Levine (1989b), is "much more than a physical experience of the whole body, although it is unquestionably a part of that awareness" (p. 334). Personal integrity emphasizes individuals' perseverance in retaining their identities. "Everyone seeks to defend his or her identity as a self, in both that hidden, intensely private person that dwells within and in the public faces assumed as individuals move through their relationships with others" (Levine, 1989b, p. 334).

Conservation of social integrity, Levine (1988b) noted, "refers to the acknowledgment of the patient as a social being. It involves the recognition and presentation of human interaction, particularly with the patient's significant others" (p. 227). That conservation principle emphasizes the fact that "selfhood needs definition beyond the individual . . . [and that] the individual is created by the environment and in turn creates within it" (Levine, 1989b, p. 335). The principle states that each individual's identity places him or her "in a family, a community, a cultural heritage, a religious belief, a socioeconomic slot, an educational background, a vocational choice" (Levine, 1989b, p. 335). Social context is a necessity of wholeness. Indeed, Levine (1991) maintained that "it is impossible to acknowledge the wholeness of the individual without placing him into his social context" (p. 9).

Levine (1988b) noted that the four conservation principles "apply equally to living things, and the derivative meaning of 'conservation' as a 'keeping together' function seemed entirely appropriate as the essential goal of nursing care" (p. 227). She also pointed out that the conservation principles do not operate singly but rather are "joined within the individual as a cascade of life events, churning and changing as the environmental challenge is confronted and resolved in each individual's unique way" (Levine, 1989b, p. 336). The integration of conservation principles is exemplified in the following quotation:

> The conservation principles address the integrity of the individual . . . from birth to death. Every activity requires an energy supply because nothing works without it. Every activity must respect the structural wholeness of the individual because well-being depends upon it. Every activity is chosen out of the abilities, life experience and desires of the "self" who makes the choices. Every activity is a product of the dynamic social systems to which the individual belongs. (Levine, 1991, p. 10)

Use of the four conservation principles is outlined in Table 5–2.

The nursing process phase of **evaluation** can be inferred from Levine's (1966b) discussion of revisions in the trophicognosis. She commented:

> Like any hypothesis, the trophicognosis is continually evaluated in the light of the results of the action, and revised and changed in response to new information signalling the necessity for change. In the very nature of the disease process, the daily flux of events causes a continuing pattern of change, and to adequately reflect the dynamics of the events the nurse is witnessing, the system used to design patient care must be equally susceptible to revision. (p. 58)

Content of the Model: Propositions

The propositions of the Conservation Model link the metaparadigm concepts of person, environment, health, and nursing. The person is

TABLE 5-2. **LEVINE'S CONSERVATION PRINCIPLES**

I. Principle of Conservation of Energy: Nursing intervention is based on the conservation of the individual patient's energy—balancing energy output and energy input by preventing excessive fatigue and promoting adequate rest, nutrition, and exercise
  A. Relevant scientific considerations
   1. The ability of the human body to perform work is dependent upon its energy balance—the supply of energy-producing nutrients measured against the rate of energy-using activities
   2. The energy required by alterations in physiological function during illness represents an additional demand made on the energy production systems
   3. Fatigue, often experienced with illness, is an empiric measure of the additional energy demand
  B. Nursing intervention
   1. General considerations
    a. Nursing intervention is based on the balancing of energy input with energy output
    b. Assessment of patient's ability to perform necessary activities without producing excessive fatigue
     (1) Vital signs
     (2) Patient's general condition
     (3) Patient's behavior
     (4) Patient's tolerance of nursing activities required by his or her condition
    c. Allowable activity for patient based on his or her energy resources
    d. Interventions designed to provide an adequate deposit of energy resource and regulate expenditure of energy
   2. Examples of specific interventions
    a. Provision for rest
    b. Maintenance of adequate nutrition
II. Principle of Conservation of Structural Integrity: Nursing intervention is based on the conservation of the individual patient's structural integrity—maintaining or restoring the structure of the body by preventing physical breakdown and promoting healing
  A. Relevant scientific considerations
   1. Structural change results in a change of function
   2. Pathophysiological processes present a threat to structural integrity
   3. Healing processes restore structural integrity
   4. Surgical procedures are designed to restore structural integrity
   5. Structural integrity is restored when the scar is organized and integrated in the continuity of the part affected
  B. Nursing intervention
   1. General considerations
    a. Limit amount of tissue involvement in infection and disease
    b. Prevent trophicogenic (nurse-induced) disease
   2. Examples of specific nursing interventions
    a. Anatomical positioning of patient
    b. Physiological positioning of patient
    c. Maintenance of patient's personal hygiene
    d. Assist patient with range of motion exercises and passive exercises
III. Principle of Conservation of Personal Integrity: Nursing intervention is based on the conservation of the patient's personal integrity—maintaining or restoring the patient's sense of identity, self-worth, and acknowledgment of uniqueness
  A. Relevant scientific considerations
   1. There is always a privacy to individual life
   2. Assumption of responsibility for one's own decisions develops with maturation

Continued

TABLE 5–2. **LEVINE'S CONSERVATION PRINCIPLES** (Continued)

3. Self-identity and self-respect are the foundations of a sense of personal integrity
4. Illness threatens self-identity and self-respect
5. Hospitalization may compound and exaggerate the threat to personal integrity
6. Individuals possess a lifetime commitment to the value systems and social patterns of their subcultural affiliations

  B. Nursing intervention

    1. General considerations

      a. Respect from the nurse is essential to the patient's self-respect
      b. Accept the patient the way he or she is
      c. Foster patient participation in decision making within safe limits
      d. Determine and take into account patient's moral and ethical values

    2. Examples of specific nursing interventions

      a. Recognize and protect patient's space needs
      b. Assure privacy during performance of body functions and therapeutic procedures
      c. Respect importance patient places on personal possessions
      d. Use appropriate mode of address when dealing with patient
      e. Support patient's defense mechanisms as appropriate

IV. Principle of Conservation of Social Integrity: Nursing intervention is based on the conservation of the individual patient's social integrity — acknowledging the patient as a social being

  A. Relevant scientific considerations

    1. The social integrity of individuals is tied to the viability of the entire social system
    2. Individual life has meaning only in the context of social life
    3. The way in which individuals relate to various social groups influences their behavior
    4. Individual recognition of wholeness is measured against relationships with others
    5. Interactions with others become more important in times of stress
    6. The patient's family may be deeply affected by the changes resulting from illness
    7. Hospitalization is characterized by isolation from family and friends

  B. Nursing intervention

    1. General considerations

      a. A failure to consider the patient's family and friends is a failure to provide excellent nursing care
      b. The social system of the hospital is artificial
      c. Concern for holistic well-being of individuals demands attention to community attitudes, resources, and provision of health care in the community
      d. The nurse-patient interaction is a social relationship which is disciplined and controlled by the professional role of the nurse

    2. Examples of specific nursing interventions

      a. Consider patients' social needs when placing them in the nursing unit
      b. Position patient in bed to foster social interaction with other patients
      c. Avoid sensory deprivation for the patient
      d. Promote the patient's use of newspapers, magazines, radio, and television as appropriate
      e. Provide family with knowledgeable support and assistance
      f. Teach family members to perform functions for the patient as necessary

Constructed from Levine, M.E. (1967). The four conservation principles of nursing. *Nursing Forum, 6,* 47–59; Levine, M.E. (1973). *Introduction to clinical nursing* (2nd ed., pp. 13–18). Philadelphia: FA Davis; and Levine, M.E. (1988). Myra Levine. In T.M. Schoor & A. Zimmerman, *Making choices. Taking chances: Nurse leaders tell their stories* (p. 227). St. Louis: CV Mosby.

repeatedly placed in the context of the environment, as illustrated in the following quotations:

> The individual is always within an environmental milieu, and the consequences of his awareness of his environment persistently influence his behavior at any given moment. (Levine, 1973, p. 444)

> [The person's] presence in the environment also influences it and thereby the kind of information available from it. (Levine, 1973, p. 446)

> The individual protects and defends himself within his environment by gaining all the information he can about it. (Levine, 1973, p. 451)

The linkages among all four metaparadigm concepts are stated in the following quotations.

> The nurse participates actively in every patient's environment, and much of what she does supports his adaptations as he struggles in the predicament of illness. (Levine, 1973, p. 13)

> But even in the presence of disease, the organism responds wholly to the environmental interaction in which it is involved, and a considerable element of nursing care is devoted to restoring the symmetry of response—symmetry that is essential to the well-being of the organism. (Levine, 1969b, p. 98)

EVALUATION OF LEVINE'S CONSERVATION MODEL

This section presents an evaluation of the Conservation Model. The evaluation is based on the results of the analysis of the model as well as on publications and presentations by Levine and by others who have used or commented on the Conservation Model.

Explication of Origins

Levine explicated the origins of the Conservation Model clearly and concisely, and she identified the motivation for development of the model. In addition, Levine articulated her philosophical claims in the form of a reasoned discussion of assumptions, beliefs, and values. Levine's presentation of the Conservation Model indicates that she values a holistic approach to the nursing care of all people, well or sick. She also values the unique individuality of each person, as noted in comments such as:

> Ultimately, decisions for nursing intervention must be based on the unique behavior of the individual patient. . . . A theory of nursing must recognize the importance of unique detail of care for a single patient within an empiric framework which successfully describes the requirements of all patients. (Levine, 1973, p. 6)

> Patient centered nursing care means individualized nursing care. It is predicated on the reality of common experience: every man is a

unique individual, and as such he requires a unique constellation of skills, techniques, and ideas designed specifically for him. (Levine, 1973, p. 23)

Furthermore, although Levine (1973) commented that human beings are dependent on their relationships with other human beings, she values the patient's participation in nursing care. This is attested to by the following comment.

"To keep together" means to maintain a proper balance between active nursing intervention coupled with patient participation on the one hand and the safe limits of the patient's ability to participate on the other. (p. 13)

Levine carefully cited the many scholars and scientists from nursing and adjunctive disciplines whose work has influenced her thinking. Indeed, she has followed her own mandate to provide proper bibliographic references to influential works and to interpret those works accurately (Levine, 1988a).

Comprehensiveness of Content

The Conservation Model is sufficiently comprehensive with regard to depth of content. Levine's descriptions of the person, the environment, health, and nursing are comprehensive and essentially complete.

Clarity could, however, be enhanced with regard to the most appropriate description of the internal environment. Despite Levine's (personal communication, August 13, 1987) comment that homeostasis best reflects congruence of the person with the environment, she continues to imply that homeorrhesis is the more appropriate descriptor of the internal environment (Levine, 1989b, 1991).

Clarity could also be enhanced with regard to the assessment phase of the nursing process. Levine has never explicitly identified the parameters of nursing assessment. Many of the practice applications of the model, which are discussed in the following section on social utility, reflect use of the conservation principles as the framework for nursing assessment; some include the elements of the perceptual, operational, and conceptual environments as well. The levels of organismic response, which Schaefer (1991b) uses in the evaluation phase of the nursing process, could also be a part of the assessment phase.

Levine repeatedly emphasized the importance of deriving trophicognoses and interventions from scientific knowledge, as well as from the messages given by the patient. This is illustrated in the following quotations:

The modern nurse has available rich knowledge of human anatomy, physiology, and adaptability. (Levine, 1966a, p. 2453)

Ultimately, decisions for nursing intervention must be based on the unique behavior of the individual patient. It is the nurse's task to bring a body of scientific principles on which decisions depend into the precise situation which she shares with the patient. (Levine, 1966a, p. 2452)

The integrated response of the individual to any stimulus results in a realignment of his very substance, and in a sense this creates a message which others may learn to understand. Each message, in turn, is the result of observation, selection of relevant data, and assessment of the priorities demanded by such knowledge. . . . Understanding the message and responding to it accurately constitute the substance of nursing science. (Levine, 1967, pp. 46–47)

The dynamic nature of the nursing process is evident in Levine's (1973) statement that nursing care plans "must allow for progress and change and project into the future the patient's response to treatment" (p. 46), as well as in Levine's (1989b) description of nursing care as use of a "cascading repertoire of skill, knowledge, and compassion" (p. 326). Given Levine's explanation of cascades as nonlinear interacting and evolving processes, the nursing process clearly is dynamic.

Levine's explication of her own value system, with its emphasis on the patient's freedom to make decisions attest to her exceptional concern for ethical standards for nursing practice. This concern is evident in the following statements:

The wholeness which is part of our awareness of ourselves is shared best with others when no act diminishes another person, and no moment of indifference leaves him with less of himself. Every moment of moral injustice extracts a price from both patient and nurse, just as every moment of moral responsibility gives each strength to grow in his wholeness. (Levine, 1977, p. 849)

Nursing intervention must deal with the rights and privileges of the individual in tangible ways. . . . The emphasis on patient teaching recognizes the individual's right to be assisted in understanding the implications of his disease, his treatment, and his care. He must also be assured that his medical and social problems will remain privileged and confidential. (Levine, 1967, p. 54)

True conservation demands that the nurse accept the patient the way he is. (Levine, 1967, p. 55)

The propositions of the Conservation Model link all four metaparadigm concepts. In addition, the integral nature of the four conservation principles is clearly specified.

The Conservation Model is also sufficiently comprehensive in breadth of content. Levine has repeatedly and emphatically explained that her conceptual model is equally applicable for the nursing care of sick and healthy individuals. She stated:

> I have described energy conservation and the wholeness embodied
> in the integrity of structure, person, and society in broad terms in order
> to emphasize that the Conservation Principles are *not* limited only to the
> care of the sick in the hospital. I have borne the burden of that naive and
> foolish criticism for several years — ever since two misinformed gradu-
> ate students wrote a chapter in which they made clear they knew more
> about what was in my mind than I did (Esposito & Leonard, 1980). They
> chose my textbook of medical-surgical nursing, *Introduction to Clinical
> Nursing* (Levine, 1969[a], 1973) as the text from which to critique my
> work. That text . . . was begun in 1963. I was not writing a nursing
> theory. I was teaching medical-surgical nursing to students whose prac-
> tice was in a hospital. That is the way it was in the early 60s. (Levine,
> 1990, p. 195)

In fact, the Conservation Model represents a broad organizing framework "within which nursing practice in every environment can be anticipated, predicted, and performed. In acute care institutions, nursing
homes, clinics, and community health programs and in their management
and administration — everywhere nursing is essential — the rules of conservation and integrity hold" (Levine, 1990, p. 195).

Furthermore, the Conservation Model permits a focus on prevention
through the principle of social integrity (Levine, 1990). Schaefer (1991b)
maintained that the principle of social integrity "provides a basis for the
nurse to consider environmental factors that affect the patient and may
indeed be far removed from the immediate environment. It is within this
framework that nurses could consider more of the social, cultural, environmental, and political factors that might affect the human condition
and over which they could have some control" (p. 220).

The comprehensiveness of the breadth of the Conservation Model is
further supported by the direction it provides for nursing research, education, administration, and practice. Although all the rules are not explicit
in Levine's writings, many can be extracted from the focus and content of
the model and from the publications of nurses who have used the model.

The rules for research indicate that the phenomena to be studied are
the conservation principles. Levine (1991) noted that although a particular study might focus on one principle, all four principles must be considered. She stated, "The conservation principles may be addressed singly.
Indeed, research and scholarly study must focus on discrete issues. But
the integrity of the whole person cannot be violated. However narrowed
the study problem may be, the influence of all four conservation principles must be acknowledged, and the wholeness of the person sustained"
(p. 10). Other relevant phenomena are the various levels of organismic
response and the elements of the perceptual, operational, and conceptual
environments.

The problems to be studied are those dealing with the maintenance of
the individual's wholeness and the interface between the internal and
external environments of the person (Levine, 1978a). The purpose of

research is to identify nursing interventions that will "maintain whole-ness and support adaptation, given the unique predicament of the individual, the family, or both" (Schaefer, 1991b, p. 222) through conservation of energy, structural integrity, personal integrity, and social integrity (Schaefer, 1991d). Subjects can be healthy or sick in virtually any setting, ranging from homes to shelters for the homeless to ambulatory clinics to emergency departments to critical care units. Schaefer (1991d) maintained that research designed to study phenomena identified by the Conservation Model should combine qualitative and quantitative methodologies. She went on to identify the specific variables listed in Table 5–3 that represent each of the conservation principles at the middle-range theory level. In addition, Schaefer (1991d) noted that change, wholeness, and adaptation are variables that cross the four conservation principles.

Specific empirical indicators that measure all relevant variables in a manner that is consistent with the Conservation Model need to be identified. Schaefer (1991d) did, however, identify a question that could be used as an empirical indicator in Conservation Model–based qualitative studies. The question is: "How has this predicament (illness, life-style change, new baby, marriage, change in job) affected your normal life-style?" (p. 52). She maintained that that question "will help to identify those aspects of care that can be directed toward the whole person" (p. 52).

TABLE 5–3. **VARIABLES THAT REPRESENT THE CONSERVATION PRINCIPLES**

Conservation of Energy	Conservation of Structural Integrity	Conservation of Personal Integrity	Conservation of Social Integrity
Anxiety	White blood cell count	Loneliness	Socialization
Oxygen saturation	Healing (granulation tissue)	Boredom	Moral development
Blood glucose	Skin integrity	Helplessness	Group process
Pulse	Sedimentation rate	Fear	Interaction
Temperature	Body density	Self-esteem	Social isolation
Respirations	Muscle strength	Privacy	
Blood pressure	End-organ damage (renal	Listening	
Hemoglobin	function, liver function)	Empathy	
Hematocrit		Control	
Skin turgor		Meaning	
Fluid and electrolytes		Teaching	
Heat		Learning	
Energy exchange		Role	
Diarrhea		Self-concept	
Blood loss			
Body weight			
Wound drainage			

Adapted from Schaefer, K.M. (1991). Levine's conservation principles and research. In K.M. Schaefer & J.B. Pond (Eds.), *Levine's conservation model: A framework for nursing practice* (p. 52). Philadelphia: FA Davis.

Techniques for data analysis should be appropriate to the particular qualitative and quantitative methodologies used. Conservation Model–based research enhances understanding of factors and interventions that promote adaptation and the maintenance of wholeness (Schaefer, 1991d).

Some rules for nursing education can be extracted from the content of the Conservation Model and descriptions of nursing education programs based on the model. The conservation principles provide the distinctive focus for the curriculum. The purpose of nursing education is to "prepare the student for the practice of holistic nursing and for lifelong learning" (Grindley & Paradowski, 1991, p. 200). The content encompasses nursing courses that focus on the conservation principles, as well as those courses in such adjunctive disciplines as philosophy, the humanities, and the biological, behavioral, and social sciences that "emphasize modes of thought that focus on critical thinking and the ability to engage in analysis of concepts" (Grindley & Paradowski, 1991, p. 201).

A definitive rule for the sequence of content has not yet been formulated. Barnum (1994) offered two alternatives. One approach would be to develop separate, sequential courses for each of the four conservation principles. Another approach would be to organize the curriculum along the health-illness continuum and include appropriate content from all four conservation principles in each course. Nursing education can occur in a variety of settings. A rule regarding the specific characteristics of students remains to be developed. Schaefer (1991c) indicated that teaching-learning strategies should encourage students "to respond to their intuitive thoughts and to take the risks needed to be creative" (p. 210). She went on to identify specific techniques that foster those skills, including free association, in-class summaries of reactions to class discussions and required readings, videotapes of oral presentations, descriptions of responses to abstract art, and validating hypotheses in practice.

Rules for nursing administration also can be extracted from the Conservation Model. The distinctive focus and purpose of Conservation Model–based nursing services is the conservation of the patient's wholeness. More specifically, the goal of the clinical agency is to maintain "the integrity of the system and the integrity of the individuals who function within the system (the employees and the patients)" (Schaefer, 1991b, p. 223). Nursing personnel must understand that patients are in a temporary state of dependence and, therefore, must be committed to fostering the patient's freedom and encouraging decision making. Nursing services may be delivered in virtually any setting. Levine (1969b) indicated that the patient's perceptual system could serve as the basis for organization of hospital units. She explained that the patient's ability to receive information and interpret it must be taken into account, as well as territorial needs. The administrator is directed to identify "alternative strategies to promote adaptation of the organization for social good" (Schaefer, 1991b, p. 223). The four conservation principles can serve as a basis for specific management strategies and administrative policies. As Schaefer (1991b) explained,

> The conservation of energy focuses the administrator on productive issues, which have a direct effect on cost. *Structural* issues address the equipment (technology) and supplies, as well as human resources, needed for the organization to function in a cost-effective manner. *Personal* issues focus the administrator on the need to run an organization that considers the individual needs of the employee, measures to ensure job satisfaction, and the need for a management style (decentralized versus centralized; shared governance) that supports the human element of an organization. *Social* issues help focus the administrator on how well the organization is meeting the needs of the community or the social system, while at the same time considering the effect of the community and the social system on the organization. (pp. 222–223)

Rules for Conservation Model–based nursing practice are evident. The purpose of nursing practice is conservation of the patient's wholeness. More specifically, "every nursing act is dedicated to the conservation, or 'keeping together,' of the wholeness of the individual" (Levine, 1991, p. 3). Furthermore, "the practice of conservation in nursing is dedicated to providing the best possible health status available to the individual" (Levine, 1990, p. 198). Clinical problems encompass conditions of health and disability reflected in the four conservation principles. Levine (1990) explained, "Every patient displays some problems in each of the areas [that] the Conservation Principles describe. Concerns for energy conservation and structural, personal, and social integrity are always present—though one area may present a more demanding problem than another. These areas can be explored individually, but they cannot be separated from the person" (p. 199).

Nursing practice can occur in both ambulatory and inpatient settings. Legitimate recipients of nursing care are individuals who are sick and those who are healthy. In fact, the conservation principles "have implications for every nursing situation" (Levine, 1990, p. 199). More specifically, legitimate recipients of nursing care are "Individuals enter into a state of patienthood when they require the expert services that physicians and nurses can provide. The fundamental moral responsibility of patient care is the limitation and relief of suffering. Once individuals are restored, the dependent but willing partnership is dissolved. Their privacy restored to them, individuals cease to be patients" (Levine, 1989c, pp. 4–5). The nursing process associated with the Conservation Model involves formulation of a trophicognosis, implementation of interventions derived from the four conservation principles, and evaluation of the consequences of care. Schaefer (1991b) maintained that the success of nursing interventions "is measured by observing the patient's organismic response" (p. 222). Conservation Model–based nursing practice contributes to the well-being of individuals by promoting wholeness.

Logical Congruence

The Conservation Model is logically congruent. The content of the model flows directly from Levine's philosophical claims. The overriding world view is that of reciprocal interaction. There is no evidence of the reaction world view in the Conservation Model. In fact, Levine (1971) explicitly rejected mechanism, stating "The mechanistic view of the body and mind does little to restore to the individual the wholeness he recognizes in himself" (p. 254). Although Levine (1966a) stated that "The human being responds to the forces in his environment in a singular yet integrated fashion" (p. 2452), she successfully translated the mechanistic idea of reaction to the environment by bringing in the idea of a more holistic, integrated response. However, Levine did cite Selye's mechanistic approach to stress within her description of the levels of organismic response. This potential threat to the logical consistency of the Conservation Model could be eliminated by the selection of a formulation of the stress response that reflects the reciprocal interaction world view.

Generation of Theory

Levine (1978a) stated that she was trying to develop two theories, which she called Therapeutic Intention and Redundancy. Work on the **Theory of Therapeutic Intention** began in the early 1970s. Levine (personal communication to L. Criddle, July 22, 1987) indicated that she "was seeking a way of organizing nursing intervention growing out of the reality of the *biological* realities which nurses had to confront." Her thinking about therapeutic intention is summarized in the following statements, which describe broad areas of therapeutic intervention and create parameters of nursing intervention.

1. Therapeutic regimens that support the integrated healing processes of the body and permit optimal restoration of structure and function through natural response to disease.

2. Therapeutic regimens that substitute an external servomechanism for a failure of autoregulation of an essential integrating system.

3. Therapeutic regimens that focus on specific causes, and by surgical restructuring or drug therapy, restore individual integrity and well-being.

4. Therapeutic regimens that cannot alter or substitute for the pathology so that only supportive measures are possible to promote comfort and humane concern.

5. Therapeutic regimens that balance a significant toxic risk against the threat of the disease process.

6. Therapeutic regimens that simulate physiological processes and reinforce or antagonize usual responses in order to create a therapeutic change in function.

7. Therapeutic regimens that provide manipulation of diet and activity to correct metabolic imbalances related to nutrition and/or exercise. (Levine, personal communication to L. Criddle, July 22, 1987)

Levine (personal communication, August 13, 1987) regarded the seven areas of therapeutic intention as an "imperfect list that is not yet complete."

Although the Theory of Therapeutic Intention seems to extend the nursing process component of the Conservation Model, Levine (personal communication to L. Criddle, July 22, 1987) stated that she never associated the idea of therapeutic intention with the conservation principles. She explained, "I suppose it would be a claim to some greater wisdom to suggest that every idea I ever had was in some way associated with the Conservation Principles — but that is simply not true. My thought habits are fairly consistent but I have devoted them to many areas which are not organically related."

Schaefer (1991b) regards the Theory of Therapeutic Intention as "very exciting" (p. 223). She commented, "Not only will the nurse have a repertoire of tested interventions, given that a theory provides specific information about care delivery, but also the nurse should have information about the expected organismic responses. With this in mind the theory provides direction for quality-assurance activities and measures of cost effectiveness" (p. 223).

Levine (1978a) noted that she and a colleague had been working on the **Theory of Redundancy** for some time. This "completely untested, completely speculative" theory has "redefined aging and almost everything else that has to do with human life." She proposed that "aging is the diminished availability of redundant systems necessary for effective maintenance of physical and social well-being" (Levine, 1978b). The theory seems to extend the discussion of redundancy related to specificity of adaptation and organismic responses. Indeed, Levine (1991) recently noted that "the possibility exists that aging itself is a consequence of failed redundancy of physiological and psychological processes" (p. 6).

Schaefer (1991b) commented that the Theory of Redundancy "may also explain the compensatory responses found in patients with congestive heart failure" (p. 223). She went on to say that the theory "is less clear than therapeutic intention because the thinking has not been related successfully to nursing practice. Continued work is needed before it can be considered for use" (p. 223). Citing a personal communication (September 21, 1989), Schaefer (1991b) reported that Levine "would like to continue to work on the development of [the] Theories [of Therapeutic Intention and Redundancy] but is unsure of the direction she will take" (p. 223).

Levine (1991) denied that the so-called models included in her textbook, *Introduction to Clinical Nursing* (vital signs, body movement and positioning, personal hygiene, pressure gradient systems—fluids, nutrition, pressure gradient systems—gases, heat and cold, medications, and asepsis) are a theory, as Pieper (1983) asserted. Rather, these so-called models "were intended to direct the nursing fundamentals essential to a beginning student of nursing. They were part of the textbook but were completely unrelated to the [Conservation Model], and only by stretching far beyond the text could they be construed as germane to the conservation principles" (Levine, 1991, p. 3).

Credibility

Social Utility

The utility of the Conservation Model for nursing research, education, administration, and practice is documented by the publication of the book, *Levine's Conservation Model: A Framework for Nursing Practice* (Schaefer & Pond, 1991), and several journal articles. The Conservation Model has a distinctive and extensive vocabulary that requires some study for mastery. Levine was, however, careful to provide adequate definitions of most terms, so that there should be minimal confusion about the meaning of her ideas.

A thorough understanding of the extensive and rich base of knowledge on which the Conservation Model is grounded requires considerable study in diverse adjunctive disciplines. Schaefer (1991c) pointed out that "a strong background in physiology and research is required" (p. 210). Levine (1990) maintained that safe and effective nursing care can be provided only with a firm grasp of physiology, microbiology, biochemistry, psychology, sociology, education, history, anthropology, and mathematics. Grindley and Paradowski (1991) added philosophy and theology to the list and also underscored the importance of English courses in learning to communicate accurately in both oral and written forms.

Conservation Model–based nursing practice is feasible for many different patient populations in many different settings. Cox's (1991) description of the use of the Conservation Model at the Alverno Health Care Facility provides glimpses of the human and material resources needed to implement the model at the agency level. The Alverno is a 136-bed intermediate care facility, which provides long-term care to a patient population with an average age of 85 years. Staff members are taught to structure all care according to the conservation principles, and nursing goals have been established for each conservation principle. Parameters have been identified to determine the need to terminate activities because of excessive energy expenditure (conservation of energy) and to assess functional capability (structural integrity). Staff learn to show respect for the residents by asking them how they wish to be addressed, and time is taken to learn the residents' former routines and to incorporate as much of that routine as possible into the plan of care (personal integrity).

Residents and staff negotiate their roles and goals, and efforts are made to help the residents to maintain ties with the local community (social integrity). Moreover, Cox (1991) commented that the conservation principles "allow each level of practitioner (nurse's aide, LPN, RN) to provide care based upon the knowledge appropriate for the level of practice" (p. 196).

NURSING RESEARCH. The utility of the Conservation Model for nursing research is documented by several studies. The doctoral dissertation research that has been guided by the Conservation Model and was retrieved from *Dissertation Abstracts International* is listed in the bibliography at the end of this chapter.

Cooper (1991) reported the development and testing of an instrument to assess the status of open, soft tissue wounds healing by secondary intention. The instrument was directly derived from the principle of the conservation of structural integrity.

Winslow and associates have conducted a series of studies, derived from the principle of the conservation of energy (Lane & Winslow, 1987; Winslow, 1983; Winslow, Lane, & Gaffney, 1984, 1985). Although the Conservation Model was not cited in the reports of some of the studies, Winslow (personal communication to M.E. Levine, October 6, 1982) indicated that her research on energy utilization during toileting and bathing was based on the principle of conservation of energy. Lane and Winslow (1987) explicitly identified this conservation principle as the guide for their study of energy expenditure during rest, occupied bedmaking, and unoccupied bedmaking.

Hanson et al. (1991) reported the results of their Conservation Model-based study of the prevalence and incidence of pressure ulcers in hospice patients. The principle of the conservation of structural integrity guided the prospective and retrospective approaches to data collection. The principle of conservation of structural integrity also influenced the multisite study conducted by Dibble et al. (1991) on the incidence of and factors associated with intravenous site symptoms.

The principles of the conservation of energy and structural integrity guided MacLean's (1987, 1988) study, which was designed to identify cues used by nurses for diagnosing activity intolerance related to an imbalance between oxygen supply and demand. Those two principles also guided Hader and Sorensen's (1988) study of the effect of different body positions on transcutaneous oxygen tension. The study subjects were infants between the ages of 2 weeks and 2 years who had been admitted to a pediatric intensive care unit.

The principles of conservation of energy and social integrity provided the basis for Newport's (1984) research. She compared the body temperatures of infants who had been placed on their mothers' chest immediately after birth with those of infants who were placed in a warmer. No difference was found between the two groups of infants.

All four conservation principles guided Yeates and Roberts' (1984) research, which compared the effects of two bearing-down techniques during the second stage of labor on labor progress. Roberts, Fleming, and Yeates-Giese (1991) integrated the findings of their earlier studies (Fleming, 1988; Yeates & Roberts, 1984) in a comprehensive discussion of the perineal integrity of the childbearing woman.

All four conservation principles also provided the framework for Schaefer's (1990; Schaefer & Shober-Potylycki, 1993) descriptive studies of fatigue associated with congestive heart failure. The first study (Schaefer, 1990) employed quantitative methods; the second employed both qualitative and quantitative methods.

Foreman (1987, 1989, 1991) linked the Conservation Model with a theory of information processing to study the development of confusion in elderly patients. Nagley (1986) tested the effects of a Conservation Model–based nursing intervention on the prevention of confusion in elderly hospitalized patients. She found that few patients were confused, and that there were no statistically significant differences in mental status scores between the experimental and control groups.

Geden's (1982) report of her study of energy expenditure during lifting cited notions of energy mentioned in a few nursing models, including Levine's. There is no evidence, however, that that research was an explicit test of Levine's principle of conservation of energy. In fact, Geden (1985) interpreted her work within the context of Orem's general theory of nursing.

Tompkins (1980) cited a few conceptual models of nursing, including Levine's, in the discussion of findings from her study of the effect of restricted mobility and leg dominance on perceived duration of time. This research was not, however, directly derived from Levine's model.

NURSING EDUCATION. The utility of the Conservation Model for nursing education also is documented. Barnum (1994) offered a hypothetical curriculum design based on Levine's model. Findings from surveys of baccalaureate nursing programs conducted by Hall (1979) and Riehl (1980) revealed that the Conservation Model was used as a guideline for curriculum development. In particular, Riehl found that Levine's model was "popular with faculty, especially in the Chicago area" (p. 396). The names of the schools of nursing using the Conservation Model were not given in the survey reports. However, Cox (1991) noted that the Conservation Model was used as a basis for course work in the master's degree medical-surgical nursing program at Loyola University of Chicago in the late 1960s.

Grindley and Paradowski (1991) presented a detailed description of the use of the Conservation Model as the curriculum guide for the baccalaureate nursing program at Allentown College of St. Francis de Sales in Center Valley, Pennsylvania. Schaefer (1991c) described the Conservation Model-based curriculum for the master's program in nursing at the same college.

In addition, L. Zwanger (personal communication, June 4, 1982) reported that Levine's Conservation Model was used in nursing education programs sponsored by Kapat-Holim, the Health Insurance Institution of the General Federation of Labour in Israel, based in Tel-Aviv. Moreover, M.J. Stafford (personal communication, June 2, 1982) stated that she used the model "in teaching formal and informal classes such as the Critical Care Nursing course, Pacemaker Therapy, and The Nurse's Role in Electrocardiography" at the Hines Veterans Administration Medical Center in Hines, Illinois.

NURSING ADMINISTRATION. Levine's Conservation Model has documented utility for nursing service administration. Taylor (1974) developed a form for evaluation of the quality of nursing care of neurological patients. The conservation principles served as the goals of nursing care and were used as the frame of reference for "defining commonly recurring nursing problems on the neurological service" (p. 342). In two later papers, Taylor (1987, 1989) described an assessment guide that directs data collection for neurological patients. The guide yields data regarding the four conservation principles and is used as the basis for the development of a comprehensive nursing care plan that lists the nursing diagnoses, expected outcomes, and interventions for each conservation principle. Taylor (1987) explained, "From the collected data a nurse can isolate the provocative facts that indicate the presence of a nursing diagnosis. The facts can then be summarized and used to develop a nursing care plan" (p. 106).

McCall (1991) described the use of an assessment tool that she developed to identify the nursing care needs of patients with epilepsy. The tool contains open-ended questions that yield data regarding the four conservation principles. Assessment of energy deals with the description of the seizures and other medical problems. Assessment of structural integrity focuses on safety measures during seizures. Assessment of personal integrity addresses the effects of the seizures on the patient's feelings and functioning. Assessment of social integrity deals with the patients' interactions with significant others, visitors during hospitalization, and other patients.

Lynn-McHale and Smith (1991) extended the Conservation Model to the care of families with their innovative family assessment tool. The tool, which was designed for families of patients in the critical care setting, contains open-ended questions that yield a comprehensive family assessment structured according to the four conservation principles. Assessment of energy focuses on perception of the event, coping mechanisms, and such logistics as transportation to the hospital and needs for assistance with lodging during a family member's hospitalization. Assessment of structural integrity addresses type of illness (acute or chronic), family functioning, and current and future health needs. Assessment of personal integrity deals with past experiences, life events, ethnic and religious factors, and additional family needs with regard to information from the health care team. Assessment of social integrity emphasizes support systems, visitation, and family members' work patterns.

In addition, M.J. Stafford (personal communication, June 2, 1982) commented that she used Levine's Conservation Model to identify process and outcome criteria in the nursing care of patients with cardiovascular problems. Furthermore, the utility of Levine's conceptual model for nursing administration is documented by its use at The Alverno Health Care Facility in Clinton, Iowa (Cox, 1991). Here, the conservation principles structure the format of the nursing care plan and provide guidelines for staff development. The nursing care plan contains an extensive summary of the patient's trophicognosis, and care is organized according to the four conservation principles.

NURSING PRACTICE. The utility of the Conservation Model for nursing practice in many different settings and for patients with many different medical conditions has been documented. Herbst (1981) linked the principles of conservation with knowledge of the pathophysiology of cancer and presented a comprehensive description of nursing that takes into account the wholeness of the cancer patient, the nurse, and the disease process. Brunner (1985) and Schaefer (1991a) used the conservation principles and knowledge of cardiac pathology to formulate comprehensive nursing care plans for patients with cardiac disease. Fawcett et al. (1987) used knowledge of end-stage cardiac disease and critical care unit environments to formulate trophicognoses for a 57-year-old man. In another publication, Fawcett et al. (1992) explained how the Conservation Model guided the nursing care of two critically ill patients. Levine's (1973) textbook includes nursing processes appropriate for patients who have a failure of nervous system integration, hormonal disturbances, fluid and electrolyte imbalances, aberrant cellular growth, and several other pathological states.

Crawford-Gamble (1986) described the use of the four conservation principles, linked with knowledge of the effects of surgery, in care of a woman undergoing reimplantation of digits of her hand. Webb (1993) also used the four conservation principles to guide the postoperative care of a man who had undergone extensive bowel surgery resulting in a colostomy. Cooper (1990) underscored the importance of the principle of structural integrity in planning nursing interventions to enhance wound healing. Pasco and Halupa (1991) discussed management of patients in pain.

Dever (1991) discussed the perceptual, operational, and conceptual environments of children and explained how the four conservation principles guided her nursing care of an infant hospitalized with pneumonia. Savage and Culbert (1989) described the role and distinctive contributions of the nurse in the care of infants and toddlers at risk for developmental delay. Bayley (1991) discussed the care of a teenager with severe burn injuries based on all four conservation principles. Bayley also discussed the patient's perceptual, operational, and conceptual environments.

Hirschfeld (1976) linked the conservation principles with theories of pathophysiology, aging, and cognitive impairment to develop nursing interventions for several patients who were cognitively impaired as a result of illness. Gingrich (1971) explained how the haptic system can be used as a substitute information-gathering system by elderly people when other perceptual systems are compromised. Foreman (1991) described the care of the confused elderly using all four conservation principles. Furthermore, Cox (1991) described the use of the Conservation Model to guide nursing care of elderly residents of The Alverno Health Care Facility in Clinton, Iowa. Her discussion underscored the utility of Levine's model for health promotion and illness prevention.

Pond and Taney (1991) reported their use of the Conservation Model in the Emergency Department of the Hospital of the University of Pennsylvania in Philadelphia. Pond (1990, 1991) explained how the Conservation Model guided her nursing care of the homeless at a clinic, shelters, day programs, feeding sites, and on the streets in Philadelphia, Pennsylvania.

Social Congruence

Although the Conservation Model was initially formulated many years ago, it is congruent with the present-day emphasis on holistic approaches to health care and consideration of the person as a unique individual. Levine developed her conceptual model at a time when nursing activities in acute care settings were becoming more mechanical, owing to the rapid increase in medical technology. In fact, she spoke out against the growing functionalism of nursing and reoriented nurses to the patient as a whole being:

> Discovering ways to perceive and cherish the essential wholeness of man becomes imperative with the rapid growth of automation in modern disciplines which possess a technology. Nursing is one of them, and nurses will not escape the sweeping changes that automation promises. But nurses do know that the integrated human being is not merely "programmed" to respond to life in automatic ways. . . . It is the task of nursing to recognize and value the wondrous variety of all mankind while offering ministrations that conserve the unique and special integrity of every man. (Levine, 1966a, p. 2453)

Levine (1973) noted that "the whole man is the focus of nursing intervention — in health and sickness, in tragedy and joy, in hospitals and clinics and in the community" (p. vii). Although little discussion of the use of the Conservation Model in health promotion and illness prevention situations is available, its broad focus is congruent with society's increasing interest in promotion of health and prevention of illness.

The Conservation Model is acceptable to all members of the health care team. Pond and Taney (1991) reported that the use of the Conservation Model effectively highlighted the nursing components of collaborative nurse-physician practice in an emergency department. Cox (1991) indicated that she has continued to use the conservation principles for more than 20 years in her work in the long-term care setting "because they are a natural fit for [that] setting. She also pointed out that the Conservation Model

> provides direction for nursing practice and staff development. The conservation principles provide an organizing framework, and easy-to-remember guide, for promoting wholeness within the limits imposed by the aging process and the consequences of chronic illness. . . . The model allows for the contributions made by all of the members of the interdisciplinary team. (p. 196)

Social Significance

The evidence supporting the social significance of the Conservation Model is largely anecdotal. Hirschfeld (1976) noted, "Myra Levine's four principles of conservation are useful in deciding what will help the cognitively impaired aged person and determining what the priorities should be in his or her care" (p. 1981). She went on to describe application of the conservation principles to the care of several patients who had cognitive impairments. In concluding her article, Hirschfeld stated:

> Surely, nursing care that incorporates Levine's four conservation principles can make a difference to the individual and family equilibrium that are disturbed by events as devastating as mental impairment. (p. 1984)

V.G. Lathrop (personal communication, May 5, 1982) used the Conservation Model to guide the nursing care of patients in the Intensive Treatment Unit for Mentally Ill Offenders at Saint Elizabeth's Hospital in Washington, DC. She stated that nursing audits based on the American Nurses' Association Psychiatric/Mental Health Standards of Nursing Practice revealed that "treatment provided was more holistic in nature."

Cox (1991) reported that the four conservation principles provide a comprehensive focus for care and that "the identification of common recurring nursing problems and goals in long-term care gives direction and unity to nursing practice that fosters quality care" (p. 196). Webb (1993) commented that the Conservation Model was useful in guiding postoperative nursing care "because of the emphasis it places on psychosocial nursing intervention, an area that is often neglected" (p. 128). Webb went on to say that "Nurses everywhere must redefine their attitude to psychological support and participate in truly holistic care that acknowledges all elements of the patient's environment" (p. 128).

Savage and Culbert (1989) pointed out that use of the conservation principles "allows the nurse to take a flexible, creative approach to caring for the family with a developmentally disabled child. Various approaches are incorporated into the nurse's role, moving the nurse from a peripheral position to a more central one on the early intervention multidisciplinary team. In turn, the nurse can contribute to the family's process of successful adaptation, which is the ultimate goal in the early intervention setting" (p. 345).

Pond and Taney (1991) maintained that the use of the Conservation Model "strengthens communication among health care providers and improves the way nursing care is transmitted to and received by patients. In an atmosphere of collaboration each participant — health care provider and patient — is rewarded with respect and active contribution to the adaptation process. Both the internal and external environments of the patient are affected in such a way as to provide a move toward homeostasis. This is the goal called conservation or, from the medical model point of view, health maintenance" (p. 166).

Finally, Pond (1991) noted the difficulty of working with homeless patients but pointed to the success of Conservation Model–based nursing care. She commented, "As the conservation principles are used to assess each patient, a comprehensive picture develops. . . . Many of our patients are easily managed and are integrated into the existing health care resources. Although it is never easy, many patients become independent in their health care and less dependent on our outreach services. We consider these many successes as reflective of the dedicated nursing interventions with these challenging situations" (p. 178).

Contributions to the Discipline of Nursing

The Conservation Model makes a substantial contribution to the discipline of nursing by focusing attention on the whole person. Levine moved beyond the idea of the total person to the concept of the person as a holistic being. Pointing to the limitations of the so-called total person approach, she noted:

> Nurses have long known that patients are complete persons, not groups of parts. It is out of this realization that the attempts toward "comprehensive care" and "total care" have come, and it is because we have been frustrated by failing to achieve the ideal of completion that the search for a more definitive approach to bedside care has continued. (Levine, 1969b, p. 94)

The Conservation Model is consistent in its approach to the person as a holistic being. Physiological and behavioral responses are regarded as one and the same, and conservation principles are joined. Moreover, the conservation principles provide a comprehensive framework for holistic nursing care. These principles focus attention on the patient as a unique individual.

Grindley and Paradowski (1991) maintained that "The adaptability of the model is one of its greatest strengths. The conservation principles have easily stood the test of time and the impact of technology" (p. 207). They went on to say,

> Individuals continue to be unique; they cope with ever-increasing assaults on their energies. The constant barrage on their integrities by the world around them reinforces the fact that the nurse must be ever alert to the potential and actual impact of these assaults. Holistic care touches the individual, the family, and the community. Levine's principles are applicable not only to individuals but also to a larger group, the others who are significant to them. (pp. 207–208)

A hallmark of Levine's Conservation Model is the accurate use of knowledge from what Levine (1988a) called adjunctive disciplines. She has credited the scholars of other disciplines from whose works she has drawn for the development of her conceptual model, and she has used that knowledge appropriately.

Although documentation of the utility of the Conservation Model for nursing activities is increasing, its credibility must be empirically established. Systematic evaluations of the use of the model in various clinical situations are needed, as are studies that test conceptual-theoretical-empirical structures directly derived from the conservation principles. Perhaps the most important need is for valid and reliable empirical indicators to measure the phenomena encompassed by the Conservation Model. The assessment tools that have already been developed require systematic testing to determine intrarater and interrater reliability. Schaefer (1991b) pointed out, "An assessment tool is perhaps the most important measure of wholeness. Using the elements of trophicognosis, practitioners and researchers are encouraged to develop assessment measures based on Levine's Conservation Model and to test for a reliable and valid data base common to all patients presenting with a need for nursing care" (p. 221).

In conclusion, Levine's Conservation Model provides nursing with a logically congruent, holistic view of the person. Two theories related to the model have been formulated, but they require further development and empirical testing. The lack of major limitations suggests that the Conservation Model may be an effective guide for nursing actions.

REFERENCES

Barnum, B.J.S. (1994). Nursing theory: Analysis, application, evaluation (4th ed.). Philadelphia: JB Lippincott.

Bates, M. (1967). A naturalist at large. Natural History, 76(6), 8–16.

Bayley, E.W. (1991). Care of the burn patient. In K.M. Schaefer & J.B. Pond (Eds.), Levine's conservation model: A framework for nursing practice (pp. 91–99). Philadelphia: FA Davis.

Beland, I. (1971). Clinical nursing: Pathophysiological and psychosocial implications (2nd ed.). New York: Macmillan.

Bernard, C. (1957). An introduction to the study of experimental medicine. New York: Dover.

Brunner, M. (1985). A conceptual approach to critical care nursing using Levine's model. Focus on Critical Care, 12(2), 39–44.

Cannon, W.B. (1939). *The wisdom of the body.* New York: Norton.

Cooper, D.M. (1990). Optimizing wound healing: A practice within nursing's domain. *Nursing Clinics of North America, 25,* 165–180.

Cooper, D.M. (1991). Development and testing of an instrument to assess the visual characteristics of open, soft tissue wounds. *Dissertation Abstracts International, 51,* 3320B. (University Microfilms No. ADG90-26541)

Cox, R.A., Sr. (1991). A tradition of caring: Use of Levine's model in long-term care. In K.M. Schaefer & J.B. Pond (Eds.), *Levine's conservation model: A framework for nursing practice* (pp. 179–197). Philadelphia: FA Davis.

Crawford-Gamble, P.E. (1986). An application of Levine's conceptual model. *Perioperative Nursing Quarterly, 2*(1), 64–70.

Dever, M. (1991). Care of children. In K.M. Schaefer & J.B. Pond (Eds.), *Levine's conservation model: A framework for nursing practice* (pp. 71–82). Philadelphia: FA Davis.

Dibble, S.L., Bostrom-Ezrati, J., & Bizzuto, C. (1991). Clinical predictors of intravenous site symptoms. *Research in Nursing and Health, 14,* 413–420.

Dubos, R. (1961). *Mirage of health.* New York: Doubleday.

Dubos, R. (1965). *Man adapting.* New Haven: Yale University Press.

Erikson, E.H. (1964). *Insight and responsibility.* New York: Norton.

Erikson, E.H. (1968). *Identity: Youth and crisis.* New York: Norton.

Esposito, C.H., & Leonard, M.K. (1980). Myra Estrin Levine. In Nursing Theories Conference Group, *Nursing theories: The base for professional nursing practice* (pp. 150-163). Englewood Cliffs, NJ: Prentice-Hall.

Fawcett, J., Archer, C.L., Becker, D., Brown, K.K., Gann, S., Wong, M.J. & Wurster, A.B. (1992). Guidelines for selecting a conceptual model of nursing: Focus on the individual patient. *Dimensions of Critical Care Nursing, 11,* 268–277.

Fawcett, J., Cariello, F.P., Davis, D.A., Farley, J., Zimmaro, D.M., & Watts, R.J. (1987). Conceptual models of nursing: Application to critical care nursing practice. *Dimensions of Critical Care Nursing, 6,* 202–213.

Feiblemann, J.K. (1959). The logical structure of the scientific method. *Dialectica, 13,* 209.

Feynman, R. (1965). *The character of physical law.* Cambridge, MA: MIT Press.

Fleming, N. (1988). Comparison of women with different perineal conditions after childbirth. *Dissertation Abstracts International, 48,* 2924B.

Foreman, M. (1987). A causal model for making decisions about confusion in the hospitalized elderly. In K.J. Hannah, M. Reimer, W.C. Mills, & S. Letourneau (Eds.), *Clinical judgment and decision making: The future with nursing diagnosis* (pp. 427–429). New York: John Wiley & Sons.

Foreman, M. (1989). Confusion in the hospitalized elderly: Incidence, onset, and associated factors. *Research in Nursing and Health, 12,* 21–29.

Foreman, M. (1991). Conserving cognitive integrity of the hospitalized elderly. In K.M. Schaefer & J.B. Pond (Eds.), *Levine's conservation model: A framework for nursing practice* (pp. 133–149). Philadelphia: FA Davis.

Geden, E. (1982). Effects of lifting techniques on energy expenditure: A preliminary investigation. *Nursing Research, 31,* 214–218.

Geden, E. (1985). The relationship between self-care theory and empirical research. In J. Riehl-Sisca, *The science and art of self-care* (pp. 265–270). Norwalk, CT: Appleton-Century-Crofts.

Gibson, J.E. (1966). *The senses considered as perceptual systems.* Boston: Houghton-Mifflin.

Gingrich, B. (1971). The use of the haptic system as an information-gathering system. In M. Duffey, E.H. Anderson, B.S. Bergersen, M. Lohr, & M.H. Rose (Eds.), *Current concepts in clinical nursing* (Vol. 3, pp. 235–246). St. Louis: CV Mosby.

Goldstein, K. (1963). *The organism.* Boston: Beacon Press.

Grindley, J., & Paradowski, M. (1991). Developing an undergraduate program using Levine's model. In K.M. Schaefer & J.B. Pond (Eds.), *Levine's conservation model: A framework for nursing practice* (pp. 199–208). Philadelphia: FA Davis.

Hader, C.F., & Sorensen, E.R. (1988). The effects of body position on transcutaneous oxygen tension. *Pediatric Nursing, 14,* 469–473.

Hall, E. (1959). *Silent language.* Greenwich, CT: Fawcett.

Hall, E. (1966). *The hidden dimension.* Garden City, NY: Doubleday.

Hall, K.V. (1979). Current trends in the use

of conceptual frameworks in nursing education. *Journal of Nursing Education, 18*(4), 26–29.

Hanson, D., Langemo, D.K., Olson, B., Hunter, S., Sauvage, T.R., Burd, C., & Cathcart Silberberg, T. (1991). The prevalence and incidence of pressure ulcers in the hospice setting: Analysis of two methodologies. *American Journal of Hospice and Palliative Care, 8*(5), 18–22.

Herbst, S. (1981). Impairments as a result of cancer. In N. Martin, N. Holt & D. Hicks (Eds.), *Comprehensive rehabilitation nursing* (pp. 553–578). New York: McGraw-Hill.

Hirschfeld, M.J. (1976). The cognitively impaired older adult. *American Journal of Nursing, 76*, 1981–1984.

Lane, L.D., & Winslow, E.H. (1987). Oxygen consumption, cardiovascular response, and perceived exertion in healthy adults during rest, occupied bedmaking, and unoccupied bedmaking activity. *Cardiovascular Nursing, 23*(6), 31–36.

Levine, M.E. (1966a). Adaptation and assessment: A rationale for nursing intervention. *American Journal of Nursing, 66*, 2450–2453.

Levine, M.E. (1966b). Trophicognosis: An alternative to nursing diagnosis. In *American Nurses' Association Regional Clinical Conference* (Vol. 2, pp. 55–70). New York: American Nurses' Association.

Levine, M.E. (1967). The four conservation principles of nursing. *Nursing Forum, 6*, 45–59.

Levine, M.E. (1969a). *Introduction to clinical nursing*. Philadelphia: FA Davis.

Levine, M.E. (1969b). The pursuit of wholeness. *American Journal of Nursing, 69*, 93–98.

Levine, M.E. (1971). Holistic nursing. *Nursing Clinics of North America, 6*, 253–264.

Levine, M.E. (1973). *Introduction to clinical nursing* (2nd ed.). Philadelphia: FA Davis.

Levine, M.E. (1977). Nursing ethics and the ethical nurse. *American Journal of Nursing, 77*, 845–849.

Levine, M.E. (1978a, December). *The four conservation principles of nursing*. Paper presented at the Second Annual Nurse Educator Conference, New York. (Cassette recording).

Levine, M.E. (1978b, December). *Application to education and practice*. Paper presented at the Second Annual Nurse Educator Conference, New York. (Cassette recording).

Levine, M.E. (1984a, August). *Myra Levine*. Paper presented at the Nurse Theorist

Conference, Edmonton, Alberta, Canada. (Cassette recording).

Levine, M.E. (1984b, August). *Concurrent sessions. M. Levine*. Discussion at the Nurse Theorist Conference, Edmonton, Alberta, Canada. (Cassette recording).

Levine, M.E. (1985, August). *Myra Levine*. Paper presented at conference on Nursing Theory in Action, Edmonton, Alberta, Canada. (Cassette recording).

Levine, M.E. (1986, August). *Myra Levine*. Paper presented at Nursing Theory Congress: Theoretical Pluralism: Direction for a Practice Discipline, Toronto, Ontario, Canada. (Cassette recording).

Levine, M.E. (1987). *The nurse theorists: Portraits of excellence: Myra Levine*. Oakland, CA: Studio Three (Videotape).

Levine, M.E. (1988a). Antecedents from adjunctive disciplines: Creation of nursing theory. *Nursing Science Quarterly, 1* 16–21.

Levine, M.E. (1988b). Myra Levine. In T.M. Schorr & A. Zimmerman, *Making choices. Taking chances: Nurse leaders tell their stories* (pp. 215–228). St. Louis: CV Mosby.

Levine, M.E. (1989a). Beyond dilemma. *Seminars in Oncology Nursing, 5*, 124–128.

Levine, M.E. (1989b). The conservation principles of nursing: Twenty years later. In J.P. Riehl, *Conceptual models for nursing practice* (3rd ed., pp. 325–337). Norwalk, CT: Appleton & Lange.

Levine, M.E. (1989c). The ethics of nursing rhetoric. *Image: Journal of Nursing Scholarship, 21*, 4–6.

Levine, M.E. (1989d). Ration or rescue: The elderly patient in critical care. *Critical Care Nursing Quarterly, 12*(1), 82–89.

Levine, M.E. (1990). Conservation and integrity. In M.E. Parker (Ed.), *Nursing theories in practice* (pp. 189–201). New York: National League for Nursing.

Levine, M.E. (1991). The conservation principles: A model for health. In K.M. Schaefer & J.B. Pond (Eds.), *Levine's conservation model: A framework for nursing practice* (pp. 1–11). Philadelphia: FA Davis.

Levine, M.E. (1992). Nightingale redux. In F.N. Nightingale, *Notes on nursing: What it is, and what it is not* (Commemorative edition, pp. 39–43). Philadelphia: JB Lippincott.

Lynn-McHale, D.J., & Smith, A. (1991). Comprehensive assessment of families of the critically ill. *AACN Clinical Issues in Critical Care Nursing, 2*, 195–209.

MacLean, S.L. (1987). Description of cues

used by nurses when diagnosing activity intolerance. In K.J. Hannah, M. Reimer, W.C. Mills, & S. Letourneau (Eds.), *Clinical judgment and decision making: The future with nursing diagnosis* (pp. 161–163). New York: John Wiley & Sons.

MacLean, S.L. (1988). Activity intolerance: Cues for diagnosis. In R.M. Carroll-Johnston (Ed.), *Classification of nursing diagnoses: Proceedings of the eighth conference: North American Nursing Diagnosis Association* (pp. 320–327). Philadelphia: JB Lippincott.

Marriner-Tomey, A. (1989). *Nursing theorists and their work* (2nd ed.). St. Louis: CV Mosby.

McCall, B.H. (1991). Neurological intensive monitoring system: Unit assessment tool. In K.M. Schaefer & J.B. Pond (Eds.), *Levine's conservation model: A framework for nursing practice* (pp. 83–90). Philadelphia: FA Davis.

Meleis, A.I. (1991). *Theoretical nursing: Development and progress* (2nd ed.). Philadelphia: JB Lippincott.

Nagley, S.J. (1986). Predicting and preventing confusion in your patients. *Journal of Gerontological Nursing, 12*(3), 27–31.

Newman, M.A. (1972). Nursing's theoretical evolution. *Nursing Outlook, 20,* 449–453.

Newport, M.A. (1984). Conserving thermal energy and social integrity in the newborn. *Western Journal of Nursing Research, 6,* 176–197.

Nightingale, F. (1859). *Notes on nursing: What it is, and what it is not.* London: Harrison & Sones.

Pasco, A., & Halupa, D. (1991). Chronic pain management. In K.M. Schaefer & J.B. Pond (Eds.), *Levine's conservation model: A framework for nursing practice* (pp. 101–117). Philadelphia: FA Davis.

Pieper, B.A. (1983). Levine's nursing model. In J.J. Fitzpatrick & A.L. Whall, *Conceptual models of nursing: Analysis and application* (pp. 101–115). Bowie, MD: Brady.

Pond, J.B. (1990). Application of Levine's conservation model to nursing the homeless community. In M.E. Parker (Ed.), *Nursing theories in practice* (pp. 203–215). New York: National League for Nursing.

Pond, J.B. (1991). Ambulatory care of the homeless. In K.M. Schaefer & J.B. Pond (Eds.), *Levine's conservation model: A framework for nursing practice* (pp. 167–178). Philadelphia: FA Davis.

Pond, J.B., & Taney, S.G. (1991). Emergency care in a large university emergency department. In K.M. Schaefer & J.B. Pond (Eds.), *Levine's conservation model: A framework for nursing practice* (pp. 151–166). Philadelphia: FA Davis.

Riehl, J.P. (1980). Nursing models in current use. In J.P. Riehl & C. Roy, *Conceptual models for nursing practice* (2nd ed., pp. 393–398). New York: Appleton-Century-Crofts.

Riehl-Sisca, J.P. (1989). *Conceptual models for nursing practice* (3rd ed.). Norwalk, CT: Appleton & Lange.

Roberts, J.E., Fleming, N., & Yeates-Giese, D. (1991). Perineal integrity. In K.M. Schaefer & J.B. Pond (Eds.), *Levine's conservation model: A framework for nursing practice* (pp. 61–70). Philadelphia: FA Davis.

Savage, T.A., & Culbert, C. (1989). Early intervention: The unique role of nursing. *Journal of Pediatric Nursing, 4,* 339–345.

Schaefer, K.M. (1990). A description of fatigue associated with congestive heart failure: Use of Levine's conservation model. In M.E. Parker (Ed.), *Nursing theories in practice* (pp. 217–237). New York: National League for Nursing.

Schaefer, K.M. (1991a). Care of the patient with congestive heart failure. In K.M. Schaefer & J.B. Pond (Eds.), *Levine's conservation model: A framework for nursing practice* (pp. 119–131). Philadelphia: FA Davis.

Schaefer, K.M. (1991b). Creating a legacy. In K.M. Schaefer & J.B. Ponds (Eds.), *Levine's conservation model: A framework for nursing practice* (pp. 219–224). Philadelphia: FA Davis.

Schaefer, K.M. (1991c). Developing a graduate program in nursing: Integrating Levine's philosophy. In K.M. Schaefer & J.B. Pond (Eds.), *Levine's conservation model: A framework for nursing practice* (pp. 209–217). Philadelphia: FA Davis.

Schaefer, K.M. (1991d). Levine's conservation principles and research. In K.M. Schaefer & J.B. Pond (Eds.), *Levine's conservation model: A framework for nursing practice* (pp. 45–59). Philadelphia: FA Davis.

Schaefer, K.M., & Pond, J.B. (1991). *Levine's conservation model: A framework for nursing practice.* Philadelphia: FA Davis.

Schaefer, K.M., & Shober-Potylycki, M.J. (1993). Fatigue associated with congestive health failure: Use of Levine's Conservation Model. *Journal of Advanced Nursing, 18,* 260–268.

Selye, H. (1956). *The stress of life.* New York: McGraw-Hill.

Sherrington, A. (1906). *Integrative function of the nervous system.* New York: Scribner's.

Taylor, J.W. (1974). Measuring the outcomes of nursing care. *Nursing Clinics of North America, 9,* 337–340.

Taylor, J.W. (1987). Organizing data for nursing diagnoses using conservation principles. In A.M. McLane (Ed.), *Classification of nursing diagnoses: Proceedings of the seventh conference: North American Nursing Diagnosis Association* (pp. 103–111). St. Louis: CV Mosby.

Taylor, J.W. (1989). Levine's conservation principles: Using the model for nursing diagnosis in a neurological setting. In J.P. Riehl-Sisca, *Conceptual models for nursing practice* (3rd ed., pp. 349–358). Norwalk, CT: Appleton & Lange.

Tillich, P. (1961). The meaning of health. *Perspectives in Biology and Medicine, 5,* 92–100.

Tompkins, E.S. (1980). Effect of restricted mobility and dominance on perceived duration. *Nursing Research, 29,* 333–338.

Waddington, C.H. (Ed.). (1968). *Towards a theoretical biology. I. Prolegomena.* Chicago: Aldine.

Webb, H. (1993). Holistic care following a palliative Hartmann's procedure. *British Journal of Nursing, 2,* 128–132.

Winslow, E.H., Lane, L.D., & Gaffney, F.A. (1984). Oxygen consumption and cardiovascular response in patients and normal adults during in-bed and out-of-bed toileting. *Journal of Cardiac Rehabilitation, 4,* 348–354.

Winslow, E.H., Lane, L.D., & Gaffney, F.A. (1985). Oxygen consumption and cardiovascular response in control adults and acute myocardial infarction patients during bathing. *Nursing Research, 34,* 164–169.

Wolf, S. (1961). Disease as a way of life: Neural integration in systemic pathology. *Perspectives in Biology and Medicine, 4,* 288–305.

Yeates, D.A., & Roberts, J.E. (1984). A comparison of two bearing-down techniques during the second stage of labor. *Journal of Nurse-Midwifery, 29,* 3–11.

BIBLIOGRAPHY

PRIMARY SOURCES

Levine, M.E. (1966). Adaptation and assessment: A rationale for nursing intervention. *American Journal of Nursing, 66,* 2450–2453.

Levine, M.E. (1966). Trophicognosis: An alternative to nursing diagnosis. In *American Nurses' Association Regional Clinical Conference* (Vol. 2, pp. 55–70). New York: American Nurses' Association.

Levine, M.E. (1967). The four conservation principles of nursing. *Nursing Forum, 6,* 45–59.

Levine, M.E. (1969). The pursuit of wholeness. *American Journal of Nursing, 69,* 93–98.

Levine, M.E. (1969). *Introduction to clinical nursing.* Philadelphia: FA Davis.

Levine, M.E. (1971). Holistic nursing. *Nursing Clinics of North America, 6,* 253–264.

Levine, M.E. (1971). *Renewal for nursing.* Philadelphia: FA Davis.

Levine, M.E. (1973). *Instructor's guide to introduction to clinical nursing* (2nd ed.). Philadelphia: FA Davis. Reprinted 1991, In K.M. Schaefer & J.B. Pond (Eds.), *Levine's conservation model: A framework for nursing practice* (pp. 225–237). Philadelphia: FA Davis.

Levine, M.E. (1973). *Introduction to clinical nursing* (2nd ed.). Philadelphia: FA Davis.

Levine, M.E. (1988). Myra Levine. In T.M. Schorr & A. Zimmerman, *Making choices. Taking chances: Nurse leaders tell their stories* (pp. 215–228). St. Louis: CV Mosby.

Levine, M.E. (1989). The conservation principles: Twenty years later. In J.P. Riehl, *Conceptual models for nursing practice* (3rd ed., pp. 325–337). Norwalk, CT: Appleton & Lange.

Levine, M.E. (1990). Conservation and integrity. In M.E. Parker (Ed.), *Nursing theories in practice* (pp. 189–201). New York: National League for Nursing.

Levine, M.E. (1991). The conservation principles: A model for health. In K.M. Schaefer & J.B. Pond (Eds.), *Levine's conservation model: A framework for nursing practice* (pp. 1–11). Philadelphia: FA Davis.

Levine, M.E. (1992). Nightingale redux. In F.N. Nightingale, *Notes on nursing: What it is, and what it is not* (Commemorative edition, pp. 39–43). Philadelphia: JB Lippincott.

Schaefer, K.M., & Pond, J.B. (Eds.). (1991). *Levine's conservation model: A framework* for nursing practice. Philadelphia: FA Davis.

COMMENTARY

Artigue, G.S., Foli, K.J., Johnson, T., et al. Myra Estrin Levine: Four conservation principles. In Marriner-Tomey, A., (Ed.), Nursing theorists and their work (3rd ed., pp. 199–210). St. Louis: Mosby-Year Book.

Esposito, C.H., & Leonard, M.K. (1980). Myra Estrin Levine. In Nursing Theories Conference Group, Nursing theories: The base for professional nursing practice (pp. 150–163). Englewood Cliffs, NJ: Prentice-Hall.

Fawcett, J. (1991). Analysis and evaluation of Levine's conservation model. In K.M. Schaefer & J.B. Pond (Eds.), Levine's conservation model: A framework for nursing practice (pp. 13–43). Philadelphia: FA Davis.

Foli, K.J., Johnson, T., Marriner, A., Poat, M.C., Poppa, L., & Zoretich, S.T. (1986). Myra Estrin Levine: Four conservation principles. In A. Marriner, Nursing theorists and their work (pp. 335–344). St. Louis: CV Mosby.

Foli, K.J., Johnson, T., Marriner-Tomey, A., Poat, M.C., Poppa, L., Woeste, R., & Zoretich, S.T. (1989). Myra Estrin Levine: Four conservation principles. In A. Marriner-Tomey, Nursing theorists and their work (2nd ed., pp. 391–401). St. Louis: CV Mosby.

Glass, J.L. (1989). Levine's theory of nursing: A critique. In J.P. Riehl-Sisca, Conceptual models for nursing practice (3rd ed., pp. 339–348). Norwalk, CT: Appleton & Lange.

Leonard, M.K. (1985). Myra Estrin Levine. In Nursing Theories Conference Group, Nursing theories: The base for professional nursing practice (2nd ed., pp. 180–194). Englewood Cliffs, NJ: Prentice-Hall.

Leonard, M.K. (1990). Myra Estrin Levine. In J.B. George (Ed.), Nursing theories: The base for professional nursing practice (3rd ed., pp. 181–192). Norwalk, CT: Appleton & Lange.

Levine, M.E. (1988). Antecedents from adjunctive disciplines: Creation of nursing theory. Nursing Science Quarterly, 1, 16–21.

Levine, M.E. (1989). Beyond dilemma. Seminars in Oncology Nursing, 5, 124–128.

Levine, M.E. (1989). The ethics of nursing rhetoric. Image: Journal of Nursing Scholarship, 21, 4–6.

Levine, M.E. (1989). Ration or rescue: The elderly patient in critical care. Critical Care Nursing Quarterly, 12(1), 82–89.

Meleis, A.I. (1991). Theoretical nursing: Development and progress (2nd ed.). Philadelphia: JB Lippincott.

Pieper, B.A. (1983). Levine's nursing model. In J.J. Fitzpatrick & A.L. Whall, Conceptual models of nursing: Analysis and application (pp. 101–115). Bowie, MD: Brady.

Pieper, B.A. (1989). Levine's nursing model: The conservation principles. In J.J. Fitzpatrick & A.L. Whall, Conceptual models of nursing: Analysis and application (2nd ed., pp. 137–146). Norwalk, CT: Appleton & Lange.

Rafferty, C. (1987–1988). An apologist's theories for the nursing profession: Adaptation and art. Nursing Forum, 23, 124–126.

Schaefer, K.M. (1991). Creating a legacy. In K.M. Schaefer & J.B. Pond (Eds.), Levine's conservation model: A framework for nursing practice (pp. 219–224). Philadelphia: FA Davis.

Schaefer, K.M., & Pond, J.B. (1990). Re: Effects of waterbed flotation on indicators of energy expenditure in preterm infants [Letter to the editor]. Nursing Research, 39, 293.

RESEARCH

Dibble, S.L., Bostrom-Ezrati, J., & Bizzuto, C. (1991). Clinical predictors of intravenous site symptoms. Research in Nursing and Health, 14, 413–420.

Foreman, M. (1987). A causal model for making decisions about confusion in the hospitalized elderly. In K.J. Hannah, M. Reimer, W.C. Mills, & S. Letourneau (Eds.), Clinical judgment and decision making: The future with nursing diagnosis (pp. 427–429). New York: John Wiley & Sons.

Foreman, M. (1989). Confusion in the hospitalized elderly: Incidence, onset, and associated factors. Research in Nursing and Health, 12, 21–29.

Foreman, M. (1991). Conserving cognitive integrity of the hospitalized elderly. In K.M. Schaefer & J.B. Pond (Eds.), Levine's conservation model: A framework for nursing practice (pp. 133–149). Philadelphia: FA Davis.

Hader, C.F., & Sorensen, E.R. (1988). The effects of body position on transcutaneous oxygen tension. *Pediatric Nursing, 14,* 469–473.

Hanson, D., Langemo, D.K., Olson, B., Hunter, S., Sauvage, T.R., Burd, C., & Cathcart-Silberberg, T. (1991). The prevalence and incidence of pressure ulcers in the hospice setting: Analysis of two methodologies. *American Journal of Hospice and Palliative Care, 8*(5), 18–22.

Lane, L.D., & Winslow, E.H. (1987). Oxygen consumption, cardiovascular response, and perceived exertion in healthy adults during rest, occupied bedmaking, and unoccupied bedmaking activity. *Cardiovascular Nursing, 23*(6), 31–36.

MacLean, S.L. (1987). Description of cues used by nurses when diagnosing activity intolerance. In K.J. Hannah, M. Reimer, W.C. Mills, & S. Letourneau (Eds.), *Clinical judgment and decision making: The future with nursing diagnosis* (pp. 161–163). New York: John Wiley & Sons.

MacLean, S.L. (1988). Activity intolerance: Cues for diagnosis. In R.M. Carroll-Johnston (Ed.), *Classification of nursing diagnoses: Proceedings of the eighth conference: North American Nursing Diagnosis Association* (pp. 320–327). Philadelphia: JB Lippincott.

Nagley, S.J. (1986). Predicting and preventing confusion in your patients. *Journal of Gerontological Nursing, 12*(3), 27–31.

Newport, M.A. (1984). Conserving thermal energy and social integrity in the newborn. *Western Journal of Nursing Research, 6,* 176–197.

Roberts, J.E., Fleming, N., & Yeates-Giese, D. (1991). Perineal integrity. In K.M. Schaefer & J.B. Pond (Eds.), *Levine's conservation model: A framework for nursing practice* (pp. 61–70). Philadelphia: FA Davis.

Schaefer, K.M. (1990). A description of fatigue associated with congestive heart failure: Use of Levine's conservation model. In M.E. Parker (Ed.), *Nursing theories in practice* (pp. 217–237). New York: National League for Nursing.

Schaefer, K.M. (1991). Levine's conservation principles and research. In K.M. Schaefer & J.B. Pond (Eds.), *Levine's conservation model: A framework for nursing practice* (pp. 45–59). Philadelphia: FA Davis.

Schaefer, K.M., & Shober-Potylycki, M.J. (1993). Fatigue associated with congestive health failure: Use of Levine's Conservation Model. *Journal of Advanced Nursing, 18,* 260–268.

Winslow, E.H., Lane, L.D., & Gaffney, F.A. (1984). Oxygen consumption and cardiovascular response in patients and normal adults during in-bed and out-of-bed toileting. *Journal of Cardiac Rehabilitation, 4,* 348–354.

Winslow, E.H., Lane, L.D., & Gaffney, F.A. (1985). Oxygen consumption and cardiovascular response in control adults and acute myocardial infarction patients during bathing. *Nursing Research, 34,* 164–169.

Yeates, D.A., & Roberts, J.E. (1984). A comparison of two bearing-down techniques during the second stage of labor. *Journal of Nurse-Midwifery, 29,* 3–11.

DOCTORAL DISSERTATIONS

Blasage, M.C. (1987). Toward a general understanding of nursing education: A critical analysis of the work of Myra Estrin Levine. *Dissertation Abstracts International, 47,* 4467B.

Cooper, D.M. (1991). Development and testing of an instrument to assess the visual characteristics of open, soft tissue wounds. *Dissertation Abstracts International, 51,* 3320B.

Cox, B. (1988). Pregnancy, anxiety, and time perception. *Dissertation Abstracts International, 48,* 2260B.

Fleming, N. (1988). Comparison of women with different perineal conditions after childbirth. *Dissertation Abstracts International, 48,* 2924B.

Foreman, M. (1988). The development of confusion in the hospitalized elderly. *Dissertation Abstracts International, 48,* 2261B–2262B.

MacLean, S. (1988). Description of cues nurses use for diagnosing activity intolerance. *Dissertation Abstracts International, 48,* 2264B.

Winslow, E.N. (1983). Oxygen consumption and cardiovascular response in normal subjects and in acute myocardial infarction patients during basin bath, tub bath, and shower. *Dissertation Abstracts International, 43,* 2856B.

EDUCATION

Grindley, J., & Paradowski, M. (1991). Developing an undergraduate program using Levine's model. In K.M. Schaefer & J.B. Pond (Eds.), *Levine's conservation model: A framework for nursing practice* (pp. 199–208). Philadelphia: FA Davis.

Schaefer, K.M. (1991). Developing a graduate program in nursing: Integrating Levine's philosophy. In K.M. Schaefer & J.B. Pond (Eds.), *Levine's conservation model:*

A framework for nursing practice (pp. 209–217). Philadelphia: FA Davis.

ADMINISTRATION

Lynn-McHale, D.J., & Smith, A. (1991). Comprehensive assessment of families of the critically ill. *AACN Clinical Issues in Critical Care Nursing, 2,* 195–209.

McCall, B.H. (1991). Neurological intensive monitoring system: Unit assessment tool. In K.M. Schaefer & J.B. Pond (Eds.), *Levine's conservation model: A framework for nursing practice* (pp. 83–90). Philadelphia: FA Davis.

Taylor, J.W. (1974). Measuring the outcomes of nursing care. *Nursing Clinics of North America, 9,* 337–340.

Taylor, J.W. (1987). Organizing data for nursing diagnoses using conservation principles. In A.M. McLane (Ed.), *Classification of nursing diagnoses: Proceedings of the seventh conference: North American Nursing Diagnosis Association* (pp. 103–111). St. Louis: CV Mosby.

Taylor, J.W. (1989). Levine's conservation principles. Using the model for nursing diagnosis in a neurological setting. In J.P. Riehl-Sisca, *Conceptual models for nursing practice* (3rd ed., pp. 349–358). Norwalk, CT: Appleton & Lange.

PRACTICE

Bayley, E.W. (1991). Care of the burn patient. In K.M. Schaefer & J.B. Pond (Eds.), *Levine's conservation model: A framework for nursing practice* (pp. 91–99). Philadelphia: FA Davis.

Brunner, M. (1985). A conceptual approach to critical care nursing using Levine's model. *Focus on Critical Care, 12*(2), 39–44.

Cooper, D.M. (1990). Optimizing wound healing: A practice within nursing's domain. *Nursing Clinics of North America, 25,* 165–180.

Cox, R.A., Sr. (1991). A tradition of caring: Use of Levine's model in long-term care. In K.M. Schaefer & J.B. Pond (Eds.), *Levine's conservation model: A framework for nursing practice* (pp. 179–197). Philadelphia: FA Davis.

Crawford-Gamble, P.E. (1986). An application of Levine's conceptual model. *Perioperative Nursing Quarterly, 2*(1), 64–70.

Dever, M. (1991). Care of children. In K.M. Schaefer & J.B. Pond (Eds.), *Levine's conservation model: A framework for nursing practice* (pp. 71–82). Philadelphia: FA Davis.

Fawcett, J., Archer, C.L., Becker, D., Brown, K.K., Gann, S., Wong, M.J., & Wurster, A.B. (1992). Guidelines for selecting a conceptual model of nursing: Focus on the individual patient. *Dimensions of Critical Care Nursing, 11,* 268–277.

Fawcett, J., Cariello, F.P., Davis, D.A., Farley, J., Zimmaro, D.M., & Watts, R.J. (1987). Conceptual models of nursing: Application to critical care nursing practice. *Dimensions of Critical Care Nursing, 6,* 202–213.

Gingrich, B. (1971). The use of the haptic system as an information-gathering system. In M. Duffey, E.H. Anderson, B. S. Bergersen, M. Lohr, & M.M. Rose (Eds.), *Current concepts in clinical nursing* (Vol. 3, pp. 235–246). St. Louis: CV Mosby.

Herbst, S. (1981). Impairments as a result of cancer. In N. Martin, N. Holt & D. Hicks (Eds.), *Comprehensive rehabilitation nursing* (pp. 553–578). New York: McGraw-Hill.

Hirschfeld, M.H. (1976). The cognitively impaired older adult. *American Journal of Nursing, 76,* 1981–1984.

Pasco, A., & Halupa, D. (1991). Chronic pain management. In K.M. Schaefer & J.B. Pond (Eds.), *Levine's conservation model: A framework for nursing practice* (pp. 101–117). Philadelphia: FA Davis.

Pond, J.B. (1990). Application of Levine's conservation model to nursing the homeless community. In M.E. Parker (Ed.), *Nursing theories in practice* (pp. 203–215). New York: National League for Nursing.

Pond, J.B. (1991). Ambulatory care of the homeless. In K.M. Schaefer & J.B. Pond (Eds.), *Levine's conservation model: A framework for nursing practice* (pp. 167–178). Philadelphia: FA Davis.

Pond, J.B., & Taney, S.G. (1991). Emergency care in a large university emergency department. In K.M. Schaefer & J.B. Pond (Eds.), *Levine's conservation model: A framework for nursing practice* (pp. 151–166). Philadelphia: FA Davis.

Savage, T.A., & Culbert, C. (1989). Early intervention: The unique role of nursing. *Journal of Pediatric Nursing, 4,* 339–345.

Schaefer, K.M. (1991). Care of the patient with congestive heart failure. In K.M. Schaefer & J.B. Pond (Eds.), *Levine's conservation model: A framework for nursing practice* (pp. 119–131). Philadelphia: FA Davis.

Webb, H. (1993). Holistic care following a palliative Hartmann's procedure. *British Journal of Nursing, 2,* 128–132.

CHAPTER

6

Neuman's Systems Model

This chapter presents an analysis and evaluation of Betty Neuman's Systems Model. Neuman's work clearly fits the definition of a conceptual model of nursing. In fact, Neuman (1989a) explicitly referred to her work as a model or conceptual framework.

The concepts of the Neuman Systems Model and their dimensions are listed below. Each concept and its dimensions are defined and described later in this chapter.

KEY CONCEPTS

CLIENT/CLIENT SYSTEM
Individual
Family
Groups
Community
Social Issues
INTERACTING VARIABLES
Physiological
Psychological
Sociocultural
Developmental
Spiritual
CENTRAL CORE
FLEXIBLE LINE OF DEFENSE
NORMAL LINE OF DEFENSE
LINES OF RESISTANCE
ENVIRONMENT
Internal
External
Created
STRESSORS
Intrapersonal

Interpersonal
Extrapersonal
HEALTH/WELLNESS/OPTIMAL
    CLIENT SYSTEM STABILITY
Wellness to Illness
Negentropy and Entropy
Variances from Wellness
Reconstitution
GOAL OF NURSING
Retain, Attain, and Maintain Optimal
    Client Wellness
NURSING PROCESS FORMAT
Nursing Diagnosis
Nursing Goals
Nursing Outcomes
    Primary Prevention
    Secondary Prevention
    Tertiary Prevention
THEORY OF OPTIMAL CLIENT
    SYSTEM STABILITY
THEORY OF PREVENTION AS
    INTERVENTION

ANALYSIS OF NEUMAN'S SYSTEMS MODEL

This section presents an analysis of the Neuman Systems Model. The analysis draws heavily from the second edition of Neuman's (1989c) book, *The Neuman Systems Model*, as well as from recent refinements in the model presented in the journal article, "Health as a continuum based on the Neuman systems model" (Neuman, 1990a), and the book chapter, "The Neuman systems model: A theory for practice" (Neuman, 1990b).

Origins of the Model

Historical Evolution and Motivation

Neuman (1989a) traced the evolution of the Neuman Systems Model from its inception in 1970 to its then current form. The Neuman Systems Model was first published in 1972, in an article entitled, "A model for teaching total person approach to patient problems" (Neuman & Young, 1972). A refinement of the model was published in the 1974 edition of Riehl and Roy's book, *Conceptual Models for Nursing Practice* and reprinted in their 1980 edition (Neuman, 1974, 1980). Further refinements were presented in a chapter (Neuman, 1982a) of the first edition of Neuman's (1982b) book, *The Neuman Systems Model: Application to Nursing Education and Practice*. Other refinements are included in the second edition of Neuman's (1989c) book, *The Neuman Systems Model*. Still other refinements in the Neuman Systems Model are presented in a journal article (Neuman, 1990a) that is based on Neuman's presentation at the 1989 Nurse Theorist Conference and a book chapter (Neuman, 1990b) that is based on Neuman's presentation at a Spring 1990 conference sponsored by Cedars Medical Center in Miami, Florida. The most recent refinements are presented in the third edition of Neuman's (in press) book.

The development of the Neuman Systems Model was motivated by Neuman's desire to respond to the expressed needs of graduate students at the School of Nursing, University of California, Los Angeles (UCLA), for course content that would present the breadth of nursing problems prior to content, emphasizing specific nursing problem areas (Neuman & Young, 1972). Neuman (1989a) claimed that she had no intention of creating a specific conceptual model for the nursing community when she developed her model. She commented, "It is important to state that I was neither knowledgeable about nursing models nor had the trend yet begun in nursing for developing models. The Neuman Systems Model was strictly developed as a teaching aid" (p. 456). It is interesting to note that the Neuman Systems Model was formulated at approximately the same time as other conceptual models of nursing (e.g., King, 1971; Orem, 1971; Rogers, 1970) and at the time when the criteria for National League for Nursing accreditation first stipulated that nursing education programs should be based on conceptual models (Peterson, 1977).

Neuman's conceptual model has undergone changes in its title since its inception. The model was originally published under the title, "A Model for Teaching Total Person Approach to Nursing Care" (Neuman & Young, 1972). The title was changed to "The Betty Neuman Health-Care Systems Model: A Total Person Approach to Patient Problems" in Neuman's 1974 and 1980 publications. Neuman's 1982a chapter carried the title, "The Neuman Health-Care Systems Model: A Total Approach to Client Care," although her book (1982b) title was The Neuman Systems Model. In her 1985b journal article, Neuman referred to the model as "The Neuman Systems Model," and this title has been retained in subsequent publications.

Philosophical Claims

Neuman has presented the philosophical claims undergirding the Neuman Systems Model in the form of a basic philosophy; beliefs about holism, reality, wellness, and the person; and basic assumptions about the person, the environment, and nursing. Neuman (1989a) revealed that her own basic philosophy is "helping each other live" (p. 458). Neuman believes in holism, which she spelled with a "w" in her 1989a, 1989d, and 1990a publications. She stated, "Wholism, implicit within the Neuman Systems Model, is both a philosophical and a biological concept, implying relationships and processes arising from wholeness, dynamic freedom, and creativity in adjusting to stress in the internal and external environments" (1989d, p. 10).

Neuman's (1990a) recent work indicates that she believes in a true reality but recognizes that the true reality may be subjectively distorted. She states:

> For a workable health creating philosophy based on systemic and holistic client perspectives, wellness can be defined in terms of the interrelationship of (a) system available energy, (b) influence of the client created-environment, and (c) caregiver clarification of client health perception. These factors all coalesce into the true reality of the client's health experience and define the nature and quality of his or her life in the process, as related to socially and culturally accepted standards. Health, then, is more than the reality of client perceived experience, inasmuch as subjectivity usually distorts true reality. (p. 130)

Neuman (1990a) further believes that wellness is an "experienced energy based reality" that is "illusive" (p. 130). She assumes that the perception of wellness "is best defined and negotiated holistically between the client and the caregiver" (pp. 130–131). She went on to state the assumption, "Nurses as healers (wholistic themselves) have as a goal conservation of client energy in keeping the system harmonious, while facilitating change toward optimal wellness. Based on this assumption, causal factors must be discovered and carefully negotiated with clients for accountable health management" (p. 131).

Neuman has referred to the person as a client since 1982. She uses the term client because she believes that the term reflects "respect for newer client, caregiver collaborative relationships, and wellness perspectives of the model" (Neuman, 1989d, p. 27).

Neuman (1990a) indicated that she assumes that "provided support factors are in place, the client, as a system, constantly monitors self by making adjustments as needed to retain, attain, and maintain stability for an optimal health state" (p. 129).

Neuman (1989d) noted that the following statements are the basic assumptions "inherent within the Neuman Systems Model" (p. 17):

1. Though each individual client or group as a client system is unique, each system is a composite of common known factors or innate characteristics within a normal, given range of response, contained within a basic structure.

2. Many known, unknown, and universal environmental stressors exist. Each differs in its potential for disturbing a client's usual stability level, or normal line of defense. The particular interrelationships of client variables — physiological, psychological, sociocultural, developmental, and spiritual — at any point in time can affect the degree to which a client is protected by the flexible line of defense against possible reaction to a single stressor or a combination of stressors.

3. Each individual client/client system, over time, has evolved a normal range of response to the environment that is referred to as a normal line of defense, or usual wellness/stability state.

4. When the cushioning, accordion-like effect of the flexible line of defense is no longer capable of protecting the client/client system against an environmental stressor, the stressor breaks through the normal line of defense. The interrelationships of variables — physiological, psychological, sociocultural, developmental, and spiritual — determine the nature and degree of the system reaction or possible reaction to the stressor.

5. The client, whether in a state of wellness or illness, is a dynamic composite of the interrelationships of variables — physiological, psychological, sociocultural, developmental, and spiritual. Wellness is on a continuum of available energy to support the system in its optimal state.

6. Implicit within each client system is a set of internal resistance factors known as lines of resistance, which function to stabilize and return the client to the usual wellness state (normal line of defense) or possibly to a higher level of stability following an environmental stressor reaction.

7. Primary prevention relates to general knowledge that is applied in client assessment and intervention in identification and reduction or mitigation of risk factors associated with environmental stressors to prevent possible reaction.

8. Secondary prevention relates to symptomatology following a reaction to stressors, appropriate ranking of intervention priorities, and treatment to reduce their noxious effects.

9. Tertiary prevention relates to the adjustive processes taking place as reconstitution begins and the maintenance factors move the client back in a circular manner toward primary prevention.

10. The client is in dynamic constant energy exchange with the environment. (pp. 17, 21–22)

In her 1990b book chapter, Neuman presented another set of statements that she labeled as philosophical. Those statements are:

The client is an open system that interacts with the environment in order to promote harmony and balance between the internal and external environment. The client is a composite of physiologic, psychologic, sociocultural, developmental, and spiritual variables that are viewed as parts of the whole. Ideally the client as a system adjusts successfully to internal and external environmental stressors retaining the normal wellness level or system stability.

Environment contains both internal and external stressors and resistance factors. Lines of resistance in the client (internal and external resources) are activated to combat potential or actual stressor reactions. The flexible line of defense protects the normal line of defense or usual wellness condition while the lines of resistance protect the basic structure and support return to wellness. Stressors are considered neutral; client encounter determines either a beneficial or noxious outcome.

Health represents a usual dynamic stability state of the normal line of defense. A reaction to stressors is caused as the normal line of defense is penetrated, causing illness symptoms. The client's position on his or her own wellness-illness continuum is related to the amount of available energy stored and/or used by the system in retaining, attaining, and maintaining system stability.

Nursing is concerned with reduction of potential or actual stressor reaction through use of primary, secondary, or tertiary prevention as intervention to retain, attain, and maintain an optimal wellness level. The goal of nursing is optimal client system stability or wellness. Perceptual distortions between client and nurse, as well as goal plans, are mutually negotiated and resolved. (p. 259)

Strategies for Knowledge Development

The Neuman Systems Model arose from Neuman's observations, her clinical and teaching experiences in mental health nursing, and her synthesis of knowledge from several adjunctive disciplines. As is evident in Neuman's (1989a) description of the development of the model, both inductive and deductive strategies were used. She explained:

The development of the wholistic systemic perspective of the Neuman Systems Model was facilitated by my own basic philosophy of *helping each other live*, many diverse observations and clinical experiences in teaching and encouraging positive aspects of human variables in a wide variety of settings, and theoretical perspectives of stress related to the interactive, interrelated, interdependent, and wholistic nature of systems theory. The significance of perception and behavioral consequences [also] cannot be overestimated. (pp. 457–458)

Influences from Other Scholars

Neuman acknowledged the influences of colleagues and other scholars on the development of the Neuman Systems Model. She noted that the UCLA School of Nursing Curriculum Committee members selected her to develop and coordinate the course for which the model was initially formulated in 1970. She acknowledged the assistance of Rae Jean Young with the evaluation of the effectiveness of the model as a teaching tool and noted that their collaboration led to the first publication about the model (Neuman & Young, 1972). Neuman (1989a) also paid tribute to UCLA School of Nursing Dean Lulu Wolfe Hassenplug and Nurse Continuing Education Director Marjorie Squaires "for offering many opportunities combined with a lack of constraints related to my functioning" (p. 457). In addition, Neuman expressed her "most sincere appreciation for all the fine people who in various ways have facilitated the mature status of the Neuman Systems Model" (p. 466).

Neuman (1974, 1989d) has also identified the knowledge from adjunctive disciplines that contributed to the content of the Neuman Systems Model. Scholars and works that were particularly influential include Chardin's (1955) philosophical beliefs about the wholeness of life, Marxist philosophical views of the oneness of man and nature (Cornu, 1957), Gestalt and field theories of the interaction between person and environment (Edelson, 1970), general system theory of the nature of living open systems (Bertalanffy, 1968), Putt's (1972) ideas of entropy and evolution in systems, Selye's (1950) conceptualization of stress, and Caplan's (1964) articulation of levels of prevention.

World View

The Neuman Systems Model primarily reflects the *reciprocal interation* world view. This world view is represented by Neuman's use of Gestalt and field theories, as well as philosophies that emphasize the unity of the person. Neuman's holistic, multidimensional approach (Neuman, 1990b) also reflects the reciprocal interaction world view. Furthermore, although Neuman identified five different variables constituting the client (physiological, psychological, sociocultural, developmental, and spiritual), she emphasized the need to consider all of the variables at any given time. To underscore that point, Neuman (1974) stated, "the wholeness concept . . . is based upon the appropriate interrelationship of variables" (p. 103).

Moreover, Neuman views the client system as active. In fact, Neuman (1989d) characterized client system-environment exchanges as "reciprocal" and noted that "both client and environment may be positively or negatively affected by each other" (p. 11).

In keeping with the reciprocal interaction world view, the Neuman Systems Model incorporates elements of both persistence and change.

Neuman's emphasis on client system stability and her focus on protection of the central core of the client system by the various lines of defense and resistance reflect persistence. Change is also evident. Indeed, Neuman (1989d) contends that "the client is in constant change" (p. 12). Persistence and change are linked in Neuman's (1989d) statement that "A system implies dynamic energy exchange [with the environment], moving toward or away from stability" (p. 10). Persistence and change, then, appear to be on a dual continuum of more or less persistence and more or less change at any time in the life of the client system. That interpretation of Neuman's work requires validation.

Though the primary world view of the Neuman Systems Model is reciprocal interaction, the *reaction world view* is introduced in Neuman's description of the created-environment as an unconscious structure, which implies a psychoanalytic orientation. The reaction world view is also evident in Neuman's use of Selye's (1950) mechanistic theory of stress and adaptation and her view of illness as entropy.

Unique Focus of the Model

The unique focus of the Neuman Systems Model is the wellness of the client/client system in relation to environmental stress and reactions to stress. The model is "a structure that depicts the parts and subparts and their interrelationship for the whole of the client as a complete system . . . [that applies] equally well to [the individual,] a small group or community, a larger aggregate, or the universe" (Neuman, 1989d, p. 16). Particular attention is given to "wellness retention and optimal client/ client system wellness attainment and maintenance" (Neuman, 1989d, p. 25) in the face of problems that originate in client system reactions to the intrapersonal, interpersonal, and extrapersonal stressors arising in the internal and external environments. Attention is also focused on variances from wellness and on nursing interventions directed toward retention, attainment, and maintenance of client system stability.

The Neuman Systems Model has always been classified as a systems model (Barnum, 1994; Marriner-Tomey, 1989; Riehl & Roy, 1974, 1980; Riehl-Sisca, 1989). Neuman (personal communications, November 6 and 13, 1980) commented that she did not take classification into account when formulating her model but that she now agrees that it is the appropriate category. In fact, she has stated, "The Neuman Systems Model is an open systems model that views nursing as being primarily concerned with defining appropriate action in stress-related situations or possible reactions of the client/client system" (Neuman, 1989d, p. 11).

The Neuman Systems Model addresses system in the discussion of the person. The definition of person as an interacting open client system that is a dynamic composite of the interrelationship of physiological, psychological, sociocultural, developmental, and spiritual variables fits the requirement that a systems view treats phenomena as organized, integrated entities.

The model addresses environment in detail, with descriptions of the internal, external, and created environments. Moreover, the internal and external environments are regarded as the sources of stressors that influence the client system.

Neuman (1989d) considers client system boundaries to be "dynamic and constantly changing, presenting different appearances according to time, place, and the significance of events" (p. 8). The lines of defense and resistance form boundaries between the central core of the client system and the environment. "The outer boundary for the client as a system," Neuman (1989d) explained, "is designated by the protective flexible line of defense" (p. 27). Boundary permeability is considered in Neuman's discussion of factors that influence stressor invasion and reactions to stressors.

Neuman's discussion of environmental stressors encompasses the systems models characteristic of tension, stress, strain, and conflict. Neuman (1989d) explicitly identified stressors as the disruptive forces that operate within or upon the system. She also stated that stressors are "tension-producing stimuli with the potential for causing disequilibrium" (p. 23).

Neuman (1989d) has referred to a dynamic equilibrium, a steady state, and to homeostasis. She depicts client system-environment interaction as a dynamic equilibrium, commenting that "A dynamic equilibrium should exist within the system. . . . Stability implies a state of balance requiring energy exchange between the system and environment to cope adequately with imposing stressors" (pp. 12–13). Neuman (1989d) also refers to system-environment interaction as a steady state. She stated, "At the simplest level a steady state, governed by a dynamic interaction of parts and subparts, is one of stability over time. This is analogous to the Neuman Systems Model's concept of normal line of defense" (p. 13).

In addition, Neuman (1989d) refers to homeostasis, which she seems to equate with stability. She stated, "Homeostasis (stability) preserves the character of the system. An adjustment in one direction is countered by a movement in the opposite direction, both movements being approximately rather than precisely compensatory. With opposing forces in effect, the process of stability is an example of the regulatory capacity of a system" (p. 14).

The systems characteristic of feedback is addressed in Neuman's (1989d) discussion of client system processes. She stated, "Feedback of output into input makes the system self-regulated in relation to either maintenance of a desired health state or goal outcome" (p. 14).

Meleis (1991) regarded the Neuman Systems model as client-focused. Barnum (1994) considered the model within the systems category; she did not place it within her classification scheme of intervention, substitution, conservation, sustenance, and enhancement categories.

Content of the Model: Concepts

Person

The person in the Neuman Systems Model is defined as a **client/ client system**. The client or client system can be an *individual*, a *family or other group*, the *community*, or even a *social issue*. The client system is "a composite of **interacting variables** — *physiological, psychological, sociocultural, developmental,* and *spiritual* [emphasis mine]" (Neuman, 1989d, p. 22). The *physiological variable* refers to bodily structure and function; the *psychological variable*, to mental processes and relationships; the *sociocultural variable*, to social and cultural functions; the *developmental variable*, to the developmental processes of life; and the *spiritual variable*, to the influences of spiritual beliefs.

The five variables are interrelated in each client system. The interrelationships "determine the amount of resistance [a client system] has to any environmental stressor" (Neuman, 1989d, p. 23). Moreover, although all five variable areas are contained within each client system, each exhibits "varying degrees of development and a wide range of interactive styles and potential" (Neuman, 1989d, p. 29). Variability in development of the spiritual variable is especially noted. Indeed, Neuman (1989d) maintained that the client may never recognize or develop the spiritual variable, although it permeates all other client system variables. More specifically, the spiritual variable is viewed as a continuum from complete unawareness or denial of its presence and potential to a consciously developed high level of spiritual understanding.

The client/client system is depicted as a **central core** surrounded by concentric rings (Figure 6-1). The central core is a basic structure of survival factors "common to the species, such as variables contained within it, innate or genetic factors, and strength and weakness of the system parts" (Neuman, 1989d, p. 27). When the client is the individual, the basic survival factors are exemplified by temperature range, genetic response patterns, ego structure, and strengths and weaknesses of body organs. Certain unique features or baseline characteristics, such as cognitive ability, also are contained within the central core (Neuman, 1989d). Thus, the five variables — physiological, psychological, sociocultural, developmental, and spiritual — are part of the basic structure (Neuman, 1985a).

The five variables also are considered to be part of the three mechanisms that protect the central core of the client system. These mechanisms are depicted as concentric rings in Figure 6-1. The outermost ring is the **flexible line of defense**. This mechanism is a protective buffer for the client's normal or stable state. Ideally, it prevents invasion of stressors and keeps the client system free from stressor reactions or symptomatology. The flexible line of defense is thought of as a dynamic accordion-like mechanism, rapidly expanding away from or drawing closer to the normal line of defense. When the flexible line has expanded away from the

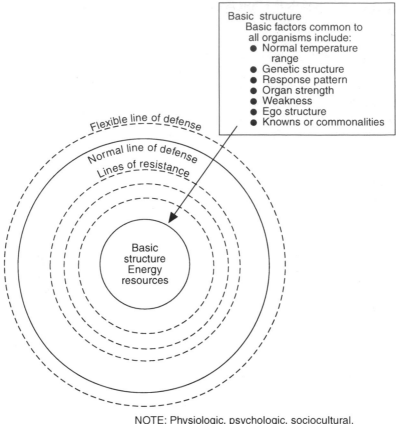

FIGURE 6-1. Diagram of the client system. (From Neuman, B: The Neuman Systems Model. Appleton & Lange, Norwalk, CT, 1989, p 28, with permission.)

normal line of defense, it provides greater protection against stressor invasion; when it draws closer to the normal line, it provides less protection. Neuman (1989d) explained that "the [five] variables contained within the flexible line of defense . . . protect the client system from possible instability caused by stressors. Determining factors . . . include the client's physiologic condition, sociocultural influences, developmental state, cognitive skills, and spiritual considerations" (p. 23).

The **normal line of defense** lies between the flexible line of defense and the lines of resistance. This second protective mechanism is the client/client system's normal or usual wellness level. The normal line of defense represents "what the client has become, the state to which the client has evolved to over time" (Neuman, 1989d, p. 30). It is the result of adjustment of the client system to environmental stressors. In effect, the normal line of defense is a standard against which variances from wellness can be judged. The normal line of defense, like the flexible line, can expand or contract but apparently does so more slowly. Expansion of the normal line of defense reflects an enhanced wellness state; contraction, a diminished state of wellness (Neuman, 1989d).

The normal line of defense is penetrated by one or more stressors when the flexible line of defense cannot withstand the stressor impact. A reaction, in the form of client system instability or illness, occurs when the normal line of defense is rendered ineffective in relation to the impact of the stressor(s) (Neuman, 1989d).

The innermost concentric rings are the **lines of resistance**. This third protective mechanism is involuntarily activated when a stressor invades the normal line of defense. The lines of resistance attempt to stabilize the client system and foster a return to the normal line of defense. These lines contain such internal factors that support the basic structure and the normal line of defense as mobilization of white blood cells or activation of the immune system mechanisms. If the lines of resistance are effective, the system can reconstitute; if they are ineffective, energy depletion occurs, and death may ensue (Neuman, 1985a, 1989d).

Neuman (1985a) explained that the flexible line of defense protects the normal line of defense, and the lines of resistance protect the basic structure. The flexible line of defense is immediately called into action when the client system encounters a stressor and attempts to maintain stability. If the flexible line of defense is not effective, the normal line of defense breaks down and a stressor reaction, or symptoms, occurs. The lines of resistance then are activated and, if effective, pull the client back toward wellness. The condition of the flexible line of defense, then, determines whether a reaction is likely when a stressor is encountered.

More specifically, the client/client system's reaction to a stressor is determined in part by natural and learned resistance, which is manifested by the strength of the flexible and normal lines of defense and the lines of resistance. The amount of resistance, in turn, is determined by the interrelationship of the five variables of the client system. Reaction also is determined by the time of encounter with a stressor, as well as by its nature and intensity. Other factors influencing reaction to a stressor include idiosyncrasies in the basic structure, past and present conditions of the client system, available energy resources, the amount of energy required for adaptation, and the client system's perception of the stressor (Neuman, 1974, 1985a, 1989d).

Environment

Environment is defined as "all factors affecting and affected by the system" (Neuman, 1989d, p. 12) and as "all internal and external factors or influences surrounding the identified client or client system" (p. 31).

Neuman (1989d, 1990a) has identified three relevant environments. The *internal environment* "consists of all forces or interactive influences internal to or contained solely within the boundaries of the defined client/ client system" (1989d, p. 31). It is intrapersonal in nature. The *external environment* "consists of all forces or interaction influences external to or existing outside the defined client/client system" (1989d, p. 31) and is interpersonal and extrapersonal in nature. The *created-environment* is subconsciously developed by the client as "a symbolic expression of system wholeness" (1989d, p. 32). It is intrapersonal, interpersonal, and extrapersonal in nature. The created-environment supersedes and encompasses both internal and external environments. Neuman (1989d) went on to explain that the created-environment

> acts as an immediate or long range safe reservoir for existence or the maintenance of system integrity expressed consciously, unconsciously, or both simultaneously. The created-environment is dynamic and represents the client's unconscious mobilization of all system variables, including the basic structure energy factors, toward system integration, stability and integrity. It is inherently purposeful, though unconsciously developed, since its function is to offer a protective shield or safe arena for system function. It pervades all systems, large and small, at least to some degree; it is either spontaneously created, increased, or decreased as warranted by a special condition of need. . . . All basic structure factors and system variables influence or are influenced by the created-environment, which is developed and maintained, in varying degrees of protectiveness, at any given place or point in time. . . . The created-environment is based on unseen, unconscious knowledge, as well as self-esteem, beliefs, energy exchanges, system variables, and predisposition; it is a process-based concept of perpetual adjustment within which a client may either increase or decrease the wellness state. (pp. 32–33)

Neuman (1990a) went on to explain that the created-environment "is a self-help phenomenon that can reflect a temporary health state as a response to situational stressors on the client's flexible [and normal] line[s] of defense [and lines of resistance]" (p. 130). Although the client may be conscious of "the environmental reality that inexorably shapes the health condition" (p. 130), the created-environment functions as a subjective safety mechanism that "may block conscious awareness of the true reality of the environment and the health experience [by structuring] a semblance or illusion of harmony in wellness" (p. 130) for the client system.

Neuman (1989d) drew from Selye's (1950) work to define **stressors** as "tension producing stimuli or forces occurring both within the internal and external environmental boundaries of the client/client system" (p. 23). She classified stressors as *intrapersonal, interpersonal,* and *extrapersonal. Intrapersonal stressors* are within the internal environment of the client/client system and include such forces as conditioned and autoimmune responses. *Interpersonal stressors* are in the external environment. They occur at the boundary between the client/client system and the proximal external environment and include such forces as role expectations and communication patterns. *Extrapersonal stressors* also are in the external environment. They occur at the boundary of the client/client system and the distal external environment and include such forces as financial concerns or social policies.

Neuman (1985a, 1989d) maintained that stressors are inert or neutral, but the outcome of a reaction to a stressor may be beneficial or noxious, positive or negative. The nature and extent of the reaction to a stressor is influenced by such factors as "the time of stressor occurrence, past and present condition of the client, nature and intensity of the stressor, and the amount of energy required by the client to adjust . . . [as well as] past coping behavior or patterns in a similar situation" (1989d, p. 24).

Person and Environment

Neuman (1989d) identified the client and the environment as basic nursing phenomena. Accordingly, the connection between the two in the Neuman Systems Model merits examination. The client/client system is an open system "in interaction and total interface with the environment" (p. 23). Neuman explained that as a system, the client is "capable of both input and output related to intra-, inter-, and extrapersonal environmental influences, interacting with the environment by adjusting to it, or . . . adjusting the environment to itself" (p. 23). The relationship between the client/client system and the environment, then, is reciprocal. In particular, "Input, output and feedback between the client and the environment is of a circular nature; client and environment have a reciprocal relationship, the outcome of which is corrective or regulative for the system" (p. 31). The reciprocal relationship may have a positive or a negative effect on either the client or the environment. Neuman (1989d) explained, "The process of interaction and adjustment results in varying degrees of harmony, stability, or balance between the client and the environment. Ideally, there is optimal client system stability" (p. 23).

Health

Neuman (1989d) equated **health** with **wellness**, defining those terms together as "the condition or the degree of system stability, that is, the condition in which all parts and subparts (variables) are in balance or harmony with the whole of the client/client system" (p. 12). The essential connection between health and wellness is reinforced in Neuman's (1989d) comment that health "is reflected in the level of wellness: when system needs are met, a state of optimal wellness exists. Conversely, unmet needs reduce the wellness state" (p. 12).

In addition, Neuman (1990b) equated health, or wellness, with **optimal client system stability**. "Optimal," Neuman (1990a) explained, "means the highest possible health condition achievable at a given point in time" (p. 129).

In keeping with the open systems perspective of the conceptual model, Neuman (1989d) conceptualized health as "a continuum from *wellness to illness*" (p. 14) but regards the end states of the continuum as dichotomous. She states, "Wellness is a state of saturation or inertness, one free of disrupting needs; illness is a state of insufficiency (disrupting needs are yet to be satisfied)" (p. 14).

Neuman (1989d, 1990a) has also described health "as living energy" (1989d, p. 33) and stated that "Health . . . is energy as a result of system balance" (1990a, p. 129). She defined energy as "the pervasive forces within the client that empowers and regulates all systemic functions from cellular to motor" (1990a, p. 129). She went on to explain that energy, which acts as a "primary and basic power resource for the client as a system" (1990a, p. 129), is innately or genetically acquired, generated and stored, used or spent, available or bound. The health condition reflects "the amount of energy remaining following efforts made by the system to achieve balance during periods of instability" (1990a, p. 129).

Within the context of health as energy, Neuman (1990a) stated, "Health on a continuum is the degree of client wellness that exists at any point in time, ranging from an optimal wellness condition, with available energy at its maximum, to death, which represents total energy depletion" (p. 129). Neuman (1989d) further described the dichotomous end states of the health continuum in terms of the flow of energy between the client system and the environment. She explained, "Wellness is determined by the amount of energy required to return to and maintain system stability. When more energy is available than is being used, the system is stable" (p. 13). Optimal wellness is "the greatest possible degree of system stability at a given point in time" (p. 25). Wellness as energy "is a manifestation of the highest possible level of system stability, implying that energy is sufficient for necessary system function from the cellular level to gross motor participation in the life processes of adjustment and change" (Neuman, 1990a, p. 129). Illness is viewed as an excessive expenditure of energy. Neuman (1989d) explained, "A violent energy flow occurs when a system is disrupted from its normal or stable state; that is, it expends energy to cope with disorganization. When more energy is used by the system in its state of disorganization than is built and stored, the outcome may be death" (pp. 12–13).

Neuman (1989d) has also described energy flow in terms of the systems notions of *negentropy and entropy*—sufficient energy is regarded as the condition of negentropy, and energy depletion is regarded as entropy. "Client movement is toward negentropy when more energy is being generated than used; when more energy is required than is being generated, movement is toward entropy, or illness—and possible death" (pp. 33–34).

Although Neuman (1989d) used the term illness repeatedly, she also spoke of *variances from wellness*, which she has described as "the difference from the normal or usual wellness condition" (p. 41). From that perspective, wellness is for Neuman (1989d) "a matter of degree, a point on a continuum running from greatest negentropy to maximum entropy" (p. 25). A variance from wellness is determined by comparing the normal health state with that which is taking place at a given time (Neuman, 1985a).

Reconstitution occurs after the client system reacts to stressors. More specifically, reconstitution "is the determined energy increase related to the degree of reaction [to a stressor]" (Neuman, 1989d, pp. 36–37) and represents the return and maintenance of system stability following treatment of stressor reactions. Reconstitution depends on "the successful mobilization of client resources to prevent further stressor reaction or regression; it represents a dynamic state of adjustment to stressors and integration of all necessary factors toward optimal use of existing resources for client system stability or wellness maintenance" (Neuman, 1989d, p. 37).

Accordingly, reconstitution leads to client system stability and a level of wellness that is the same as it was prior to the stressor reaction, at a higher than usual wellness level, or at a lower than usual wellness level. Health of the client/client system, therefore, "is envisioned as being at various and changing levels within normal range, rising or falling throughout the life span because of basic structure factors and the satisfactory or unsatisfactory adjustment to environmental stressors" (Neuman, 1989d, p. 33). If reconstitution does not occur, death ensues.

Nursing

Neuman (1974) viewed nursing as a "unique profession [that] is concerned with all the variables affecting an individual's response to stressors" (p. 102). The major concern for nursing is "keeping the client system stable through accuracy both in the assessment of effects and possible effects of environmental stressors and in assisting client adjustments required for an optimal wellness level" (Neuman, 1989d, p. 34).

The **goal of nursing**, according to Neuman (1989d), is "*to facilitate optimal wellness for the client through retention, attainment, or maintenance of client system stability*" (p. 25). More specifically, the goal of nursing actions is to "assist the client in creating and shaping reality in a desired direction, related to retention, attainment, or maintenance of optimal system wellness, or a combination of these, through purposeful interventions [that should] mitigate or reduce stress factors and adverse conditions which affect or could affect optimal client functioning, at any given point in time" (p. 17).

Neuman (1989d) presented a **nursing process format** that is made up of three steps or categories: nursing *diagnosis*, nursing *goals*, and nursing *outcomes*. The first step, nursing *diagnosis*, encompasses the collection of data about the dynamic interactions among the physiological, psychological, sociocultural, developmental, and spiritual variables making up the client system. This step of the nursing process takes into account the perceptions of both the client and the caregiver. Underscoring this point, Neuman (1989d) maintained that proper assessment requires consideration of both the client's and the caregiver's perceptions of the basic structure, the lines of resistance and defense, and the internal and external environments.

In addition, the client's created-environment must be discovered. Neuman (1990a) pointed out that although the identification of the relevant factors in the client's internal and external environments is relatively easy, determination of the created-environment can be challenging. She explained:

> The familiar conscious level of internal (intrapersonal) and external (interpersonal and extrapersonal) environment factors of the model can be easily determined, whereas those of the unconsciously derived created-environment are more illusive and fragile, requiring discovery of causal as well as defining factors. These created-environment factors can best be identified and defined as client patterned responses through caregiver use of intuition, empathy, inference, and clustering of response patterns to form mini-hypotheses for careful informal testing in client-nurse interaction. (p. 130)

The first step of the nursing process concludes with the formulation of a nursing diagnostic statement, formulation and prioritization of possible goals, and identification of hypothetical interventions. The nursing diagnosis "must be a comprehensive statement that encompasses the client's general condition or circumstances" (Neuman, 1989b, p. 57), including identification of actual or potential variances from wellness and available resources. The diagnostic statement is based on a synthesis of client data and relevant theory from nursing and adjunctive disciplines. Neuman (1989d) recommended that the diagnostic statement use "available and relevant diagnostic nomenclature, adding to it as required" (p. 39). The diagnostic statement serves as the basis for the formulation and prioritization of client needs as well as identification of hypothetical interventions postulated to assist the client reach the highest possible level of system stability or wellness.

The second step of the nursing process is the negotiation of actual *nursing goals* with the client for desired prescriptive changes to correct variances from wellness. Specific intervention strategies postulated to retain, attain, and/or maintain client system stability are also negotiated with the client. The second step, then, encompasses specification of actual outcome goals and intervention strategies designed to achieve the goals.

The third nursing process step is nursing *outcomes*. Intervention strategies, using one or more prevention as intervention modalities, are implemented during this step. Neuman's (1989d) prevention as intervention format specifies three modalities. Primary prevention is described as the action required to retain client system stability. Intervention involving primary prevention is selected when the risk of or hazard from a stressor is known, but a reaction has not yet occurred. Interventions attempt to reduce the possibility of the client's encounter with the stressor or strengthen the flexible line of defense to decrease the possibility of a reaction when the stressor is encountered. Neuman (1989d) regards health promotion as a component of primary prevention, noting that it "relates to activities that optimize the client wellness potential or condition" (p. 39). She explained that "intervention can begin at any point at which a stressor is either suspected or identified" (p. 35).

Secondary prevention is the action required to attain system stability. Intervention involving secondary prevention is selected when a reaction to a stressor has already occurred. Interventions deal with existing symptoms and attempt to strengthen the lines of resistance through use of the client's internal and external resources. Neuman (1974) introduced the idea of priorities in secondary prevention by stating, "ranking of need priority can occur . . . only by proper assessment of internal as well as external resources, that is, getting at the total meaning of the experience for the individual" (p. 105). If secondary prevention interventions are effective, reconstitution occurs. If they are not effective, "death occurs as a result of failure of the basic structure" (Neuman, 1989d, p. 36).

Tertiary prevention is the action required to maintain system stability. Intervention involving tertiary prevention is selected when some degree of client system stability and reconstitution has occurred following secondary prevention interventions. Tertiary prevention interventions maintain reconstitution when client resources are mobilized to prevent additional reactions to stressors or regression from the current wellness level. Neuman (1989d) noted that "tertiary prevention tends to lead back, in circular fashion, toward primary prevention" (p. 37).

Neuman (1989d) pointed out that the prevention as intervention modalities represent a typology of nursing actions that identifies the client's entry point into the health care system as well as the type of intervention needed. She also pointed out that more than one prevention modality may be used simultaneously if the client's condition warrants such multilevel intervention. Specific functions or actions taken as part of primary, secondary, and tertiary prevention include but are not limited to initiating, planning, organizing, monitoring, coordinating, implementing, integrating, advocating, supporting, and evaluating (Neuman, 1989d).

The final step of the nursing process concludes when the results of intervention, termed outcome goals, are evaluated to confirm their attainment or to guide reformulation of the goals. Consequently, the client outcome acts as feedback for additional system input.

The entire nursing process format for Neuman's model is outlined in Table 6–1. The outline incorporates two Neuman Systems Models "tools" for model implementation, the Neuman Nursing Process Format and the Prevention as Intervention Format. The Nursing Process Format provided details about the specific components of each step of the Neuman Systems Model nursing process. The Prevention as Intervention Format provided specific interventions for the three interventions as intervention modalities.

TABLE 6–1. THE NEUMAN SYSTEMS MODEL: NURSING PROCESS FORMAT

I. Nursing diagnosis
  A. Establish data base that includes the simultaneous consideration of the dynamic interactions of physiological, psychological, sociocultural, developmental, and spiritual variables
    1. Identify client/client system's perceptions
      a. Assess condition and strength of basic structure factors and energy resources
      b. Assess characteristics of the flexible and normal lines of defense, lines of resistance, degree of potential or actual reaction, and potential for reconstitution following a reaction
      c. Asess internal and external environments
        (1) Identify and evaluate potential or actual stressors that pose a threat to the stability of the client/client system
        (2) Classify stressors that threaten stability of client/client system
          (a) Deprivation
          (b) Excess
          (c) Change
          (d) Intolerance
      d. Identify, classify, and evaluate potential and/or actual intrapersonal, interpersonal, and extrapersonal interactions between the client/client system and the environment, considering all five variables
      e. Assess the created-environment
        (1) Discover nature of client/client system's created-environment
          (a) Assess client/client system's perception of stressors
          (b) Identify client/client system's major problem, stress areas, or areas of concern
          (c) Identify client/client system's perceptions of how present circumstances differ from usual pattern of living
          (d) Identify ways in which client/client system handled similar problems in the past
          (e) Identify what client/client system anticipates for self in the future as a consequence of the present situation
          (f) Determine what client/client system is doing and what he or she can do to help himself or herself
          (g) Determine what client/client system expects caregivers, family, friends, or others to do for him or her
        (2) Determine degree of protection provided
        (3) Uncover cause of client/client system's created environment
      f. Evaluate influence of past, present, and possible future life process and coping patterns on client/client system stability
      g. Identify and evaluate actual and potential internal and external resources for optimal state of wellness
    2. Identify caregiver's perceptions (repeat 1 a,b,c,d,f,g from caregiver's perspective)
    3. Compare client/client system's and caregiver's perceptions
      a. Identify similarities and differences in perceptions
      b. Facilitate client awareness of major perceptual distortions
      c. Resolve perceptual differences

TABLE 6–1. **THE NEUMAN SYSTEMS MODEL: NURSING PROCESS FORMAT**
(Continued)

B. Variances from wellness
    1. Synthesize client data base with relevant theories from nursing and adjunctive disciplines
    2. State a comprehensive nursing diagnosis
    3. Prioritize goals
        a. Consider client/client system wellness level
        b. Consider system stability needs
        c. Consider total available resources
    4. Postulate outcome goals and interventions that will facilitate the highest possible level of client/client system stability or wellness, i.e., maintain the normal line of defense and retain the flexible line of defense

II. Nursing goals
  A. Negotiate desired prescriptive change or outcome goals to correct variances from wellness with the client/client system
    1. Consider needs identified in I.B.3.b.
    2. Consider resources identified in I.B.3.c.
  B. Negotiate prevention as intervention modalities and actions with client/client system

III. Nursing outcomes
  A. Implement nursing interventions through use of one or more of three prevention modalities
    1. Primary prevention nursing actions to retain system stability
        a. Prevent stressor invasion
        b. Provide information to retain or strengthen existing client/client system strengths
        c. Support positive coping and functioning
        d. Desensitize existing or possible noxious stressors
        e. Motivate toward wellness
        f. Coordinate and integrate interdisciplinary theories and epidemiological input
        g. Educate or reeducate
        h. Use stress as a positive intervention strategy
    2. Secondary prevention nursing actions to attain system stability
        a. Protect basic structure
        b. Mobilize and optimize internal/external resources to attain stability and energy conservation
        c. Facilitate purposeful manipulation of stressors and reactions to stressors
        d. Motivate, educate, and involve client/client system in health care goals
        e. Facilitate appropriate treatment and intervention measures
        f. Support positive factors toward wellness
        g. Promote advocacy by coordination and integration
        h. Provide primary preventive intervention as required
    3. Tertiary prevention nursing actions to maintain system stability
        a. Attain and maintain highest possible level of wellness and stability during reconstitution
        b. Educate, reeducate, and/or reorient as needed
        c. Support client/client system toward appropriate goals
        d. Coordinate and integrate health service resources
        e. Provide primary and/or secondary preventive intervention as required
  B. Evaluate outcome goals
    1. Confirm attainment of outcome goals
    2. Reformulate goals
  C. Set intermediate and long-range goals for subsequent nursing action that are structured in relation to short-term goal outcomes

Adapted from Neuman, B. (1989). *The Neuman systems model* (pp. 18–21). Norwalk, CT: Appleton & Lange, © 1980, rev. 1987 Betty Neuman; and Neuman, B.M. (1990). Health as a continuum based on the Neuman Systems Model. *Nursing Science Quarterly, 3,* 129–135, with permission.

Content of the Model: Propositions

The relationship between the person and the environment is mentioned repeatedly in the Neuman Systems Model. The reciprocal nature of that relationship is articulated in the following quotations:

> The client is an interacting open system in total interface with both internal and external environmental forces or stressors; the client is in constant change, with reciprocal environmental interaction, at all times moving either toward a dynamic state of wellness or toward one of illness in varying degrees. (Neuman 1989d, p. 12)

> The client is a system capable of both input and output related to the intra-, inter-, and extrapersonal environmental influences, interacting with the environment by adjusting to it or adjusting the environment to itself. (Neuman 1989d, p. 23)

The linkage between health and nursing is evident in the following statement:

> Nursing acts to conserve energy to impede or arrest movement toward the entropic (illness) state and to facilitate movement toward the negentropic (wellness) state. (Neuman 1989d, p. 14)

The four metaparadigm concepts are linked in Neuman's statements about primary, secondary, and tertiary prevention. Although environment is more implicit than explicit in those statements, it is taken into account. Indeed, as Neuman (1989d) pointed out, "In keeping the systems stable, the nurse creates a linkage between the client, environment, health and nursing" (p. 34). Those linkages are reflected in the following quotations:

> The primary prevention as intervention . . . modality is used for primary prevention as wellness retention, that is, to protect the client system's normal line of defense or usual wellness state by strengthening the flexible line of defense. The goal is to promote client wellness by stress prevention and reduction of risk factors. (Neuman 1989d, p. 35)

> The secondary prevention as intervention modality is used for secondary prevention as wellness attainment, that is, to protect the basic structure by strengthening the internal lines of resistance. The goal is to provide appropriate treatment of symptoms to attain optimal client system stability or wellness and energy conservation. (Neuman 1989d, p. 36)
> The tertiary prevention as intervention modality is used for tertiary prevention as wellness maintenance, that is, to protect client system reconstitution or return to wellness following treatment. Reconstitution may be viewed as feedback from the input and output of secondary intervention. The goal is to maintain an optimal wellness level by supporting existing strengths and conserving client system energy. (Neuman 1989d, p. 37)

The integral relationship of person, environment, health, and nursing is especially evident in the following statement, which includes environment in an explicit manner:

> The major concern for nursing is in keeping the client system stable through accuracy both in the assessment of effects and possible effects of environmental stressors and in assisting client adjustments required for an optimal wellness level. (Neuman 1989d, p. 34)

EVALUATION OF NEUMAN'S SYSTEMS MODEL

This section presents an evaluation of the Neuman Systems Model. The evaluation is based on the results of the analysis, as well as on publications and presentations by Neuman and by others who have used or commented on the model.

Explication of Origins

Neuman explicated the origins of the Neuman Systems Model clearly and concisely. She traced her own background and the evolution of the model from a teaching aid to a fully developed conceptual model of nursing in a concise yet richly detailed manner (Neuman, 1989a), and she made clear the forces and circumstances that motivated her work. Furthermore, Neuman explicitly identified the philosophical claims undergirding the model. These beliefs and assumptions indicate that Neuman values a holistic, systems-based approach to the care of clients. Neuman's choice of a systems approach to health care reflects her assumption that systems thinking is a comprehensive way of viewing clients and their environments. Neuman also values intervention prior to manifestations of variances from wellness, as well as after they occur. She emphasized the need to consider both the client's and the caregiver's perceptions of stressors. Furthermore, she assumes that nursing goals are established effectively when negotiated with the client. These aspects of the Neuman Systems Model indicate her respect for the perceptions and rights of each client. In fact, she deliberately labeled the person as a client to denote her respect for those for whom nurses care and her concern for collaborative goal setting. Furthermore, Neuman values wellness. In fact, Neuman has always regarded her work as a wellness model. Neuman assumes that the environment is the source of stressors, but she regards stressors as neutral. The outcome of encounters with stressors is what has a negative or positive valence.

It must be noted that the 10 statements Neuman (1989d) identified as the assumptions of the Neuman Systems Model and the statements about the client, the environment, health, and nursing that she labeled as philosophical statements (Neuman, 1990b) actually are the propositions that define, describe, and link the concepts of the model. Strictly speaking, then, those assumptions and statements are not philosophical claims.

Neuman explicitly acknowledged nursing colleagues who influenced her thinking and supported her work, and she cited the knowledge she drew on from adjunctive disciplines for the development of the Neuman Systems Model. Neuman has always cited the influence of systems thinking and has become increasingly clear about how she has integrated ideas from general system theory into the model.

Comprehensiveness of Content

The Neuman Systems Model is sufficiently comprehensive with regard to depth of content. However, although the revisions and refinements evident in Neuman's (1989d, 1990a) current version of the model have clarified several areas of confusion found in earlier versions and have improved the adequacy of concept definitions and descriptions, some points require additional clarification. The revisions and refinements to date certainly suggest that Neuman has been responsive to critiques of her work, such as the chapter on analysis and evaluation of the model by Fawcett et al. (1982) published in the first edition of The Neuman Systems Model (Neuman, 1982b). Indeed, Stevens (1982) commended Neuman for the scholarly attitude and scientific detachment demonstrated by inclusion of that critique in the book.

Given the abstract and general nature of conceptual models, Neuman's descriptions of the person, the environment, health, and nursing are generally adequate. The concept of health could, however, be clarified with regard to Neuman's (1989d) view of wellness and illness as a continuum with dichotomous end points. Given Neuman's apparent emphasis on a continuum, it would be more appropriate to identify wellness and illness as the polar ends of the continuum, rather than dichotomous conditions. Another aspect of health that could be clarified is Neuman's view of wellness as negentropy and illness as entropy. Clarification is needed because general system theory, upon which Neuman based a substantial portion of her model, views the living open system as negentropic. Entropy, according to Bertalanffy (1968), is a characteristic only of closed systems.

Furthermore, Neuman's explicit characterization of client system-environment interactions as a dynamic equilibrium, a steady state, and homeostasis requires clarification. In particular, a decision as to which of those three possible but logically incompatible views of system-environment interactions represents Neuman's conceptualization of the client system and the environment is required.

Neuman's (1989d) approach to the nursing process reflects systems thinking. She stated, "Using a wholistic systems approach to protect and promote client welfare, nursing action must be skillfully related to the meaningful and dynamic organization of . . . the whole" (p. 10). She went on to say, "Both system processes and nursing actions are purposeful and goal directed. That is, nursing vigorously attempts to control variables affecting client care" (p. 15).

The Neuman Systems Model is based on reputable scientific findings from several disciplines. Neuman has continuously emphasized the importance of basing nursing diagnoses on knowledge derived from a synthesis of theory with the data base of client factors. The nursing process is dynamic in that there is ongoing establishment of nursing goals, negotiation between nurse and client with regard to the goals and intervention strategies, and feedback from client outcomes to confirm goals or serve as a basis for reformulation of new goals. Dynamism also is evident in the circularity of the prevention as intervention modalities. Neuman (1989d) noted that "tertiary prevention tends to lead back, in circular fashion, toward primary prevention" (p. 37). Neuman's emphasis on the client's view of the situation and the negotiation needed for identification of appropriate goals and interventions reflects a concern for ethical standards.

The Neuman Systems Model propositions that link person, environment, health, and nursing leave no gaps among those concepts. Neuman's statements about primary, secondary, and tertiary prevention provide the required general linkages among the concepts of the model.

The Neuman Systems Model is comprehensive in breadth of content. "The major goal for nursing," Neuman (1989d) asserted, "is to reduce stressor impact, whether actual or potential, and to increase client resistance" (p. 39). She went on to point out that the Neuman Systems Model encompasses health promotion and illness care, commenting:

> Ideally, health promotion goals should work in concert with both secondary and tertiary preventions as interventions to prevent recidivism and to promote optimal wellness, since the Neuman Systems Model is wellness oriented. Health promotion, in general, and within the primary prevention concept, relates to activities that optimize the client wellness potential or condition. (p. 39)

The comprehensiveness of the breadth of the Neuman Systems Model is further supported by the direction it provides for research, education, administration, and practice. Many rules for each area have already been developed, and others can be extracted from publications about the model.

The rules for nursing research were extracted from the content of the Neuman Systems Model and the literature based on the model, including a recent article by Grant, Kinney, and Davis (1993), and discussion with the Neuman Systems Model Trustees Group (personal communication, April 24, 1993). The first research rule states that the phenomena to be studied encompass (a) physiological, psychological, sociocultural, developmental, and spiritual variables; (b) properties of the central core of the client system; (c) properties of the flexible and normal lines of defense as well as of the lines of resistance; (d) characteristics of the internal, external, and created environments; (e) characteristics of intrapersonal, interpersonal, and extrapersonal stressors; and (f) elements of primary, secondary, and tertiary prevention interventions.

The second rule states that the clinical problems to be studied are those that deal with the impact of stressors on client system stability with regard to physiological, psychological, sociocultural, developmental, and spiritual variables, as well as the lines of defense and resistance. One purpose of Neuman Systems Model–based research is to predict the effects of primary, secondary, and tertiary prevention interventions on retention, attainment, and maintenance of client system stability. Another purpose is to determine the cost, benefit, and utility of prevention interventions.

The third rule states that subjects can be the client systems of individuals, families, groups, communities, organizations, or collaborative relationships between two or more individuals. Data encompass both client system and investigator perceptions and strategies for negotiated goal setting and may be collected in inpatient, ambulatory, home, and community settings.

The fourth rule indicates that the Neuman Systems Model is an appropriate base for inductive and deductive research using both qualitative and quantitative research designs and associated instrumentation. The fifth rule states that data analysis techniques associated with both qualitative and quantitative research designs are appropriate. The sixth rule states that research will advance understanding of the influence of prevention interventions on the relationship between stressors and client system stability.

Rules for education are being formulated. The distinctive focus of the curriculum is on the client/client system's reaction to environmental stressors. The purpose of nursing education is to teach students to design and use primary, secondary, and tertiary prevention as intervention modalities to assist client systems to retain, attain, and maintain optimal wellness.

Mirenda's (1986) description of the use of the Neuman Systems Model to guide curriculum development indicates that the curriculum content may be based on categories of stressors (intrapersonal, interpersonal, and extrapersonal); the physiological, psychological, sociocultural, developmental, and spiritual variables; and primary, secondary, and tertiary prevention as intervention modalities. Mirenda's discussion also indicates that the prevention as intervention modalities may guide the sequence of content.

The Neuman Systems Model is appropriate at all levels of nursing education, including hospital-based diploma programs, associate degree programs, baccalaureate programs, and graduate programs (Neuman, 1985a). Specific characteristics of students remain to be identified. Some teaching-learning strategies that facilitate understanding of the content and processes of the Neuman Systems Model are a visual representation of the five variables, the Neuman Wheel (Johnson, 1989), and a core course offered in the first semester of the nursing program that includes in-depth lecture and discussion of each concept of the model, as well as engaging in small group activities and keeping a journal of thoughts and questions about the model (Lowry, 1988). Other teaching-learning strategies include lectures about the individual as client, the family as client, and the community as client; case studies of simulated client situations to test students' assessment and decision-making skills; clinical experiences in various hospital-, home-, and community-based settings; and clinical papers focusing on a client from a hospital-based setting, assessment of families and their health status; the health assessment of a community; and the relevance of the Neuman Systems Model to community nursing (Ross, Bourbonnais, & Carroll 1987).

Rules for administration were formulated by Fawcett, Botter, Burritt, Crossley, and Frink (1989). They stipulated that the distinctive focus of and purpose to be fulfilled by nursing in the clinical agency is the provision of nursing services designed to help client systems retain, attain, or maintain stability by means of primary, secondary, and tertiary prevention. The collective nursing staff is thought of as a client system that is a composite of physiological, psychological, sociocultural, developmental, and spiritual variables. The department of nursing or the larger health care institution could also be viewed as the client system. The settings for nursing services are those in which primary, secondary, and tertiary prevention are appropriate, including but not limited to ambulatory clinics, acute care medical centers, and rehabilitation units. Management strategies focus on the staff, the department of nursing, or the total institution as the client system of the administrator, who uses management practices that promote system stability.

Rules for Neuman Systems Model–based nursing practice are evident. The purpose of nursing practice is to assist clients to retain, attain, or maintain optimal system stability. Clinical problems of interest are those related to actual or potential reactions to stressors. Neuman Systems Model–based nursing practice can occur in virtually any health care or community-based setting, such as clinics, hospitals, hospices, homes, and the streets and sidewalks of the community. Legitimate recipients of Neuman Systems Model–based nursing care are individuals, families, groups, and communities who are faced with actual or potential environmental stressors. The nursing process is described as the three-step format of nursing diagnosis, nursing goals, and nursing outcomes. Interventions take the form of primary, secondary, and tertiary prevention. The nursing process is facilitated by the use of the Neuman Nursing Process Format and the Prevention as Intervention Format (Neuman, 1989d). Neuman Systems Model–based nursing practice contributes to client well-being by facilitating "the highest possible health condition achievable at a given point in time" (Neuman, 1990a, p. 129).

Logical Congruence

The content of the Neuman Systems Model is not completely logically congruent. The model was developed primarily within the tradition of the reciprocal interaction world view. However, despite refinements in content, elements of the reaction world view remain in Neuman's conceptualization of the created-environment and in the reliance on Selye's work for her view of stress and stressors. To her credit, Neuman (1990a) has attempted to translate the created-environment in such a way that it reflects the reciprocal interaction world view. She explained that although the created-environment is functionally at the unconscious level, "it exchanges energy with and encompasses the internal and external environments, making it congruent with the open system concept . . . of the Neuman Systems Model" (pp. 129–130). Still, however, the emphasis on the unconscious reflects a mechanistic, psychoanalytic orientation to the concept. The logical problem with Neuman's view of stress could be resolved by incorporating a more dynamic view of stress than Selye's, such as Lazarus' (1981) notions of stress and coping.

Furthermore, logical congruence would be enhanced if illness were defined within an open systems perspective, rather than as a reflection of a closed, entropic system. In particular, Neuman's (1989d) statement, "Movement toward energy depletion (entropy) signals closure of the system as available energy fails to sustain life" (p. 14), is not logically consistent with Bertalanffy's (1968) view that the living system is never a closed system.

The Neuman Systems Model clearly represents the systems category of nursing knowledge. Although the model includes a developmental variable, it is viewed as change in the client system over time. Thus, there is no evidence of logical incompatibility with regard to different categories of nursing knowledge.

Generation of Theory

Neuman (1989a, 1989d) recently stated that she and her colleague, Audrey Koertvelyessy, collaborated to identify a major theory for the model, which they called the **Theory of Optimal Client System Stability**. She did not, however, identify the concepts and propositions of that theory.

The **Theory of Prevention as Intervention** is also being generated from the Neuman Systems Model. Citing a personal communication in the fall of 1987 with Koertvelyessy, Neuman (1989d) stated:

> [Koertvelyessy] views the concept of prevention, whether primary,
> secondary, or tertiary, as prevalent and significant in the Neuman Sys-
> tems Model, linked to each of the broad concepts of the model, that is,
> man (client), environment, health, and nursing. Since the prevention
> strategies are the modes instituted to retain, attain, or maintain stability
> of the client's health status, she considers the development of a theory
> statement linking these concepts a necessary next step. (p. 38)

Neuman (1989d) also noted, "Several other theories inherent within
the model could be identified and clarified with the goal of optimizing
health for the client," (p. 34). She did not, however, provide any direction
for the generation of such theories.

Hoffman (1982) began the task of operationally defining the concepts
of the Neuman Systems Model. For example, she proposed that one possible definition of internal environment could be strength or weakness of
various body parts or organs. Hoffman's attempt is a noteworthy first step,
but it stops short of identifying the methods needed to empirically measure the concepts. Measurement of strength or weakness of body parts, for
example, must be described in observable terms if the concept of internal
environment is to be empirically tested.

Credibility

Social Utility

The social utility of the Neuman Systems Model is thoroughly documented. Two editions of *The Neuman Systems Model* (Neuman, 1982b,
1989c), which contain numerous examples of the use of the model in
nursing education, practice, administration, and research, have already
been published, and the third edition is due in 1994. The periodic literature dealing with applications of the model has burgeoned in recent years.
The model is being used by nurses throughout the United States, and in
Canada, Iceland, England, Wales, Denmark, Finland, Norway, Sweden,
Portugal, Australia, Puerto Rico, Costa Rica, Brazil, Taiwan, and South
Korea, among other countries. Furthermore, International Neuman Sys-
tems Model Symposia have been held biennially since 1986.

Although the content of the Neuman Systems Model comprises many
terms, most are familiar; therefore, use of the model does not require
mastery of an extensive new vocabulary. Extensive study of the model
content is, however, required prior to knowledgeable application in nursing research, education, administration, and practice. Indeed, Neuman
Systems Model-based nursing practice requires "a synthesis of comprehensive client data and relevant theory [from nursing and adjunctive
disciplines] that is appropriate to the client's perception of need and is
related to functional competence or possibility within the client's environmental context" (Neuman 1989d, pp. 25, 27). Moreover,

It is assumed that the professional nurse operates from a theoretical perspective as client data are gathered. It is most often in the interpretation of client data that theory is either not explicitly used or improperly related to client data, resulting in confusing and often faulty diagnoses. It is more common for theory to be related to interventions than to diagnoses. Professional nurses should (to be considered truly professional) be able to justify their diagnostic statement based upon specific theoretical relationships with available client data. [In addition,] when client data are specifically related to [nursing and] social sciences theories in developing the nursing diagnosis, nurses can present themselves as professional in a knowledgeable manner. It is a responsibility to one's self, profession, clients, colleagues, and other health disciplines to be able to present a logical and rational justification for such decision making. Unless nurses can clearly articulate to others, particularly to the client, the *why* and *how* for arriving at a particular nursing diagnosis, they cannot claim the validity of their position; nor can they be certain of appropriate subsequent interventions. (Neuman, 1989b, pp. 57–58)

Neuman Systems Model–based nursing practice is feasible for the health promotion and illness care of individuals, families and other groups, and communities with many different conditions. Caramanica and Thibodeau (1987) identified some of the human and material resources needed to implement the model at the clinical agency level. They cited the need for a formal action plan, a task force made up of nurses from all levels, and a consultant. Moreover, they maintained that the use of a conceptual model of nursing is especially important when resources are limited, commenting that

In times of rapid change, a theory-based model which reflects staff's beliefs gives purpose, direction and organization to a department of nursing. It profiles desired nursing practice and facilitates unified, goal-directed nursing care behaviors so vital in times of reduced resources and increased acuity. (p. 71)

Capers, O'Brien, Quinn, Kelly, and Fenerty (1985) underscored the importance of thorough planning for the implementation of the Neuman Systems Model at the clinical agency level. Their strategies include the appointment of a planning committee to oversee the entire implementation project, with philosophy, nursing process, and implementation subcommittees and the establishment of a timetable for implementation and evaluation, with target dates for a pilot implementation project, subsequent adoption of the model by several units, and evaluation of the project. Other strategies are a formal staff education program with collegiate course, continuing education, and independent study options along with use of nurse preceptors, planning unit conferences, patient-centered unit conferences, and nursing grand rounds. Capers et al. cited the importance of including representatives from head nurse, coordinator, and staff nurse levels on the subcommittees and ascertaining that nurses from all three shifts are included in all aspects of the project. Other strategies are hiring a project facilitator to coordinate the planning, implementation, and evaluation phases of the project and seeking consultation from the faculty of a nearby college that uses the Neuman Systems Model. Capers et al. also emphasized the importance of developing a comprehensive documentation package that is congruent with the Neuman Systems Model, including a nursing assessment form, a nursing care plan format, a nursing flow sheet, nursing progress notes, and a nursing discharge summary. They also noted the importance of adequate funding for the project and encouraged solicitation of funds from foundations or other extramural sources.

Moynihan (1990) cited the utility of a forced-choice Neuman Systems Model–based assessment tool for decreasing the missing data that frequently occur when an open-ended format is used and noted the effectiveness of self-directed learning using an educational booklet. Moreover, she highlighted the need for a surveillance or oversight committee to track progress toward full implementation of the model at the clinical agency level.

NURSING RESEARCH. Neuman Systems Model–based research is rapidly increasing. Citations and abstracts for several unpublished studies conducted by graduate students and faculty, obtained from a survey of schools of nursing in the United States, Canada, and Europe, are given in Louis and Koertvelyessy (1989). The bibliography at the end of this chapter includes citations for theses and dissertations that were obtained from *Master's Abstracts International* and *Dissertation Abstracts International*.

The full reports of many studies have been published in journal articles and book chapters. A review of the research revealed that the Neuman Systems Model has guided a range of study designs, from qualitative descriptions of relevant phenomena to quantitative experiments that tested effects of preventive interventions on a variety of client system outcomes.

Several Neuman Systems Model–based descriptive studies have been conducted. Radwanski (1992) described the use of alcohol, marijuana, over-the-counter drugs, and prescription drugs by 15 men and 1 woman who had traumatic spinal cord injuries and who experienced chronic pain. Bueno, Redeker, and Norman (1992) examined the incidence of the risk behaviors of safety restraint use and alcohol use and the demographic characteristics of motor vehicle crash victims. Bowdler and Barrell (1987) described the health needs of the homeless population of Richmond, Virginia. Gries and Fernsler (1988) described clients' perceptions of mechanical ventilation during hospitalization in a critical care unit. Bass (1991) identified the needs of parents whose infants were in a neonatal intensive care unit. Kahn (1992) studied the needs of family members of critically ill clients. She noted few differences in needs of the families of clients who had a "Do Not Resuscitate" order and those who did not. Clark, Cross, Deane, and Lowry (1991) ascertained the spiritual needs of a sample of 15 adults who had experienced surgery due to cancer or cardiac disease within 6 months of the study.

Loescher, Clark, Atwood, Leigh, and Lamb (1990) examined the changes, problems, concerns, and needs of adult cancer survivors related to long-term and late effects of cancer and cancer therapy. Cava (1992) studied the coping strategies used by adult cancer survivors. Grant and Bean (1992) described the self-identified needs of the informal caregivers of head-injured adults in the home setting. Decker and Young (1991) identified self-perceived needs of the primary caregivers of terminally ill home-hospice clients. Blank, Clark, Longman, and Atwood (1989) identified the home care needs of both metastatic cancer patients and their significant other caregivers.

A few Neuman Systems Model–based correlational studies have been conducted. Capers (1991) studied the relationship between cultural variables and perceptions of problematical behavior held by lay black adults and black and white registered nurses. Wilson (1987) examined the relationship between patients' psychological responses to the surgical intensive care unit and their identification of stressors. Hinds (1990) reported that prognosis, surgery, current radiation therapy, performance status, self-control skills, preference for information, and age were associated with quality of life in a sample of 87 men and women with lung cancer.

Several Neuman Systems Model–based quasi-experimental and experimental studies have been conducted. Waddell and Demi (1993) reported that post-test fear of fear, severity of psychological impairment, and general emotional distress scores were lower than pretest scores in a sample of 32 participants in a 5-week partial psychiatric hospitalization program. Freiberger, Bryant, and Marino (1992) found no differences in bacterial growth on the skin of four groups of hospitalized children who had central venous line sites treated with different combinations of antiseptics and dressings. Heffline (1991) found no meaningful differences in the use of the nursing intervention of radiant heat alone or in combination with pharmacological intervention on postanesthesia shivering.

The results of some studies support the effectiveness of preventive interventions. Ali and Khalil (1989) found that a preoperative primary prevention psychoeducational intervention reduced postoperative state anxiety in a sampling of men and women who had bladder cancer. Hoch (1987) studied the effects of a treatment protocol derived from the Neuman Systems Model on depression and life satisfaction in a sample of retired individuals. She found that the Neuman protocol group had lower depression scores and higher life satisfaction scores than a control group who received a nursing intervention that was not based on an explicit conceptual model. Vaughn, Cheatwood, Sirles, and Brown (1989) reported that a group of insurance company clerical workers who received the primary and secondary prevention intervention of progressive muscle relaxation had a lower mean stress response score than the control group. Sirles, Brown, and Hilyer (1991) found that an experimental Back School exercise regimen had a beneficial effect on back strength, back flexibility, psychological well-being, and anxiety levels in a sample of municipal workers who had experienced back injuries.

In contrast, the results of other studies did not support the hypothesized effectiveness of preventive interventions. Koku (1992) was unable to support the hypothesized effectiveness of the secondary and tertiary prevention intervention of counseling regarding low back pain on municipal workers' reports of the severity of back pain. Ziemer (1983) was unable to demonstrate the expected beneficial effects of primary prevention in the form of preoperative information on postoperative complications. Gavigan, Kline-O'Sullivan, and Klump-Lybrand (1990) found no differences in atelectasis, other postoperative complications, or length of stay in the surgical critical care unit and in the hospital between clients who received the primary prevention intervention of changes in body position every 2 hours following coronary artery bypass graft surgery and those who received the standard treatment of maintenance of the supine position for the first 24 hours. Leja (1989) found no differences in depression scores 1 week after hospital discharge between a group of older adults who received the experimental treatment of guided imagery discharge teaching and a control group.

Other studies have used students and practicing nurses as study subjects. Ziegler (1982) reported preliminary work using graduate students to generate Neuman Systems Model–based nursing diagnoses. Lowry and Jopp (1989) reported the results of their study of the development of an instrument to evaluate the use of the Neuman Systems Model by graduates of an associate degree nursing program. Preliminary results from the use of the instrument indicate that although the Neuman Systems Model is well internalized by the time of graduation, "the degree to which the model is used in practice settings appears to vary according to the encouragement and recognition of model usage by the graduates' supervisors in agencies where they are employed" (p. 84). Speck (1990) found that a group of baccalaureate nursing students who received a guided imagery experimental treatment prior to performing their first injections had lower anxiety levels than those of the control group. No group differences, however, were found for stress, performance times, or performance scores.

Carroll (1989) reported that the role deprivation scores of senior generic baccalaureate nursing students in a Neuman Systems Model–based curriculum were greater than the scores of students in the same school when the curriculum was medical model-based. Nortridge, Mayeux, Anderson, and Bell (1992) found that elements of diploma nursing program students' cognitive style were related to their first semester final grade.

Cantin and Mitchell (1989) assessed the smoking rate of 612 Canadian registered nurses, registered psychiatric nurses, and licensed practical nurses. They found no difference in the smoking rates of the nurses and the Canadian population as a whole. Louis (1989) reported that the nurses who participated in a short-term (four 1-hour meetings) low-intensity nurse-led mutual help group had lower anxiety scores than nurses who did not participate in the group. She concluded that the mutual help group can strengthen the lines of defense and resistance of nurses who work with long-term care clients in public health and rehabilitation settings. Courchene, Patalski, and Martin (1991) found that nurses who regularly handled Cyclosporin A (CyA) were more likely to experience constipation, tinnitus, and headache than nurses who did not administer the drug. The two groups of nurses were similar, however, in experiences of nine other symptoms that could be linked to CyA exposure.

NURSING EDUCATION. The utility of the Neuman Systems Model for nursing education is well documented in the literature. Bower (1982) presented a blueprint for curriculum development based on the model. This blueprint "is consistent with the model and . . . gives direction for the generation of terminal and level outcomes of the curriculum, the content and its organization, and the course configuration of the program" (p. 99).

The Neuman Systems Model has been used as a basis for curriculum construction and revision in associate degree, baccalaureate, and master's programs. Associate degree nursing programs that are based on the model include Cecil Community College in North East, Maryland (Johnson, 1989; Lowry, 1986, 1988; Lowry & Jopp, 1989); the University of Nevada in Las Vegas, Santa Fe Community College in Gainesville, Florida, and Indiana University-Purdue University in Fort Wayne (Lowry & Green, 1989).

Sipple and Freese (1989) described the transition from an associate degree program to a Neuman Systems Model–based baccalaureate program at Lander College in Greenwood, South Carolina. Lebold and Davis (1980, 1982) described use of the Neuman Systems Model in the baccalaureate nursing curriculum at St. Xavier College in Chicago. They noted that the model

> supported the development of a holistic curriculum that focuses on primary, secondary, and tertiary prevention of individuals, families, and communities in multiple and diverse systems. The resultant curriculum design facilitates learning and role induction into the profession by providing students with a structure for integrating new knowledge and skills during the program and upon its completion. (1980, p. 157)

Mirenda (1986) described use of the Neuman Systems Model for the baccalaureate nursing program at Neumann College in Aston, Pennsylvania. She commented, "The nursing faculty at Neumann College have reported their satisfaction with this systems approach to the curriculum and to client care, and nursing students have demonstrated both professional growth and personal maturity" (p. 148).

Nichols, Dale, and Turley (1989) described the use of the Neuman

Systems Model in the baccalaureate program at the University of Wyoming in Laramie. Dale and Savala (1990) described a collaborative demonstration project between the University of Wyoming and the Veterans Administration Medical Center in Cheyenne for a baccalaureate nursing program senior practicum. They reported that the staff, who acted as preceptors, became more aware of documentation, holistic nursing care, and the rationale for nursing practice, and students gained confidence, became responsible and self-motivated, and became more proficient with time management and decision making.

Beitler, Tkachuck, and Aamodt (1980) described lesson plans for care of clients with personality disorders and for working with low-income families that are part of the baccalaureate program at Union College in Lincoln, Nebraska. Knox, Kilchenstein, and Yakulis (1982) and Kilchenstein and Yakulis (1984) discussed the use of the model in the baccalaureate nursing program at the University of Pittsburgh in Pennsylvania. Story and Ross (1986) described the use of Neuman's conceptual model as a guide to content for the junior year family-centered community health nursing course at the University of Ottawa in Ontario, Canada. Bourbonnais and Ross (1985) and Ross, Bourbonnais, and Carroll (1987) described how Neuman's model guides content for the final senior year nursing course at the University of Ottawa.

The Neuman Systems Model has also guided baccalaureate program curriculum construction for the Minnesota Intercollegiate Nursing Consortium (Mrkonich, Hessian, & Miller, 1989; Mrkonich, Miller, & Hessian, 1989) and the North Dakota-Minnesota Nursing Education Consortium (Nelson, Hansen, & McCullagh, 1989). Other baccalaureate nursing programs in the United States and abroad that use Neuman's model include Saint Anselm College in Manchester, New Hampshire (Beyea & Matzo, 1989; Bruton & Matzo, 1989); Simmons College in Boston, Massachusetts (Edwards & Kittler, 1991); the University of Missouri-Kansas City (Conners, 1982, 1989); the University of Saskatchewan in Canada (Dyck, Innes, Rae, & Sawatzky, 1989); Queens University in Kingston, Ontario, Canada (Laschinger, Maloney, Trammer, 1989); and Aarhus University in Aarhus, Denmark (Johansen, 1989).

In addition to its use in the associate degree program, the Neuman Systems Model also guided curriculum development for the baccalaureate degree completion program and the master's degree program at the University of Nevada, Las Vegas (Louis, Witt, & LaMancusa, 1989). The model was also used to guide curriculum development for the baccalaureate and master's degree programs at California State University in Fresno (Stittich, Avent, & Patterson, 1989).

Johnson, Vaughn-Wrobel, Ziegler, Hough, Bush, and Kurtz (1982) described the development of the master's program curriculum from the Neuman Systems Model at Texas Woman's University College of Nursing. Other Texas Woman's University faculty members further described the development of various courses using the model (Conners, Harmon, & Langford, 1982; Tollett, 1982). Moxley and Allen (1982) outlined the use of Neuman's model in the master's degree program at Northwestern State University in Shreveport, Louisiana. Neuman and Wyatt (1980) described the master's program in nursing service administration at Ohio University School of Nursing in Athens, Ohio. The curriculum for that program was developed from the Neuman Nursing Administration Stress/Adaptation Systems Model, a modification of Neuman's original model. Arndt (1982b) also described a curriculum for nursing administration.

Gunter (1982) described a comprehensive curriculum for gerontic nursing. The curriculum includes specific content that is appropriate for various levels of nursing personnel including aides and technicians, licensed practical nurses, registered nurses, master's prepared clinical specialists, and doctorally prepared nurse gerontologists. Gunter noted that the Neuman Systems Model "is compatible with our overall design of a structure or framework for the total assessment of an older person" (p. 207).

The Neuman Systems Model also has documented utility for continuing education in nursing. Harty (1982) demonstrated the use of the model as "a facilitating framework for accomplishing continuing education in nursing's primary goal: maintenance and reinforcement of the theoretical knowledge and clinical competence of the professional nurse" (p. 101). Baker (1982a) outlined a continuing education program for nurses in a psychiatric mental health hospital. Story and DuGas (1988) presented a detailed description of a successful 1-day workshop designed to help nurses apply the Neuman Systems Model in a simulated clinical setting. They credited the success of the workshop to the use of simple terminology, a focus on acute care, and the use of practical examples to facilitate the transfer of learning to the clinical setting. Teaching strategies included didactic presentation of the model content, use of a simulated clinical situation and case study, a programmed live interview with a mock patient, and small group work.

A timely and innovative addition to the use of the Neuman Systems Model in nursing education is computer-assisted learning. Reed-Sorrow, Harmon, and Kitundu (1989) described one computer program that uses creative graphics to present the content of the Neuman Systems Model and another program that deals with Neuman Systems Model–based health assessment.

NURSING ADMINISTRATION. The utility of the Neuman Systems Model in nursing service administration is also documented. Arndt (1982a) combined the concepts of the model with organizational theory to outline areas to consider in the analysis of nursing service organizations. Kelly, Sanders, and Pierce (1989) explained how the Neuman Systems Model can be adapted for use by the nurse administrator in either education or nursing service. They presented an innovative Neuman Systems-Management Tool that can be used by the administrator to document analysis of management situations, implementation of preventive management interventions, and evaluation of outcomes. An especially attractive feature of the tool is that it takes just 3 minutes to complete. Vokaty (1982) briefly described the role of the clinical nurse specialist within the context of the Neuman Systems Model. Simmons and Borgdon (1991) displayed a grid that shows the relationship between the Neuman Systems Model levels of prevention and the various activities associated with the clinical nurse specialist roles of educator, consultant, researcher, and manager.

The Neuman Systems Model has proved useful for development of assessment tools, a diagnostic taxonomy, documentation formats, and nursing care plans. Quayhagen and Roth (1989) developed an extremely innovative approach to Neuman Systems Model–based assessment. They identified psychometrically sound clinical research instruments that are appropriate measures of the physiological, psychological, sociocultural, developmental, and spiritual variables and the external environment. The result is a comprehensive assessment protocol for individuals and families.

Breckenridge, Cupit, and Raimondo (1982) described a tool for assessment of continuous ambulatory peritoneal dialysis (CAPD) clients. Neuman Systems Model–based family health assessment was described in detail by Mischke-Berkey et al. (Mischke-Berkey & Hanson, 1991; Mischke-Berkey, Warner, & Hanson, 1989). They developed the Family Systems Stressor-Strength Inventory (FS3I), which permits comprehensive assessment of family stressors and family strengths. In addition, they identified interventions that can facilitate restoration of normal family functioning. Flannery (1991) described the FAMLI-RESCUE, an assessment tool for the collection and evaluation of family data that can be used by neuroscience nurses in acute care settings. Beddome (1989) described the development and use of a Neuman Systems Model-based community-as-client assessment tool.

Ziegler (1982) described the development of a computerized taxonomy of nursing diagnoses deduced from the Neuman Systems Model. The following category sets were used for the taxonomy:

1. The responding subsystem: psychological, physiological, sociocultural.
2. The system being diagnosed: individual, family, group or community.
3. The level of response: primary, secondary, and tertiary.
4. The source of the stressor etiology: intrasystem, intersystem, and extrasystem.
5. The type of stressor etiology: physiological, psychological, and sociocultural. (p. 57)

Schlentz (1993) described the innovative use of the Neuman Systems Model as the conceptual base for the Minimum Data Set to document nursing practice at the Francis Ashbury Manor United Methodist Homes in Ocean Grove, New Jersey. The result is the Minimum Data Set Resident Assessment Protocol Summary (MDS RAPS). Each RAPS problem area is structured according to the Neuman Systems Model levels of prevention, with appropriate nursing actions.

Mayers and Watson (1982) described the adaptation of their basic nursing care planning format to accommodate the Neuman Systems Model. Neal (1982) and Capers and Kelly (1987) also described nursing care plans derived from the Neuman Systems Model.

The Neuman Systems Model has been adopted at the agency level in the United States, Canada, England, and Wales. Pinkerton (1974) described the organization of services provided by the Allied Home Health Association of San Diego, California, according to Neuman's model. Capers et al. (1985) and Burke, Capers, O'Connell, Quinn, and Sinnott (1989) presented detailed descriptions of the project undertaken to implement the Neuman Systems Model at Mercy Catholic Medical Center, Fitzgerald Mercy Division in Darby, Pennsylvania. Caramanica and Thibodeau (1987) and Moynihan (1990) described the progress toward implementation of the Neuman Systems Model at Mount Sinai Hospital in Hartford, Connecticut. Hinton-Walker and Raborn (1989) explained how the Neuman Systems Model was adopted as an organizing framework for nursing administration and delivery of nursing care at Jefferson Davis Memorial Hospital in Natchez, Mississippi.

The Neuman Systems Model is used to guide nursing practice at the Manitoba Department of Health (Drew, Craig, & Beynon, 1989). The model has also served as the basis of standards for community health nursing practice for the Province of Ontario and as a guide for practice at the Middlesex-London Health Unit in southwestern Ontario (Drew et al., 1989), as well as an organizational guide for the Regional Neonatal Education Program of Eastern Ontario in Ottawa, Ontario, Canada (Dunn & Trépaniér, 1989). Furthermore, the model is used at the Hospice of Windsor in Ontario, Canada (Echlin, 1982).

Johns (1991) described the model for nursing practice used at Burford Community Hospital in Oxfordshire, England. The Neuman Systems Model levels of prevention serve as the framework for nursing intervention. In addition, the Neuman Systems Model was selected to guide community psychiatric nursing practice in Breconshire, Powys, Wales (Davies, 1989).

NURSING PRACTICE. The utility of Neuman's conceptual model for nursing practice is exceedingly well documented. Nursing practice targeted to the individual as the client system has been described in several publications. Some of those papers describe the application of the Neuman Systems Model to the care of clients who are HIV-positive (Pierce & Hutton, 1992) and to the care of adults with such diverse acute and chronic conditions as hypermetabolism in multisystem organ failure

(Bergstrom, 1992), myocardial infarction and other cardiac disease (Fawcett et al., 1987, 1992; McInerney, 1982; Ross & Bourbonnais, 1985; Smith, 1989), cerebral aneurysm (Fawcett et al., 1987), gangrene (Baerg, 1991), acute and chronic phase spinal cord injuries (Foote, Piazza, & Schultz, 1990; Hoeman & Winters, 1990; Sullivan, 1986), orthopedic problems (Shaw, 1991), colon cancer (Weinberger, 1991), chronic obstructive pulmonary disease (Baker, 1982b; Hiltz, 1990), kidney disease (Breckenridge, 1982, 1989), multiple sclerosis (Knight, 1990), and hypertension (Johnson, 1983; Utz, 1980). Furthermore, the model has been used to assess the nutritional status of an infant (Torkington, 1988), to guide the care of a child with leukemia (Piazza, Foote, Wright, & Holcombe, 1992), and to assess children who require psychiatric services (Herrick, Goodykoontz, Herrick, & Hackett, 1991).

Other papers describe the use of the Neuman Systems Model to assess nutritional status across the life process (Gavan, Hastings-Tolsma, & Troyan, 1988), as the basis for a framework to guide combined oral contraceptive counseling (Lindell & Olsson, 1991) and to guide development of interventions for cardiovascular risk factor reduction (Brown, 1988) and as preventive interventions for the elderly (Davis, 1982), and to care for patients in pain (Cunningham, 1982). In addition, Sohier (1989) explained how the sociocultural variable of the Neuman Systems Model can be expanded to provide a comprehensive assessment of individuals' culturally based beliefs and values. Still other papers describe the application of the Neuman Systems Model to clients in such diverse settings as psychiatric and mental health units (Beitler et al., 1980; Clark, 1982; Moore & Munro, 1990), medical and surgical units (Beitler et al., 1980; Rice, 1982; Robichaud-Ekstrand & Delisle, 1989), an orthopedic practice (Shaw, 1991), critical care or intensive care units (Biley, 1989; Dunbar, 1982; Fulbrook, 1991; Kido, 1991), rehabilitation units (Cardona, 1982; Cunningham, 1983), an emergency department (Redheffer, 1985), a hospice (Echlin, 1982), a children's day-care center (Bowman, 1982), and clients' homes (Millard, 1992).

Galloway (1993) shifted the focus from clients to nurses in her Neuman Systems Model–based self-analysis of her care of a mentally and physically impaired infant. She stated:

> Through analyzing my role as a student nurse in a difficult clinical situation, I learned that I not only adapted well but also experienced personal growth. I did not avoid the reality of my situation; rather, I worked within the difficulties it presented. Understanding the importance of identifying and expressing emotions, I did not deny my positive and negative feelings. By using effective coping mechanisms and introducing alternative methods as necessary to deal with stressors, I achieved a positive result. Although my flexible line of defense contracted slightly due to the influence of specific negative variables, it buffered effectively so that my underlying normal line of defense was not penetrated. (p. 36)

Neuman Systems Model–based nursing practice with the family as the client system has been described by Neuman (1983a, 1983b, 1989b) and Reed (1982, 1989, 1993). Moreover, Ross and Helmer (1988) identified the similarities and differences of Neuman Systems Model–based nursing of the individual as a client and of the family as the client. Herrick and Goodykoontz (1989) described a Neuman Systems Model–based framework to guide the assessment and intervention of a dysfunctional family. Goldblum-Graff and Graff (1982) adapted the model to family therapy by linking its concepts and propositions to those of a theory of contextual family therapy. In addition, the Neuman Systems Model guided the development of family-focused practice frameworks for the care of a terminally ill neurologically impaired child (Wallingford, 1989), for the prevention of elder abuse (Delunas, 1990), and for use with elderly families in crisis (Beckingham & Baumann, 1990). Buchanan (1987) modified Neuman's model for use with aggregates, families, and the community.

Neuman Systems Model–based nursing practice with the community as the client system has been discussed by Benedict and Sproles (1982). They applied the model to general nursing health care delivery in community settings by adding the following basic premise to Neuman's assumptions:

> A population possesses characteristics reflective of the community as an entity in itself. These characteristics usually are represented as group-specific tendencies. They define a population-at-risk or determine a priority high-risk group. Just as there are common "knowns" for all individuals and their response ranges, so too there are separate sets of commonalities for health risk populations and/or subgroups such as the aged, the worker, or the handicapped. (p. 224)

Spradley (1990) offered a brief explanation of how the model can be used for community health nursing practice. Balch (1974), Beitler et al. (1980), and Craddock and Stanhope (1980) all described the use of the Neuman Systems Model in community health nursing practice. Anderson, McFarlane, and Helton (1986) adapted the Neuman Systems Model for the development of their community-as-client model, which reflects a synthesis of nursing and public health.

Social Congruence

Although Neuman (1974, 1989d) has asserted for many years that nursing is a unique profession, she has always also considered her model to be appropriate for use by members of other health care disciplines as well. In fact, the multidimensional nature of the Neuman Systems Model is attractive to the many health care workers who recognize the complex nature of humans and their interactions with the environment. The adoption of the model by other health care disciplines is, however, a two-edged sword, because the applicability of the model to all health care disciplines can foster a common perspective, but in doing so may fail to point out the distinctive contribution of nursing to health care.

The Neuman Systems Model is generally congruent with current societal expectations of nursing care. The present emphasis on primary prevention and health promotion seen in the news media and in numerous self-help books and articles is increasing consumers' awareness of the contributions of all health care workers, including nurses, to promotion of wellness and prevention of illness. As more nurses move into ambulatory care settings, their roles in primary prevention should become a typical expectation of consumers. Indeed, Neuman (1989d) commented, "Primary Prevention as intervention with inherent health promotion is an expanding futuristic, proactive concept with which the nursing field must become increasingly concerned. It has unlimited potential for major role development that could shape the future image of nursing" (p. 39).

The fact that the Neuman Systems Model emphasizes consideration of the client's perspective and negotiation of nursing goals and interventions between client and caregiver enhances its congruence with those members of society who desire input into their care. Neuman (1989d) commented, "These characteristics follow current mandates within the health care system for client rights in health care issues" (p. 40). Paradoxically, however, the emphasis on client participation may limit the congruence of Neuman Systems Model–based practice with the expectations for care held by individuals whose personal or culturally-derived beliefs lead to the lack of desire to play a part in their care, such as people of some Middle Eastern cultures (Meleis, 1991).

Some anecdotal evidence of the congruence of Neuman Systems Model–based nursing practice exists. In general, the authors of papers describing the use of the Neuman Systems Model in nursing practice have indicated their own satisfaction with the resultant nursing care in terms of comprehensiveness. Millard (1992), for example, indicated that use of the model facilitated achievement of the primary health care team's short and medium-term objectives for an elderly couple. Knight's (1990) comment that the outcomes of a client- and nurse-negotiated plan of care were "found to be largely congruent with the expected outcomes" (p. 455) suggests that satisfaction with Neuman Systems Model–based care extends to the client.

Social Significance

Neuman (1989a) noted that she foresees increased utilization of the Neuman Systems Model "well into the twenty-first century" (p. 466). She went on to point out that the model "has either preceded or complemented changing trends in nursing, and in health care in general, since its inception. . . . Its utilization is basically unlimited because of its wholistic systemic base and perspective" (p. 466). In addition, Neuman maintained that use of the model may resolve cross-cultural differences and improve health care in the many countries where it has been successfully applied.

The empirical evidence related to the social significance of the Neuman Systems Model is mixed. As noted above in the social utility section on nursing research, the findings of some studies support the efficacy of preventive interventions, but the results of other studies do not. Additional research is warranted. Moreover, a meta-analysis of the existing studies is recommended to determine the magnitude of effects and to identify design and other factors that might contribute to the conflicting findings (Rosenthal, 1991).

Contributions to the Discipline of Nursing

The Neuman Systems Model reflects nursing's interest in people as holistic systems, whether well or ill, and in environmental influences on health. The use of such terms as variances from wellness and primary prevention underscores the emphasis Neuman places on wellness. Furthermore, the focus on clients' perceptions of stressors and on negotiation of nursing care goals and interventions with the client underscores the importance of the person who is the client in the nursing situation.

The primary contribution of the Neuman Systems Model has been pragmatic, in that it has proved to be a useful guide for nursing education and nursing practice in various settings in several countries. The model has proved to be readily translatable to other cultures and, therefore, has the potential to facilitate important global sharing and resolution of universal nursing concerns (Neuman, 1989a). Additional systematic research guided by Neuman Systems Model–based conceptual-theoretical-empirical structures is needed to determine the credibility of the model beyond pragmatic considerations.

Neuman's (1989d) own words best summarize the overall contributions of the Neuman Systems Model. She states:

> The Neuman Systems Model fits well with the wholistic concept of optimizing a dynamic yet stable interrelationship of mind, body and spirit of the client in a constantly changing environment and society. . . . It joins the recent World Health Organization mandate for the year 2000 of desired unity in wellness states—wellness of body, mind, spirit, and environment. It is also in accord with the American Nursing Association, sharing its concern about potential stressors and its emphasis on primary prevention. (p. 10)

Neuman (1989a) has ensured the continued evolution of her conceptual model through establishment of the Neuman Systems Model Trustees Group. Members of the Trustees Group, who include nurses from the United States and other countries, have agreed "to preserve, protect, and perpetuate the integrity of the Model for the future of nursing" (p. 467).

REFERENCES

Ali, N.S., & Khalil, H.Z. (1989). Effect of psychoeducational intervention on anxiety among Egyptian bladder cancer patients. *Cancer Nursing, 12,* 236–242.

Anderson, E., McFarlane, J., & Helton, A. (1986). Community-as-client: A model for practice. *Nursing Outlook, 34,* 220–224.

Arndt, C. (1982a). Systems concepts for management of stress in complex health-care organizations. In B. Neuman, *The Neuman systems model: Application to nursing education and practice* (pp. 97–114). Norwalk, CT: Appleton-Century-Crofts.

Arndt, C. (1982b). Systems theory and educational programs for nursing service administration. In B. Neuman, *The Neuman systems model: Application to nursing education and practice* (pp. 182–187). Norwalk, CT: Appleton-Century-Crofts.

Baerg, K.L. (1991). Using Neuman's model to analyze a clinical situation. *Rehabilitation Nursing, 16,* 38–39.

Baker, N.A. (1982a). The Neuman systems model as a conceptual framework for continuing education in the work place. In B. Neuman, *The Neuman systems model: Application to nursing education and practice* (pp. 260–264). Norwalk, CT: Appleton-Century-Crofts.

Baker, N.A. (1982b). Use of the Neuman model in planning for the psychological needs of the respiratory disease patient. In B. Neuman, *The Neuman systems model: Application to nursing education and practice* (pp. 241–251). Norwalk, CT: Appleton-Century-Crofts.

Balch, C. (1974). Breaking the lines of resistance. In J.P. Riehl & C. Roy, *Conceptual models for nursing practice* (pp. 130–134). New York: Appleton-Century-Crofts.

Barnum, B.J.S. (1994). *Nursing theory: Analysis, application, evaluation* (4th ed.). Philadelphia: JB Lippincott.

Bass, L.S. (1991). What do parents need when their infant is a patient in the NICU? *Neonatal Network, 10*(4), 25–33.

Beckingham, A.C., & Baumann, A. (1990). The ageing family in crisis: Assessment and decision-making models. *Journal of Advanced Nursing, 15,* 782–787.

Beddome, G. (1989). Application of the Neuman systems model to the assessment of community-as-client. In B. Neuman, *The Neuman systems model* (2nd ed., pp. 363–374). Norwalk, CT: Appleton & Lange.

Beitler, B., Tkachuck, B., & Aamodt, D. (1980). The Neuman model applied to mental health, community health, and medical-surgical nursing. In J.P. Riehl & C. Roy, *Conceptual models for nursing practice* (2nd ed., pp. 170–178). New York: Appleton-Century-Crofts.

Benedict, M.B., & Sproles, J.B. (1982). Application of the Neuman model to public health nursing practice. In B. Neuman, *The Neuman systems model: Application to nursing education and practice* (pp. 223–240). Norwalk, CT: Appleton-Century-Crofts.

Bergstrom, D. (1992). Hypermetabolism in multisystem organ failure: A Neuman systems perspective. *Critical Care Nursing Quarterly, 15*(3), 63–70.

Bertalanffy, L. (1968). *General system theory.* New York: Braziller.

Beyea, S., & Matzo, M. (1989). Assessing elders using the functional health pattern assessment model. *Nurse Educator, 14*(5), 32–37.

Biley, F.C. (1989). Stress in high dependency units. *Intensive Care Nursing, 5,* 134–141.

Blank. J.J., Clark, L., Longman, A.J., & Atwood, J.R. (1989). Perceived home care needs of cancer patients and their caregivers. *Cancer Nursing, 12,* 78–84.

Bourbonnais, F.F., & Ross, M.M. (1985). The Neuman systems model in nursing education: Course development and implementation. *Journal of Advanced Nursing, 10,* 117–123.

Bowdler, J.E., & Barrell, L.M. (1987). Health needs of homeless persons. *Public Health Nursing, 4,* 135–140.

Bower, F.L. (1982). Curriculum development and the Neuman Model. In B. Neuman, *The Neuman systems model: Application to nursing education and practice* (pp. 94–99). Norwalk, CT: Appleton-Century-Crofts.

Bowman, G.E. (1982). The Neuman assessment tool adapted for child day-care centers. In B. Neuman, *The Neuman systems model: Application to nursing education and practice* (pp. 324–334). Norwalk, CT: Appleton-Century-Crofts.

Breckenridge, D.M. (1982). Adaptation of the Neuman systems model for the renal client. In B. Neuman, *The Neuman systems model: Application to nursing education and practice* (pp. 267–277). Norwalk, CT: Appleton-Century-Crofts.

Breckenridge, D.M. (1989). Primary prevention as an intervention modality for the renal client. In B. Neuman, *The Neuman systems model* (2nd ed., pp. 397–406). Norwalk, CT: Appleton & Lange.

Breckenridge, D.M., Cupit, M.C., & Raimondo, J.M. (1982). Systematic nursing assessment tool for the CAPD client. *Nephrology Nurse*, (January/February), 24, 26–27, 30–31.

Brown, M.W. (1988). Neuman's systems model in risk factor reduction. *Cardiovascular Nursing*, 24(6), 43.

Bruton, M.R., & Matzo, M. (1989). Curriculum revisions at Saint Anselm College: Focus on the older adult. In B. Neuman, *The Neuman systems model* (2nd ed., pp. 201–210). Norwalk, CT: Appleton & Lange.

Buchanan, B.F. (1987). Human-environment interaction: A modification of the Neuman systems model for aggregates, families, and the community. *Public Health Nursing*, 4, 52–64.

Bueno, M.N., Redeker, N., & Norman, E.M., (1992). Analysis of motor vehicle crash data in an urban trauma center: Implications for nursing practice and research. *Heart and Lung*, 21, 558–567.

Burke, M.E. Sr., Capers, C.F., O'Connell, R.K., Quinn, R. M., & Sinnott, M. (1989). Neuman-based nursing practice in a hospital setting. In B. Neuman, *The Neuman systems model* (2nd ed., pp. 423–444). Norwalk, CT: Appleton & Lange.

Cantin, B., & Mitchell, M. (1989). Nurses' smoking behavior. *The Canadian Nurse*, 85(1), 20–21.

Capers, C.F. (1991). Nurses' and lay African Americans' views about behavior. *Western Journal of Nursing Research*, 13, 123–135.

Capers, C.F., & Kelly, R. (1987). Neuman nursing process: A model of holistic care. *Holistic Nursing Practice*, 1(3), 19–26.

Capers, C.F., O'Brien, C., Quinn, R., Kelly, R., & Fenerty, A. (1985). The Neuman systems model in practice: Planning phase. *Journal of Nursing Administration*, 15(5), 29–39.

Caplan, G. (1964). *Principles of preventive psychiatry*. New York: Basic Books.

Caramanica, L., & Thibodeau, J. (1987). Nursing philosophy and the selection of a model for practice. *Nursing Management*, 10(10), 71.

Cardona, V.D. (1982). Client rehabilitation and the Neuman model. In B. Neuman, *The Neuman systems model: Application to nursing education and practice* (pp. 278–290). Norwalk, CT: Appleton-Century-Crofts.

Carroll, T.L. (1989). Role deprivation in baccalaureate nursing students pre and post

curriculum revision. *Journal of Nursing Education*, 28, 134–139.

Cava, M.A. (1992). An examination of coping strategies used by long-term cancer survivors. *Canadian Oncology Nursing Journal*, 2, 99–102.

Chardin, P.T. (1955). *The phenomenon of man*. London: Collins.

Clark, C.C., Cross, J.R., Deane, D.M., & Lowry, L.W. (1991). Spirituality: Integral to quality care. *Holistic Nursing Practice*, 5, 67–76.

Clark, F. (1982). The Neuman systems model: A clinical application for psychiatric nurse practitioners. In B. Neuman, *The Neuman systems model: Application to nursing education and practice* (pp. 335–353). Norwalk, CT: Appleton-Century-Crofts.

Clark, J. (1982). Development of models and theories on the concept of nursing. *Journal of Advanced Nursing*, 7, 129–134.

Conners, V.L. (1982). Teaching the Neuman systems model: An approach to student and faculty development. In B. Neuman, *The Neuman systems model: Application to nursing education and practice* (pp. 176–181). Norwalk, CT: Appleton-Century-Crofts.

Conners, V.L. (1989). An empirical evaluation of the Neuman systems model: The University of Missouri-Kansas City. In B. Neuman, *The Neuman systems model* (2nd ed., pp. 249–258). Norwalk, CT: Appleton & Lange.

Conners, V., Harmon, V.M., & Langford, R.W. (1982). Course development and implementation using the Neuman systems model as a framework: Texas Woman's University (Houston Campus). In B. Neuman, *The Neuman systems model: Application to nursing education and practice* (pp. 153–158). Norwalk, CT: Appleton-Century-Crofts.

Cornu, A. (1957). *The origins of Marxian thought*. Springfield, IL: Charles C Thomas.

Courchene, V.S., Patalski, E., & Martin, J. (1991). A study of the health of pediatric nurses administering Cyclospirine A. *Pediatric Nursing*, 17, 497–500.

Craddock, R.B., & Stanhope, M.K. (1980). The Neuman Health-Care Systems Model: Recommended adaptation. In J.P. Riehl & C. Roy, *Conceptual models for nursing practice* (2nd ed., pp. 159–169). New York: Appleton-Century-Crofts.

Cunningham, S.G. (1982). The Neuman

model applied to an acute care setting: Pain. In B. Neuman, *The Neuman systems model: Application to nursing education and practice* (pp. 291–296). Norwalk, CT: Appleton-Century-Crofts.

Cunningham, S.G. (1983). The Neuman systems model applied to a rehabilitation setting. *Rehabilitation Nursing, 8*(4), 20–22.

Dale, M.L., & Savala, S.M. (1990). A new approach to the senior practicum. *Nursing Connections, 3*(1), 45–51.

Davies, P. (1989). In Wales: Use of the Neuman systems model by community psychiatric nurses. In B. Neuman, *The Neuman systems model* (2nd ed., pp. 375–384). Norwalk, CT: Appleton & Lange.

Davis, L.H. (1982). Aging: A social and preventive perspective. In B. Neuman, *The Neuman systems model: Application to nursing education and practice* (pp. 211–214). Norwalk, CT: Appleton-Century-Crofts.

Decker, S.D., & Young, E. (1991). Self-perceived needs of primary caregivers of home-hospice clients. *Journal of Community Health Nursing, 8*, 147–154.

Delunas, L.R. (1990). Prevention of elder abuse: Betty Neuman health care systems approach. *Clinical Nurse Specialist, 4*, 54–58.

Drew, L.L., Craig, D.M., & Beynon, C.E. (1989). The Neuman systems model for community health administration and practice: Provinces of Manitoba and Ontario, Canada. In B. Neuman, *The Neuman systems model* (2nd ed., pp. 315–342). Norwalk, CT: Appleton & Lange.

Dunbar, S.B. (1982). Critical care and the Neuman model. In B. Neuman, *The Neuman systems model: Application to nursing education and practice* (pp. 297–307). Norwalk, CT: Appleton-Century-Crofts.

Dunn, S.I., & Trépaniér, M.J. (1989). Application of the Neuman model to perinatal nursing. In B. Neuman, *The Neuman systems model* (2nd ed., pp. 407–422). Norwalk, CT: Appleton & Lange.

Dyck, S.M., Innes, J.E., Rae, D.I., & Sawatzky, J.E. (1989). The Neuman systems model in curriculum revision: A baccalaureate program, University of Saskatchewan. In B. Neuman, *The Neuman systems model* (2nd ed., pp. 225–236). Norwalk, CT: Appleton & Lange.

Echlin, D.J. (1982). Palliative care and the Neuman model. In B. Neuman, *The Neuman systems model: Application to nurs-ing education and practice* (pp. 257–259). Norwalk, CT: Appleton-Century-Crofts.

Edelson, M. (1970). *Sociotherapy and psychotherapy*. Chicago: University of Chicago Press.

Edwards, P.A., & Kittler, A.W. (1991). Integrating rehabilitation content in nursing curricula. *Rehabilitation Nursing, 16*, 70–73.

Fawcett, J., Archer, C.L., Becker, D., Brown, K.K., Gann, S., Wong, M.J., & Wurster, A.B. (1992). Guidelines for selecting a conceptual model of nursing: Focus on the individual patient. *Dimensions of Critical Care Nursing, 11*, 268–277.

Fawcett, J., Botter, M.L., Burritt, J., Crossley, J.D., & Fink, B.B. (1989). Conceptual models of nursing and organization theories. In B. Henry, M. DiVincenti, C. Arndt, & A. Marriner (Eds.), *Dimensions of nursing administration: Theory, research, education, and practice* (pp. 143–154). Boston: Blackwell Scientific Publications.

Fawcett, J., Cariello, F.P., Davis, D.A., Farley, J., Zimmaro, D.M., & Watts, R.J. (1987). Conceptual models of nursing: Application to critical care nursing practice. *Dimensions of Critical Care Nursing, 6*, 202–213.

Fawcett, J., Carpenito, J.J., Efinger, J., Goldblum-Graff, D., Groesbeck, M.J.V., Lowry, L.W., McCreary, C.S., & Wolf, Z.R. (1982). A framework for analysis and evaluation of conceptual models of nursing with an analysis and evaluation of the Neuman systems model: In B. Neuman, *The Neuman systems model: Application to nursing education and practice* (pp. 30–43). Norwalk: CT: Appleton-Century Crofts.

Flannery, J. (1991). FAMLI-RESCUE: A family assessment tool for use by neuroscience nurses in the acute care setting. *Journal of Neuroscience Nursing, 23*, 111–115.

Foote, A.W., Piazza, D., & Schultz, M. (1990). The Neuman Systems Model: Application to a patient with a cervical spinal cord injury. *Journal of Neuroscience Nursing, 22*, 302–306.

Freiberger, D., Bryant, J., & Marino, B. (1992). The effects of different central venous line dressing changes on bacterial growth in a pediatric oncology population. *Journal of Pediatric Oncology Nursing, 9*, 3–7.

Fulbrook, P.R. (1991). The application of the Neuman Systems Model to intensive care. *Intensive Care Nursing, 7*, 28–39.

Galloway, D.A. (1993). Coping with a mentally and physically impaired infant: A self-analysis. *Rehabilitation Nursing, 18,* 34–36.

Gavan, C.A.S., Hastings-Tolsma, M.T., & Troyan, P.J. (1988). Explication of Neuman's model: A holistic systems approach to nutrition for health promotion in the life process. *Holistic Nursing Practice, 3*(1), 26–38.

Gavigan, M., Kline-O'Sullivan, C., & Klumpp-Lybrand, B. (1990). The effect of regular turning on CABG patients. *Critical Care Nursing Quarterly, 12*(4), 69–76.

Goldblum-Graff, D., & Graff, H. (1982). The Neuman model adapted to family therapy. In B. Neuman, *The Neuman systems model: Application to nursing education and practice* (pp. 217–222). Norwalk, CT: Appleton-Century-Crofts.

Grant, J.S., & Bean, C.A. (1992). Self-identified needs of informal caregivers of head-injured adults. *Family and Community Health, 15*(2), 49–58.

Grant, J.S., Kinney, M.R., & Davis, L.L. (1993). Using conceptual frameworks of models to guide nursing research. *Journal of Neuroscience Nursing, 25,* 52–56.

Gries, M., & Fernsler, J. (1988). Patient perceptions of the mechanical ventilation experience. *Focus on Critical Care, 15,* 52–59.

Gunter, L.M. (1982). Application of the Neuman systems model to gerontic nursing. In B. Neuman, *The Neuman systems model: Application to nursing education and practice* (pp. 196–210). Norwalk, CT: Appleton-Century-Crofts.

Harty, M.B. (1982). Continuing education in nursing and the Neuman model. In B. Neuman, *The Neuman systems model: Application to nursing education and practice* (pp. 100–106). Norwalk, CT: Appleton-Century-Crofts.

Heffline, M.S. (1991). A comparative study of pharmacological versus nursing interventions in the treatment of postanesthesia shivering. *Journal of Post Anesthesia Nursing, 6,* 311–320.

Herrick, C.A., & Goodykoontz, L. (1989). Neuman's systems model for nursing practice as a conceptual framework for a family assessment. *Journal of Child and Adolescent Psychiatric and Mental Health Nursing, 2,* 61–67.

Herrick, C.A., Goodykoontz, L., Herrick, R.H., & Hackett, B. (1991). Planning a continuum of care in child psychiatric nursing: A collaborative effort. *Journal of Child and Adolescent Psychiatric and Mental Health Nursing, 4,* 41–48.

Hiltz, D. (1990). The Neuman systems model: An analysis of a clinical situation. *Rehabilitation Nursing, 15,* 330–332.

Hinds, C. (1990). Personal and contextual factors predicting patients' reported quality of life: Exploring congruency with Betty Neuman's assumptions. *Journal of Advanced Nursing, 15,* 456–462.

Hinton-Walker, P., & Raborn, M. (1989). Application of the Neuman model in nursing administration and practice. In B. Henry, C. Arndt, M. DiVincenti, & A. Marriner-Tomey (Eds.), *Dimensions of nursing administration: Theory, research, education, and practice* (pp. 711–723). Boston: Blackwell Scientific Publications.

Hoch, C.C. (1987). Assessing delivery of nursing care. *Journal of Gerontological Nursing, 13,* 1–17.

Hoeman, S.P., & Winters, D.M. (1990). Theory-based case management: High cervical spinal cord injury. *Home Healthcare Nurse, 8,* 25–33.

Hoffman, M.K. (1982). From model to theory construction: An analysis of the Neuman Health-Care systems model: In B. Neuman, *The Neuman systems model: Application to nursing education and practice* (pp. 45–54). Norwalk, CT: Appleton-Century-Crofts.

Johansen, H. (1989). Neuman model concepts in joint use—community health practice and student teaching—School of Advanced Nursing Education, Aarhus University, Aarhus, Denmark. In B. Neuman, *The Neuman systems model* (2nd ed., pp. 334–362). Norwalk, CT: Appleton & Lange.

Johns, C. (1991). The Burford Nursing Development Unit holistic model of nursing practice. *Journal of Advanced Nursing, 16,* 1090–1098.

Johnson, M.N., Vaughn-Wrobel, B., Ziegler, S., Hough, L., Bush, H.A., & Kurtz, P. (1982). Use of the Neuman Health-Care systems model in the master's curriculum: Texas Woman's University. In B. Neuman, *The Neuman systems model: Application to nursing education and practice* (pp. 130–152). Norwalk, CT: Appleton-Century-Crofts.

Johnson, P. (1983). Black hypertension: A transcultural case study using the Betty Neuman model of nursing care. *Issues in Health Care of Women, 4,* 191–210.

Johnson, S.E. (1989). A picture is worth a thousand words: Helping students visualize a conceptual model. *Nurse Educator*, 14(3), 21–24.

Kahn, E.C. (1992). A comparison of family needs based on the presence or absence of DNR orders. *Dimensions of Critical Care Nursing*, 11, 286–292.

Kelly, J.A., Sanders, N.F., & Pierce. J.D. (1989). A systems approach to the role of the nurse administrator in education and practice. In B. Neuman, *The Neuman systems model* (2nd ed., pp. 115–138). Norwalk, CT: Appleton & Lange.

Kido, L.M. (1991). Sleep deprivation and intensive care unit psychosis. *Emphasis: Nursing*, 4(1), 23–33.

Kilchenstein, L., & Yakulis, I. (1984). The birth of a curriculum: Utilization of the Betty Neuman health care systems model in an integrated baccalaureate program. *Journal of Nursing Education*, 23, 126–127.

King, I.M. (1971). *Toward a theory for nursing*. New York: John Wiley & Sons.

Knight, J.B. (1990). The Betty Neuman systems model applied to practice: A client with multiple sclerosis. *Journal of Advanced Nursing*, 15, 447–455.

Knox, J.E., Kilchenstein, L., & Yakulis, I.M. (1982). Utilization of the Neuman model in an integrated baccalaureate program: University of Pittsburgh. In B. Neuman, *The Neuman systems model: Application to nursing education and practice* (pp. 117–123). Norwalk, CT: Appleton-Century-Crofts.

Koku, R.V. (1992). Severity of low back pain: A comparison between participants who did and did not receive counseling. *American Association of Occupational Health Nurses Journal*, 40, 84–89.

Laschinger, S.J., Maloney, R., & Tramer, J.E. (1989). An evaluation of student use of the Neuman systems model: Queen's University, Canada. In B. Neuman, *The Neuman systems model* (2nd ed., pp. 211–224). Norwalk, CT: Appleton & Lange.

Lazarus, R. (1981). The stress and coping paradigm. In C. Eisdorfer, D. Cohen, A. Kleinman, & P. Maxim (Eds.), *Models for clinical psychopathology* (pp. 177–214). New York: SP Medical and Scientific Books.

Lebold, M., & Davis, L. (1980). A baccalaureate nursing curriculum based on the Neuman health systems model. In J.P. Riehl & C. Roy, *Conceptual models for nursing practice* (2nd ed., pp. 151–158). New York: Appleton-Century-Crofts.

Lebold, M.M., & Davis, L.H. (1982). A bacca-

laureate nursing curriculum based on the Neuman systems model: Saint Xavier College. In B. Neuman, *The Neuman systems model: Application to nursing education and practice* (pp. 124–129). Norwalk, CT: Appleton-Century-Crofts.

Leja, A.M. (1989). Using guided imagery to combat postsurgical depression. *Journal of Gerontological Nursing*, 15(4), 6–11.

Lindell, M., & Olsson, H. (1991). Can combined oral contraceptives be made more effective by means of a nursing care model? *Journal of Advanced Nursing*, 16, 475–479.

Loescher, L.J., Clark, L., Atwood, J.R., Leigh, S., & Lamb, G. (1990). The impact of the cancer experience on long-term survivors. *Oncology Nursing Forum*, 17, 223–229.

Louis, M. (1989). An intervention to reduce anxiety levels for nursing working with long-term care clients using Neuman's model. In J.P. Riehl-Sisca, *Conceptual models for nursing practice* (3rd ed., pp. 95–103). Norwalk, CT: Appleton & Lange.

Louis, M., & Koertvelyessy, A. (1989). The Neuman model in research. In B. Neuman, *The Neuman systems model* (2nd ed., pp. 93–114). Norwalk, CT: Appleton & Lange.

Louis, M., Witt, R., & LaMancusa, M. (1989). The Neuman systems model in multilevel nurse education programs: University of Nevada, Las Vegas. In B. Neuman, *The Neuman systems model* (2nd ed., pp. 237–248). Norwalk, CT: Appleton & Lange.

Lowry, L. (1986). Adapted by degrees. *Senior Nurse*, 5(3), 25–26.

Lowry, L.W. (1988). Operationalizing the Neuman systems model: A course in concepts and process.. *Nurse Educator*, 13(3), 19–22.

Lowry, L.W., & Green, G.H. (1989). Four Neuman-based associate degree programs: Brief description and evaluation. In B. Neuman, *The Neuman systems model* (2nd ed., pp. 283–312). Norwalk, CT: Appleton & Lange.

Lowry, L.W., & Jopp, M.C. (1989). An evaluation instrument for assessing an associate degree nursing curriculum based on the Neuman systems model. In J.P. Riehl-Sisca, *Conceptual models for nursing practice* (3rd ed., pp. 73–85). Norwalk, CT: Appleton & Lange.

Mayers, M.A., & Watson, A.B. (1982). Nursing care plans and the Neuman systems model: In B. Neuman, *The Neuman systems model: Application to nursing education and practice (pp. 69–84). Norwalk, CT: Appleton-Century-Crofts.

Marriner-Tomey, A. (1982). Nursing theorists and their work (2nd ed.). St. Louis: CV Mosby.

McInerney, K.A. (1982). The Neuman systems model applied to critical care nursing of cardiac surgery clients. In B. Neuman, The Neuman systems model: Application to nursing education and practice (pp. 308–315). Norwalk, CT: Appleton-Century-Crofts.

Meleis, A.I. (1991). Theoretical nursing: Development and progress (2nd ed.). Philadelphia: JB Lippincott.

Millard, J. (1992). Health visiting an elderly couple. British Journal of Nursing, 1, 769–773.

Mirenda, R.M. (1986). The Neuman systems model: Description and application. In P. Winstead-Fry (Ed.), Case studies in nursing theory (pp. 127–166). New York: National League for Nursing.

Mischke-Berkey, K., & Hanson, S.M.H. (1991). Pocket guide to family assessment and intervention. St. Louis: Mosby-Year Book.

Mischke-Berkey, K., Warner, P., & Hanson, S. (1989). Family health assessment and intervention. In P.J. Bomar (Ed.), Nurses and family health promotion: Concepts, assessment, and interventions (pp. 115–154). Baltimore: Williams & Wilkins.

Moore, S.L., & Munro, M.F. (1990). The Neuman systems model applied to mental health nursing of older adults. Journal of Advanced Nursing, 15, 293–299.

Moxley, P.A., & Allen, L.M.H. (1982). The Neuman systems model approach in a master's degree program: Northwestern State University. In B. Neuman, The Neuman systems model: Application to nursing education and practice (pp. 168–175). Norwalk, CT: Appleton-Century-Crofts.

Moynihan, M.M. (1990). Implementation of the Neuman systems model in an acute care nursing department. In M.E. Parker (Ed.), Nursing theories in practice (pp. 263–273). New York: National League for Nursing.

Mrkonich, D.E., Hessian, M., & Miller, M.W. (1989). A cooperative process in curriculum development using the Neuman health-care systems model. In J.P. Riehl-Sisca, Conceptual models for nursing practice (3rd ed., pp. 87–94). Norwalk, CT: Appleton & Lange.

Mrkonich, D., Miller, M., & Hessian, M. (1989). Cooperative baccalaureate education: The Minnesota intercollegiate nursing consortium. In B. Neuman, The Neu-

man systems model (2nd ed., pp. 175–182). Norwalk, CT: Appleton & Lange.

Neal, M.C. (1982). Nursing care plans and the Neuman Systems Model: II. In B. Neuman, The Neuman systems model: Application to nursing education and practice (pp. 85–93). Norwalk, CT: Appleton-Century-Crofts.

Nelson, L.F., Hansen, M., & McCullagh, M. (1989). A new baccalaureate North Dakota-Minnesota nursing education consortium. In B. Neuman, The Neuman systems model (2nd ed., pp. 183–192). Norwalk, CT: Appleton & Lange.

Neuman, B. (1974). The Betty Neuman Health-Care Systems Model: A total person approach to patient problems. In J.P. Riehl & C. Roy, Conceptual models for nursing practice (pp. 99–114). New York: Appleton-Century-Crofts.

Neuman, B. (1980). The Betty Neuman Health-Care Systems Model: A total person approach to patient problems. In J.P. Riehl & C. Roy, Conceptual models for nursing practice (2nd ed., pp. 119–134). New York: Appleton-Century-Crofts.

Neuman, B. (1982a). The Neuman health-care systems model: A total approach to client care. In B. Neuman, The Neuman systems model: Application to nursing education and practice (pp. 8–29). Norwalk, CT: Appleton-Century-Crofts.

Neuman, B. (1982b). The Neuman systems model. Application to nursing education and practice. Norwalk, CT: Appleton-Century-Crofts.

Neuman B. (1983a). Family intervention using the Betty Neuman health care systems model. In I.W. Clements & F.B. Roberts, Family health: A theoretical approach to nursing care (pp. 239–254). New York: John Wiley & Sons.

Neuman, B. (1983b). The family experiencing emotional crisis: Analysis and application of Neuman's health care systems model. In I.W. Clements & F.B. Roberts, Family health: A theoretical approach to nursing care (pp. 353–367). New York: John Wiley & Sons.

Neuman, B. (1985a, August). Betty Neuman. Paper presented at conference on Nursing Theory in Action, Edmonton, Alberta, Canada. (Cassette recording).

Neuman B. (1985b). The Neuman systems model. Senior Nurse, 3(3), 20–23.

Neuman, B. (1989a). In conclusion—in transition. In B. Neuman, The Neuman systems model (2nd ed., pp. 453–470). Norwalk, CT: Appleton & Lange.

Neuman, B. (1989b). The Neuman nursing

process format: Family. In J.P. Riehl-Sisca, *Conceptual models for nursing practice* (3rd ed., pp. 49–62). Norwalk, CT: Appleton & Lange.

Neuman, B. (1989c). *The Neuman systems model* (2nd ed.). Norwalk, CT: Appleton & Lange.

Neuman, B. (1989d). The Neuman systems model. In B. Neuman, *The Neuman systems model* (2nd ed., pp. 3–63). Norwalk, CT: Appleton & Lange.

Neuman, B.M. (1990a). Health as a continuum based on the Neuman Systems Model. *Nursing Science Quarterly, 3,* 129–135.

Neuman, B. (1990b). The Neuman systems model: A theory for practice. In M.E. Parker (Ed.), *Nursing theories in practice* (pp. 241–261). New York: National League for Nursing.

Neuman, B. (in press). *The Neuman systems model* (3rd ed.). Norwalk, CT: Appleton & Lange.

Neuman, B., & Wyatt, M. (1980). The Neuman stress/adaptation systems approach to education for nurse administrators. In J.P. Riehl & C. Roy, *Conceptual models for nursing practice* (2nd ed., pp. 142–150). New York: Appleton-Century-Crofts.

Neuman, B., & Young, R.J. (1972). A model for teaching total person approach to patient problems. *Nursing Research, 21,* 264–269.

Nichols, E.G., Dale, M.L., & Turley, J. (1989). The University of Wyoming evaluation of a Neuman-based curriculum. In B. Neuman, *The Neuman systems model* (2nd ed., pp. 259–282). Norwalk, CT: Appleton & Lange.

Nortridge. J.A., Mayeux, V., Anderson, S.J., & Bell, M.L. (1992). The use of cognitive style mapping as a predictor for academic success of first semester diploma nursing students. *Journal of Nursing Education, 31,* 352–356.

Orem, D. (1971). *Nursing: Concepts of practice.* New York: McGraw-Hill.

Peterson, C.J. (1977). Questions frequently asked about the development of a conceptual framework. *Journal of Nursing Education, 16*(4), 22–32.

Piazza, D., Foote, A., Wright, P., & Holcombe, J. (1992). Neuman Systems Model used as a guide for the nursing care of an 8-year-old child with leukemia. *Journal of Pediatric Oncology Nursing, 9*(1), 17–24.

Pierce, J.D., & Hutton, E. (1992). Applying the new concepts of the Neuman systems model. *Nursing Forum, 27,* 15–18.

Pinkerton, A. (1974). Use of the Neuman model in a home health-care agency. In J.P. Riehl & C. Roy, *Conceptual models for nursing practice* (pp. 122–129). New York: Appleton-Century-Crofts.

Putt, A. (1972). Entropy, evolution and equifinality in nursing. In J. Smith (Ed.), *Five years of cooperation to improve curricula in Western schools of nursing.* Boulder, CO: Western Interstate Commission for Higher Education.

Quayhagen, M.P., & Roth, P.A. (1989). From models to measures in assessment of mature families. *Journal of Professional Nursing, 5,* 144–151.

Radwanski, M. (1992). Self-medicating practices for managing chronic pain after spinal cord injury, *Rehabilitation Nursing, 17,* 312–318.

Reed, K. (1982). The Neuman systems model: A basis for family psychosocial assessment. In B. Neuman, *The Neuman systems model: Application to nursing education and practice* (pp. 188–195). Norwalk, CT: Appleton-Century-Crofts.

Reed, K.S. (1989). Family theory related to the Neuman systems model. In B. Neuman, *The Neuman systems model* (2nd ed., pp. 385–396). Norwalk, CT: Appleton & Lange.

Reed, K.S. (1993). Adapting the Neuman systems model for family nursing. *Nursing Science Quarterly, 6,* 93–97.

Reed-Sorrow, K., Harmon, R.L., & Kitundu, M.E. (1989). Computer-assisted learning and the Neuman systems model. In B. Neuman, *The Neuman systems model* (2nd ed., pp. 155–160). Norwalk, CT: Appleton & Lange.

Redheffer G. (1985). Application of Betty Neuman's Health Care Systems Model to emergency nursing practice: Case review. *Point of View, 22*(2), 4–6.

Rice, M.J. (1982). The Neuman systems model applied in a hospital medical unit. In B. Neuman, *The Neuman systems model: Application to nursing education and practice* (pp. 316–323). Norwalk, CT: Appleton-Century-Crofts.

Riehl, J.P., & Roy, C. (1974). Conceptual models for nursing practice. New York: Appleton-Century-Crofts.

Riehl, J.P., & Roy, C. (1980). *Conceptual models for nursing practice* (2nd ed.). New York: Appleton-Century-Crofts.

Riehl-Sisca, J.P. (1989). *Conceptual models for nursing practice* (3rd ed.). Norwalk, CT: Appleton & Lange.

Robichaud-Ekstrand, S., & Delisle, L. (1989). Neuman en médecine-chirurgie [The Neuman model in medical-surgical settings]. *The Canadian Nurse, 85*(6), 32–35.

Rogers, M.E. (1970). *An introduction to the*

theoretical basis of nursing. Philadelphia: FA Davis.

Rosenthal, R. (1991). Meta-analytic procedures for social research (rev. ed.). Newbury Park, CA: Sage.

Ross, M., & Bourbonnais, F. (1985). The Betty Neuman Systems Model in nursing practice: A case study approach. Journal of Advanced Nursing, 10, 199–207.

Ross, M.M., Bourbonnais, F.F., & Carroll, G. (1987). Curricular design and the Betty Neuman systems model: A new approach to learning. International Nursing Review, 34, 75–79.

Ross, M.M., & Helmer, H. (1988). A comparative analysis of Neuman's model using the individual and family as the units of care. Public Health Nursing, 5, 30–36.

Schlentz, M.D. (1993). The minimum data set and the levels of prevention in the long-term care facility. Geriatric Nursing, 14, 79–83.

Selye, H. (1950). The physiology and pathology of exposure to stress. Montreal: ACTA.

Shaw, M.C. (1991). A theoretical base for orthopaedic nursing practice: The Neuman systems model. Canadian Orthopaedic Nurses Association Journal, 13(2), 19–21.

Simmons, L., & Borgdon, C. (1991). The clinical nurse specialist in HIV care. The Kansas Nurse, 66(1), 6–7.

Sipple, J.A., & Freese, B.T. (1989). Transition from technical to professional-level nursing education. In B. Neuman, The Neuman systems model (2nd ed., pp. 193–200). Norwalk, CT: Appleton & Lange.

Sirles, A.T., Brown, K., & Hilyer, J.C. (1991). Effects of back school education and exercise in back injured municipal workers. American Association of Occupational Health Nursing Journal, 39, 7–12.

Smith, M.C. (1989). Neuman's model in practice. Nursing Science Quarterly, 2, 116–117.

Sohier, R. (1989). Nursing care for the people of a small planet: Culture and the Neuman systems model. In B. Neuman, The Neuman systems model (2nd ed., pp. 139–154). Norwalk, CT: Appleton & Lange.

Speck, B.J. (1990). The effect of guided imagery upon first semester nursing students performing their first injections. Journal of Nursing Education, 29, 346–350.

Spradley, B.W. (1990). Community health nursing: Concepts and practice. Glenview, IL: Scott, Foresman/Little, Brown Higher Education.

Stevens, B.J. (1982). Foreword. In B. Neuman, The Neuman systems model: Application to nursing education and practice (pp. xiii–xiv). Norwalk, CT: Appleton-Century-Crofts.

Stittich, E.M., Avent, C.L., & Patterson, K. (1989). Neuman-based baccalaureate and graduate nursing programs, California State University, Fresno. In B. Neuman, The Neuman systems model (2nd ed., pp. 163–174). Norwalk, CT: Appleton & Lange.

Story, E.L., & DuGas, B.W. (1988). A teaching strategy to facilitate conceptual model implementation in practice. Journal of Continuing Education in Nursing, 19, 244–247.

Story, E.L., & Ross, M.M. (1986). Family centered community health nursing and the Betty Neuman systems model. Nursing Papers, 18(2), 77–88.

Sullivan, J. (1986). Using Neuman's model in the acute phase of spinal cord injury. Focus on Critical Care, 13(5), 34–41.

Tollett, S.M. (1982). Teaching geriatrics and gerontology: Use of the Neuman systems model. In B. Neuman, The Neuman systems model: Application to nursing education and practice (pp. 1159–1164). Norwalk, CT: Appleton-Century-Crofts.

Torkington, S. (1988). Nourishing the infant. Senior Nurse, 8(2), 24–25.

Utz, S.W. (1980). Applying the Neuman model to nursing practice with hypertensive clients. Cardio-Vascular Nursing, 16, 29–34.

Vaughn, M., Cheatwood, S., Sirles, A.T., & Brown, K.C. (1989). The effect of progressive muscle relaxation on stress among clerical workers. American Association of Occupational Health Nurses Journal, 37, 302–306.

Vokaty, D.A. (1982). The Neuman systems model applied to the clinical nurse specialist role. In B. Neuman, The Neuman systems model: Application to nursing education and practice (pp. 165–167). Norwalk, CT: Appleton-Century-Crofts.

Waddell, K.L., and Demi, A.S. (1993). Effectiveness of an intensive partial hospitalization program for treatment of anxiety disorders. Archives of Psychiatric Nursing, 7, 2–10.

Wallingford, P. (1989). The neurologically impaired and dying child: Applying the Neuman systems model. Issues in Comprehensive Pediatric Nursing, 12, 139–157.

Weinberger, S.L. (1991). Analysis of a clinical situation using the Neuman System Model. Rehabilitation Nursing, 16, 278, 280–281.

Wilson, V.S. (1987). Identification of stres-

sors related to patients' psychological responses to the surgical intensive care unit.
Heart and Lung, 16, 267–273.

Ziegler, S.M. (1982). Taxonomy for nursing
diagnosis derived from the Neuman systems model. In B. Neuman, *The Neuman*

systems model: Application to nursing education and practice (pp. 55–68). Norwalk, CT: Appleton-Century-Crofts.

Ziemer, M.M. (1983). Effects of information
on postsurgical coping. *Nursing Research,
32,* 282–287.

BIBLIOGRAPHY

PRIMARY SOURCES

Neuman, B. (1974). The Betty Neuman
Health-Care Systems Model: A total per-
son approach to patient problems. In J.P.
Riehl & C. Roy, *Conceptual models for
nursing practice* (pp. 99–114). New York:
Appleton-Century-Crofts.

Neuman, B. (1980). The Betty Neuman
Health-Care Systems Model: A total per-
son approach to patient problems. In J.P.
Riehl & C. Roy, *Conceptual models for
nursing practice* (2nd ed., pp. 119–134).
New York: Appleton-Century-Crofts.

Neuman, B. (1982). The Neuman health-
care systems model: A total approach to
client care. In B. Neuman, *The Neuman
systems model: Application to nursing education and practice* (pp. 8–29). Norwalk,
CT: Appleton-Century-Crofts.

Neuman, B. (1982). *The Neuman systems
model: Application to nursing education
and practice.* Norwalk, CT: Appleton-
Century-Crofts.

Neuman, B. (1982). The systems concept
and nursing. In B. Neuman, *The Neuman
systems model: Application to nursing education and practice* (pp. 3–7). Norwalk,
CT: Appleton-Century-Crofts.

Neuman B. (1983). Family intervention
using the Betty Neuman health care systems model. In I.W. Clements & F.B. Roberts, *Family health: A theoretical approach to nursing care* (pp. 239–254).
New York: John Wiley & Sons.

Neuman, B. (1983). The family experiencing
emotional crisis: Analysis and application
of Neuman's health care systems model.
In I.W. Clements & F.B. Roberts, *Family
health: A theoretical approach to nursing
care* (pp. 353–367). New York: John Wiley
& Sons.

Neuman, B. (1985). The Neuman systems
model. *Senior Nurse, 5*(3), 20–23.

Neuman, B. (1989). The Neuman nursing
process format: Family. In J.P. Riehl-Sisca,
Conceptual models for nursing practice
(3rd ed., pp. 49–62). Norwalk, CT: Appleton & Lange.

Neuman, B. (1989). In conclusion—in transition. In B. Neuman, *The Neuman systems model* (2nd ed., pp. 453–470). Norwalk, CT: Appleton & Lange.

Neuman, B. (1989). *The Neuman systems
model* (2nd ed.). Norwalk, CT: Appleton &
Lange.

Neuman, B. (1989). The Neuman systems
model. In B. Neuman, *The Neuman systems model* (2nd ed., pp. 3–63). Norwalk,
CT: Appleton & Lange.

Neuman, B. (1990). The Neuman systems
model: A theory for practice. In M.E.
Parker (Ed.), *Nursing theories in practice*
(pp. 241–261). New York: National
League for Nursing.

Neuman, B.M. (1990). Health as a continuum based on the Neuman Systems
Model. *Nursing Science Quarterly, 3,*
129–135.

Neuman, B., & Young, R.J. (1972). A model
for teaching total person approach to patient problems. *Nursing Research, 21,*
264–269.

COMMENTARY

Aggleton, P., & Chalmers, H. (1989). Neuman's systems model. *Nursing Times,
85*(51), 27–29.

Barrett, M. (1991). A thesis is born. *Image:
Journal of Nursing Scholarship, 23,*
261–262.

Beckman, S.J., Boxley-Harges, S., Bruick-
Sorge, C., et al. (1994). Betty Neuman:
Systems model. In Marriner-Tomey (Ed.),
Nursing theorists and their work (3rd ed.
pp. 269–304). St. Louis: Mosby-Year Book.

Bigbee, J. (1984). The changing role of rural
women: Nursing and health implications.
Health Care of Women International, 5,
307–322.

Biley, F. (1990). The Neuman model: An
analysis. *Nursing (London), 4*(4), 25–28.

Burney, M.A. (1992). King and Newman: In
search of the nursing paradigm. *Journal of
Advanced Nursing, 17,* 601–603.

Campbell, V. (1989). The Betty Neuman
health care systems model: An analysis

(pp. 63–72). In J.P. Riehl-Sisca, *Conceptual models for nursing practice* (3rd ed., pp. 63–72). Norwalk, CT: Appleton & Lange.

Christensen, P.J., & Kenney, J.W. (Eds.). *Nursing process: Application of conceptual models.* St. Louis: CV Mosby.

Cross, J.R. (1985). Betty Neuman. In *Nursing Theories Conference Group, Nursing theories: The base for professional nursing practice* (pp. 258–286). Englewood Cliffs, NJ: Prentice-Hall.

Cross, J.R. (1990). Betty Neuman. In J.B. George (Ed.), *Nursing theories: The base for professional nursing practice* (3rd ed., pp. 259–278). Norwalk, CT: Appleton & Lange.

Fawcett, J. (1989). Analysis and evaluation of the Neuman systems model. In B. Neuman, *The Neuman systems model* (2nd ed., pp. 65–92). Norwalk, CT: Appleton & Lange.

Fawcett, J., Carpenito, J.J., Efinger, J., Goldblum-Graff, D., Groesbeck, M.J.V., Lowry, L.W., McCreary, C.S., & Wolf, Z.R. (1982). A framework for analysis and evaluation of conceptual models of nursing with an analysis and evaluation of the Neuman systems model: In B. Neuman, *The Neuman systems model: Application to nursing education and practice* (pp. 30–43). Norwalk, CT: Appleton-Century-Crofts.

Harris, S.M., Hermiz, M.E., Meininger, M., & Steinkeler, S.E. (1989). Betty Neuman: Systems model. In A. Marriner-Tomey, *Nursing theorists and their work* (2nd ed., pp. 361–388). St. Louis: CV Mosby.

Hermiz, M.E., & Meininger, M. (1986). Betty Neuman. Systems model. In A. Marriner, *Nursing theorists and their work* (pp. 313–331). St. Louis: CV Mosby.

Hoffman, M.K. (1982). From model to theory construction: An analysis of the Neuman Health-Care systems model. In B. Neuman, *The Neuman systems model: Application to nursing education and practice* (pp. 44–54). Norwalk, CT: Appleton-Century-Crofts.

Huch, M.H. (1991). Perspectives on health. *Nursing Science Quarterly, 4,* 33–40.

Lancaster, D.R., & Whall, A.L. (1989). The Neuman systems model. In J.J. Fitzpatrick & A.L. Whall, *Conceptual models of nursing: Analysis and application* (2nd ed., pp. 255–270). Bowie, MD: Brady.

Meleis, A.I. (1991). *Theoretical nursing: Development and progress* (2nd ed.). Philadelphia: JB Lippincott.

Mirenda, R.M., & Wright, C. (1987). Using nursing model to affirm Catholic identity. *Health Progress, 68*(2), 63–67, 94.

Reed, K.S. (1993). *Betty Neuman: The Neuman systems model.* Newbury Park, CA: Sage.

Salvage, J., & Turner, C. (1989). Brief abstracts: The Neuman model use in England. In B. Neuman, *The Neuman systems model* (2nd ed., pp. 445–450). Norwalk, CT: Appleton & Lange.

Stevens, B.J. (1982). Forward. In B. Neuman, *The Neuman systems model: Application to nursing education and practice* (pp. xiii–xiv). Norwalk, CT: Appleton-Century-Crofts.

Thibodeau, J.A. (1983). *Nursing models: Analysis and evaluation.* Monterey, CA: Wadsworth.

Venable, J.F. (1974). The Neuman Health-Care Systems Model: An analysis. In J.P. Riehl & C. Roy, *Conceptual models for nursing practice* (pp. 115–122). New York: Appleton-Century-Crofts. Reprinted in J.P. Riehl & C. Roy (1980), *Conceptual models for nursing practice* (2nd ed., pp. 135–141). New York: Appleton-Century-Crofts.

Walker, L.O., & Avant, K.C. (1983). *Strategies for theory construction in nursing.* Norwalk, CT: Appleton-Century-Crofts.

Whall, A.L. (1983). The Betty Neuman Health Care System Model. In J.J. Fitzpatrick & A.L. Whall, *Conceptual models of nursing: Analysis and application* (pp. 203–219). Bowie, MD: Brady.

RESEARCH

Ali, N.S., & Khalil, H.Z. (1989). Effect of psychoeducational intervention on anxiety among Egyptian bladder cancer patients. *Cancer Nursing, 12,* 236–242.

Bass, L.S. (1991). What do parents need when their infant is a patient in the NICU? *Neonatal Network, 10*(4), 25–33.

Blank. J.J., Clark, L., Longman, A.J., & Atwood, J.R. (1989). Perceived home care needs of cancer patients and their caregivers. *Cancer Nursing, 12,* 78–84.

Bowdler, J.E., & Barrell, L.M. (1987). Health needs of homeless persons. *Public Health Nursing, 4,* 135–140.

Bueno, M.N., Redeker, N., & Norman, E.M. (1992). Analysis of motor vehicle crash data in an urban trauma center: Implications for nursing practice and research. *Heart and Lung, 21,* 558–567.

Burke, S.O., & Maloney, R. (1986). The Women's Value Orientation Questionnaire: An instrument revision study. *Nursing Papers, 18*(1), 32–44.

Cantin, B., & Mitchell, M. (1989). Nurses'

smoking behavior. *The Canadian Nurse*, *85*(1), 20–21.

Capers, C.F. (1991). Nurses' and lay African Americans' views about behavior. *Western Journal of Nursing Research*, *13*, 123–135.

Carroll, T.L. (1989). Role deprivation in baccalaureate nursing students pre and post curriculum revision. *Journal of Nursing Education*, *28*, 134–139.

Cava, M.A. (1992). An examination of coping strategies used by long-term cancer survivors. *Canadian Oncology Nursing Journal*, *2*, 99–102.

Clark, C.C., Cross, J.R., Deane, D.M., & Lowry, L.W. (1991). Spirituality: Integral to quality care. *Holistic Nursing Practice*, *5*, 67–76.

Courchene, V.S., Patalski, E., & Martin, J. (1991). A study of the health of pediatric nurses administering Cyclosporine A. *Pediatric Nursing*, *17*, 497–500.

Decker, S.D., & Young, E. (1991). Self-perceived needs of primary caregivers of home-hospice clients. *Journal of Community Health Nursing*, *8*, 147–154.

Freiberger, D., Bryant, J., & Marino, B. (1992). The effects of different central venous line dressing changes on bacterial growth in a pediatric oncology population. *Journal of Pediatric Oncology Nursing*, *9*, 3–7.

Gavigan, M., Kline-O'Sullivan, C., & Klumpp-Lybrand, B. (1990). The effect of regular turning on CABG patients. *Critical Care Nursing Quarterly*, *12*(4), 69–76.

Grant, J.S., & Bean, C.A. (1992). Self-identified needs of informal caregivers of head-injured adults. *Family and Community Health*, *15*(2), 49–58.

Grant, J.S., Kinney, M.R., & Davis, L.L. (1992). Using conceptual frameworks of models to guide nursing research. *Journal of Neuroscience Nursing*, *25*, 52–56.

Gries, M., & Fernsler, J. (1988). Patient perceptions of the mechanical ventilation experience. *Focus on Critical Care*, *15*, 52–59.

Heffline, M.S. (1991). A comparative study of pharmacological versus nursing interventions in the treatment of postanesthesia shivering. *Journal of Post Anesthesia Nursing*, *6*, 311–320.

Hinds, C. (1990). Personal and contextual factors predicting patients' reported quality of life: Exploring congruency with Betty Neuman's assumptions. *Journal of Advanced Nursing*, *15*, 456–462.

Hoch, C.C. (1987). Assessing delivery of nursing care. *Journal of Gerontological Nursing*, *13*, 1–17.

Johnson, P. (1983). Black hypertension: A transcultural case study using the Betty Neuman model of nursing care. *Issues in Health Care of Women*, *4*, 191–210.

Kahn, E.C. (1992). A comparison of family needs based on the presence or absence of DNR orders. *Dimensions of Critical Care Nursing*, *11*, 286–292.

Koku, R.V. (1992). Severity of low back pain: A comparison between participants who did and did not receive counseling. *American Association of Occupational Health Nurses Journal*, *40*, 84–89.

Leja, A.M. (1989). Using guided imagery to combat postsurgical depression. *Journal of Gerontological Nursing*, *15*(4), 6–11.

Loescher, L.J., Clark, L., Atwood, J.R., Leigh, S., & Lamb, G. (1990). The impact of the cancer experience on long-term survivors. *Oncology Nursing Forum*, *17*, 223–229.

Louis, M. (1989). An intervention to reduce anxiety levels for nursing working with long-term care clients using Neuman's model. In J.P. Riehl-Sisca, *Conceptual models for nursing practice* (3rd ed., pp. 95–103). Norwalk, CT: Appleton & Lange.

Louis, M., & Koertvelyessy, A. (1989). The Neuman model in research. In B. Neuman, *The Neuman systems model* (2nd ed., pp. 93–114). Norwalk, CT: Appleton & Lange.

Lowry, L.W., & Jopp, M.C. (1989). An evaluation instrument for assessing an associate degree nursing curriculum based on the Neuman systems model. In J.P. Riehl-Sisca, *Conceptual models for nursing practice* (3rd ed., pp. 73–85). Norwalk, CT: Appleton & Lange.

Nortridge, J.A., Mayeux, V., Anderson, S.J., & Bell, M.L. (1992). The use of cognitive style mapping as a predictor for academic success of first semester diploma nursing students. *Journal of Nursing Education*, *31*, 352–356.

Radwanski, M. (1992). Self-medicating practices for managing chronic pain after spinal cord injury. *Rehabilitation Nursing*, *17*, 312–318.

Sirles, A.T., Brown, K., & Hilyer, J.C. (1991). Effects of back school education and exercise in back injured municipal workers. *American Association of Occupational Health Nursing Journal*, *39*, 7–12.

Speck, B.J. (1990). The effect of guided imagery upon first semester nursing students performing their first injections. *Journal of Nursing Education*, *29*, 346–350.

Vaughn, M., Cheatwood, S., Sirles, A.T., & Brown, K.C. (1989). The effect of progressive muscle relaxation on stress among clerical workers. *American Association of Occupational Health Nurses Journal, 37*, 302–306.

Waddell, K.L., & Demi, A.S. (1993). Effectiveness of an intensive partial hospitalization program for treatment of anxiety disorders. *Archives of Psychiatric Nursing, 7*, 2–10.

Wilson, V.S. (1987). Identification of stressors related to patients' psychological responses to the surgical intensive care unit. *Heart and Lung, 16*, 267–273.

Ziegler, S.M. (1982). Taxonomy for nursing diagnosis derived from the Neuman systems model. In B. Neuman, *The Neuman systems model: Application to nursing education and practice* (pp. 55–68). Norwalk, CT: Appleton-Century-Crofts.

Ziemer, M.M. (1983). Effects of information on postsurgical coping. *Nursing Research, 32*, 282–287.

DOCTORAL DISSERTATIONS

Burritt, J.E. (1988). The effects of perceived social support on the relationship between job stress and job satisfaction and job performance among registered nurses employed in acute care facilities. *Dissertation Abstracts International, 49*, 2123B.

Capers, C.F. (1987). Perceptions of problematic behavior as held by lay black adults and registered nurses. *Dissertation Abstracts International, 47*, 4467B.

Collins, A.S. (1992). Effects of positional changes on selected physiological and psychological measurements in clients with atrial fibrillation. *Dissertation Abstracts International, 53*, 200B.

Flannery, J.C. (1988). Validity and reliability of Levels of Cognitive Functioning Assessment Scale for adults with closed head injuries. *Dissertation Abstracts International, 48*, 3248B.

Fulton, B.J. (1993). Evaluation of the effectiveness of the Neuman systems model as a theoretical framework for baccalaureate nursing programs. *Dissertation Abstracts International, 53*, 5641B.

Goble, D.S. (1991). A curriculum framework for the prevention of child sexual abuse. *Dissertation Abstracts International, 52*, 2004A.

Harbin, P.D.O. (1990). A Q-analysis of the stressors of adult female nursing students enrolled in baccalaureate schools of nursing. *Dissertation Abstracts International, 50*, 3919B.

Heaman, D.J. (1992). Perceived stressors and coping strategies of parents with develop-

mentally disabled children. *Dissertation Abstracts International, 52*, 6316B.

Lancaster, D.R.N. (1992). Coping with appraised threat of breast cancer: Primary prevention coping behaviors utilized by women at increased risk. *Dissertation Abstracts International, 53*, 202B.

McDaniel, G.M.S. (1990). The effects of two methods of dangling on heart rate and blood pressure in postoperative abdominal hysterectomy patients. *Dissertation Abstracts International, 50*, 3923B.

Moody, N.B. (1991). Selected demographic variables, organizational characteristics, role orientation, and job satisfaction among nurse faculty. *Dissertation Abstracts International, 52*, 1356B.

Norman, S.E. (1991). The relationship between hardiness and sleep disturbances in HIV-infected men. *Dissertation Abstracts International, 51*, 4780B.

Norris, E.W. (1990). Physiologic response to exercise in clients with mitral valve prolapse syndrome. *Dissertation Abstracts International, 50*, 5549B.

Peoples, L.T. (1991). The relationship between selected client, provider, and agency variables and the utilization of home care services. *Dissertation Abstracts International, 51*, 3782B.

Poole, V.L. (1992). Pregnancy wantedness, attitude toward pregnancy, and use of alcohol, tobacco, and street drugs during pregnancy. *Dissertation Abstracts International, 52*, 5193B.

Pothiban, L. (1993). Risk factor prevalence, risk status, and perceived risk for coronary heart disease among Thai elderly. *Dissertation Abstracts International, 54*, 1337B.

Rowe, M.L. (1990). The relationship of commitment and social support to the life satisfaction of caregivers to patients with Alzheimer's disease. *Dissertation Abstracts International, 51*, 1747B.

Rowles, C.J. (1993). The relationship of selected personal and organizational variables and the tenure of directors of nursing in nursing homes. *Dissertation Abstracts International, 53*, 4593B.

Schlosser, S.P. (1985). The effect of anticipatory guidance on mood state in primiparas experiencing unplanned cesarean delivery (metropolitan area, Southeast). *Dissertation Abstracts International, 46*, 2627B.

Sipple, J.E.A. (1989). A model for curriculum change based on retrospective analysis. *Dissertation Abstracts International, 50*, 1927A.

Tennyson, M.G. (1992). Becoming pregnant:

Perceptions of black adolescents. *Dissertation Abstracts International, 52,* 5196B.

Terhaar, M.F. (1989). The influence of physiologic stability, behavioral stability and family stability on the preterm infant's length of stay in the neonatal intensive care unit. *Dissertation Abstracts International, 50,* 1328B.

Vincent, J.L.M. (1988). A Q analysis of the stressors of fathers with an infant in an intensive care unit. *Dissertation Abstracts International, 49,* 3111B.

Watson, L.A. (1991). Comparison of the effects of usual, support, and informational nursing interventions on the extent to which families of critically ill patients perceived their needs were met. *Dissertation Abstracts International, 52,* 2999B.

Webb, C.A. (1988). A cross-sectional study of hope, physical status, cognitions and meaning and purpose of pre- and post-retirement adults. *Dissertation Abstracts International, 49,* 1922A.

Whatley, J.H. (1989). Effects of health locus of control and social network on risk-taking in adolescents. *Dissertation Abstracts International, 50,* 129B.

MASTER'S THESES

Anderson, R.R. (1992). Indicators of nutritional status as a predictor of pressure ulcer development in the critically ill adults. *Masters Abstracts International, 30,* 92.

Averill, J.B. (1989). The impact of primary prevention as an intervention strategy. *Masters Abstracts International, 27,* 89.

Baskin-Nedzelski, J. (1992). Job stressors among visiting nurses. *Masters Abstracts International, 30,* 79.

Besseghini, C. (1990). Stressful life events and angina in individuals undergoing exercise stress testing. *Masters Abstracts International, 28,* 569.

Blount, K.R. (1989). The relationship between the parents' and five to six-year-old child's perception of life events as stressors within the Neuman health care system framework. *Master Abstracts International, 27,* 487.

Elgar, S.J. (1992). The influence of companion animals on perceived social support and perceived stress among family caregivers. *Masters Abstracts International, 30,* 732.

Fields, W.L. (1988). The effects of the 12-hour shift on fatigue and critical thinking performance in critical care nurses. *Masters Abstracts International, 26,* 237.

Finney, G.A.H. (1990). Spiritual needs of patients. *Masters Abstracts International, 28,* 272.

Goldstein, L.A. (1988). Needs of spouses of hospitalized cancer patients. *Masters Abstracts International, 26,* 105.

Harper, B. (1993). Nurses' beliefs about social support and the effect of nursing care on the cardiac clients' attitudes in reducing cardiac risk status. *Masters Abstracts International, 31,* 273.

Haskill, K.M. (1988). Sources of occupational stress of the community health nurse. *Masters Abstracts International, 26,* 106.

Morris, D.C. (1991). Occupational stress among home care first line managers. *Masters Abstracts International, 29,* 443.

Murphy, N.G. (1990). Factors associated with breastfeeding success and failure: A systematic integrative review (infant nutrition). *Masters Abstracts International, 28,* 275.

Petock, A.M. (1991). Decubitus ulcers and physiological stressors. *Masters Abstracts International, 29,* 267.

Sammarco, C.C.A. (1990). The study of stressors of the operating room nurse versus those of the intensive care unit nurse. *Masters Abstracts International, 28,* 276.

Scarpino, L.L. (1988). Family caregivers' perceptions associated with the chemotherapy treatment setting for the oncology client. *Masters Abstracts International, 26,* 424.

Sullivan, M.M. (1991). Comparisons of job satisfaction scores of school nurses with job satisfaction normative scores of hospital nurses. *Masters Abstracts International, 29,* 652.

Wilkey, S.F. (1990). The effects of an eight-hour continuing education course on the death anxiety levels of registered nurses. *Masters Abstracts International, 28,* 480.

EDUCATION

Arndt, C. (1982). Systems theory and educational programs for nursing service administration. In B. Neuman, *The Neuman systems model: Application to nursing education and practice* (pp. 182–187). Norwalk, CT: Appleton-Century-Crofts.

Baker, N.A. (1982). The Neuman systems model as a conceptual framework for continuing education in the work place. In B. Neuman, *The Neuman systems model: Application to nursing education and practice* (pp. 260–264). Norwalk, CT: Appleton-Century-Crofts.

Bourbonnais, F.F., & Ross, M.M. (1985). The Neuman systems model in nursing education: Course development and implementation. *Journal of Advanced Nursing, 10,* 117–123.

Bower, F.L. (1982). Curriculum development and the Neuman Model. In B. Neuman, *The Neuman systems model: Application to nursing education and practice* (pp. 94–99). Norwalk, CT: Appleton-Century-Crofts.

Bruton, M.R., & Matzo, M. (1989). Curriculum revisions at Saint Anselm College: Focus on the older adult. In B. Neuman, *The Neuman systems model* (2nd ed., pp. 201–210). Norwalk, CT: Appleton & Lange.

Capers, C.F. (1986). Some basic facts about models, nursing conceptualizations, and nursing theories. *Journal of Continuing Education, 16,* 149–154.

Conners, V.L. (1982). Teaching the Neuman systems model: An approach to student and faculty development. In B. Neuman, *The Neuman systems model: Application to nursing education and practice* (pp. 176–181). Norwalk, CT: Appleton-Century-Crofts.

Conners, V.L. (1989). An empirical evaluation of the Neuman systems model: The University of Missouri-Kansas City. In B. Neuman, *The Neuman systems model* (2nd ed., pp. 249–258). Norwalk, CT: Appleton & Lange.

Conners, V., Harmon, V.M., & Langford, R.W. (1982). Course development and implementation using the Neuman systems model as a framework: Texas Woman's University (Houston Campus). In B. Neuman, *The Neuman systems model: Application to nursing education and practice* (pp. 153–158). Norwalk, CT: Appleton-Century-Crofts.

Dale, M.L., & Savala, S.M. (1990). A new approach to the senior practicum. *Nursing-Connections, 3*(1), 45–51.

Dyck, S.M., Innes, J.E., Rae, D.I., & Sawatzky, J.E. (1989). The Neuman systems model in curriculum revision: A baccalaureate program, University of Saskatchewan. In B. Neuman, *The Neuman systems model* (2nd ed., pp. 225–236). Norwalk, CT: Appleton & Lange.

Edwards, P.A. & Kittler, A.W. (1991). Integrating rehabilitation content in nursing curricula. *Rehabilitation Nursing, 16,* 70–73.

Harty, M.B. (1982). Continuing education in nursing and the Neuman model. In B. Neuman, *The Neuman systems model:* *Application to nursing education and practice* (pp. 100–106). Norwalk, CT: Appleton-Century-Crofts.

Johansen, H. (1989). Neuman model concepts in joint use—community health practice and student teaching—School of Advanced Nursing Education, Aarhus University, Aarhus, Denmark. In B. Neuman, *The Neuman systems model* (2nd ed., pp. 334–362). Norwalk, CT: Appleton & Lange.

Johnson, M.N. Vaughn-Wrobel, B., Ziegler, S., Hough, L., Bush, H.A., & Kurtz, P. (1982). Use of the Neuman Health-Care systems model in the master's curriculum: Texas Woman's University. In B. Neuman, *The Neuman systems model: Application to nursing education and practice* (pp. 130–152). Norwalk, CT: Appleton-Century-Crofts.

Johnson, S.E. (1989). A picture is worth a thousand words: Helping students visualize a conceptual model. *Nurse Educator, 14*(3), 21–24.

Kilchenstein, L., & Yakulis, I. (1984). The birth of a curriculum: Utilization of the Betty Neuman health care systems model in an integrated baccalaureate program. *Journal of Nursing Education, 23,* 126–127.

Knox, J.E., Kilchenstein, L., & Yakulis, I.M. (1982). Utilization of the Neuman model in an integrated baccalaureate program: University of Pittsburgh. In B. Neuman, *The Neuman systems model: Application to nursing education and practice* (pp. 117–123). Norwalk, CT: Appleton-Century-Crofts.

Laschinger, S.J., Maloney, R., & Tranmer, J.E. (1989). An evaluation of student use of the Neuman systems model: Queen's University, Canada. In B. Neuman, *The Neuman systems model* (2nd ed., pp. 211–224). Norwalk, CT: Appleton & Lange.

Lebold, M., & Davis, L. (1980). A baccalaureate nursing curriculum based on the Neuman health systems model. In J.P. Riehl & C. Roy, *Conceptual models for nursing practice* (2nd ed., pp. 151–158). New York: Appleton-Century-Crofts.

Lebold, M.M., & Davis, L.H. (1982). A baccalaureate nursing curriculum based on the Neuman systems model: Saint Xavier College. In B. Neuman, *The Neuman systems model: Application to nursing education and practice* (pp. 124–129). Norwalk, CT: Appleton-Century-Crofts.

Louis, M., Witt, R., & LaMancusa, M. (1989). The Neuman systems model in multilevel nurse education programs: University of

Nevada, Las Vegas. In B. Neuman, *The Neuman systems model* (2nd ed., pp. 237–248). Norwalk, CT: Appleton & Lange.

Lowry, L. (1985). Adapted by degrees. *Senior Nurse, 5*(3), 25–26.

Lowry, L.W. (1988). Operationalizing the Neuman systems model: A course in concepts and process. *Nurse Educator, 13*(3), 19–22.

Lowry, L.W., & Green, G.H. (1989). Four Neuman-based associate degree programs: Brief description and evaluation. In B. Neuman, *The Neuman systems model* (2nd ed., pp. 283–312). Norwalk, CT: Appleton & Lange.

Mirenda, R.M. (1986). The Neuman systems model: Description and application. In P. Winstead-Fry (Ed.), *Case studies in nursing theory* (pp. 127–166). New York: National League for Nursing.

Moxley, P.A., & Allen, L.M.H. (1982). The Neuman systems model approach in a master's degree program: Northwestern State University. In B. Neuman, *The Neuman systems model: Application to nursing education and practice* (pp. 168–175). Norwalk, CT: Appleton-Century-Crofts.

Mrkonich, D.E., Hessian, M., & Miller, M.W. (1989). A cooperative process in curriculum development using the Neuman health-care systems model. In J.P. Riehl-Sisca, *Conceptual models for nursing practice* (3rd ed., pp. 87–94). Norwalk, CT: Appleton & Lange.

Mrkonich, D., Miller, M., & Hessian, M. (1989). Cooperative baccalaureate education: The Minnesota intercollegiate nursing consortium. In B. Neuman, *The Neuman systems model* (2nd ed., pp. 175–182). Norwalk, CT: Appleton & Lange.

Nelson, L.F., Hansen, M., & McCullagh, M. (1989). A new baccalaureate North Dakota-Minnesota nursing education consortium. In B. Neuman, *The Neuman systems model* (2nd ed., pp. 183–192). Norwalk, CT: Appleton & Lange.

Nichols, E.G., Dale, M.L. & Turley, J. (1989). The University of Wyoming evaluation of a Neuman-based curriculum. In B. Neuman, *The Neuman systems model* (2nd ed., pp. 259–282). Norwalk, CT: Appleton & Lange.

Reed-Sorrow, K., Harmon, R.L., & Kitundu, M.E. (1989). Computer-assisted learning and the Neuman systems model. In B. Neuman, *The Neuman systems model* (2nd ed., pp. 155–160). Norwalk, CT: Appleton & Lange.

Ross, M.M., Bourbonnais, F.F., & Carroll, G.

(1987). Curricular design and the Betty Neuman systems model: A new approach to learning. *International Nursing Review, 34,* 75–79.

Sipple, J.A., & Freese, B.T. (1989). Transition from technical to professional-level nursing education. In B. Neuman, *The Neuman systems model* (2nd ed., pp. 193–200). Norwalk, CT: Appleton & Lange.

Stittich, E.M., Avent, C.L., & Patterson, K. (1989). Neuman-based baccalaureate and graduate nursing programs, California State University, Fresno. In B. Neuman, *The Neuman systems model* (2nd ed., pp. 163–174). Norwalk, CT: Appleton & Lange.

Story, E.L., & DuGas, B.W. (1988). A teaching strategy to facilitate conceptual model implementation in practice. *Journal of Continuing Education in Nursing, 19,* 244–247.

Story, E.L., & Ross, M.M. (1986). Family centered community health nursing and the Betty Neuman systems model. *Nursing Papers, 18*(2), 77–88.

Tollett, S.M. (1982). Teaching geriatrics and gerontology: use of the Neuman systems model. In B. Neuman, *The Neuman systems model: Application to nursing education and practice* (pp. 1159–1164). Norwalk, CT: Appleton-Century-Crofts.

ADMINISTRATION

Arndt, C. (1982). Systems concepts for management of stress in complex health-care organizations. In B. Neuman, *The Neuman systems model: Application to nursing education and practice* (pp. 97–114). Norwalk, CT: Appleton-Century-Crofts.

Bowman, G.E. (1982). The Neuman assessment tool adapted for child day-care centers. In B. Neuman, *The Neuman systems model: Application to nursing education and practice* (pp. 324–334). Norwalk, CT: Appleton-Century-Crofts.

Breckenridge, D.M., Cupit, M.C., & Raimondo, J.M. (1982). Systematic nursing assessment tool for the CAPD client. *Nephrology Nurse,* (January/February), *24,* 26–27, 30–31.

Burke, M.E. Sr., Capers, C.F., O'Connell, R.K., Quinn, R.M., & Sinnott, M. (1989). Neuman-based nursing practice in a hospital setting. In B. Neuman, *The Neuman systems model* (2nd ed., pp. 423–444). Norwalk, CT: Appleton & Lange.

Capers, C.F., & Kelly, R. (1987). Neuman nursing process: A model of holistic care. *Holistic Nursing Practice, 1*(3), 19–26.

Capers, C.F., O'Brien, C., Quinn, R., Kelly, R., & Fenerty, A. (1985). The Neuman systems model in practice: Planning phase. *Journal of Nursing Administration, 15*(5), 29–39.

Caramanica, L., & Thibodeau, J. (1987). Nursing philosophy and the selection of a model for practice. *Nursing Management, 10*(10), 71.

Davies, P. (1989). In Wales: Use of the Neuman systems model by community psychiatric nurses. In B. Neuman, *The Neuman systems model* (2nd ed., pp. 375–384). Norwalk, CT: Appleton & Lange.

Drew, L.L., Craig, D.M., & Beynon, C.E. (1989). The Neuman systems model for community health administration and practice: Provinces of Manitoba and Ontario, Canada. In B. Neuman, *The Neuman Systems model* (2nd ed., pp. 315–342). Norwalk, CT: Appleton & Lange.

Fawcett, J., Botter, M.L., Burritt, J., Crossley, J.D., & Fink, B.B. (1989). Conceptual models of nursing and organization theories. In B. Henry, M. DiVincenti, C. Arndt, & A. Marriner (Eds.), *Dimensions of nursing administration: Theory, research, education, and practice* (pp. 143–154). Boston: Blackwell Scientific Publications.

Flannery, J. (1991). FAMLI-RESCUE: A family assessment tool for use by neuroscience nurses in the acute care setting. *Journal of Neuroscience Nursing, 23,* 111–115.

Hinton-Walker, P., & Raborn, M. (1989). Application of the Neuman model in nursing administration and practice. In B. Henry, C. Arndt, M. DiVincenti, & A. Marriner (Eds.), *Dimensions of nursing administration. Theory, research, education, and practice* (pp. 711–723). Boston: Blackwell Scientific Publications.

Johns, C. (1991). The Burford Nursing Development Unit holistic model of nursing practice. *Journal of Advanced Nursing, 16,* 1090–1098.

Kelly, J.A., Sanders, N.F., & Pierce, J.D. (1989). A systems approach to the role of the nurse administrator in education and practice. In B. Neuman, *The Neuman systems model* (2nd ed., pp. 115–138). Norwalk, CT: Appleton & Lange.

Mayers, M.A., & Watson, A.B. (1982). Nursing care plans and the Neuman systems model: In B. Neuman, *The Neuman systems model: Application to nursing education and practice* (pp. 69–84). Norwalk, CT: Appleton-Century-Crofts.

Mischke-Berkey, K., & Hanson, S.M.H. (1991). *Pocket guide to family assessment and intervention.* St. Louis: Mosby-Year Book.

Mischke-Berkey, K., Warner, P., & Hanson, S. (1989). Family health assessment and intervention. In P.J. Bomar (Ed.), *Nurses and family health promotion: Concepts, assessment, and interventions* (pp. 115–154). Baltimore: Williams & Wilkins.

Moynihan, M.M. (1990). Implementation of the Neuman systems model in an acute care nursing department. In M.E. Parker (Ed.), *Nursing theories in practice* (pp. 263–273). New York: National League for Nursing.

Neal, M.C. (1982). Nursing care plans and the Neuman Systems Model: II. In B. Neuman, *The Neuman systems model: Application to nursing education and practice* (pp. 85–93). Norwalk, CT: Appleton-Century-Crofts.

Neuman, B., & Wyatt, M. (1980). The Neuman stress/adaptation systems approach to education for nurse administrators. In J.P. Riehl & C. Roy, *Conceptual models for nursing practice* (2nd ed., pp. 142–150). New York: Appleton-Century-Crofts.

Pinkerton, A. (1974). Use of the Neuman model in a home health-care agency. In J.P. Riehl & C. Roy, *Conceptual models for nursing practice* (pp. 122–129). New York: Appleton-Century-Crofts.

Quayhagen, M.P., & Roth, P.A. (1989). From models to measures in assessment of mature families. *Journal of Professional Nursing, 5,* 144–151.

Schlentz, M.D. (1993). The minimum data set and the levels of prevention in the long-term care facility. *Geriatric Nursing, 14,* 79–83.

Simmons, L., & Borgdon, C. (1991). The clinical nurse specialist in HIV care. *The Kansas Nurse, 66*(1), 6–7.

Vokaty, D.A. (1982). The Neuman systems model applied to the clinical nurse specialist role. In B. Neuman, *The Neuman systems model: Application to nursing education and practice* (pp. 165–167). Norwalk, CT: Appleton-Century-Crofts.

PRACTICE

Anderson, E., McFarlane, J., & Helton, A. (1986). Community-as-client: A model for practice. *Nursing Outlook, 34,* 220–224.

Baerg, K.L. (1991). Using Neuman's model to analyze a clinical situation. *Rehabilitation Nursing, 16,* 38–39.

Baker, N.A. (1982). Use of the Neuman model in planning for the psychological needs of the respiratory disease patient. In B. Neuman, *The Neuman systems model: Application to nursing education and practice* (pp. 241–251). Norwalk, CT: Appleton-Century-Crofts.

Balch, C. (1974). Breaking the lines of resistance. In J.P. Riehl & C. Roy, *Conceptual models for nursing practice* (pp. 130–134). New York: Appleton-Century-Crofts.

Beckingham, A.C., & Baumann, A. (1990). The ageing family in crisis: Assessment and decision-making models. *Journal of Advanced Nursing, 15,* 782–787.

Beddome, G. (1989). Application of the Neuman systems model to the assessment of community-as-client. In B. Neuman, *The Neuman systems model* (2nd ed., pp. 363–374). Norwalk, CT: Appleton & Lange.

Beitler, B., Tkachuck, B., & Aamodt, D. (1980). The Neuman model applied to mental health, community health, and medical-surgical nursing. In J.P. Riehl & C. Roy, *Conceptual models for nursing practice* (2nd ed., pp. 170–178). New York: Appleton-Century-Crofts.

Benedict, M.B., & Sproles, J.B. (1982). Application of the Neuman model to public health nursing practice. In B. Neuman, *The Neuman systems model: Application to nursing education and practice* (pp. 223–240). Norwalk, CT: Appleton-Century-Crofts.

Bergstrom, D. (1992). Hypermetabolism in multisystem organ failure: A Neuman systems perspective. *Critical Care Nursing Quarterly, 15*(3), 63–70.

Beyea, S., & Matzo, M. (1989). Assessing elders using the functional health pattern assessment model. *Nurse Educator, 14*(5), 32–37.

Biley, F.C. (1989). Stress in high dependency units. *Intensive Care Nursing, 5,* 134–141.

Breckenridge, D.M. (1982). Adaptation of the Neuman systems model for the renal client. In B. Neuman, *The Neuman systems model: Application to nursing education and practice* (pp. 267–277). Norwalk, CT: Appleton-Century-Crofts.

Breckenridge, D.M. (1989). Primary prevention as an intervention modality for the renal client. In B. Neuman, *The Neuman systems model* (2nd ed., pp. 397–406). Norwalk, CT: Appleton & Lange.

Brown, M.W. (1988). Neuman's systems model in risk factor reduction. *Cardiovascular Nursing, 24*(6), 43.

Buchanan, B.F. (1987). Human-environment interaction: A modification of the Neuman systems model for aggregates, families, and the community. *Public Health Nursing, 4,* 52–64.

Cardona, V.D. (1982). Client rehabilitation and the Neuman model. In B. Neuman, *The Neuman systems model: Application to nursing education and practice* (pp. 278–290). Norwalk, CT: Appleton-Century-Crofts.

Clark, F. (1982). The Neuman systems model: A clinical application for psychiatric nurse practitioners. In B. Neuman, *The Neuman systems model: Application to nursing education and practice* (pp. 335–353). Norwalk, CT: Appleton-Century-Crofts.

Clark, J. (1982). Development of models and theories on the concept of nursing. *Journal of Advanced Nursing, 7,* 129–134.

Craddock, R.B., & Stanhope, M.K. (1980). The Neuman Health-Care Systems Model: Recommended adaptation. In J.P. Riehl & C. Roy, *Conceptual models for nursing practice* (2nd ed., pp. 159–169). New York: Appleton-Century-Crofts.

Cunningham, S.G. (1982). The Neuman model applied to an acute care setting: Pain. In B. Neuman, *The Neuman systems model: Application to nursing education and practice* (pp. 291–296). Norwalk, CT: Appleton-Century-Crofts.

Cunningham, S.G. (1983). The Neuman systems model applied to a rehabilitation setting. *Rehabilitation Nursing, 8*(4), 20–22.

Davis, L.H. (1982). Aging: A social and preventive perspective. In B. Neuman, *The Neuman systems model: Application to nursing education and practice* (pp. 211–214). Norwalk, CT: Appleton-Century-Crofts.

Delunas, L.R. (1990). Prevention of elder abuse: Betty Neuman health care systems approach. *Clinical Nurse Specialist, 4,* 54–58.

Dunbar, S.B. (1982). Critical care and the Neuman model. In B. Neuman, *The Neuman systems model: Application to nursing education and practice* (pp. 297–307). Norwalk, CT: Appleton-Century-Crofts.

Dunn, S.I., & Trépaniér, M.J. (1989). Application of the Neuman model to perinatal nursing. In B. Neuman, *The Neuman systems model* (2nd ed., pp. 407–422). Norwalk, CT: Appleton & Lange.

Eclin, D.J. (1982). Palliative care and the Neuman model. In B. Neuman, *The Neuman systems model: Application to nursing education and practice (pp. 257–259). Norwalk, CT: Appleton-Century-Crofts.

Fawcett, J., Archer, C.L., Becker, D., Brown, K.K., Gann, S., Wong, M.J., & Wurster, A.B. (1992). Guidelines for selecting a conceptual model of nursing: Focus on the individual patient. Dimensions of Critical Care Nursing, 11, 268–277.

Fawcett, J., Cariello, F.P. Davis, D.A., Farley, J., Zimmaro, D.M., & Watts, R.J. (1987). Conceptual models of nursing: Application to critical care nursing practice. Dimensions of Critical Care Nursing, 6, 202–213.

Foote, A.W., Piazza, D., & Schultz, M. (1990). The Neuman Systems Model: Application to a patient with a cervical spinal cord injury. Journal of Neuroscience Nursing, 22, 302–306.

Fulbrook, P.R. (1991). The application of the Neuman Systems Model to intensive care. Intensive Care Nursing, 7, 28–39.

Galloway, D.A. (1993). Coping with a mentally and physically impaired infant: A self-analysis. Rehabilitation Nursing, 18, 34–36.

Gavan, C.A.S., Hastings-Tolsma, M.T., & Troyan, P.J. (1988). Explication of Neuman's model: A holistic systems approach to nutrition for health promotion in the life process. Holistic Nursing Practice, 3(1), 26–38.

Goldblum-Graff, D., & Graff, H. (1982). The Neuman model adapted to family therapy. In B. Neuman, The Neuman systems model: Application to nursing education and practice (pp. 217–222). Norwalk, CT: Appleton-Century-Crofts.

Gunter, L.M. (1982). Application of the Neuman systems model to gerontic nursing. In B. Neuman, The Neuman systems model: Application to nursing education and practice (pp. 196–210). Norwalk, CT: Appleton-Century-Crofts.

Herrick, C.A., & Goodykoontz, L. (1989). Neuman's systems model for nursing practice as a conceptual framework for a family assessment. Journal of Child and Adolescent Psychiatric and Mental Health Nursing, 2, 61–67.

Herrick, C.A., Goodykoontz, L., Herrick, R.H., & Hackett, B. (1991). Planning a continuum of care in child psychiatric nursing: A collaborative effort. Journal of Child and Adolescent Psychiatric and Mental Health Nursing, 4, 41–48.

Hiltz, D. (1990). The Neuman systems model: An analysis of a clinical situation. Rehabilitation Nursing, 15, 330–332.

Hoeman, S.P., & Winters, D.M. (1990).

Theory-based case management: High cervical spinal cord injury. Home Healthcare Nurse, 8, 25–33.

Kido, L.M. (1991) Sleep deprivation and intensive care unit psychosis. Emphasis: Nursing, 4(1), 23–33.

Knight, J.B. (1990). The Betty Neuman systems model applied to practice: A client with multiple sclerosis. Journal of Advanced Nursing, 15, 447–455.

Lindell, M., & Olsson, H. (1991). Can combined oral contraceptives be made more effective by means of a nursing care model? Journal of Advanced Nursing, 16, 475–479.

McInerney, K.A. (1982). The Neuman systems model applied to critical care nursing of cardiac surgery clients. In B. Neuman, The Neuman systems model: Application to nursing education and practice (pp. 308–315). Norwalk, CT: Appleton-Century-Crofts.

Millard, J. (1992). Health visiting an elderly couple. British Journal of Nursing, 1, 769–773.

Mirenda, R.M. (1986). The Neuman model in practice. Senior Nurse, 5(3), 26–27.

Mirenda, R.M. (1986). The Neuman systems model: Description and application. In P. Winstead-Fry (Ed.), Case studies in nursing theory (pp. 127–166). New York: National League for Nursing.

Moore, S.L., & Munro, M.F. (1990). The Neuman systems model applied to mental health nursing of older adults. Journal of Advanced Nursing, 15, 293–299.

Piazza, D., Foote, A., Wright, P., & Holcombe, J. (1992). Neuman Systems Model used as a guide for the nursing care of an 8-year-old child with leukemia. Journal of Pediatric Oncology Nursing, 9(1), 17–24.

Pierce, J.D., & Hutton, E. (1992). Applying the new concepts of the Neuman systems model. Nursing Forum, 27, 15–18.

Reed, K. (1982). The Neuman systems model: A basis for family psychosocial assessment. In B. Neuman, The Neuman systems model: Application to nursing education and practice (pp. 188–195). Norwalk, CT: Appleton-Century-Crofts.

Reed, K.S. (1989). Family theory related to the Neuman systems model. In B. Neuman, The Neuman systems model (2nd ed., pp. 385–396). Norwalk, CT: Appleton & Lange.

Reed, K.S. (1993). Adapting the Neuman systems model for family nursing. Nursing Science Quarterly, 6, 93–97.

Redheffer G. (1985). Application of Betty Neuman's Health Care Systems Model to emergency nursing practice: Case review. *Point of View, 22*(2), 4–6.

Rice, M.J. (1982). The Neuman systems model applied in a hospital medical unit. In B. Neuman, *The Neuman systems model: Application to nursing education and practice* (pp. 316–323). Norwalk, CT: Appleton-Century-Crofts.

Robichaud-Ekstrand, S., & Delisle, L. (1989). Neuman en médecine-chirurgie [The Neuman model in medical-surgical settings]. *The Canadian Nurse, 85*(6), 32–35.

Ross, M., & Bourbonnais, F. (1985). The Betty Neuman Systems Model in nursing practice: A case study approach. *Journal of Advanced Nursing, 10,* 199–207.

Ross, M.M., & Helmer, H. (1988). A comparative analysis of Neuman's model using the individual and family as the units of care. *Public Health Nursing, 5,* 30–36.

Shaw, M.C. (1991). A theoretical base for orthopaedic nursing practice: The Neuman systems model. *Canadian Orthopaedic Nurses Association Journal, 13*(2), 19–21.

Smith, M.C. (1989). Neuman's model in practice. *Nursing Science Quarterly, 2,* 116–117.

Sohier, R. (1989). Nursing care for the people of a small planet: Culture and the Neuman systems model. In B. Neuman, *The Neuman systems model* (2nd ed., pp. 139–154). Norwalk, CT: Appleton & Lange.

Spradley, B.W. (1990). *Community health nursing: Concepts and practice.* Glenview, IL: Scott, Foresman/Little, Brown Higher Education.

Sullivan, J. (1986). Using Neuman's model in the acute phase of spinal cord injury. *Focus on Critical Care, 13*(5), 34–41.

Torkington, S. (1988). Nourishing the infant. *Senior Nurse, 8*(2), 24–25.

Utz, S.W. (1980) Applying the Neuman model to nursing practice with hypertensive clients. *Cardio-Vascular Nursing, 16,* 29–34.

Wallingford, P. (1989). The neurologically impaired and dying child: Applying the Neuman systems model. *Issues in Comprehensive Pediatric Nursing, 12,* 139–157.

Weinberger, S.L. (1991). Analysis of a clinical situation using the Neuman System Model. *Rehabilitation Nursing, 16, 278,* 280–281.

7

Orem's Self-Care Framework

This chapter presents an analysis and evaluation of Dorothea Orem's Self-Care Framework, which has also been called the Self-Care Deficit Theory of Nursing and the Self-Care Nursing Theory. In a recent explication of the structure of her work, Orem (1990, 1991) stated that the Self-Care Deficit Theory is a frame of reference that contains three parts — the Theory of Self-Care, the Theory of Self-Care Deficit, and the Theory of Nursing System. The concepts and propositions of the Self-Care Deficit Theory are at the level of abstraction and generality usually seen in a conceptual model. Because of this and to avoid confusion with grand and middle-range theories, Orem's work is called the Self-Care Framework in this chapter.

The concepts of the Self-Care Framework and their dimensions are listed below. Each concept and its dimensions are defined and described later in this chapter.

KEY CONCEPTS

SELF-CARE/DEPENDENT-CARE
SELF-CARE AGENT/DEPENDENT-
  CARE AGENT
Power Components
Basic Conditioning Factors
THERAPEUTIC SELF-CARE DEMAND
Universal Self-Care Requisites
Developmental Self-Care Requisites
Health-Deviation Self-Care Requisites
SELF-CARE DEFICIT/DEPENDENT-
  CARE DEFICIT
NURSING AGENCY
GOAL OF NURSING AGENCY
To Help People Meet Their Own

Therapeutic Self-Care Demands
PROFESSIONAL AND CASE
  MANAGEMENT OPERATIONS OF
  NURSING PRACTICE
Nursing Diagnosis
Nursing Prescription
Nursing System Design
  *Wholly Compensatory Nursing
  System*
  *Partly Compensatory Nursing
  System*
  *Supportive-Educative Nursing
  System*
  Methods of Helping

Planning	THEORY OF SELF-CARE DEFICIT
Regulatory Care	THEORY OF NURSING SYSTEM
Controlling	GENERAL THEORY OF NURSING
DEPENDENT-CARE SYSTEMS	ADMINISTRATION
THEORY OF SELF-CARE	

ANALYSIS OF OREM'S SELF-CARE FRAMEWORK

This section presents an analysis of the Self-Care Framework. The analysis draws primarily from the fourth edition of Orem's (1991) book, *Nursing: Concepts of Practice*, and a book chapter entitled "A nursing practice theory in three parts, 1956–1989" (Orem, 1990).

Origins of the Model

Historical Evolution and Motivation

Orem began to develop the Self-Care Framework in the 1950s, a time when most nursing education programs were based on conceptual models more representative of such other disciplines as medicine, psychology, and sociology than of nursing (Phillips, 1977). Thus, Orem may be considered a pioneer in the development of distinctive nursing knowledge.

The development of the Self-Care Framework has been described in considerable detail (Nursing Development Conference Group, 1979; Orem & Taylor, 1986; Orem, 1991). The initial impetus for public articulation of the Self-Care Framework apparently was the need to develop a curriculum for a practical nursing program (Orem, 1959). Orem (1978) commented that that task required identification of the domain and boundaries of nursing as a science and an art. Continued work on the Self-Care Framework was motivated by "dissatisfaction and concern due to the absence of an organizing framework for nursing knowledge and . . . the belief that a concept of nursing would aid in formalizing such a framework" (Nursing Development Conference Group, 1973, p. ix). In particular, the Self-Care Framework was formulated as a solution to the problem of

> the lack of specification of, and agreement about, the general elements of nursing that give direction to (1) the isolation of problems that are specifically nursing problems and (2) the organization of knowledge accruing from research in problem areas. (Nursing Development Conference Group, 1973, p. 6)

Ideas that helped to shape the Self-Care Framework were formulated as Orem experienced a period of intensive exposure to nurses and their endeavors from 1949 to 1957, during her tenure as a nursing consultant in the Division of Hospital and Institutional Services of the Indiana State Board of Health. Her observations led to the idea that "nursing involved both a mode of thinking and a mode of communication" (Orem & Taylor, 1986, p. 41). In 1956, Orem prepared a report that contained the following definition of nursing:

1. Nurses as practitioners of nursing give specialized assistance to individuals.

2. Persons to whom nurses give specialized assistance have limitations for action of such a character that more than ordinary assistance from family or friends is necessary to meet daily needs for self-care and to intelligently participate in their medical care.

3. Nurses practice their art through their use of distinct modes of helping: by doing for persons under care, helping them do for themselves, or by helping a family member learn how to help persons with care limitations. (p. 85)

Orem's "interest in and insights about the domain and boundaries of nursing" progressed from a global focus on "preventive health care" to a formal search "to know nursing in a way that would enlarge and deepen its meaning" and to identify "a proper nursing focus" (Orem, 1991, p. 60; Orem & Taylor, 1986, p. 39). Her search for the meaning of nursing was structured by three questions:

1. What do nurses do and what should nurses do as practitioners of nursing?

2. Why do nurses do what they do?

3. What results from what nurses do as practitioners of nursing? (Orem & Taylor, 1986, p. 39)

The answers to those questions began to emerge when Orem introduced elements of her Self-Care Framework in the 1959 publication, *Guides for Developing Curricula for the Education of Practical Nurses*. In this report, Orem maintained that human limitations for self-care associated with health situations give rise to a requirement for nursing. She then identified areas of daily self-care, conditions that limit individuals' self-care capabilities, and methods of assisting those whose self-care abilities are limited.

The questions were answered more fully as Orem and other members of the Nursing Model Committee of The Catholic University Nursing Faculty began their work in 1965. The final report of this committee was submitted to the School of Nursing in May 1968. Orem continued her work on the Self-Care Framework with a group of colleagues who formed the Nursing Development Conference Group in September 1968. In 1971, Orem published the first edition of her book, *Nursing: Concepts of Practice*. The next publication dealing with the Self-Care Framework was authored by the Nursing Development Conference Group and appeared in 1973 under the title, *Concept Formalization in Nursing: Process and Product*. Revisions in the Self-Care Framework, with more comprehensive answers to the questions, were presented by Orem in her 1978 speech at the Second Annual Nurse Educator Conference, as well as in the second editions of the books by the Nursing Development Conference Group (1979) and Orem (1980). Three theories connected to the Self-Care Framework were presented by Orem in her 1980 book. Refinements in the Self-Care Framework and the three theories were evident in the third edition of Orem's (1985) book and in the Orem and Taylor (1986) book chapter. Further refinements are evident in the fourth edition of Orem's (1991) book.

The structure and components of the Self-Care Framework have undergone various interpretations over time. Orem (1991) explained, "All of the conceptual elements [of the Self-Care Framework] were formalized and validated as static concepts by 1970. Since then, some refinement of expression and further development of substantive structure and continued validation have occurred, but no substantive changes have been made" (p. 65). In the first edition of her book, *Nursing: Concepts of Practice*, Orem (1971) referred to dimensions of self-care and dimensions of nursing. By the second edition, she regarded her work as a "general comprehensive theory of nursing," which was made up of three "theoretical constructs" or theories — self-care deficit, self-care, and nursing system (Orem, 1980, p. 26). This structure was maintained in the third edition of Orem's (1985) book. A slight digression from the structure was noted in Orem and Taylor's 1986 book chapter, in which the theory of nursing system was referred to as "the general theory of nursing, because it explains the product made by nurses in nursing practice situations in relation to two conceptualized properties of individuals who need nursing, as these properties are expressed and related in the theory of self-care deficit" (p. 44).

Returning to the earlier structure in the fourth edition of her book, Orem (1991) gave a title to the general theory and provided a hierarchical structure for the Theories of Self-Care, Self-Care Deficit, and Nursing System. She stated, "Together the three theories [self-care deficit, self-care, and nursing system] constitute a general theory of nursing, named the self-care deficit theory of nursing" (p. 66). She went on to explain that "the theory of nursing system subsumes the theory of self-care deficit, which subsumes the theory of self-care" (p. 66).

Further refinements in the structure of the Self-Care Framework are anticipated. Orem (1991) noted, "Each concept continues to undergo development through the identification and organization of secondary concepts that constitute its substantive structure" (p. 65).

Philosophical Claims

Orem has presented the philosophical claims undergirding the Self-Care Framework in the form of assumptions, premises, and presuppositions. Orem's early search for the meaning of nursing led to the formulation of the following assumptions about nursing:

1. Nursing is a form of help or assistance given by nurses to persons with a legitimate need for it.

2. Nurses are characterized by their knowledge of nursing and their capabilities to use their knowledge and specialized skills to produce nursing for others in a variety of types of situations.

3. Persons with a legitimate need for nursing are characterized (a) by a demand for discernible kinds and amounts of self-care or dependent-care and (b) by health-derived or health-related limitations for the continuing production of the amount and kind of care required. In dependent-care situations the limitations of dependent-care givers are associated with the health state and the care requirements of the dependent person.

4. Results of nursing are associated with the characterizing conditions of persons in need of nursing and include (a) the meeting of existent and emerging demands for self-care and dependent care and (b) the regulation of the exercise or development of capabilities for providing care. (Orem, 1985, p. 31)

Furthermore, Orem (1991) assumes that nursing is deliberate action. She states, "Nursing in every instance of its practice is action deliberately performed by some members of a social group to bring about events and results that benefit others in specified ways. Thinking about and conceptualizing nursing as *deliberate action* is the most general approach that one can take to understand nursing" (p. 79).

Orem (1991) expanded the assumption of nursing as deliberate action to include reflection. She explained, "The agent, the person performing the actions, has incoming *sensory knowledge and awareness* of the reality of the situation of action. The agent *reflects* on the meaning of existent conditions and circumstances for the set or series of actions in process and for attainment of results toward purpose achievement. Reflection terminates in a particular productive situation with the agent's *decision* about the action that will be taken" (p. 80).

Orem (1991) noted that the acceptance of the assumption of nursing as deliberate action involving reflection in turn "requires the acceptance of [the assumption of] human beings as having intrinsic activity rather than passivity or strict reactivity to stimuli" (p. 80). That basic assumption about human beings led to the following additional assumptions that Orem drew from Arnold's (1960) work:

1. Human beings know and appraise objects, conditions, and situations in terms of their effects on ends being sought.

2. Human beings know directly by sensing, but they also reflect, reason, and understand.

3. Human beings are capable of self-determined actions, even when they feel an emotional pull in the opposite direction.

4. Human beings can prolong reflection indefinitely in deliberations about what action to take by raising questions about and directing attention to different aspects of a situation and different possibilities for action.

5. In order to act, human beings must concentrate on a suitable course of action and exclude other courses of action.

6. Purposive action requires not only that human beings be aware of objects, conditions, and situations but also that they have the ability to contend with them and treat them in some way.

7. Persons, as unitary beings, are the agents who act deliberately to attain ends or goals. (Orem, 1991, pp. 80–81)

Orem (1991) went on to point out that if these seven assumptions about human beings are accepted, additional assumptions must be made with regard to the "human and environmental conditions and factors that must be developed and operational if individuals are to appraise, select, and proceed with courses of action" (p. 81). Drawing again from Arnold (1960), Orem (1991) assumed that the following six general conditions "may encourage action tendencies for self-care" (p. 81):

1. Persons must have available the knowledge necessary to distinguish something as good or desirable from bad and undesirable and to reflect on its desirability or undesirability. The goal and ways to achieve it must be conceptualized or imagined.

2. Reasons for selecting certain actions to attain what has been appraised as good or desirable and afforded the tentative status of a goal should be known.

3. Time as well as knowledge is required for persons to form ideas about particular actions or to form images of how each action relates to the goal.

4. Reflection should be directed to these questions: Is this way of acting good or desirable? Is it more desirable or less desirable than other ways of acting to achieve the goal?

5. Reflection about choosing a way of action could go on indefinitely; therefore, reflection should be brought to a close with a decision when the ways of action have been conceived as clear ideas or clear images are formed.

6. A person owns his or her appraisal of possible ways of action to attain a goal and his or her decision to act according to one or a combination of these ways, when this way of acting is formalized and incorporated into the person's self-image or self-concept. (p. 81)

Orem (1991) further explained that five premises about human beings served as "guiding principles throughout the process of conceptualizing nursing" (p. 66). She commented that although the statements were referred to as assumptions in her earlier publications, "they are more properly referred to as premises since they were and are advanced as true and not merely assumed" (p. 67). The premises are:

1. Human beings require continuous deliberate inputs to themselves and their environments in order to remain alive and function in accord with natural human endowments.

2. Human agency, the power to act deliberately, is exercised in the form of care of self and others in identifying needs for and in making needed inputs.

3. Mature human beings experience privations in the form of limitations for action in care of self and others involving the making of life-sustaining and function-regulating inputs.

4. Human agency is exercised in discovering, developing, and transmitting to others ways and means to identify needs for and make inputs to self and others.

5. Groups of human beings with structured relationships cluster tasks and allocate responsibilities for providing care to group members who experience privations for making required deliberate input to self and others. (p. 67)

The foregoing assumptions about nursing and assumptions and premises about human beings led to additional assumptions about nursing. One assumption is expressed in the following proposition: "Not all people under health care, for example, from physicians, are under nursing care nor does it follow that they should be" (Orem, 1991, p. 61).

The answer to the question, "What condition exists in a person when that person or a family member or the attending physician or a nurse makes the judgment that the person should be under nursing care?" (Orem, 1985, p. 19), represents another, and crucial, assumption undergirding the Self-Care Framework. This assumption identifies the proper object of nursing. Orem (1991) explained that proper refers to "that which belongs to the field" (p. 3). Object "is used in the philosophic or scientific sense as that which is studied or observed, that to which action is directed to obtain information about it or to bring about some new condition. Object is not used in the sense of something tangible" (p. 3). The proper object of nursing for Orem is "human beings as subject to health-derived or health-related limitations for engagement in self-care or dependent care" (p. 70).

Stated more elaborately, Orem (1991) assumes that the proper object of nursing is expressed in the conditions of adults and children that validate a requirement for nursing. "The condition . . . in an adult is the *absence of the ability to maintain continuously that amount and quality of self-care which is therapeutic in sustaining life and health, in recovering from disease or injury, or in coping with their effects.* With children, the condition is the *inability of the parent (or guardian) to maintain continuously for the child the amount and quality of care that is therapeutic"* (p. 41). Orem went on to explain that "therapeutic is used to mean supportive of life processes, remedial or curative when related to malfunction due to disease processes, and contributing to personal development and maturing" (p. 41).

Orem (1991) assumes that nursing is a helping service and a human service. The following three statements represent assumptions about nursing as a helping and human service:

1. Nursing relationships in society are based on a state of imbalance between the *abilities of nurses to prescribe, design, manage, and maintain systems* of therapeutic self-care for individuals and the *abilities of*

these individuals or their families to do so. In other words the nurses' abilities exceed those of other individuals. When the imbalance is in the opposite direction or when there is no imbalance, there is no valid basis for a nursing relationship.

2. Nursing practice has not only technologic aspects but also moral aspects, since nursing decisions affect the lives, health, and welfare of human beings. Nurses must ask [if it is] right for the patient as well as will it work.

3. Solutions proposed to problems of the management and maintenance of therapeutic self-care for patients and families with limited ability to maintain their own care may give rise to other problems, solutions to which may be difficult if not impossible. (pp. 54–55)

Orem (1991) summarized her philosophical claims about nursing and human beings in the following statement: "The [Self-Care Framework] assumes that nursing is a response of human groups to one recurring type of incapacity for action to which human beings are subject, namely, the incapacity to care for oneself or one's dependents when action is limited because of health state or health care needs of the care recipient. From a nursing point of view, human beings are viewed as needing continuous self-maintenance and self-regulation through a type of action named *self-care*" (p. 73).

Orem (1991) also identified premises about self-care. They are:

1. Self-care is conduct. It is ego-processed. It is learned activity, learned through interpersonal relations and communications.

2. Adult persons have the right and responsibility to care for themselves to maintain rational life and health; they may have such responsibility for other persons.

   a. Infant and child care, care of the aged, and care of adolescents include the giving, assisting with, or supervising the self-care of another.

   b. Social assistance will be needed by adult persons whenever they are unable to obtain needed resources and maintain conditions necessary for the preservation of life and promotion of health for themselves or for their dependents; such assistance may be needed for the accomplishment or the supervision of self-care. (p. 119)

Orem went on to claim that "self-care as conduct reflects the essence of the concept: self-care is behavior, it exists in reality situations" (p. 119).

Furthermore, Orem (1991) explained that the concept of self-care requisites is based on the following three assumptions:

1. Human beings, by nature, have common needs for the intake of materials (air, water, foods) and for bringing about and maintaining living conditions that support life processes, the formation and mainte-nance of structural integrity, and the maintenance and promotion of functional integrity.

2. Human development, from intrauterine life to adult maturation, re-quires the formation and maintenance of conditions that promote known developmental processes at each period of the life cycle.

3. Genetic and constitutional defects and deviations from normal structural and functional integrity and well-being bring about requirements for [a] their prevention and [b] regulatory action to control their extension and to control and mitigate their effects. (p. 121)

Additional philosophical claims undergird the Theory of Self-Care, the Theory of Self-Care Deficit, and the Theory of Nursing System and are stated in the form of presuppositions. The four presuppositions for the Theory of Self-Care are:

1. All things being equal, human beings have the potential to develop intellectual and practical skills and maintain the motivation essential for self-care and care of dependent family members.

2. Ways of meeting self-care requisites are culture elements and vary with individuals and larger social groups.

3. Self-care and care of dependent family members are forms of deliberative action, dependent for performance on individuals' action repertoires, and their predilection for taking action under certain circumstances.

4. Identifying and describing recurring requisites for self-care and the care of dependent family members lead to investigating and developing ways to meet known requisites and to form care habits. (Orem, 1991, p. 69)

Orem (1991) presented the presuppositions for the Theory of Self-Care Deficit in two sets. The first set is made up of the following four statements:

1. Engagement in self-care requires ability to manage self within a stable or changing environment.

2. Engagement in self-care or dependent-care is affected by persons' valuation of care measures with respect to life, development, health, and well-being.

3. The quality and completeness of self-care and dependent-care in families and communities rests on the culture, including scientific attainments of social groups and the educability of group members.

4. Engagement in self-care and dependent-care are affected, as is engagement in all forms of practical endeavor, by persons' limitations in knowing what to do under existent conditions and circumstances or how to do it. (Orem, 1991, pp. 70–71)

The second set of presuppositions is made up of the following five statements:

1. Societies provide for the human state of social dependency by instituting ways and means to aid persons according to the nature of and the reasons for their dependency.

2. When they are institutionalized, direct helping operations of members of social groups become the means for aiding persons in states of social dependency.

3. The direct helping operations of members of social groups may be classified into those associated with states of age-related dependency and those not so associated.

4. Direct helping services instituted in social groups to provide assistance to persons irrespective of age include the health services.

5. Nursing is one of the health services of Western civilization. (Orem, 1991, p. 71)

Two presuppositions undergird the Theory of Nursing System. They are:

1. Nursing is the practical endeavors of nurses engaged in for some duration of time for individuals in time-place localizations whenever their action limitations for engagement in self-care or dependent-care are health related or derived.

2. Nursing is an institutionalized human health service with a domain and boundaries defined by its proper object or specialized focus in society. (Orem, 1991, p. 72)

Still other philosophical claims, also in the form of presuppositions, undergird the rudimentary General Theory of Nursing Administration that was developed by Orem (1989). These presuppositions are:

1. Health service institutions or health units of other types of institutions have purposes or missions that can be fulfilled at least in part through the provision of nursing to persons served by the institution.

2. Health service institutions or units serve persons who constitute describable changing populations.

3. Nursing administration is an organizational body, a component part of a health service institution or a unit of another type of institution.

4. Nursing administration in organized enterprises receives its managerial power from persons charged with institutional governance or with institutional administration.

5. Health-service institutions where nursing is provided as a continuously available service employ nursing practitioners or contract with them for their services, or grant them the privilege of practicing nursing within the institution. (Orem, 1989, pp. 58–59)

Strategies for Knowledge Development

Orem's description of the development of the Self-Care Framework indicates that she made extensive use of inductive reasoning. She explained that "The answer to the question [regarding conditions that exist in a person when a judgment is made of the need for nursing care] came spontaneously with images of situations where such judgments were made and the idea that a nurse is 'another self' in a figurative sense, for the person under nursing care" (Orem, 1991, p. 61). Orem (1978) added that she looked to her personal and professional experiences for examples of judgments regarding the need for nursing care and the conditions of the persons when these judgments were made. The answer, she stated, finally came as a "flash of insight, an understanding that the reason why individuals could benefit from nursing was the existence of . . . self-care limitations." Inductive reasoning is also evident in the comment that the Self-

Care Framework is "successful . . . because it is constituted from conceptualizations of the constant elements and relationships of nursing practice situations" (Orem & Taylor, 1986, p. 38).

Deductive reasoning is evident in Orem's (1991) discussion of her use of knowledge from adjunctive disciplines. For example, she explained, "Arnold's position about deliberate action and motivation led in 1987 to the expression of six conditions that may encourage action tendencies for self-care" (p. 81).

Influences from Other Scholars

Orem has always cited the works of scholars in several adjunctive disciplines and has acknowledged the contributions to her thinking from her educational experiences. In fact, she read in a

> wide range of fields, from organization and administration to social philosophy, including the philosophic notions of points of order in wholes composed of parts and different kinds of wholes; from hygiene and sanitation to cultural anthropology; from the philosophic notion of human acts to action theory as developed in sociology, psychology, and philosophy; and from action theory to a concept of systems and the constructs of cybernetics. (Orem & Taylor, 1986, p. 43)

Orem (1991) explicitly acknowledged the influences of Arnold (1960) and Kotarbinski (1965) on her ideas about deliberate human action and of Parsons (1937, 1951) on her ideas about the context of action. She also acknowledged Lonergan's (1958) influence on her thinking. She commented that her ability to express her ideas "required self-knowledge toward clarification of my own reality of knowing nursing in a dynamic way. B.J.F. Lonergan's work, Insight (1958), was a helpful though difficult guide to self-knowledge" (Orem & Taylor, 1986, p. 43).

In addition, Orem (1991) acknowledged the contributions of the members of the Nursing Development Conference Group to the development and refinement of much of the content of the Self-Care Framework. Over the years of its existence, the group membership list included Sarah E. Allison, Joan E. Backscheider, Cora S. Balmat, Judy Crews, Mary B. Collins, M. Lucille Kinlein, Janina B. Lapniewski, Melba Anger Malatesta, Sheila M. McCarthy, Joan Nettleton, Louise Hartnett Rauckhorst, Helen A. St. Denis, and Dorothea Orem. The product of their combined effort to formalize a concept of nursing was the publication of two editions of the book, Concept Formalization in Nursing: Process and Product (Nursing Development Conference Group, 1973, 1979).

There is no evidence to support contentions that the Self-Care Framework is based on earlier works by Frederick and Northam (1938) or Henderson (1955). Indeed, although the idea of patient as care agent was put forth by Frederick and Northam, the idea of self-care originated with and was formalized by Orem (Nursing Development Conference Group, 1979). Moreover, Orem explicitly denied that her Self-Care Framework was derived from Henderson's 1955 definition of nursing, although she recognized the similarities between it and her own 1956 definition of nursing (Orem & Taylor, 1986).

World View

Orem's (1991) view of the relationship between the person and the environment clearly reflects the *reciprocal interaction* world view. She indicated that human beings exist in and are never isolated from their environments, claiming that "Person and environment are identified as a unity characterized by human-environmental interchanges and by the impact of one on the other. Person-environment constitutes a functional type of unity with a concrete existence" (p. 143).

The person is viewed as holistic. In fact, although Orem (1991) indicated that human beings have structural parts (e.g., arms, legs, stomach, lungs) and functional parts (e.g., urinary system, neuroendocrine system, neural circuits), she viewed the parts within the unity of human structure and functioning. She stated, "If there is acceptance of the real unity of individual human beings, there should be no difficulty in recognizing structural and functional differentiations within the unity" (p. 185). Moreover, the person is viewed as an active agent who maintains self-care and seeks health care when faced with an imbalance between the current therapeutic demand for self-care or dependent-care and existing self-care agency or dependent-care agency.

In keeping with the reciprocal interaction world view, the Self-Care Framework reflects elements of persistence and change. Orem's emphasis on maintenance of self-care agency represents persistence. In particular, stability of therapeutic self-care agency is the desired goal in the Self-Care Framework. Loss of self-care results from health-derived or health-related limitations and is not considered desirable. Change is evident in the developmental and health-related changes that occur in the demand for continuing therapeutic care and in self-care agency and dependent-care agency. These changes are necessary for survival as the person matures.

Unique Focus of the Model

The unique focus of the Self-Care Framework is the nurse's deliberate action related to the diagnosis, prescription, design, planning, implementation, management, and maintenance of systems of therapeutic self-care for individuals who have limitations in their abilities to provide continuing therapeutic self-care or care of dependent others. Limitations in the individual's abilities to provide complete and effective self-care or dependent-care stem from the individual's or the dependent other's health state or developmental stage.

The Self-Care Framework was classified as a systems model by Riehl and Roy (1980). Riehl-Sisca (1989) changed the classification to the interaction category. No rationale for its classification in either category was provided. Close examination of the Self-Care Framework failed to reveal any evidence of a match between its content and the characteristics of systems or interaction models as those categories of nursing knowledge are interpreted in this book.

The Self-Care Framework is more appropriately classified as a developmental model. The characteristics of growth, development, and maturation are addressed by the notion of developmental self-care requisites and by the consideration of the individual's self-care agency adjusted for age and developmental state.

The developmental model characteristic of change is addressed in terms of changes in self-care agency that occur throughout life. Direction of change is viewed as toward higher levels of integration and assumption of self-care and dependent-care agency, which is reflected in the following statement of Orem's (1991) position about human beings as persons with regard to health and well-being:

> The point of view of human beings as persons is a moving rather than a static one. It is the view of personalization of the individual, that is, moving toward maturation and achievement of the individual's human potential. This process of coming to be a person involves individuals in communications with their worlds; in action; in the exercise of the human desire to know, to seek the truth; and in the giving of themselves in the doing of good for themselves and others. . . . Personalization proceeds as individuals live under conditions favorable or unfavorable to human developmental processes. . . . There is a striving by individuals to achieve the potential of their natural endowments for physical and rational functioning while living a life of faith with respect to things hoped for and to perfect themselves as responsible human beings who raise questions, seek answers, reflect, and come to awareness of the relationship between what they know and what they do. (p. 185)

Orem addressed the characteristic of identifiable state through her discussion of the differences in self-care agency throughout life. The child is viewed as being in the stage of dependent-care, and the healthy adult is in a stage of total self-care and dependent-care agency. Socially dependent adults, including ill and disabled persons, are in a stage of dependent-care. Orem (1991) explained:

> Infants and children require care from others because they are in the early stages of development physically, psychologically, and psychosocially. The aged person requires total care or assistance whenever declining physical and mental abilities limit the selection or performance of self-care actions. The ill or disabled person requires partial or total care from others (or assistance in the form of teaching or guidance) depending on his or her health state and immediate or future requirements for self-care. Self-care is an adult's continuous contribution to his

or her own continued existence, health, and well-being. Care of others is an adult's contribution to the health and well-being of dependent members of the adult's social group. (p. 117)

The Self-Care Framework addresses form of progression of development as cycles of change in self-care agency. Although the overall direction is toward increasing ability for self-care and dependent-care, loss of some agency does occur at various times throughout life, such as when illness or disability imposes limitations on self-care and dependent-care agency.

The characteristic of forces that produce growth and development is viewed in the Self-Care Framework as a natural component of human development. That is, self-care and dependent-care agency naturally increase as the person matures. Indeed, Orem assumed that people have an inherent, overt potential for development of self-care agency.

Meleis (1991) regarded the Self-Care Framework as an example of the needs category of models and also placed it in her nursing therapeutics category. Marriner-Tomey (1989) placed Orem's work in her humanistic category. Barnum (1994) regarded the Self-Care Framework as a good example of the substitution category of her classification scheme.

Content of the Model: Concepts

Orem and Taylor (1986) explained that "the general theory of nursing [i.e., the Self-Care Framework] is relatively simple, as it is constituted from six central or core concepts and one peripheral concept" (p. 45). The six central concepts are self-care, self-care agency, therapeutic self-care demand, self-care deficit, nursing agency, and nursing system. The peripheral concept is basic conditioning factors. These concepts, along with dependent-care, dependent-care agency, and dependent-care system, are discussed within the context of the nursing metaparadigm concepts of person, environment, health, and nursing.

Person

Orem (1991) described the person as "a human being . . . a unity that can be viewed as functioning biologically, symbolically, and socially" (p. 181). The person of particular interest in the Self-Care Framework is the nurse's patient, that is, the person who receives help and care from a nurse. Patient is used in the sense of "a receiver of care, someone who is under the care of a health care professional at this time, in some place or places" (p. 30).

The Self-Care Framework focuses on the person's ability to perform **self-care,** which is defined as "behavior that exists in concrete life situations directed by persons to self or to the environment to regulate factors that affect their own development and functioning in the interests of life, health, or well-being" (Orem, 1991, p. 64).

Orem (1991) uses the word self to denote "one's whole being" and pointed out that self-care "carries the dual connotation of 'for oneself' and 'given by oneself'" (p. 117). Self-care is regarded as a goal-oriented activity that is learned. "The provider of self-care," Orem (1991) explained, "is referred to as a **self-care agent**" (p. 117). She went on to say that "The term agent is used in the sense of the person taking action" (p. 117). Self-care agents, then, are "mature or maturing persons who have developed the [requisite action] capabilities to take care of themselves in their environmental situations . . . [and] have . . . the power to act deliberately to regulate factors that affect their own functioning and development" (p. 117). More specifically, self-care agents have the capability to

(1) determine the presence and characteristics of specific requirements for regulating their own functioning and development, including prevention and amelioration of disease processes and injuries (identification and particularization of self-care requisites); (2) make judgments and decisions about what to do; and (3) perform care measures to meet specific self-care requisites in time and over time. (Orem & Taylor, 1986, p. 52)

Adults care for themselves, but infants, children, and socially dependent adults require varying degrees of assistance with self-care activities. When assistance that encompasses the range of actions constituting self-care is given to infants, children, and socially dependent adults by such responsible adults as family members or significant others, it is called **dependent-care** (Orem, 1991). The provider of this care is referred to as a **dependent-care agent.**

The person's ability to perform self-care is influenced by 10 *power components*. The power components refer specifically to human powers that enable the performance of actions required for self-care (Orem, 1991). They are:

1. Ability to maintain attention and exercise requisite vigilance with respect to self as self-care agent and internal and external conditions and factors significant for self-care

2. Controlled use of available physical energy that is sufficient for the initiation and continuation of self-care operations

3. Ability to control the position of the body and its parts in the execution of the movements required for the initiation and completion of self-care operations

4. Ability to reason within a self-care frame of reference

5. Motivation (i.e., goal orientations for self-care that are in accord with its characteristics and its meaning for life, health, and well-being)

6. Ability to make decisions about care of self and to operationalize these decisions

7. Ability to acquire technical knowledge about self-care from authoritative sources, to retain it, and to operationalize it

8. A repertoire of cognitive, perceptual, manipulative, communication, and interpersonal skills adapted to the performance of self-care operations

9. Ability to order discrete self-care actions or action systems into relationships with prior and subsequent actions toward the final achievement of regulatory goals of self-care

10. Ability to consistently perform self-care operations, integrating them with relevant aspects of personal, family, and community living (Orem, 1991, p. 155)

The person's ability to perform self-care as well as the kind and amount of self-care that is required are influenced by internal and external factors that are called *basic conditioning factors.* The 10 basic conditioning factors identified to date are:

1. Age
2. Gender
3. Developmental state
4. Health state
5. Sociocultural orientation
6. Health care system factors; for example, medical diagnostic and treatment modalities
7. Family system factors
8. Patterns of living including activities regularly engaged in
9. Environmental factors
10. Resource availability and adequacy (Orem, 1991, p. 136)

The purpose of self-care and dependent-care is to meet what Orem (1991) calls the **therapeutic self-care demand,** which is defined as "the self-care actions to be performed for some duration in order to meet known self-care requisites [that are] particularized for individuals in relation to their conditions and circumstances" (Orem, 1991, pp. 65, 123). It follows that each person's therapeutic self-care demand varies throughout life.

Self-care requisites are "expressions of action to be performed by or for individuals in the interest of controlling human and environmental factors that affect human functioning and human development" (Orem, 1991, p. 121). Self-care requisites, Orem (1991) explained, "have their origins in the anatomic and functional features of human beings" (p. 139). Three types of self-care requisites constitute the therapeutic self-care demand: *universal self-care requisites, developmental self-care requisites,* and *health-deviation self-care requisites.*

Universal self-care requisites are actions that need to be performed to maintain life processes, the integrity of human structure and function, and general well-being. These requisites are "common to all human beings during all stages of the life cycle, adjusted to age, developmental state, and environmental and other factors" (Orem, 1991, p. 125). Universal self-care requisites encompass the maintenance of a sufficient intake of air, water, and food; provision of care associated with elimination and excrements; maintenance of a balance between activity and rest and between solitude and social interaction; prevention of hazards to human life, functioning, and well-being; and promotion of human functioning and development within social groups in accord with human potential, known limitations, and the desire to be normal. "Normalcy," Orem (1991) explained, "is used in the sense of that which is essentially human and that which is in accord with the genetic and constitutional characteristics and the talents of individuals" (p. 126).

Developmental self-care requisites are actions that need to be performed in relation to human developmental processes, conditions, and events and in relation to events that may adversely affect development. More specifically, one category of developmental self-care requisites is made up of specialized expressions of the universal self-care requisites particularized for each developmental stage of life. The second category of developmental self-care requisites consists of new action requirements that arise from a condition or an event that could adversely affect human development.

Health-deviation self-care requisites are actions that need to be performed in relation to genetic and constitutional defects, human structural and functional deviations and their effects, and medical diagnostic and treatment measures prescribed or performed by physicians. Health-deviation self-care requisites "exist for persons who are ill or injured, have specific forms of pathology including defects and disabilities, and who are under medical diagnosis and treatment" (Orem, 1991, p. 132). More specifically, one category of health-deviation self-care requisites arises directly from disease, injury, disfigurement, and disability. Another category arises from the medical care measures that physicians perform or prescribe. A list of the categories of all three types of self-care requisites is presented in Table 7–1.

The universal and developmental self-care requisites, "particularized for the person by age, gender, developmental stage, pattern of living, and environmental conditions and circumstances," represent the baseline of the therapeutic self-care demand (Orem, 1991, p. 138). Any health-deviation self-care requisites are then added to the therapeutic self-care demand.

When the person's ability to perform self-care, that is, self-care agency, is not sufficient to meet his or her therapeutic self-care demand, a **self-care deficit** exists. Similarly, when the person's ability to perform dependent-care (i.e., dependent-care agency) is not sufficient to meet the socially dependent person's therapeutic self-care demand, a **dependent-care deficit** exists. Self-care deficits and dependent-care deficits may be associated with functional and structural disorders, but they are not disorders per se. Rather, a deficit signifies that the action demand for self-care or dependent-care is greater than the person's current capability for self-care or dependent-care (Orem, 1991).

Self-care deficits and dependent-care deficits are, then, relational entities; they express relationships of inadequacy between self-care

TABLE 7-1. **SELF-CARE REQUISITES**

Universal Self-Care Requisites

1. The maintenance of a sufficient intake of air
2. The maintenance of a sufficient intake of water
3. The maintenance of a sufficient intake of food, in the form of nutrients
   a. Proteins and amino acids
   b. Fats and fatty acids
   c. Carbohydrates
   d. Minerals
   e. Vitamins
4. The provision of care associated with elimination processes and excrements
5. The maintenance of a balance between activity and rest
6. The maintenance of a balance between solitude and social interaction
7. The prevention of hazards to human life, human functioning, and human well-being
8. The promotion of human functioning and development within social groups in accord with human potential, known human limitations, and the human desire to be normal

Developmental Self-Care Requisites

1. Bringing about and maintaining conditions that support life processes and promote the processes of development, i.e., human progress toward higher levels of the organization of human structures and toward maturation during:
   a. The intrauterine stages of life and the process of birth
   b. The neonatal stage of life
      (1) Premature or term birth
      (2) Normal or low birth weight
   c. Infancy
   d. The developmental stages of childhood, including adolescence and entry into adulthood
   e. The developmental stages of adulthood
   f. Pregnancy in either childhood or adulthood
2. Provision of care associated with effects of conditions that can adversely affect human development
   a. Provision of care to prevent the occurrence of deleterious effects of conditions that can adversely affect human development
   b. Provision of care to mitigate or overcome existent deleterious effects of conditions that adversely affect human development
   c. Conditions that can adversely affect human development include:
      (1) Educational deprivation
      (2) Problems of social adaptation
      (3) Failures of healthy individuation
      (4) Loss of relatives, friends, associates
      (5) Loss of possessions, loss of occupational security
      (6) Abrupt change of residence to an unfamiliar environment
      (7) Status-associated problems
      (8) Poor health or disability
      (9) Oppressive living conditions
      (10) Terminal illness and impending death

Health-Deviation Self-Care Requisites

1. Seeking and securing appropriate medical assistance when there is exposure to specific physical or biological agents or environmental conditions associated with human pathological events and states, or when there is evidence of genetic, physiological, or psychological conditions known to produce or to be associated with human pathology
2. Being aware of and attending to the effects and results of pathological conditions and states, including effects on development
3. Effectively carrying out medically prescribed diagnostic, therapeutic, and rehabilitative measures directed to preventing specific types of pathology, the pathology itself, the regulation of human integrated functioning, the correction of deformities or abnormalities, or compensation for disabilities

TABLE 7-1. **SELF-CARE REQUISITES** (Continued)

4. Being aware of and attending to or regulating the discomforting or deleterious effects of medical care measures performed or prescribed by the physician, including effects on development
5. Modifying the self-concept and self-image in accepting oneself as being in a particular state of health and in need of specific forms of health care
6. Learning to live with the effects of pathological conditions and states and the effects of medical diagnostic and treatment measures in a lifestyle that promotes continued personal development

Adapted from Orem, D.E. (1991). *Nursing: Concepts of practice* (4th ed., pp. 126, 131, 134). St. Louis: Mosby-Year Book, with permission.

agency or dependent-care agency—the action capabilities—and the therapeutic self-care demand—the set of action requirements for engaging in self-care or dependent-care (Orem & Taylor, 1986). A deficit exists if the person does not yet have the ability to perform required self-care or dependent-care actions or if the person cannot perform those actions because of health-related or situational circumstances. Self-care and dependent-care deficits may be complete or partial. Orem (1991) explained that a complete deficit "means no capability to meet a therapeutic self-care demand" (p. 173). In contrast, partial deficits "may be extensive or may be limited to an incapacity for meeting one or several self-care requisites within a therapeutic self-care demand" (p. 173).

Environment

Orem (1991) described human environments in terms of "physical, chemical, biologic, and social features . . . [which] may be interactive" (p. 38). Physicochemical features that are particularly relevant to the values and presence of self-care requisites include the earth's atmosphere, the gaseous composition of the air, solid and gaseous pollutants, smoke, weather conditions, and the geographic stability of the earth's crust. Relevant biological features include pets, wild animals, and infectious organisms or agents along with their human and animal hosts. Relevant social features encompass family factors and community factors.

The family factors include composition by roles and ages of members; cultural prescriptions of authority, responsibilities, and rights; positions and culturally prescribed relationships among members; time-place localization of members; family dynamics; the nature of relationships; the system of family living; the resources of the family as a unit and of the individual members; cultural prescriptions related to resources; and cultural elements regarding patterns of self-care and dependent-care and selection and use of self-care measures.

The community factors include the population; composition by type of unit; availability of resources for daily living for community members and the community as a whole; the kind, location, and availability of health services; openness to individuals and families; accessibility; cultural practices and associated prescriptions; and methods of financing (Orem, 1991).

Orem (1991) underscored the potential contribution of the environment to the person's development. She explained, "It is the total environment, not any single part of it, that makes it developmental" (p. 11). A developmental environment is one that contains closely related physical and psychosocial environmental conditions "that motivate the person being helped to establish appropriate goals and adjust behavior to achieve results specified by the goals" (Orem, 1991, p. 11).

Health

Orem (1991) defined health as a "state of the person that is characterized by soundness or wholeness of developed human structures and of bodily and mental functioning" (p. 184). "Integrated human functioning," Orem (1991) asserted, "[requires] continuous self-care that has therapeutic quality" (p. 181).

Health encompasses inseparable physical, psychological, interpersonal, and social aspects. It includes "that which makes a person human (form of mental life), operating in conjunction with psychologic and psychophysiologic mechanisms and a material structure (biologic life) and in relation to coexistence with other human beings (interpersonal and social life)" (p. 180).

Well-being, which Orem (1991) differentiated from health, focuses on the person's "perceived condition of existence" (p. 184). It is defined as "a state characterized by experiences of contentment, pleasure, and kinds of happiness; by spiritual experiences; by movement toward fulfillment of one's self-ideal; and by continuing personalization" (p. 184). Orem went on to explain that although well-being is associated with health, the experience of well-being may occur for an individual under adverse conditions, including disorders in human structure and function.

Orem (1991) also differentiated health from disease, which is defined as "an abnormal biologic process with characteristic symptoms" (p. 252). The distinction between disease and health is evident in Orem's classification of nursing situations by health focus. Three categories are proposed:

1. The presence or absence of disease, injury, disability, or disfigurement

2. The quality of general health state described in the general sense as excellent, good, fair, poor, or in terms of the values of sets of selected characteristics that together define the person's health state

3. The life-cycle-oriented events and circumstances that indicate current changes and existing needs for health care. (p. 199)

Furthermore, Orem (1991) made a distinction between illness, which she variously referred to as acute, chronic, and disabling, and health. Along with well-being, general health state, and injury, illness is a critical factor in nursing situations. Together, all of these factors "are the determinants of the appropriate health care focus and the types of health results sought" (p. 246).

Finally, Orem (1991) differentiated between sickness or poor health and injury or disability. She noted, however, that "any deviation from normal structure or functioning is properly referred to as an absence of health in the sense of wholeness or integrity" (p. 179).

Orem's discussion of the various health-related terms and her categories of health-related nursing situations suggest that she views health both as a continuum from excellent to poor and as a dichotomy of presence or absence. In addition, Orem apparently views disease, illness, sickness, injury, and disability as separate dichotomies of presence or absence.

Nursing

Orem (1991) noted that the word nursing "is used as a noun, as an adjective, and as a verbal auxiliary derived from the verb to nurse" (p. 2). She further explained:

> Used as a noun and an adjective nursing signifies the kind of care or service that nurses provide. It is the work that persons who are nurses do. The word nursing as used in the statement *I am nursing* is a verbal auxiliary, a participle. To nurse literally means (1) to attend to and serve and (2) to provide close care of a person, an infant or a sick or disabled person, unable to care for self with the goal of helping the person become sound in health and "self-sufficient." (pp. 2–3)

Orem (1985, 1991) has characterized nursing as a human service and a helping service. As a human service, nursing "has its foundations, on the one hand, in persons with needs for self-care of a positive, therapeutic quality and limitations for its management or maintenance and, on the other, in the specialized knowledge, skills, and attitudes of persons prepared as nurses" (1991, p. 42). As a helping service, nursing is "a creative effort of one human being to help another human being" (1985, p. 132).

Orem (1991) distinguished nursing from medicine by noting that the physician focuses on the patient's life processes as they have been disrupted by injury or illness, and the nurse focuses on the patient's continuing therapeutic care. More specifically, the nurse's focus encompasses six components:

1. The patient's perspective of his or her own health situation
2. The physician's perspective of the patient's health situation
3. The patient's state of health
4. The health results sought for the patient, which may be life, normal or near normal functioning, or effective living despite disability

5. The therapeutic self-care demand emanating from universal, developmental, and health-deviation self-care requisites

6. The patient's present abilities to engage in self-care and his or her health-related disabilities in giving self-care.

The special concern of nursing is "the continuing therapeutic care the patient requires" (Orem, 1991, p. 190). More specifically, nursing's special concern is "the individual's need for self-care action and the provision and management of it on a continuous basis in order to sustain life and health, recover from disease or injury, and cope with their effects" (Orem, 1985, p. 54).

The ability to nurse is termed **nursing agency,** which is described as a "complex property or attribute of persons educated and trained as nurses that is enabling when exercised for knowing and helping others know their therapeutic self-care demands, for helping others meet or in meeting their therapeutic self-care demands, and in helping others regulate the exercise or development of their self-care agency or their dependent care-agency" (Orem, 1991, pp. 64–65). Nursing agency is developed and activated by individual nurses.

The **goal of nursing agency** is to *help people meet their own and their dependent others' therapeutic self-care demands.* This goal has three components:

1. Helping the patient accomplish therapeutic self-care

2. Helping the patient move toward responsible self-care, which may take the form of (a) steadily increasing independence in self-care actions, (b) adjustment to interruptions in self-care capabilities, or (c) steadily declining self-care capacities

3. Helping members of the patient's family or other person who attends the patient become competent in providing and managing the patient's care using appropriate nursing supervision and consultation. (Orem, 1985)

Orem (1991) identified social, interpersonal, and technological components of nursing practice. The social component encompasses the role of the nurse and the role of the patient. Legitimate patients of nurses "are persons whose self-care agency or dependent-care agency, because of their own or their dependents' health states or health care requirements, is not adequate or will become inadequate for knowing or meeting their own or their dependents' therapeutic self-care demands" (Orem, 1991, p. 64). Legitimate nurses "are persons who have the sets of qualities symbolized by the term nursing agency to the degree that they have the capability and the willingness to exercise it in knowing and meeting the existent and emerging nursing requirements of persons with health-associated, self-care or dependent-care deficits" (Orem, 1991, p. 64).

A contractual relationship is established between the nurse and the patient for the purpose of obtaining nursing care when an actual or potential self-care or dependent-care deficit is evident. The contract specifies that "the relation of the nurse to the patient is complementary. This means that nurses act to help patients act responsibly for their health-related self-care [or dependent-care] by (1) making up for existent health-related deficiencies in the patients' capabilities for self-care [or dependent-care] and (2) supplying the necessary conditions for the patients to withhold, for therapeutic reasons, the exercise of capabilities or to maintain or increase capabilities for self-care in order to maintain, protect, and promote their functioning as human beings" (Orem, 1991, p. 49).

The interpersonal component of nursing practice highlights the interpersonal relationship between the nurse and the patient, which is necessary for establishment of the social contract and for the provision of care. The essential elements of the interpersonal relationship are contact, association, and communication. Orem (1991) explained: "Interpersonal contact and communication require effort and energy expenditure by both patient and nurse. . . . Patients vary in their tolerance for contact and associations in accord with their temperament, their degree of illness, and their available energy" (p. 230). Orem went on to say, "Ideally, the interpersonal relationship between a nurse and a patient contributes to the alleviation of the patient's stress and that of the family, enabling the patient and the family to act responsibly in matters of health and health care. A relationship that permits a patient to develop and maintain confidence in the nurse and in himself or herself is the foundation for a deliberate process of nursing that contributes positively to the patient's achievement of present and future health goals" (p. 230).

The technological component of nursing practice refers to nurses' actions that are "designed for the attainment of nursing results for patients, [which] occur within the frame of a social-contractual relationship and an interpersonal relationship or in some instances intergroup relationships" (Orem, 1991, p. 234). Thus, the social, interpersonal, and technological components of nursing practice are linked.

The technological component encompasses the **professional and case management operations of nursing practice.** Orem (1991) explained that "The professional operations are collectively referred to as the nursing process. The [case] management operations of planning and controlling (including evaluation) are interspersed with the [professional] operations of nursing diagnosis, nursing prescription, [design of nursing systems,] and nursing regulation or treatment" (p. 235).

There are, then, six operations that describe and give direction to nursing practice — nursing *diagnosis, nursing prescription, nursing system design, planning, nursing regulation or treatment,* and *controlling.* The professional operation of nursing *diagnosis* focuses on determining why the person needs nursing care. This requires calculation of the person's therapeutic self-care demand through assessment of the self-care requisites, assessment of self-care agency or dependent-care agency, including determination of the influence of the power components and the basic conditioning factors, and identification of the self-care deficit or dependent-care deficit. The elements of nursing diagnosis are more fully specified in Table 7–2.

Four levels of nursing diagnosis are appropriate within the Self-Care Framework (Taylor, 1991). The first level focuses on health and well-being, with emphasis on the relationship of self-care and self-care management to the overall life situation. The second level deals with the relationship between the therapeutic self-care demand and self-care agency. The third level expresses the relationship of the action demand by particular self-care requisites to particular self-care operations as influenced by the power components. The fourth level expresses the influence of the basic conditioning factors on the therapeutic self-care demand and self-care agency. Nursing diagnoses may be developed when the individual is the unit of service or when a dependent unit, family, or community is the unit of service.

TABLE 7–2. **ELEMENTS OF NURSING DIAGNOSIS PERTAINING TO SELF-CARE AND DEPENDENT-CARE**

I. Calculate the present and future therapeutic self-care demand
   A. Identify, formulate, and express each universal, developmental, and health-deviation self-care requisite in its relation to some aspect(s) of human functioning and development, including particularizing the values and frequency with which each requisite should be met
   B. Identify the presence of human and environmental conditions
      1. Identify conditions that are enabling for meeting each requisite
      2. Identify conditions that are not enabling and constitute obstacles to or interference with meeting each requisite
   C. Determine the methods or technologies that are known or hypothesized to have validity and reliability in meeting each requisite under prevailing human and environmental conditions and circumstances
   D. Specify the sets and sequences of actions to be performed when a particular method or technology or some combination is selected for use as the means through which each particularized requisite will be met under existent and emerging conditions and circumstances
II. Determine self-care agency or dependent-care agency
   A. Determine the person's self-care or dependent-care abilities by ascertaining the degree of development, the operability, and the adequacy of his or her ability to:
      1. Attend to specific things and exclude other things
      2. Understand the characteristics and meaning of the characteristics of specific things
      3. Apprehend the need to change or regulate the things observed
      4. Acquire knowledge of appropriate courses of action for regulation
      5. Decide what to do
      6. Act to achieve change or regulation
   B. Determine the influence of power components on the exercise and operability of self-care or dependent-care agency
      1. Determine the person's ability to maintain attention and exercise requisite vigilance with respect to self as self-care or dependent-care agent and internal and external conditions and factors significant for self-care or dependent-care

TABLE 7–2. **ELEMENTS OF NURSING DIAGNOSIS PERTAINING TO SELF-CARE AND DEPENDENT-CARE** (Continued)

2. Determine the person's use of available physical energy for the initiation and continuation of self-care or dependent-care operations
3. Determine the person's ability to control body position and parts in the execution of the movements required for the initiation and completion of self-care or dependent-care operations
4. Determine the person's ability to reason within a self-care or dependent-care frame of reference
5. Determine the person's motivation for self-care or dependent-care
6. Determine the person's ability to make decisions about self-care or dependent-care and to operationalize those decisions
7. Determine the person's ability to acquire technical knowledge about self-care or dependent-care from authorative sources, to retain it, and to operationalize it
8. Determine the person's repertoire of cognitive, perceptual, manipulative, communication, and interpersonal skills for self-care or dependent-care operations
9. Determine the person's ability to order discrete self-care or dependent-care actions systems into relationships with prior and subsequent actions
10. Determine the person's ability to consistently perform self-care or dependent-care operations, integrating them with relevant aspects of personal, family, and community living

C. Determine the influence of basic conditioning factors on the exercise and operability of self-care or dependent-care agency
1. Determine the influence of the person's age, gender, developmental state, and health state
2. Determine the influence of sociocultural orientation
3. Determine the influence of health care system, family system, and environmental factors
4. Determine the influence of the pattern of activities of daily living
5. Determine the influence of resource availability and adequacy

D. Determine whether the person should be helped to refrain from self-care actions or dependent-care actions for therapeutic purposes

E. Determine whether the person should be helped to protect already developed self-care or dependent-care capabilities for therapeutic purposes

F. Determine the person's potential for self-care or dependent-care agency in the future
1. Determine the person's ability to increase or deepen self-care or dependent-care knowledge
2. Determine the person's ability to learn techniques of care
3. Determine the person's willingness to engage in self-care or dependent-care
4. Determine the person's ability to effectively and consistently incorporate essential self-care or dependent-care measures into daily living

III. Calculate the self-care deficit or dependent-care deficit
A. Determine the qualitative or quantitative inadequacy of self-care agency or dependent-care agency in relation to the calculated therapeutic self-care demand
B. Determine the nature of and reasons for the existence of the self-care deficit or dependent-care deficit
C. Determine the extent of the self-care deficit or dependent-care deficit
1. Complete
2. Partial

Constructed from Orem, D.E. (1985). *Nursing: Concepts of practice* (3rd ed.) New York: McGraw-Hill; and Orem, D.E. [1991]. *Nursing: Concepts of practice* (4th ed.). St. Louis: Mosby-Year Book.

The professional operation of *nursing prescription* specifies the means to be used to meet particular self-care requisites, all care measures needed to meet the entire therapeutic self-care demand, and the roles to be played by the nurse(s), patient, and dependent-care agent(s) in meeting the patient's therapeutic self-care demand and in regulating the patient's exercise or development of self-care agency. The professional operation of *nursing system design* follows nursing diagnosis and prescription. A nursing system is a series of coordinated deliberate practical actions performed by nurses and patients directed toward meeting the patient's therapeutic self-care demand and protecting and regulating the exercise or development of the patient's self-care agency. Orem (1991) identified three types of regulatory nursing system designs: (1) the <u>wholly compensatory nursing system</u>, (2) <u>the partly compensatory nursing system</u>, and (3) the <u>supportive-educative nursing system</u>. These three nursing system designs are defined and outlined in Table 7–3.

TABLE 7–3. **COMPONENTS OF NURSING SYSTEMS**

I. Wholly compensatory nursing system
    A. Outcomes of nursing action
        1. Accomplishes patient's therapeutic self-care
        2. Compensates for patient's inability to engage in self-care
        3. Supports and protects the patient
    B. Subtype 1
        1. Nursing systems for persons unable to engage in any form of deliberate action
            a. Persons who are unable to control their position and movement in space
            b. Persons who are unresponsive to stimuli or responsive to internal and external stimuli only through hearing and feeling
            c. Persons who are unable to monitor the environment and convey information to others because of loss of motor ability
        2. Method of helping is acting for or doing for the patient
    C. Subtype 2
        1. Nursing systems for persons who are aware and who may be able to make observations, judgments, and decisions about self-care and other matters but cannot or should not perform actions requiring ambulation and manipulative movements
            a. Persons who are aware of themselves and their immediate environment and able to communicate with others normally or in a restricted manner
            b. Persons who are unable to move about and perform manipulative movements because of pathological processes or the effects or results of injury, immobilizing measures of medical treatment, or extreme weakness or debility
            c. Persons who are under medical orders to restrict movement
        2. Methods of helping
            a. Providing a developmental environment
            b. Acting for or doing for the patient
            c. Supporting the patient psychologically
            d. Guiding the patient
            e. Teaching the patient
    D. Subtype 3
        1. Nursing systems for persons who are unable to attend to themselves and make reasoned judgments and decisions about self-care and other matters but who can be ambulatory and may be able to perform some measures of self-care with continuous guidance and supervision
            a. Persons who are conscious but unable to focus attention on themselves or others for purposes of self-care or care of others
            b. Persons who do not make rational or reasonable judgments and decisions about their own care and daily living without guidance

TABLE 7–3. **COMPONENTS OF NURSING SYSTEMS** (Continued)

---

        c. Persons who can ambulate and perform some measures of self-care with continuous guidance and supervision

    2. Methods of helping

        a. Providing a developmental environment

        b. Guiding the patient

        c. Providing support for the patient

        d. Acting for or doing for the patient

II. Partly compensatory nursing system

  A. Outcomes

    1. Nurse action

        a. Performs some self-care measures for the patient

        b. Compensates for self-care limitations of the patient

        c. Assists the patient as required

        d. Regulates self-care agency

    2. Patient action

        a. Performs some self-care measures

        b. Regulates self-care agency

        c. Accepts care and assistance from the nurse

  B. Subtype 1

    1. Patient performs universal measures of self-care; nurse performs medically prescribed measures and some universal self-care measures

    2. Methods of helping

        a. Acting for or doing for the patient

        b. Guiding the patient

        c. Supporting the patient

        d. Providing a developmental environment

        e. Teaching the patient

  C. Subtype 2

    1. Patient learns to perform some new care measures

    2. Methods of helping

        a. Acting for or doing for the patient

        b. Guiding the patient

        c. Supporting the patient

        d. Providing a developmental environment

        e. Teaching the patient

III. Supportive-educative nursing system

  A. Outcomes

    1. Nurse action: regulates the exercise and development of self-care agency

    2. Patient action

        a. Accomplishes self-care

        b. Regulates the exercise and development of self-care agency

  B. Subtype 1

    1. Patient can perform care measures

    2. Methods of helping

        a. Guiding the patient

        b. Supporting the patient

  C. Subtype 2

    1. Patient can perform care measures

    2. Method of helping is teaching the patient

  D. Subtype 3

    1. Patient can perform care measures

    2. Method of helping is providing a developmental environment

  E. Subtype 4

    1. Patient is competent in self-care

    2. Method of helping is guiding the patient periodically

Constructed from Orem, D.E. (1991). *Nursing: Concepts of practice* (4th ed.). St. Louis: Mosby-Year Book.

Orem (1991) explained that the selection of a nursing system is based on the answer to the question of who can or should perform self-care actions and the determination of the patient's role (no role, some role) in the production and management of self-care. The wholly compensatory nursing system is selected when the patient cannot or should not perform any self-care actions, and thus the nurse must perform them. The partly compensatory nursing system is selected when the patient can perform some, but not all, self-care actions. The supportive-educative nursing system is selected when the patient can and should perform all self-care actions.

A single patient may require one or a sequential combination of the three types of nursing systems. All three nursing systems are most appropriately used with individuals. Orem (1991) pointed out that such multi-person units as families usually require combinations of the partly compensatory and supportive-educative nursing systems. She went on to comment, "It is in the realm of possibility that families or residence groups would need wholly compensatory nursing systems under some circumstances, but it is advisable at this stage of the development of nursing knowledge to confine the use of the three nursing systems to situations where individuals are the units of care or service" (pp. 288–289).

The selection of the appropriate type of nursing system is followed by selection of the practical actions of nursing systems, which are referred to as <u>methods of helping</u>. Orem (1991) identified the following five methods that a person can use to give help or assistance to others:

1. Acting for or doing for another
2. Guiding and directing
3. Providing physical or psychological support
4. Providing and maintaining an environment that supports personal development
5. Teaching (Orem, 1991, p. 9)

The use of these methods of helping in the nursing systems is shown in Table 7–3.

Nurses implement nursing systems with people who have self-care or dependent-care deficits. Dependent-care agents implement **dependent-care systems.** Nurses may contribute to the design of dependent-care systems. Indeed, "nurses' contributions to the design of dependent-care systems and planning for their operation and maintenance should be an important consideration in endeavors to develop nursing services that meet needs of communities. The articulation of nursing systems with dependent-care systems is an important consideration whenever there is a need for periodic nursing that is conjoined with a wholly compensatory system of dependent-care or with combined systems of self-care and dependent-care" (Orem, 1991, pp. 293–294).

The case management operation of *planning* follows the design of the nursing system. Planning requires specification of the "time, place, environmental conditions, and equipment and supplies, . . . [as well as] the number and the qualifications of nurses or others necessary . . . to produce a designed nursing system or a portion thereof, to evaluate effects, and to make needed adjustments" (Orem, 1991, pp. 279–280). The plan also specifies the organization and timing of tasks to be performed, allocates task performance to nurse or patient, and identifies specific strategies to be used by nurses to help the patient.

The professional operation of *regulatory care* involves the production and management of the designated nursing system and methods of helping. More specifically, regulatory care operations encompass the provision of direct nursing care and decisions regarding the continuing of direct care in its present form or changing the form. Regulatory nursing systems are produced "when nurses interact with patients and take consistent action to meet their prescribed therapeutic self-care demands and to regulate the exercise or development of their capabilities for self-care" (Orem, 1991, p. 280). Actions taken by nurses to accomplish regulatory care operations are presented in Table 7–4.

TABLE 7–4. **REGULATORY CARE OPERATIONS**

I. Direct nursing care operations
  A. Perform and regulate the self-care tasks for patients or assist patients with their performance of self-care tasks
  B. Coordinate self-care task performance so that a unified system of care is produced and coordinated with other components of health care
  C. Help patients, their families, and others bring about systems of daily living for patients that support the accomplishment of self-care and are, at the same time, satisfying in relation to patients' interests, talents, and goals
  D. Guide, direct, and support patients in their exercise of, or in the withholding of the exercise of, their self-care agency
  E. Stimulate patients' interests in self-care by raising questions and promoting discussions of care problems and issues when conditions permit
  F. Support and guide patients in learning activities and provide cues for learning as well as instructional sessions
  G. Support and guide patients as they experience illness or disability and the effects of medical care measures and as they experience the need to engage in new measures of self-care or change their ways of meeting ongoing self-care requisites
II. Decision-making operations regarding direct nursing care
  A. Monitor patients and assist patients to monitor themselves to determine if self-care measures were performed and to determine the effects of self-care, the results of efforts to regulate the exercise or development of self-care agency, and the sufficiency and efficiency of nursing action directed to these ends
  B. Make characterizing judgments about the sufficiency and efficiency of self-care, the regulation of the exercise or development of self-care agency, and nursing assistance
  C. Make judgments about the meaning of the results derived from nurses' performance when monitoring patients and judging outcomes of self-care for the well-being of patients, and make or recommend adjustments in the nursing care system through changes in nurse and patient roles

Adapted from Orem, D.E. (1991). *Nursing: Concepts of practice* (4th ed., pp. 280–281). St. Louis: Mosby-Year Book, with permission.

The case management operation of *controlling* encompasses observation and appraisal of the nursing system. Emphasis is placed on determination of whether the nursing system that was designed is actually produced and whether there is a fit between the current prescription for care and the nursing system that is being produced. In addition, control operations determine "if regulation of the patient's functioning is being achieved through performance of care measures to meet the patient's therapeutic self-care demand, if the exercise of the patient's self-care agency is properly regulated, if developmental change is in process and is adequate, or if the patient is adjusting to declining powers to engage in self-care" (Orem, 1991, p. 283).

Orem (1991) noted that nursing care may occur at three levels of prevention: primary, secondary, and tertiary. Universal self-care and developmental self-care, when therapeutic, constitute the primary level of prevention. Nursing care at this level includes assisting the patient to learn self-care practices that "maintain and promote health and development and [that] prevent specific diseases" (p. 196). Health-deviation self-care, when therapeutic, constitutes the secondary or tertiary level of prevention. Nursing care at these levels focuses on helping the patient learn self-care practices that "regulate and prevent adverse effects of the disease, prevent complicating diseases, prevent prolonged disability, or adapt or adjust functioning to overcome or compensate for the adverse effects of permanent or prolonged disfigurement or dysfunction" (p. 198).

Content of the Model: Propositions

The link between the person and the environment is specified in the following propositions:

> Certain environmental features are continuously or periodically interactive with men, women, and children in their time-place localizations.

> Environmental conditions can positively or negatively affect the lives, health, and well-being of individuals, families, communities; under conditions of war or natural disaster, whole societies are subject to disruption or destruction. (Orem, 1991, p. 38)

The linkage of person, environment, and nursing is reflected in the statement, "Nurses in concrete nursing practice situations seek nursing-relevant information about both persons who seek or need nursing and their environmental situations" (Orem, 1991, p. 38).

The linkage of person, health, and nursing is evident in the following propositions:

> Nursing has as its special concern the individual's need for self-care action and the provision and management of it on a continuous basis in order to sustain life and health, recover from disease or injury, and cope with their effects. (Orem, 1985, p. 54)

> Nurses act deliberately to produce systems of nursing for persons who have health-related action deficits for knowing and continually meeting their own or their dependents' therapeutic self-care demands. (Orem, 1991, p. 82)

No statement linking person, environment, health, and nursing could be located in the fourth edition of Orem's (1991) book or in any other recent publication by Orem. The following statement, which does link the four metaparadigm concepts, was found in the second edition of Orem's (1980) book:

> Nursing is made or produced by nurses. It is a service, a mode of helping human beings. . . . Nursing's form or structure is derived from actions deliberately selected and performed by nurses to help individuals or groups under their care to maintain or change conditions in themselves or their environments. This may be done by individuals or groups through their own actions under the guidance of a nurse or through the actions of nurses when persons have health-derived or health-related limitations that cannot be immediately overcome. (p. 5)

EVALUATION OF OREM'S SELF-CARE FRAMEWORK

This section presents an evaluation of the Self-Care Framework. The evaluation is based on the results of the analysis, as well as on publications and presentations by Orem and by others who have used or commented on her work.

Explication of Origins

Orem explicated the origins of the Self-Care Framework clearly. She traced the development and refinement of her work from the 1950s to the 1990s in the fourth edition of her book (Orem, 1991). The fourth edition is especially informative in that it includes much of the content of the out-of-print text by the Nursing Development Conference Group (1979), along with the content of the Self-Care Framework and the Theory of Self-Care, the Theory of Self-Care Deficit, and the Theory of Nursing System.

Orem identified the philosophical claims undergirding her work in the form of assumptions and premises about human beings, nursing, and self-care and presuppositions for the theories of Self-Care, Self-Care Deficit, and Nursing System. Taken together, Orem's philosophical claims indicate that she values individuals' abilities to care for themselves and dependent others with intervention from health care professionals only when actual or potential self-care deficits arise. Furthermore, Orem expects people to be responsible for themselves and to seek help when they cannot maintain therapeutic self-care or dependent-care.

Orem also values the person's perspective of his or her health status, as well as that of the physician. Consequently, she does not expect nursing care to be based solely on the nurse's view of the patient's situation.

Orem acknowledged the contributions of her colleagues in the Nursing Development Conference Group to the evolution and refinement of her ideas about nursing. She also acknowledged and cited the work of scholars from adjunctive disciplines, emphasizing the importance of the work on deliberate human action to the development of the Self-Care Framework.

Comprehensiveness of Content

The Self-Care Framework is sufficiently comprehensive in depth of content. The person is fully defined and described as he or she relates to nursing. Orem (1991) was very clear about the correct label for the recipient of nursing care. She rejected the term *client* for the person, preferring instead the term *patient*. She noted, "Some nurses use the term client in place of the term patient. This effort seems to be directed toward recognition of the contractual nature of the relationships of nurses to persons under their care and to avoidance of the philosophical use of the word patient to mean that which is acted upon. It is customary to use the term client in the practice of law, in business, and trade. . . . Client also means a customer who regularly buys from another or receives services from another. . . . Persons who are regular seekers of the services of, that is who are clients of, this or that nurse may not be under nursing care at a particular time and, therefore, would not have patient status" (p. 30).

Orem's description of environment is comprehensive, although environment is never explicitly defined. Health and well-being are clearly defined, but illness is not. The person's state of health is regarded as a factor that may impose new or different demands for self-care on the person. In particular, illness, disability, and disease may impose demands that exceed the person's self-care agency or dependent-care agency and, therefore, create a self-care deficit or a dependent-care deficit.

Nursing is defined clearly and described in terms of scope and appropriate actions to be taken in relation to patients. Orem's description of the nursing process has, however, become more difficult to understand. In the first, second, and third editions of *Nursing: Concepts of Practice*, Orem (1971, 1980, 1985) presented a readily comprehensible three-step nursing process of diagnosis and prescription, designing and planning, and producing care to regulate therapeutic self-care demand and self-care agency. In the fourth edition, Orem (1991) mentioned three steps but gave an explicit number to only the third step, now called regulatory care or regulatory and treatment operations. In addition, confusion about the number of steps in the nursing process was introduced in the fourth edition with the inclusion of a section on control operations. Moreover, the language used to describe the process became obtuse in the fourth edition, with increased emphasis placed on discussion of technological operations and the dimensions of professional and case management operations. The description of the nursing practice operations given in the analysis section of this chapter was constructed only after repeated readings of Orem's fourth edition and the extraction of relevant content from different chapters of that book.

The Self-Care Framework is based on philosophical, theoretical, and scientific knowledge about human behavior, with emphasis placed on theories of deliberate action. Orem (1991) noted that nursing agency is based in large part on knowledge of nursing, sciences, arts, and humanities, and that the design of a nursing system is based on the nurse's factual knowledge about the patient, accumulated information about various therapeutic self-care demands and methods of helping, and knowledge about self-care as deliberate action (Orem, 1991).

The dynamic nature of the nursing process was evident in the third edition of Orem's (1985) book but is not addressed in the fourth edition (1991). In the third edition, Orem (1985) states:

> The degree to which designing nursing systems and planning their production can be separately performed in a block of time in between steps 1 and 3 of the nursing process varies. Factors that militate against this include (1) rapid and complex changes in the health status of patients, (2) needs for continuous adjustments in patients' therapeutic self-care demands, (3) insufficient amounts of valid and reliable factual information about patients and their environments, and (4) inability of the nurse to predict the future values of the patient variables (therapeutic self-care demand and self-care agency). (p. 231)

Orem's inclusion of the patient's perspective of health status, her emphasis on determining the extent of the patient's willingness to collaborate with nurses and participate in their care, and her emphasis on obtaining sufficient information for an accurate diagnosis all reflect her concern with ethical standards. This concern is underscored by Orem's (1991) characterization of nursing as having a moral component. She commented, "Nursing practice has not only technologic aspects but also moral aspects, since nursing decisions affect the lives, health, and welfare of human beings. Nurses must ask [if it is] right for the patient as well as will it work" (p. 55).

The criterion for the linkage of concepts requires that the propositions of the conceptual model link all four metaparadigm concepts. This criterion was met only by recourse to a quotation found in the second edition of Orem's (1980) book.

The Self-Care Framework is also sufficiently comprehensive with regard to breadth of content. The framework has been used in a wide variety of nursing situations and with patients and multiperson units with many different health states. For Orem, multiperson units include families, residence groups, work groups, self-help groups, prenatal or postnatal groups, weight control groups, and groups of patients in nursing clinics.

Despite Orem's (1991) inclusion of multiperson units as a unit of nurses' service, the emphasis is on the individual. She explained, "Persons are provided with nursing as individuals or as members of multiperson units. Nurses recognize that only individuals have self-care requisites and developing or developed powers of self-care agency. It is the societal and interpersonal relationships of individuals and their interactions that focus nurses' attention on families and groups as units of service" (p. 294).

The comprehensiveness of the breadth of the Self-Care Framework is further supported by the direction it provides for research, education, administration, and practice. Rules for each area can be extracted from the content of the framework and various publications about its use.

Some rules for nursing research can be extracted from the content of the Self-Care Framework and Orem's comments on the discipline of nursing. Orem (1991) has come to view the field of inquiry and knowledge known as nursing "as a practical science, with theoretically practical components and more practically oriented (practically practical) components" (p. 86).

Theoretically or speculatively practical knowledge "brings unity and meaning to the universe of action (action domain) of a practice field and to its elements" (p. 87). This kind of knowledge encompasses concepts and theories. Practically practical knowledge deals with "the details of cases, but always within the universal conceptualizations of the practice field, including its domain, elements, and types of results sought" (pp. 87–88). This kind of knowledge encompasses the rules and standards of practice, the knowledge necessary for taking action.

The phenomena to be studied, then, include speculatively practical and practically practical components of self-care, dependent-care, self-care agency, dependent-care agency, the therapeutic self-care demand, self-care deficits, dependent-care deficits, nursing agency, nursing systems, and methods of helping. Smith (1979) identified specific variables that make up nursing knowledge from the perspective of the Self-Care Framework in the categories of basic conditioning factors, self-care practices, self-care requisites, health state, health results sought, the therapeutic self-care demand, self-care deficits, nursing requirements, health focus, nursing situations, nursing systems, nursing technologies, ways of assisting, and outcomes of nursing.

The problems to be studied are those that reflect actual or predictable self-care or dependent-care deficits. The ultimate purpose of Self-Care Framework–based nursing research is to identify the effects of nursing systems of regulatory care on the exercise of self-care agency and dependent-care agency.

Research subjects are people who may be considered legitimate patients of nursing, that is, people "with deficit relationships between (1) their current or projected capability for providing self-care or dependent-care and (2) the qualitative and quantitative demand for care . . . [due to] the health state or health care needs of those requiring care" (Orem, 1991, p. 339). These people may be approached for research purposes in their homes; in hospitals, clinics, and resident-care institutions; and in various other settings in which nursing occurs.

Geden (1985) maintained that "at this time in the development of . . . self-care theory, all [research] approaches are appropriate and necessary" (p. 265). The development of valid and reliable measures of the phenomena encompassed by the Self-Care Framework is progressing, with emphasis to date on measures of self-care agency (e.g., Denyes, 1982; Kearney & Fleischer, 1979) and the power components (Hanson & Bickel, 1985). More definitive rules regarding methodological issues, including research designs, instruments, procedures, and data analysis techniques, remain to be developed. Self-Care Framework–based nursing research contributes to the advancement of knowledge by enhancing understanding of patient and nurse variables that affect the exercise of continuing therapeutic self-care and dependent-care.

Rules for nursing education have been formulated. The distinctive focus of the curriculum is the Self-Care Framework and associated theories. Taylor (1985a) maintained that the Self-Care Framework of nursing provides the "structured body of knowledge essential for curriculum development" (p. 27). Her claim indicates that the focus of the curriculum is on components of self-care, dependent-care, self-care agency, dependent-care agency, self-care deficits, dependent-care deficits, nursing agency, and nursing systems. The purpose of nursing education, according to Orem (1991), is to prepare nursing practitioners at the entry and advanced level of professional nursing practice.

Orem (1991) pointed out that understanding nursing as a human service and a helping service requires the following: knowledge of the arts and humanities, the history of health care and nursing in western and eastern civilizations, languages and cultural elements of specific cultural groups, foundational and basic sciences, and applied medical and public health sciences; experiential knowledge of social and interpersonal situations; development of the social and interpersonal skills needed to work with adults and children individually and in groups; knowledge of nursing as a field of knowledge and practice, including nursing's domain and boundaries as defined by the proper object of nursing, nursing's social field, the profession and occupation of nursing, nursing jurisprudence, nursing ethics, and nursing economics; speculatively and practically practical knowledge of nursing science; and "personal knowledge arising from direct insights into self and others in personal relations" (p. 337). Orem (1991) underscored the importance of basing nursing courses on "a general concept of nursing and [the] understanding of nursing as a practice or science" (p. 336), and encouraged nursing educators to avoid developing nursing courses "that are constituted primarily from content from the biologic, behavioral, and medical sciences" (p. 336).

With regard to sequence of content, Riehl-Sisca (1985a) pointed out that the focus of undergraduate nursing education should be on the operations of information giving and acquiring, reflection on the information received, making some judgments, and problem solving. At the master's level, emphasis should be placed on acquiring specialized areas of information, increasing abilities to reflect and make judgments, and developing some facility with the operations of investigation and meaning. At the doctoral level, emphasis is placed on the advanced understanding of the operations of investigation and meaning.

Education for entry to the profession of nursing "as nursing practitioners and for movement to a professional (scientific) level of practice are offered at the senior college and university level" (Orem, 1991, p. 333). Nursing students must have the ability to achieve mastery "of a general comprehensive [conceptual model] of nursing [so that they will] become able to maintain awareness of the relationship between what they know and what they do as nursing practitioners" (Orem, 1991, p. 339). More specifically, Orem (1991) maintained that nursing students must have the ability to develop themselves as persons who can:

1. Establish contacts, negotiate agreements, and maintain contacts with persons who need nursing and those who seek it for them

2. Interact and communicate with persons under nursing care and their significant others, with other nurses and care givers under ranges of conditions and circumstances that facilitate or hinder interactions and communication

3. Direct interactions and communications toward the development of interpersonal, functional unities

4. Perform with increasing developing skills professional-technologic operations of nursing, including observation, reasoning, judgment and decision-making, and production of practical results in interpersonal and group situations

5. Seek nursing consultation as needed with respect to the professional-technologic operations of nursing

6. Maintain a dynamic sense of duty in all nursing practice situations

Taylor (1985b) identified teaching-learning strategies that are effective with the Self-Care Framework. She pointed out that it is critical that the faculty "have knowledge of [the Self-Care Framework] and skill in its use in order to teach it to students" (p. 41). She suggested that students should initially be presented with an overview of the structure of the framework. Then, as students progress through the educational program, specific linkages should be made between the framework and new content. "By the completion of the program," Taylor (1985b) explained, "the student has (1) seen the overall structure [of the framework], (2) examined the elements in detail, (3) related the elements back to the overall [framework], and (4) tested these in clinical practice settings" (p. 41). Taylor emphasized the importance of developing students' abilities to process information by starting with more concrete elements of the Self-Care Framework, such as self-care requisites and basic conditioning factors, and progressing to more abstract elements, such as the power components. She recommended the development of nursing systems for various situations that students can use as examples. Finally, she highlighted the importance of providing opportunities for students to test nursing systems and to reflect on their efficacy for particular patients.

Rules for nursing administration can be extracted from two of Orem's (1989, 1991) recent publications. The distinctive focus of nursing is to provide regulatory nursing care to "individuals with diagnosed health-derived or health-associated self-care deficits in their time-place localizations" (1991, p. 305). The purpose of nursing services is to help people to enhance their abilities to provide continuing, therapeutic self-care and dependent-care.

Legitimate nurses, according to Orem and Taylor (1986) "are persons who have the sets of qualities or characteristics symbolized by the term nursing agency. To be a legitimate nurse in specific nursing practice situations, the nursing agency of a nurse must be equal to or exceed that required for knowing and meeting the existent and emergent requirements of individuals for nursing" (p. 53). Nursing personnel include nurses, nursing practitioners, and nursing administration. Orem (1991) explained that nurses are "women and men prepared either through high-level technical education or professional level education" (p. 30). Nursing practitioners are "professionally educated nurses working at the entry or advanced level of nursing practice" (p. 30). Orem further explained, "Nurses prepared through high-level technical education work with nursing practitioners or work under established nursing protocols" (p. 30). Nursing administration is "the body of persons who function in situational contexts to collectively manage courses of affairs enabling for the provision of nursing to the population currently served by an organized health service institution or agency and to populations to be served at future times" (p. 308).

Nursing services are delivered in a variety of settings. Orem (1989) commented, "Nurses may go to where patients are, in their homes, in hospitals, or other types of resident-care institutions. Or patients may come to clinics or other types of facilities where nurses are available to provide nursing" (p. 56).

Orem (1989, 1991) distinguished between the focus and actions of nurses and nursing administration. She maintained that "The object of the actions of nurses who engage in the practice of nursing is persons who seek and can benefit from nursing because of the presence of existent or predicted health derived or health related self-care or dependent-care deficits" (1989, p. 56). The object or focus of nursing administration, in contrast, is "the complement of persons for whom a health service agency has contracted to or in the process of contracting to provide nursing or agrees to admit on an ad hoc basis for purposes of receiving nursing (and other health services)" (1991, p. 305).

Orem (1989, 1991) identified two managerial tasks and several associated managerial work operations. The first managerial task is "the proper ordering of persons and material resources so that a functioning whole is continuously created as organizational members fulfill their positional role responsibilities" (1989, p. 61). Managerial work operations associated with that task include the following:

1. Objective setting in relation to the population to be served and to the health care enterprise

2. Analysis and organization of work to achieve objectives

3. Establishing standards for selection of nurses, assistants to nurses, and other support personnel

4. Motivating and communicating

5. Producing designs for measuring performance of nursing care

6. Measuring performance of nursing care and using the results for the enterprise as a whole and for each of its unitary parts. (1989, p. 61; 1991, pp. 311–312)

The second managerial task is "to ensure that the current decisions and actions incorporate or are in harmony with future requirements of the enterprise" (1989, p. 61). The following are managerial work operations associated with this task:

1. Establishing and using standards and criteria for selection of people for operational and managerial positions

2. Identifying costs of continuing operations and sources of capital to finance them

3. Finding new operational methods or extension of methods presently in use in performance of the production or distribution or financing function

4. Developing self and others within the individual's managerial domain. (1989, p. 61)

Rules for nursing practice have been formulated. The domain of nursing practice, according to Orem (1991) is "a composite of persons characterized by conditions that generate nursing requirements and the actions that nurses perform when they provide nursing to these persons" (p. 340). The domain encompasses five areas of activity:

1. Entering into and maintaining nurse-patient relationships with individuals, families, or groups until patients can legitimately be discharged from nursing

2. Determining if and how patients can be helped through nursing

3. Responding to patients' requests, desires, and needs for nurse contacts and assistance

4. Prescribing, providing, and regulating direct help to patients (and their significant others) in the form of nursing

5. Coordinating and integrating nursing with the patient's daily living, or other health care needed or being received, and social and educational services needed or being received. (p. 340)

Orem (1991) presented detailed lists of directives for nursing practice within the following five sets: (1) initial period of contact between nurse and patient, (2) continuing nurse-patient contacts, (3) the quality of interpersonal situations with patients, (4) the production of nursing, and (5) relationships of the nurse with other nurses and other health care providers. It is clear from these directives and the content of the Self-Care Framework that nursing practice is directed toward and contributes to facilitation of individuals' self-care agency and dependent-care agency, and that the clinical problems of interest are the individuals' self-care deficits and dependent-care deficits. Nursing practice occurs in homes, hospitals, resident-care facilities, clinics, and various other institutions. Legitimate recipients of nursing are persons "with deficit relationships between (1) their current or projected capability for providing self-care or dependent-care and (2) the qualitative and quantitative demand for care . . . [due to] the health state or health care needs of those requiring care" (Orem, 1991, p. 339).

Nursing involves a sequence of technological professional and case management operations that are integrated with the social, or contractual, and interpersonal components of practice. Orem (1991) identified six technological operations: diagnosis, prescription, design, planning, regulatory care, and controlling. Diagnosis is based on the calculation of the therapeutic self-care demand from assessment of universal, developmental, and health-deviation self-care requisites and of the existing self-care or dependent-care agency. Regulatory care is implemented as a wholly compensatory, partly compensatory, or supportive-educative nursing system that incorporates various methods of helping. Self-Care Framework–based nursing practice contributions to the well-being of care recipients by regulating self-care agency or dependent-care agency and meeting self-care requisites.

Logical Congruence

The Self-Care Framework is logically congruent. The content of the Self-Care Framework flows directly from Orem's philosophical claims. Just one world view—reciprocal interactionism—is evident. Despite Smith's (1987) claim to the contrary, there is no evidence of the reaction world view in the content of the Self-Care Framework. More specifically, Smith (1987) maintained that Orem's work "fits with the totality paradigm" (p. 97). To the extent that the totality paradigm reflects the reaction world view or even a bridge between the reaction and reciprocal interaction world views, that classification seems inappropriate.

Furthermore, although the framework has been classified as a systems model (Riehl & Roy, 1980) and an interaction model (Riehl-Sisca, 1989), the analysis presented in this book clearly supports its classification as a developmental model with no evidence of the characteristics of other categories of nursing knowledge.

Generation of Theory

Orem, as noted at the beginning of this chapter, views the Theory of Self-Care, the Theory of Self-Care Deficit, and the Theory of Nursing System as the constituent elements of the more general Self-Care Deficit Theory, that is, the Self-Care Framework. Accordingly, an attempt was made to incorporate the three theories into the analysis of the framework. This attempt yielded a cumbersome and confusing structure. Consequently, the decision was made to treat the broad concepts of self-care, therapeutic self-care demand, basic conditioning factors, self-care agency, self-care deficit, nursing agency, and nursing system as the concepts of the Self-Care Framework, and to discuss the central ideas and propositions of the three theories here. It is clear that continued refinement of Orem's work is required to clarify its structure with regard to the conceptual and theoretical elements.

An analysis of the **Theory of Self-Care** revealed that it may be regarded as a middle-range descriptive theory that is made up of the concept of self-care and six propositions that provide definitions and descriptions of that concept. The central idea of the Theory of Self-Care is:

> Within the context of day-to-day living in social groups and their time-place localizations, mature and maturing persons perform learned actions and sequences of actions directed toward themselves or toward environmental features known or assumed to meet identified requisites for controlling factors that either promote or adversely affect or interfere with ongoing regulation of their own functioning or development in order to contribute to continuance of life, self-maintenance, and personal health and well-being. They also perform such regulatory actions for dependent family members or others. (Orem, 1991, p. 69)

The six propositions of the Theory of Self-Care are the following:

1. Self-care is intellectualized as a human regulatory function deliberately executed with some degree of completeness and effectiveness.

2. Self-care in its concreteness is directed and deliberate action that is responsive to persons' knowing how human functioning and human development can and should be maintained within a range that is compatible with human life and personal health and well-being under existent conditions and circumstances.

3. Self-care in its concreteness involves the use of material resources and energy expenditures directed to supply materials and conditions needed for internal functioning and development and to establish and maintain essential and safe relationships with environmental factors and forces.

4. Self-care in its concreteness when externally oriented emerges as observable events resulting from performed sequences of practical ac-

tions directed by persons to themselves or their environments. Self-care that has the form of internally oriented self-controlling actions is not observable and can be known by others only by seeking subjective information. Reasons for the actions and the results being sought from them may or may not be known to the subject who performs the actions.

5. Self-care that is performed over time can be understood (intellectualized) as an action system—a self-care system—whenever there is knowledge of the complement of different types of action sequences or care measures performed and the connecting linkages among them.

6. Constituent components of a self-care system are sets of care measures or tasks necessary to use valid and selected means (i.e., technologies to meet existent and changing values of known self-care requirements). (Orem, 1991, pp. 69–70)

An analysis of the **Theory of Self-Care Deficit** revealed that it also may be regarded as a middle-range descriptive theory. The theory is made up of five concepts—self-care, basic conditioning factors, therapeutic self-care demand, self-care deficit, and nursing—and six propositions about those concepts. The central idea of the Theory of Self-Care Deficit is:

All limitations of persons for engagement in practical endeavors within the domain and boundaries of nursing are associated with subjectivity of mature and maturing individuals to health-related or health-derived action limitations that render them completely or partially unable to know existent and emerging requisites for regulatory care for themselves or their dependents and to engage in the continuing performance of care measures to control or in some way manage factors that are regulatory of their own or their dependents' functioning and development. (Orem, 1991, p. 70)

The six propositions of the Theory of Self-Care Deficit are the following:

1. Persons who take action to provide their own self-care or care for dependents have specialized capabilities for action.

2. Individuals' abilities to engage in self-care or dependent-care are conditioned by age, developmental state, life experience, sociocultural orientation, health, and available resources.

3. Relationship of individuals' abilities for self-care or dependent-care to the qualitative and quantitative self-care or dependent-care demand can be determined when the value of each is known.

4. The relationship between care abilities and care demand can be defined in terms of equal to, less than, and more than.

5. Nursing is a legitimate service when [a] care abilities are less than those required for meeting a known self-care demand (a deficit relationship); and [b] self-care or dependent-care abilities exceed or are equal to those required for meeting the current self-care demand, but a future deficit relationship can be foreseen because of predictable decreases in care abilities, qualitative or quantitative increases in the care demand, or both.

6. Persons with existing or projected care deficits are in, or can expect to be in, states of social dependency that legitimate a nursing relationship. (Orem, 1991, p. 71)

An analysis of the **Theory of Nursing System** indicated that it too may be regarded as a middle-range descriptive theory. It is made up of four concepts—patients, self-care, self-care deficit, and nursing system—and eight propositions that provide definitions and descriptions of the concepts. The central idea of the Theory of Nursing System is the following:

All systems of practical action that are nursing systems are formed by nurses through their deliberate exercise of specialized nursing capabilities (nursing agency) within the context of their interpersonal and contractual relationship with persons with health-derived and health-associated deficits for production of continuing, effective, and complete care for themselves or their dependents for purposes of ensuring that therapeutic self-care demands are known and met and self-care agency is protected or its exercise or development regulated. Nursing systems may be formed or produced for individuals, for persons who constitute a dependent-care unit, for groups whose members have therapeutic self-care demands with similar components, or who have similar limitations for engagement in self-care or dependent-care, for families, or for other multiperson units. (Orem, 1991, p. 72)

The following are the eight propositions of the Theory of Nursing System:

1. Nurses relate to and interact with persons who occupy the status of nurses' patient.

2. Legitimate patients have existent or projected self-care requisites.

3. Legitimate patients have existent or projected deficits for meeting their own self-care requirements.

4. Nurses determine the current and changing values of patients' self-care requisites, select valid and reliable processes or technologies for meeting these requisites, and formulate the courses of action necessary for using selected processes or technologies that will meet identified self-care requisites.

5. Nurses determine the current and changing values of patients' abilities to meet their self-care requisites using specific processes or technologies.

6. Nurses estimate the potential of patients to [a] refrain from engaging in self-care for therapeutic purposes or [b] develop or refine abilities to engage in care now or in the future.

7. Nurses and patients act together to allocate the roles of each in the production of patients' self-care and in the regulation of the exercise or development of patients' self-care capabilities.

8. The actions of nurses and the actions of patients (or nurses' actions that compensate for the patients' action limitations) that regulate patients' self-care capabilities and meet self-care needs constitute nursing systems. (Orem, 1991, pp. 72–73)

Moore (1993) conducted an explicit test of the Theory of Self-Care Deficit, which yielded evidence supportive of this theory. No additional evidence of explicit empirical testing of the three theories could be located. As Moore (1993) demonstrated, the propositions of each theory are, however, sound starting points for the generation of empirically testable hypotheses. Indeed, Orem (1991) regards the propositions of each theory as suggested guides for the further development of that theory.

Orem (1989) also has developed a rudimentary **General Theory of Nursing Administration.** The theory is stated as follows:

> All actions that are proper to nursing administration are actions that are produced by persons with foreknowledge of: (1) nursing as a field of knowledge and practice, (2) the purpose or mission of the institution of which they are an organic part, (3) how nursing contributes to mission fulfillment, and (4) the domain and boundaries of their received powers to manage courses of affairs that ensure the continuing provision of nursing to populations served. All actions that are proper to nursing administration regardless of situational location have a sequential order related to the purposes and the forms of the actions. Courses of action to provide continuous descriptions from a nursing perspective of populations to be provided with nursing are prior to courses of action to provide continuous calculation of what is required to provide nursing to the populations served at this time and at future times. These two courses of action are prior to and provide the substructure or foundation for as well as the linkages with the continuous management of all courses of affairs that ensure the continuing availability and provision of nursing to present and future populations served by the institution. (pp. 57–58)

Credibility

Social Utility

The social utility of the Self-Care Framework is extremely well-documented. Orem (1991) noted that "nurses provide help or care in the form of nursing for persons of different ages, in different stages of development, in different health states, and in different time-place localizations" (p. 101). The framework and theories are being used by nurses throughout the United States and in Canada, Australia, Switzerland, Denmark, and Sweden (Orem, personal communication, August 6, 1987), as well as in Brazil (Beckmann, 1987). Books related to the Self-Care Framework of nursing have been published by Munley and Sayers (1984) and Riehl-Sisca (1985c). The Self-Care Framework and the theories of Self-Care Deficit, Self-Care, and Nursing System are the focus of an annual self-care deficit theory of nursing conference, an annual self-care deficit theory of nursing institute, and research conferences sponsored by the University of Missouri-Columbia School of Nursing.

Prior to the use of the Self-Care Framework, considerable study is required to fully understand its unique focus and content. Nurses and nursing students have to learn the particular "style of thinking and communicating nursing" (Orem, 1991, p. 74) that is reflected in the Self-Care Framework. The framework has an extensive and relatively unique vocabulary that requires mastery for full understanding of its content. Orem and Taylor (1986) explained that "the terminology used to name the elements of the [framework] and the theories and their elements has its origin in the language traditionally used to describe and explain deliberate result-seeking action of human beings" (p. 49). Thus, familiarity with the language of the theories of deliberate human action enhances understanding of Orem's work. In particular, "nurses must understand the actions that constitute self-care and dependent-care, as well as the capabilities that are enabling for performing these kinds of actions" (Orem, 1991, p. 145). Confusion about the meaning and measurement of each concept of the Self-Care Framework, which was noted by Anna and associates (1978) and Foster and Janssens (1985), should be decreased as appropriate clinical and research tools are developed.

The use of the Self-Care Framework also requires understanding of various human sciences "including the concepts, values, and views by means of which data are perceived and evaluated" (p. 59). Understanding the relationships between the societal, interpersonal, and technological components of nursing practice is also required. Furthermore, nurses need to develop "the diagnostic skill of identifying the self-care deficits of adult patients in meeting their current or projected therapeutic self-care demands. A related diagnostic skill [to be developed] is that of determining the infant or child care or dependent adult care competencies of responsible adults" (Orem, 1991, p. 142).

The implementation of Self-Care Framework–based nursing practice is feasible for patients of all ages who are found in diverse clinical situations ranging from health promotion practices to critical care units. The framework may not, however, be appropriate for use in special hospitals for the criminally insane. Mason and Chandley (1990) pointed out that the framework "produces a fundamental conflict between the patient and society according to the clash of values embroiled with the special hospital setting" (p. 670).

Taylor (1990) noted that the implementation of Self-Care Framework-based nursing practice requires consideration of "the philosophy, goals, and objectives; the standards and quality assurance program; and the documentation, job description, and personnel evaluation systems" of the institution (p. 65). The array of human and material resources required for such an undertaking are evident in the comprehensive plan for the implementation of Self-Care Framework-based nursing practice described by Nunn and Marriner-Tomey (1989).

The first phase of planned change includes education of key people, including the nurse administrators, nurse educators, and quality assurance staff, along with a show of support by the nurse administrators through hiring a consultant and sponsoring a retreat devoted to the framework. Next, the key people should participate in the development of plans for implementation and provided leadership in revisions of the nursing philosophy, objectives of nursing service, care plans, standards of care, and evaluation mechanisms. The third phase involves selection of a pilot unit to begin the implementation of the framework. The fourth phase focuses on an assessment of the nursing care delivery model. Nunn and Marriner-Tomey (1989) maintained that the method of care delivery must have built-in accountability. They recommended primary nursing or collaborative practice but indicated that team nursing could be effective if a permanent team leader can assure continuity and accountability for care. They maintained that team nursing with rotating team leaders and functional nursing are not effective. The fifth phase of planned change focuses on preparation of staff on the pilot unit(s) using such strategies as structured classes, reading assignments, and discussion groups.

If the institution is affiliated with one or more schools of nursing, the faculty should be informed that Self-Care Framework–based nursing practice is being implemented. In addition, the hospital administrator, physicians, and consumers need to be "coached" regarding the change (p. 67). The plan for change must also include an evaluation phase. Nunn and Marriner-Tomey (1989) maintained that "The criterion for evaluating Orem's [Self-Care Framework] should include patient and family teaching, patient and family understanding, goal attainment, progress or lack of progress toward goals, and discharge planning to support continuing care after discharge where necessary. Patient and family satisfaction can be checked through the use of a questionnaire at the time of discharge. Patient outcomes need to be evaluated at the time of discharge and thereafter. . . . It is also appropriate to check nurse and physician satisfaction" (p. 67).

Hooten (1992) cited the value of a formal launching of the implementation plan with an "Orem Day" celebration. The celebration was in the form of a conference keynoted by a well-known nurse and featuring a demonstration of a Self-Care Framework-based computer software package. Hooten also noted that prior to the conference, articles about the framework were published in the agency's nursing newsletter. In addition, Hooten (1992) cited the value of on-going guest lectures, and Paternostro (1992) cited the value of a Self-Care Framework-based computerized documentation system, as ways to encourage continued efforts after the framework is incorporated into daily clinical practice.

Wagnild, Rodriguez, and Pritchett's (1987) survey identified factors that enhanced and inhibited the use of the Self-Care Framework by graduates of a baccalaureate program that was based on the framework. Use of the framework was enhanced in practice settings that encouraged self-care, prioritized early discharge planning, subscribed to a whole-person concept of care, and placed a high expectation on patient teaching. Factors that inhibited use included time constraints, inability to adapt the framework to the clinical setting, difficulties in communicating with other staff nurses because of the terminology of the framework, along with patient preferences for dependence on the nurse and lack of interest in self-care.

Implementation of the Self-Care Framework, like any conceptual model of nursing, can occur at the level of the clinical unit or the entire clinical agency. Taylor (1990) noted that implementation of the Self-Care Framework at the unit rather than the agency level "works well when units are decentralized and relatively independent" (p. 65).

NURSING RESEARCH. A plethora of Self-Care Framework–based studies have been conducted. Numerous master's theses and doctoral dissertations have used the Self-Care Framework as a guide. The bibliography at the end of this chapter includes citations for theses and dissertations that were obtained from *Master's Abstracts International* and *Dissertation Abstracts International*. Citations to all published full reports that could be located are also listed in this bibliography. Following the cautionary words of Orem and Taylor (1986), an attempt was made to include only those studies that were based on Orem's approach to self-care rather than self-care in a general sense.

A review of the research literature revealed that the Self-Care Framework has guided a wide range of research designs, from psychometric studies of framework-based instruments to experimental studies. A systematic review of all Self-Care Framework–based research is beyond the scope of this chapter, but many of the published full reports are discussed here.

Most of the psychometric research has focused on development of instruments to measure self-care agency. Kearney and Fleischer (1979) developed an instrument to measure exercise of self-care agency. They validated the instrument by comparing items with other instruments that measure various psychological characteristics of individuals. McBride (1987) reported additional research on the psychometric properties of that instrument.

Hanson and Bickel (1985) developed a questionnaire designed to measure the adult's perception of his or her self-care agency. The Perceived Self-Care Agency Questionnaire items reflect the 10 power components of the Self-Care Framework. Weaver (1987) found that the factor structure of the instrument was significantly different from that proposed by Hanson and Bickel. He concluded that his findings call into question the construct validity of Hanson and Bickel's instrument in noninstitutionalized adults. Cleveland (1989) recommended additional research to further investigate the psychometric properties of the instrument.

The Appraisal of Self-Care Agency Scale was developed to measure self-reported (ASA-A) and nurse-rated (ASA-B) self-care agency (van

Achterberg, Lorensen, Isenberg, Evers, Levin, & Philipsen, 1991; Lorensen, Holter, Evers, Isenberg, & van Achterberg, 1993). The emphasis is placed on assessment of whether a person can actually meet general self-care needs. Cross-cultural studies have revealed acceptable psychometric properties for appropriately translated versions of both forms of the instrument (ASA-A, ASA-B) in elderly populations in The Netherlands, Norway, and Denmark.

Denyes (1982) developed an instrument to measure the self-care agency of adolescents. Gaut and Kieckhefer (1988) examined the psychometric properties of the instrument in a sample of chronically ill adolescents.

Biggs (1990) developed the Biggs Elderly Self-Care Assessment Tool (BESCAT) to measure family caregiver-rated self-care abilities of the elderly. The BESCAT items are based on the universal, developmental, and health-related self-care requisites. Nine subscales permit assessment of breathing, water intake, food intake, bowel and bladder functioning, balancing activities and rest, balancing social interaction and solitude, safety and prevention of injuries, promotion of normalcy, and health deviation self-care requisites.

Moore and Gaffney (1989) developed the Dependent Care Agency questionnaire to measure mothers' performance of their children's self-care activities. Although a factor analysis did not confirm the three categories of universal, developmental, and health deviation self-care requisites, the factor structure did reflect various combinations of those categories of self-care requisites.

Gulick (1987) used the Self-Care Framework as the basis for the Activities of Daily Living (ADL) Self-Care Scale for use with persons diagnosed with multiple sclerosis. Factor analysis of the original 52-item scale yielded 15 items that represent universal and developmental self-care requisites. Gulick noted that the scale may be useful to assess the function of people with various chronic neurological illnesses. Gulick (1989) also developed the MS-Related Symptom Checklist from the Self-Care Framework. She noted that "one essential self-care action required to promote regulation of one's functioning and well-being is detecting and monitoring symptoms" (p. 147). Factor analysis reduced the number of items from 26 to 22. The scale scores may be used as the basis for determination of potential self-care deficits for universal self-care requisites.

McFarland et al. (1992) developed the Self-Care Assessment Tool (SCAT) as a measure of the cognitive and functional skills needed for self-care in persons with spinal cord injuries. The SCAT, which has acceptable psychometric properties, permits assessment of skills in bathing/grooming, nutritional management, taking medications, mobility/transfers/safety, skin management, bladder management, bowel management, and dressing.

Campbell (1986) developed the Danger Assessment instrument to measure the extent to which battered women are in danger of homicide. She stated that "within the Self-Care Framework," the process of completing the Danger Assessment instrument "can be considered an instance of enhancing the woman's self-care agency or her ability to take deliberate action to perform self-care" (p. 37).

Hayward et al. (1989) developed a questionnaire to measure stressors experienced by new renal transplant patients. They linked the tool to the Self-Care Framework through their conceptualization of stress as a self-care deficit, reasoning that stress "may limit a person's agency (ability) to meet some or all therapeutic self-care demands" (p. 81).

Descriptive Self-Care Framework–based research has emphasized determination of the meaning of self-care, the measurement of the level of patients' self-care practices, and self-care agency. Whetstone (1987) and Whetstone and Hansson (1989) reported the findings of cross-cultural studies of the meanings of self-care to American, German, and Swedish people. Allison (1971) explored the meaning of rest for patients. Humphreys (1991) reported the findings of her study of children's worries about their battered mothers. Degenhart-Leskosky (1989) compared the needs of adolescent and young adult mothers for information on self-care and infant care. Neil (1984) measured the self-care agency of members of an Al-Anon group. Woods (1985) and Maunz and Woods (1988) described self-care activities used by young adult women. Patterson and Hale (1985) described self-care practices related to menstruation. Hartweg (1993) described the self-care actions of middle-aged women. Baulch and associates (1992) identified factors that influence proficiency in breast self-examination in older women. Harris and Williams (1991) described universal self-care requisites identified by homeless men. Jopp, Carroll, and Waters (1993) reported the results of their study of how older adults manage self-care activities at home following hospital discharge.

Schafer (1989) described the health habits and lifestyle practices of older men and women, as well as their ideas regarding the need for dependent-care agents. Brock and O'Sullivan (1985) identified factors that distinguish newly institutionalized elderly people from elderly people able to remain in the community. Hamilton and Creason (1992) described changes in the mental status and functional abilities of institutionalized elderly women over a period of 1 year. Chang, Uman, Linn, Ware, and Kane (1984, 1985) studied factors affecting satisfaction with nursing care and adherence to health care regimens in elderly women.

Crockett (1982) studied the self-care practices for coping used by adult psychiatric and nonpsychiatric subjects. Hamera, Peterson, Young, and Schaumloffel (1992) identified indicators that people with schizophrenia use to identify their mental illness. Sandman, Norberg, Adolfsson, Alexsson, and Hedly (1986) used the Self-Care Framework to guide their analysis of the behaviors of five patients with Alzheimer-type dementia and their nurses during morning care.

Dodd (1982, 1984b, 1988a) described self-care behaviors of cancer patients who were receiving chemotherapy or radiation therapy. Kubricht (1984) described the therapeutic self-care demands of outpatients receiving radiation therapy. Robinson and Posner (1992) described the fatigue experienced by patients receiving interleukin-2, interferon alfa, or tumor necrosis factor. Hiromoto and Dungan (1991) described the outcomes of a pilot test of a clinical protocol for chemotherapy patients. They found that contract learning was associated with symptom recognition, consideration of options for self-care actions, initiation of self-care behaviors, and evaluation of the effectiveness of self-care actions in four of five patients who participated in the initial test of the learning protocol.

Hautman (1987) used Orem's definition of self-care in her study of self-care responses to respiratory illness in a sample of Vietnamese persons residing in Texas. Rew (1987) compared the self-care behaviors of children with asthma before and after a 1-week residential camping experience. Monsen (1992) compared the self-care agency of healthy adolescents with that of those who have spina bifida. Carlisle et al. (1993) described caregivers' knowledge of and self-care activities related to cardiovascular risk factors in their 2- and 3-year-old children. Utz and Ramos (1993) have conducted a series of studies of the self-care needs of people with symptomatic mitral value prolapse.

Miller (1982) identified categories of self-care needs for a sample of diabetics. Germain and Nemchik (1988) described the desires, concerns, and experiences of diabetics regarding retention of self-management during hospitalization. Storm and Baumgartner (1987) presented a case study within the context of the Self-Care Framework of a 41-year-old woman with multiple sclerosis who was discharged home with a mechanical ventilator.

Bliss-Holtz (1988) identified the extent of primiparas' concern for learning dependent-care of their infants during the three trimesters of pregnancy. She found that the pregnant women expressed little interest in learning infant care. Further analysis of her data revealed greater interest in learning about labor and delivery (Bliss-Holtz, 1991).

Geden (1985) placed her studies of oxygen consumption within the context of the Self-Care Framework. She commented that her study of 1982, and those of Hathaway and Geden (1983) and Flanagan (1983) "may be related to the universal self-care requisite of maintaining a balance between activity and rest and/or related to the power component of self-care agency" dealing with ability to control body position (p. 268).

Correlational studies have focused on the identification of variables associated with the exercise of self-care agency. Moore (1987a) found a positive relationship between autonomy and self-care agency in a sample of fifth-grade children. In a later study, Moore (1993) found that basic conditioning factors, self-care agency, and mothers' dependent-care performance were related to children's self-care performance. Frey and Fox (1990) found that diabetes self-care was related to universal self-care, health status, and metabolic control of diabetic children. Lakin (1988) found positive relationships between internal locus of control, health values, health status, and satisfaction with health and the exercise of self-care agency in a sample of working women. McDermott (1993) found evidence of an inverse relationship between learned helplessness and self-care agency in a sample of working women and men. Smits and Kee (1992) found a strong positive relationship between self-concept and exercise of self-care agency in a sample of independently living older people.

Malik (1992) studied the influence of knowledge, beliefs, and health practices about breast cancer on breast self-examination in a sample of women in Delhi, India. Weinrich (1990) examined the association between demographic and health variables and participation in fecal occult blood screening.

Oberst, Hughes, Chang, and McCubbin (1991) studied factors that are associated with self-care burden in radiotherapy patients. Hanucharurnkul (1989) found that socioeconomic status and social support were associated with self-care behaviors in a sample of Thai adults receiving radiation therapy. Rhodes, Watson, and Hanson (1988) reported that tiredness and weakness most interfered with the self-care activities performed by patients receiving chemotherapy. Gammon (1991) found a strong positive relationship between self-care and the individual's ability to cope with cancer.

Several Self-Care Framework – based experimental studies have been conducted. The findings of some of those studies provide evidence that supports the effectiveness of Self-Care Framework – based nursing interventions. McCord (1990) reported that parents who received detailed preoperative information about their children's tonsillectomies had higher knowledge scores and were more compliant with regard to postoperative instructions than parents who received the routine information. Alexander, Younger, Cohen, and Crawford (1988) found that clinical nurse specialist contact emphasizing preventive health measures resulted in fewer emergency room visits by children with chronic asthma during a 12-month follow-up period than by children in a control group. Blazek and McClellan (1983) found that an experimental treatment designed to help children become managers of their own health care had the hypothesized effect of increasing health locus of control. Moore (1987b) found that either or both assertion training and first aid instruction increased autonomy and that first aid training increased self-care agency in school-aged children.

The findings of two studies supported the beneficial effects of educational programs on self-care related to premenstrual symptomatology (Kirkpatrick, Brewer, & Stocks, 1990; Seideman, 1990). Buckley (1990) found that postpartum appointment keeping at a high-risk perinatal center was greater for women who received a pre-hospital discharge postpartum visit by a nurse practitioner than for those who did not receive the visit. Palmer and Meyers (1990) reported positive preliminary results from a demonstration project to determine the safety of outpatient chemotherapy for patients with acute lymphoblastic leukemia. Williams et al. (1988) reported that Filipina women undergoing mastectomy or hysterectomy who received an experimental preoperative and predischarge teaching program performed more self-care activities during hospitalization and after discharge than a control group.

Toth (1980) found that structured information given in preparation for transfer from the coronary care unit reduced patient anxiety more than unstructured information. Stockdale-Woolley (19984) found that group education classes improved the self-care agency of patients with chronic obstructive pulmonary disease. Gulick (1991) found that patients with multiple sclerosis who received an experimental intervention focusing on self-assessment and monitoring of functioning and symptom prevalence used fewer professional health services than a control group during a 27-month study period. Huss, Alerno, and Huss (1991) found that adult atopic asthmatics who received experimental computer-assisted instruction reported greater adherence to house dust mite avoidance techniques than a control group. Harper (1984) found that elderly black women who participated in a medication education program demonstrated greater knowledge about medications and higher levels of self-care medication behaviors than did women who did not participate in the program. Rothlis (1984) found that subjects with reactive depression who participated in a self-help group experienced decreased feelings of hopelessness and helplessness when compared with patients who did not participate in the group.

Other studies yielded conflicting findings. Arneson and Triplett (1990) found that an educational program increased preschool children's knowledge of care safety but did not increase their use of seat belts. Youssef (1987) found that experimental group subjects who received a predischarge family-patient teaching program had a greater improvement in functional level, but no difference in readmission rate, than control group subjects. Goodwin (1979) found that subjects who received a programmed instruction booklet shortly after pulmonary surgery had greater knowledge, performed more recommended self-care activities, and had better respiratory function just prior to discharge and 30 days after discharge than those who did not receive the booklet. The groups did not differ, however, on performance of potentially harmful activities, posture, range of motion, and resumption of work and social activities. Dodd (1983, 1984a) found that cancer patients on chemotherapy who received information on side effect management techniques (SEMT) initiated more self-care behaviors with a higher degree of perceived effectiveness than patients who did not receive SEMT. Two later studies of SEMT with chemotherapy and radiation therapy patients, however, revealed that although the experimental information group performed more self-care behaviors in response to experienced symptoms, they neither initiated preventive self-care behaviors sooner nor experienced less severe side effect symptoms than the control groups (Dodd, 1987, 1988b). Whetstone (1986) found limited support for the hypothesized beneficial effect of social dramatics on social skills of chronically mentally ill patients.

Still other studies failed to support the effectiveness of Self-Care Framework – based nursing interventions. Meeker, Rodriguez, and Johnson (1992) found that a structured preoperative teaching program did not have the expected beneficial effects of reducing the incidence of postoperative atelectasis and increasing patient satisfaction. Hagopian et al. (Hagopian, 1991; Hagopian & Rubenstein, 1990; Weintraub & Hagopian, 1990) were unable to establish the efficacy of nursing consultation, a weekly newsletter, or telephone calls on such outcomes as anxiety, side effects, or self-care behaviors of patients receiving radiation therapy. Porter, Youssef, Shaaban, and Ibrahim (1992) failed to find support for their hypotheses of greater self-esteem and self-care agency in high-risk Egyptian mothers who participated in a parental enhancement program when compared with that of a control group. Karl (1982) found no support for the hypothesis that an exercise program would increase independence in self-care abilities in a sample of elderly patients.

Some Self-Care Framework – based studies have focused on the nurse as the study subject. Bidigare and Oermann (1991) described nurses' attitudes toward and knowledge of organ procurement. Steele and Sterling (1992) reported a case study of nursing interventions designed to prepare family members to care for a child requiring complex care at home. Denyes, Neuman, and Villarruel (1991) reported the results of two studies of actions used by nurses to prevent and alleviate pain in hospitalized children. Barron, Ganong, and Brown (1987) described the preconception self-care practices taught to women as part of routine health maintenance.

Kerkstra, Castelein, and Philipsen (1991) identified the type and number of preventive interventions used by community nurses in The Netherlands during home visits to the elderly. Ewing (1989) found that nursing interventions did not adequately prepare stoma patients for self-care in preparation for hospital discharge. Bennett, DeMayo, and Saint Germain (1993) studied the relationship of empathy, knowledge and attitudes about sex, and homophobia to registered nurses' attitudes about AIDS care.

Harrison and Novak's (1988) evaluation of the effects of a gerontological continuing education program revealed that nurses had more knowledge of and more positive attitudes about the elderly following participation in the program. Siebert and associates (1986) found that nursing students had more positive general perceptions of preschool-aged children from two-parent families compared with those from single-parent families, but no differences in perceptions when the child was viewed as a potential patient in a hospital unit.

NURSING EDUCATION. The utility of the Self-Care Framework for nursing education is evident. Indeed, citing an unpublished survey by Karb and Von Cannon, Berbiglia (1991) noted that "of the four nursing [models] most frequently used by [National League for Nursing] accredited baccalaureate programs that adopted a single [model], the [Self-Care Framework] ranked second in use" (p. 1159). Publications have documented the use of the framework as a curriculum guide for the diploma nursing program at Methodist Medical Center of Illinois in Peoria, Illinois (Woolley, McLaughin, & Durham, 1990); the associate degree nursing program at Thornton Community College in South Holland, Illinois (Fenner, 1979); and the baccalaureate programs at George Mason University in Fairfax, Virginia (Mullin & Weed, 1980), Georgetown University in Washington, DC (Piemme & Trainor, 1977), Illinois Wesleyan University in Bloomington, Illinois (Woolley et al., 1990), the University of Missouri-Columbia (Taylor, 1985b), the University of Southern Mississippi (Herrington & Houston, 1984; Richeson & Huch, 1988), and Wichita State University in Wichita, Kansas (Kruger, 1988).

Berbiglia (1991) stated that the Self-Care Framework has guided the curriculum "for more than a decade and has emphasized educator competency in the use of this [framework in] a parochial liberal arts college in the south-west United States," but she did not identify the school by name (p. 1160). In addition, the Self-Care Framework guides aspects of the content of the junior year nursing course at the University of Ottawa in Ontario, Canada (Story & Ross, 1986).

Herrington and Houston (1984) described nursing students' use of two faculty-developed clinical nursing process tools at the University of Southern Mississippi in Hattiesburg. Laschinger (1990) described a clinical assessment tool based on the Self-Care Framework that she claimed facilitated students' development of nursing care plans and their understanding of the framework.

Mulkeen (1989) described the strategies she used to help a student district nurse at the Bolton Health Authority in England learn about self-care for a diabetic patient. She highlighted the effectiveness of the contract of teaching she established with the student, who in turn, established a contract of care with the patient.

Langland and Farrah (1990) explained how the Self-Care Framework was used as the basis for a continuing education course in gerontological nursing. They noted that the course, which was repeated over a 3-year period at nine sites in Missouri, resulted in an increase in participants' knowledge of "theory-based gerontological nursing and theory-based practice" (p. 270).

NURSING ADMINISTRATION. The utility of the Self-Care Framework for administration of nursing services is evident. Publications document the use of the framework as an administrative and management guide in several clinical agencies. One of the early uses of the Self-Care Framework was at the nurse-managed clinics at the Johns Hopkins Hospital in Baltimore, Maryland (Allison, 1973; Bachscheider, 1974; Crews, 1972). The Self-Care Framework has been the basis for structuring nursing practice and roles and functions of nurses at the Mississippi Methodist Hospital and Rehabilitation Center since 1976 (Allison, 1985). The framework also structures nursing practice at the Betty Bachrach Rehabilitation Hospital in Pomona, New Jersey (Derstine, 1992) and the National Jewish Center for Immunology and Respiratory Medicine in Denver, Colorado (Barnes, 1991). The use of the Self-Care Framework to structure nursing practice at a pediatric rehabilitation facility, Children's Seashore House, when it was located in Atlantic City, New Jersey, is documented in a videotape produced by Hale and Rhodes (1985).

Publications document the use of the framework to structure professional nursing practice at many community hospitals and medical centers, including Binghamton General Hospital in Binghamton, New York (Feldsine, 1982), the Newark Beth Israel Medical Center in Newark, New Jersey (Fernandez, Brennan, Alvarez, & Duffy, 1990), Saint Elizabeth's Hospital in Elizabeth, New Jersey (Fernandez & Wheeler, 1990), Riverview Medical Center in Red Bank, New Jersey (Fernandez et al., 1990; Brennan & Duffy, 1992), Phoenixville Hospital in Phoenixville, Pennsylvania (Husted & Strzelecki, 1985), Georgetown University Hospital in Washington, DC (Van Eron, 1985), and the Tucson Medical Center in Tucson, Arizona (Del Togno-Armanasco, Olivas, & Harter, 1989). The Self-Care Framework also serves as the basis for administration of nursing practice at the Veterans Administration Medical Centers in Fresno, California (Rossow-Sebring, Carrieri, & Seward, 1992), Indianapolis, Indiana (Nunn & Marriner-Tomey, 1989), and Salem, Virginia (McCoy, 1989).

Self-Care Framework – based cooperative care, which encourages patient self-care and family involvement in care giving, has been implemented on the Cooperative Care Unit at the Medical Center Hospital of Vermont in Burlington (Weis, 1988) and on the oncology and acute care units of the Dorn Veterans' Hospital in Columbia, South Carolina (Roach & Woods, 1993). Collaborative care, which fosters patient participation in health care during hospitalization, has been implemented at the Veterans' Administration Medical Center in Gainesville, Florida (Lott, Blazey, & West, 1992).

In addition, the Self-Care Framework is used to guide nursing practice on the renal transplant unit at the University of Tennessee, Memphis, William F. Bowld Hospital (Hathaway & Strong, 1988); at the hospice at Overlook Hospital in Summit, New Jersey (Murphy, 1981); at the Supervised Environmental Living Facility (SELF) in Waterbury, Connecticut, a supervised apartment program for chronically mentally ill people that was founded by Dibner and Murphy (1991); and at the Neighborhood Family Service Center in Scottsbluff, Nebraska (McVay, 1985). The framework also provided some guidance for the structure of nursing practice at a nurse-managed wellness center for senior citizens in New York City (Smith & Sorrell, 1989).

International use of the Self-Care Framework is documented at the Vancouver Health Department in British Columbia, Canada (Duncan & Murphy, 1988; McWilliams, Murphy, & Sobiski, 1988); Toronto General Hospital (Campbell, 1984; Harman et al., 1989; Laurie-Shaw & Ives, 1988a, 1988b; Reid, Allen, Gauthier, & Campbell, 1989), Scarborough General Hospital, and The Mississauga Hospital, all in Toronto, Ontario, Canada (Fitch et al., 1991); the Nursing Clinic for Rheumatoid Arthritis at the Sir Mortimer B. Davis-Jewish General Hospital in Montreal, Quebec, Canada (Porter & Shamian, 1983); Prince Henry Hospital in Sydney, Australia (Avery, 1992); the St. John's Dermatology Centre outpatient department of St. Thomas's Hospital in London, England (Hunter, 1992); the day hospital at Worthing Hospital in England (Dyer, 1990); and Birmingham Children's Hospital in England (Clark & Bishop, 1988).

Dier (1987) proposed a collaborative project between Canada and Thailand that "combines the Canadian experience in using Orem's Self-Care Framework with the extensive Thai knowledge about nursing in primary health settings" (p. 326). She pointed out that the Self-Care Framework and the primary health care approach "have many similarities, for example the focus on health promotion rather than illness, of working *with* clients rather than doing *for* them and of sharing information so people can make knowledgeable decisions about their own health" (p. 326). Beckmann (1987) described the influence of the Self-Care Framework on the structure of nursing practice and the perinatal health-care delivery system in Brazil. In addition, Dennis (1989) maintained that hospital-based nursing in the Soviet Union was consistent with the Self-Care Framework.

Tools for clinical assessment of self-care, self-care agency, and the therapeutic self-care demand have been developed. Three separate scales that can be used to determine the degree of development of self-care agency, degree of operability of self-care agency, and adequacy of self-care agency in relation to a known therapeutic self-care demand were described by the Nursing Development Conference Group (1979).

Snyder et al. (1991) described the development of the Self-Management Inventory, which is used to assess the universal, developmental, and health-deviation self-care requisites of older people. Taira (1991) described a tool that she developed to assess the knowledge of chronically ill independent-living older persons about their prescribed medications. Data are obtained via interviews with patients.

Johannsen (1992) described a self-assessment instrument for use by cardiac patients. The information obtained can be used to develop individualized teaching and discharge plans. Graff, Thomas, Hollingsworth, Cohen, and Rubin (1992) described a patient self-assessment form for use during recovery from surgery. The information is used to determine the need for postoperative home nursing care.

Switching the focus from self-care to dependent care, Baldwin and Davis (1989) developed the Health Education Questionnaire to assess parents' perceptions of themselves as health educators for their school-aged children. Angeles (1991) switched the focus from patients to nurses in her description of an orientation checklist that assesses nursing agency with regard to meeting the self-care demands of neonates. The checklist is used during the orientation program for the Neonatal Intensive Care Unit at the Loma Linda University Medical Center in Loma Linda, California.

Nursing diagnosis within the context of the Self-Care Framework has been discussed. Taylor (1987, 1991) developed a four-level diagnostic structure based on the relationship between action demands and agency. Jenny (1991) reported the results of a study of the fit between diagnoses from the North American Nursing Diagnosis Association (NANDA) taxonomy and Orem's self-care requisites. Jenny reported that appropriate diagnoses were found for most of the self-care requisites. McKeighen, Mehmert, and Dickel (1991) described the development of the nursing diagnosis of self-care deficit, bathing/hygiene. Aukamp (1989) described the development of the nursing diagnosis of knowledge deficit in the third trimester of pregnancy. Jenny (1988, 1989) described a schema for nursing diagnosis based on self-care and cited Orem's work. In a later publication, Jenny (1992) explained that her taxonomy was not derived from the Self-Care Framework and is, in fact, "distinctly different from Orem's concepts" (p. 44).

O'Connor (1990) outlined the steps of a comprehensive patient education program. Her article includes the form used to document patient education at the Veterans Administration Medical Center in Roseburg, Oregon.

The Self-Care Framework has been used as a basis for patient classification systems. Miller (1980) presented a model for dynamic nursing practice based on the Self-Care Framework. The model emphasizes the changes in nursing strategies as the patient's health status changes. Leatt, Bay, and Stinson (1981) used Orem's definition of self-care practices in their patient classification instrument.

The Self-Care Framework has also been used to guide development of measures of the quality of nursing care. Clinton, Denyes, Goodwin, and Koto (1977) reported their work on development of patient outcome criteria derived from self-care requisites. Fukuda (1990) outlined basic outcome standards for patients with chronic congestive heart failure. Kitson (1986) described indicators of quality for geriatric nursing care. Gallant and McLane (1979) described a process for validation of outcome criteria based on the Self-Care Framework. Horn (1978) described the Horn and

Swain (1977) measure of quality of nursing care. That instrument is based on the universal self-care requisites. Hageman and Ventura (1981) reported the results of their study of the use of an instrument designed to measure the quality of nursing care with regard to effects of medication teaching regimens. The instrument was adapted from medication-related items on the Horn and Swain instrument.

Padilla and Grant (1982) described a comprehensive quality assurance program based on the Self-Care Framework. The program includes a definition of criteria and standards, nursing care management protocols that define standards of care, continuing education courses for nursing based on management protocols, and methods to audit and record nursing processes and patient outcomes.

Perhaps the most innovative and timely use of the Self-Care Framework in nursing administration is the development of a computer software package, Professional Care System, for nursing documentation (Bliss-Holtz, Taylor, McLaughin, Sayers, & Nickle, 1992). Software development was initiated by Patricia Sayers, the founder and president of Nursing Systems International Incorporated of Bordentown, New Jersey. McLaughlin, Taylor, Bliss-Holtz, Sayers, & Nickle (1990) explained that the software package "is an information system based in nursing theory that supports nursing practice and management of nursing services" (p. 175). The input to the computer is clinical data from patients, structured within the context of the Self-Care Framework. "Output from the system includes production of individualized patient care plans, a chronological record of patient care, reports in narrative or chart form relating patient variables with nurse action and patient outcomes, quality assurance reports, and other periodic management reports. (Bliss-Holtz et al., 1990, p. 175). Placement of computers at the patient's bedside facilitates comprehensive documentation (Paternostro, 1992).

NURSING PRACTICE. The utility of the Self-Care Framework for nursing practice is fully documented. The Self-Care Framework has been used to guide the care of patients who seek care in many different inpatient and outpatient settings. Publications document the use of the framework as a guide to patient care in such inpatient settings as:

Intensive care and critical care units (Fawcett et al., 1987, 1992; Jacobs, 1990; James, 1992; Miller, 1989)

Neonatal intensive care units (Tolentino, 1990)

Operating rooms (Caradus, 1991; Kam & Werner, 1990)

Acute care units (Mullin, 1980)

Medical-surgical units (Robichaud-Ekstrand, 1990)

Obstetrical units (Fields, 1987; Wollery, 1983)

Psychiatric units and institutions (Davidhizar & Cosgray, 1990; Duffey, Miller, & Parlocha, 1993; Lacey, 1993; Moscovitz, 1984)

Rehabilitation units (Bracher, 1989; Smith, 1977)

Pediatric residential treatment facilities (Titus & Porter, 1989)

Nursing homes (Anna, Christensen, Hohon, Ord, & Wells, 1978)

Self-Care Framework – based nursing care is also documented in such outpatient settings as:

Emergency departments (Hughes, 1983)

Ambulatory clinics (Alford, 1985; Allison, 1973; Backscheider, 1974; Crews, 1972; Vasquez, 1992)

Pediatric interdisciplinary phenylketonuria clinics (Hurst & Stullenbarger, 1986)

College health programs (Hedahl, 1983)

Industry (Komulainen, 1991; Ruddick-Bracken & Mackie, 1989)

Hospices (Murphy, 1981; Walborn, 1980)

In those and other settings, the Self-Care Framework has been used to guide the nursing care of patients with conditions such as:

Asthma (Walsh, 1989)

Upper respiratory infections and gastroenteritis (Facteau, 1980)

Diabetes (Allison, 1973; Backscheider, 1974; Petrlik, 1976; Zach, 1982)

Cardiac and circulatory problems (Crews, 1972; Dumas, 1992; Flanagan, 1991)

Cerebral vascular accidents (Anna et al., 1978; Redfern, 1990)

Various neurological problems (Mitchell & Irvin, 1977)

Multiple sclerosis (MacLellan, 1989)

Parkinson's disease (MacSweeney, 1992)

Guillain-Barré syndrome (Anderson, 1992)

End-stage renal disease requiring peritoneal dialysis (Perras & Zappacosta, 1982; Turner, 1989)

Emotional problems and mental illness (MacDonald, 1991; Moore, 1989; Wright, 1988)

Terminal illness (Walborn, 1980)

In addition, Self-Care Framework-based nursing care has been described for patients who have had the following:

Elective minor surgery (Swindale, 1989)

Cataract surgery (Beed, 1991),

Head and neck surgery (Dropkin, 1981),

Coronary artery bypass surgery (Campuzano, 1982),

Renal transplant (Norris, 1991),

Hip arthroplasty (Boon & Graham, 1992; Craig, 1989)

Hysterectomy (Thomas, Graff, Hollingsworth, Cohen, & Rubin, 1992)

The Self-Care Framework has been used to design nursing care for patients of various ages and with a variety of self-care requisites. For example, Facteau (1980) described the nursing care of hospitalized infants, toddlers, and preschool-age and school-age children. Foote et al. (1993) described Self-Care Framework – based care of children with cancer. Gantz (1980) developed a health education program aimed at enhancing self-care agency for 10-year-old school children. Harrigan, Faro, Van Putte, and Stoler (1987) designed an educational program for juvenile diabetics that accounted for the children's locus of control orientation. Rew (1990) described Self-Care Framework–based nursing interventions for children who have been sexually abused. Atkins (1992) discussed issues in the care of children whose parents are mentally ill. Raven (1988–1989, 1989) discussed issues involved in the Self-Care Framework–based care of children and adults with developmental disabilities.

Nursing care guidelines for adolescent alcohol abusers were presented by Michael and Sewall (1980). Self-Care Framework–based nursing care of adults having such substance abuse problems as alcohol dependence (Dunn, 1990) and drug addiction (Compton, 1989) has also been described. Park (1989) outlined Self-Care Framework–based nursing care of homeless adults.

Harris (1980) used the Self-Care Framework to design nursing care for patients having cesarean childbirth. Oakley, Denyes, and O'Conner (1989) described nursing actions designed to promote effective use of contraceptives. Cretain (1989) discussed the promotion of breast self-examination within the content of the Self-Care Framework. Others have discussed the nursing care of patients with various cancers and cancer-related problems based on the framework (Mack, 1992; Meriney, 1990; Morse & Werner, 1988; Richardson, 1991; Whenery-Tedder, 1991). Petrlik (1976) focused on the adult with diabetic peripheral neuropathy.

Sullivan and Munroe (1986) explained how they adapted the Self-Care Framework for the elderly. Specific reports of the nursing care of the aged were offered by Garvan, Lee, Lloyd, and Sullivan (1980) and Finnegan (1986). O'Donovan (1990a, 1990b) described the Self-Care Framework–based nursing care of elderly people who are mentally ill. Blaylock (1991) and Priddy (1989) offered practical suggestions for the nursing care of elderly patients with ostomies, and Langley (1989) outlined a plan of care for an elderly, incontinent patient.

The Self-Care Framework has been extended for use with the family (Chin, 1985; Gray & Sergi, 1989; Orem, 1983a, 1983b, 1983c; Tadych, 1985). Moreover, Palmer (1993) discussed the advantages and disadvantages of Care-by-Parents units in inpatient settings. Steele et al. (1989) described how parents can provide home care for Down's syndrome children experiencing mild upper-respiratory infections. Haas (1990) identified issues involved in the dependent-care of chronically ill children.

The Self-Care Framework has also been extended for use in the community (Orem, 1984). Hanchett (1990) explained how the Self-Care Framework is used when the community is viewed as an aggregate of individuals. Taylor and McLaughlin (1991) explained that Orem's work is compatible with views of the community as an aggregate or collection, an

entity having meaning and purpose beyond the individual, and as relationships among groups of people. Nowakowski (1980) described a community health education program developed at Georgetown University.

Furthermore, the Self-Care Framework has been successfully
adapted for use in diverse cultures. Branch (1985) discussed requirements
for successful nursing care of black patients living in the United States.
Chamorro (1985) described Self-Care Framework-based nursing in Puerto
Rico. Hammonds (1985) described some of the self-care practices of Navajo Indians living in Shiprock, New Mexico. Morales-Mann and Jiang
(1993) described the use of the framework in Chinese nursing practice.

Social Congruence

The Self-Care Framework is generally congruent with contemporary
expectations regarding nursing practice. Riehl-Sisca (1985b) noted that
the self-care label associated with the Self-Care Framework is appealing
to nurses and to potential and actual patients. She pointed out that Orem's
approach to nursing "appeared on the scene when the general public was
becoming more knowledgeable about medical treatment and disen-
chanted with physicians' care and motivation. . . . In some cases, the
patient seems to know as much about his or her condition as does the
physician. This encourages the taking care of oneself" (p. 308).

The Self-Care Framework is congruent with society's expectations
that individuals should have decision-making responsibility regarding
their health care. Indeed, Bramlett, Gueldner, and Sowell (1990) noted
that Orem's assumptions about human beings and the overall focus of the
Self-Care Framework lead to the consumer-centric form of nursing advocacy. They commented, "Although Orem's framework does not explicitly
admonish paternalistically based advocacy, [it] specifies that advocacy
activities should be limited to only those instances when an individual is
incapable of complete self-care, and that such behaviors should be temporary, and clients should be provided with as much information regarding
their health as possible" (p. 160).

The emphasis on self-care agency during times of illness is, however,
not completely congruent with some people's expectations of nursing
practice. Moreover, attention must be given to expectations of people of
different regional and cultural groups. For example, Anna et al. (1978)
found that the nursing goal of self-care agency for the patient was not well
accepted by either patients or staff of a nursing home. In this situation, a
more dependent sick role view, with the nurse doing for and acting for the
patient, had been adopted by both patients and staff. Anna and associates
also noted that a Mexican-American patient in the nursing home "did not
see the relevance of performing self-care activities, and he functioned
with the expectation that the staff would do everything for him" (p. 11).
Similarly, Roach and Woods (1993) reported that although physicians and
many patients had positive responses to an Orem Self-Care Framework –

based cooperative care program, the program "was not attractive to all patients" (p. 28). They attributed the lack of acceptance of cooperative care "in part to the fact that many of our patients were older men from traditional southern backgrounds who were cared for by spouses and female relatives" even when the men were functionally able to care for themselves (p. 29).

Orem (1991) noted that when the person is able but reluctant to engage in self-care, he or she must be helped to view himself or herself as a self-care agent. Elaborating, she stated, "Self-care is performed largely out of habit, but individuals who have not thought about their self-care role may need to be helped to look at themselves as self-care agents in order to understand the values to which their habits commit them and to appraise the adequacy of their self-care abilities" (p. 147). Roach and Woods (1993) added that "In such instances, patients were encouraged to learn to care for themselves in case their spouse became unavailable or unable to do care giving" (p. 29).

Patients can be assisted to understand self-care and to become willing to participate actively in their care through the use of *The Self-Care Manual for Patients*, which was developed by Kyle and Pitzer (1990) for those purposes. They commented, "The key to the success of self-care is the transformation of individuals from passive, dependent patients to active partners" (p. 39).

In discussing the constraints on use of the Self-Care Framework of nursing in the United Kingdom, Behi (1986) stated, "Perhaps the most fundamental constraint in this country is society's attitude. Self-care as a concept, and more importantly, as a value, is stronger in American society where control of an individual's health is seen as that person's responsibility" (p. 35). Behi concluded, however, that the Self-Care Framework could be used in general wards of the National Health Service in the United Kingdom.

The primary prevention aspect of the Self-Care Framework is another area where attention to congruence with societal expectations must be given. Although consumers are becoming more aware of the value of health promotion and the nurse's role in promoting wellness, they still may need to be helped to accept that nursing role and utilize nursing services in that area.

Anecdotal and empirical evidence is beginning to support the speculative claims that the Self-Care Framework is generally congruent with the expectations of patients and health care team members for nursing care. Orem's (1991) list of nurses' reaction to use of the Self-Care Framework provides some anecdotal evidence of its social congruence. Particularly relevant points from the list are the following:

1. Nurses develop their personal styles of practice within the domain and boundaries of nursing set by the [framework].

2. Nurses (and physicians more slowly) recognize the need for nursing discharge of patients separate from medical discharge.

3. Nurses recognize that they have a theoretical base that serves them in performing the professional function of design of systems of nursing care. The design function is retained by and specific to the professional person.

4. Nurses through their design of systems of nursing bring into focus their own role responsibilities and role functions, as well as those of other nurses, their patients, and members of patients' families who are dependent-care agents. (pp. 74–75)

An addition to the anecdotal evidence comes from Doherty (1992), who commented that the Self-Care Framework made important contributions to her thinking about nursing care plans. Furthermore, Roach and Woods (1993) noted "Requests for [Orem Self-Care Framework–based] cooperative care were made by patients on repeat hospital admissions" (p. 29). Moreover, Scherer (1988) reported that use of the Self-Care Framework at the Beth Israel Medical Center in Newark, New Jersey is associated with enhanced patient satisfaction with nursing care, less staff turnover, and reduced costs. Empirical evidence was provided by Nunn and Marriner-Tomey (1989), who reported that in one survey at the Veterans Administration Medical Center in Indianapolis, Indiana, "30 out of 39 nurses perceived that [framework]-based practice would increase their job satisfaction, five said it wouldn't, and four were uncertain" (p. 67). In a survey of nursing attendants, 34 indicated that they believed patients would benefit from Self-Care Framework-based nursing practice, 2 did not believe patients would benefit, and 3 were uncertain (Nunn & Marriner-Tomey, 1989). Rossow-Sebring, Carrieri, and Seward (1992) reported that the evaluation of the implementation of the Self-Care Framework at the Veterans Administration Medical Center in Fresno, California, revealed "increase[d] staff nurses' satisfaction with nursing and enhanced [nursing] perception of the value of patient teaching" (p. 212).

Social Significance

Orem (1991) claimed that Self-Care Framework–based nursing practice compensates for or overcomes "health-associated human limitations for engagement in self-care or dependent-care" (p. 38). By doing so, nursing contributes to "health maintenance, prevention of disease and disability and to restoring and maintaining life processes" (p. 38). The empirical evidence supporting that claim is beginning to accrue. Buckwalter and Kerfoot's (1982) work suggested that psychiatric patient discharge teaching that emphasizes self-care was effective in areas such as compliance with psychotropic medication regimens and appropriate use of community resources. The emphasis on self-care agency and recognition of the person's ability to care for self could lead to more efficient use of health care services. In fact, Gulick's (1991) study findings revealed an intervention focusing on self-assessment and monitoring of functioning, and symptom prevalence resulted in less frequent use of professional health services by the experimental group of multiple sclerosis patients than by the control group during a 27-month period.

Thus, if people are helped to recognize and improve their own self-care abilities and to use health services only when they identify potential or actual self-care deficits, less inappropriate use of the services occurs. Furthermore, emphasis on self-care agency could reduce the length of time the person requires health care services. This may be especially important in the present era of cost containment.

The empirical evidence related to the social significance of the Self-Care Framework is, however, equivocal. Some study results reveal beneficial effects of framework-based nursing interventions, but other results fail to support the hypothesized benefits. Consequently, additional research is warranted. Furthermore, sufficient research now exists to support a meta-analysis that could determine the magnitude of effects and identify design and other study characteristics that may enhance understanding of the conflicting findings (Rosenthal, 1991).

Contributions to the Discipline of Nursing

The Self-Care Framework and the Theory of Self-Care Deficit, the Theory of Self-Care, and the Theory of Nursing System represent a substantial contribution to nursing knowledge by providing an explicit and specific focus for nursing actions that is different from that of other health care professions. Orem has fulfilled her goal of identifying the domain and boundaries of nursing as a science and an art.

The emphasis on self-care agency in the Self-Care Framework and the consideration given to the patient's perspective of health status underscore the importance of the person in the nursing care situation. The wide acceptance of the Self-Care Framework suggests that these features are especially attractive to nurses who view the person as capable of independent action. Moreover, the use of the model in many different settings and with different age groups suggests that that view of the person who is the patient may be an appropriate one for nursing.

Orem (personal communication, August 6, 1987) continues to develop aspects of the Self-Care Framework and the Theory of Self-Care, the Theory of Self-Care Deficit, and the Theory of Nursing System. She stated that her future work will focus specifically on "development of practice models, development of rules for practice when certain conditions prevail, continued study of 'foundational capabilities and dispositions' in their relationship to action, and development of . . . models for each of the power components of self-care agency." Although some progress on that work is evident in publications by Orem and others, much more remains to be done.

The needed Self-Care Framework–based nursing research, including systematic study of nursing practice outcomes, should be ensured by two organizations devoted to the study of self-care. The Self-Care Institute was established at George Mason University School of Nursing in Fairfax, Virginia, to develop, compile, and maintain a database consisting of individuals and organizations united across disciplines by a common interest in self-care and to promote self-care research. It should be noted that the interests of the Institute extend beyond Orem's approach to self-care to a consideration of self-care in a general manner. The International Orem Society for Nursing Science and Scholarship was founded in 1991 to "advance nursing science and scholarship through the use of Dorothea E. Orem's nursing conceptualizations in nursing education, practice, and research" (Bylaws of the International Orem Society for Nursing Science and Scholarship, April 1992, p. 1). The Society publishes a newsletter/journal that extends the *Self-Care Deficit Nursing Theory Newsletter* that had been published by the School of Nursing at the University of Missouri-Columbia. Furthermore, the volume and quality of nursing research dealing with self-care, including Orem's framework, certainly should be increased by the federally funded predoctoral and postdoctoral fellowship program that was established in 1992 at Wayne State University in Detroit, Michigan.

The Self-Care Framework has been adopted enthusiastically by many nurses. It presents an optimistic view of patients' contributions to their health care that is in keeping with currently evolving social values. Despite the many advantages of the Self-Care Framework, potential users are encouraged to continue to evaluate the effectiveness of the Self-Care Framework in nursing situations through systematic research so that its credibility may be more fully determined.

REFERENCES

Alexander, J.S., Younger, R.E., Cohen, R.M., & Crawford, L.V. (1988). Effectiveness of a nurse-managed program for children with chronic asthma. *Journal of Pediatric Nursing, 3*, 312–317.

Alford, D.M. (1985). Self-care practices in ambulatory nursing clinics for older adults. In J. Riehl-Sisca, *The science and art of self-care* (pp. 253–261). Norwalk, CT: Appleton-Century-Crofts.

Allison, S.E. (1971). The meaning of rest: An exploratory nursing study. In *ANA clinical sessions* (pp. 191–205). New York: Appleton-Century-Crofts.

Allison, S.E. (1973). A framework for nursing action in a nurse-conducted diabetic management clinic. *Journal of Nursing Administration, 3*(4), 53–60.

Allison, S.E. (1985). Structuring nursing practice based on Orem's theory of nursing: A nurse administrator's perspective.

In J. Riehl-Sisca, *The science and art of self-care* (pp. 225–235). Norwalk, CT: Appleton-Century-Crofts.

Anderson, S.B. (1992). Guillain-Barré syndrome: Giving the patient control. *Journal of Neuroscience Nursing, 24*, 158–162.

Angeles, D.M. (1991). An Orem-based NICU orientation checklist. *Neonatal Network, 9*(7), 43–48.

Anna, D.J., Christensen, D.G., Hohon, S.A., Ord, L., & Wells, S.R. (1978). Implementing Orem's conceptual framework. *Journal of Nursing Administration, 8*(11), 8–11.

Arneson, S.W., & Triplett, J.L. (1990). Riding with Bucklebear: An automobile safety program for preschoolers. *Journal of Pediatric Nursing, 5*, 115–122.

Arnold, M.B. (1960). Deliberate action. In *Emotion and personality. Vol. 11, Neurological and physiological aspects* (pp.

193–204). New York: Columbia University Press.

Atkins, F.D. (1992). An uncertain future: Children of mentally ill patients. *Journal of Psychosocial Nursing and Mental Health Services, 30*(8), 13–16.

Aukamp, V. (1988). Defining characteristics of knowledge deficit in the third trimester. In R.M. Carroll-Johnston (Ed.), *Classification of nursing diagnoses: Proceedings of the Eighth Conference: North American Nursing Diagnosis Association* (pp. 299–306). Philadelphia: JB Lippincott.

Avery, P. (1992). Self-care in the hospital setting: The Prince Henry Hospital experience. *Lamp, 49*(2), 26–28.

Backscheider, J.E. (1974). Self-care requirements, self-care capabilities and nursing systems in the diabetic nurse management clinic. *American Journal of Public Health, 64*, 1138–1146.

Baldwin, J., & Davis, L.L. (1989). Assessing parents as health educators. *Pediatric Nursing, 15*, 453–457.

Barnes, L.P. (1991). Teaching self-care to children. *American Journal of Maternal Child Nursing, 16*, 101.

Barnum, B.J.S. (1994). *Nursing theory: Analysis, application, evaluation* (4th ed.). Philadelphia: JB Lippincott.

Barron, M.L., Ganong, L.H., & Brown, M. (1987). An examination of preconception health teaching by nurse practitioners. *Journal of Advanced Nursing, 12*, 605–610.

Baulch, Y.S., Larson, P.J., Dodd, M.J., & Dietrich, C. (1992). The relationship of visual acuity, tactile sensitivity, and mobility of the upper extremities to proficient breast self-examination in women 65 and older. *Oncology Nursing Forum, 19*, 1367– 1372.

Beckmann, C.A. (1987). Maternal-child health in Brazil. *Journal of Obstetric, Gynecologic, and Neonatal Nursing, 16*, 238–241.

Beed, P. (1991). Sight restored. *Nursing Times, 87*(30), 46–48.

Behi, R. (1986). Look after yourself. *Nursing Times, 82*(37), 35–37.

Bennett, J.A., DeMayo, M., & Saint Germain, M. (1993). Caring in the time of AIDS: The importance of empathy. *Nursing Administration Quarterly, 17*(2), 46–60.

Berbiglia, V.A. (1991). A case study: Perspectives on a self-care deficit nursing theory-based curriculum. *Journal of Advanced Nursing, 16*, 1158–1163.

Bidigare, S.A., & Oermann, M.H. (1991). Attitudes and knowledge of nurses regarding organ procurement. *Heart and Lung, 20*, 20–24.

Biggs, A.J. (1990). Family care-giver versus nursing assessments of elderly self-care abilities. *Journal of Gerontological Nursing, 16*(8), 11–16.

Blaylock, B. (1991). Enhancing self-care of the elderly client: Practical teaching tips for ostomy care. *Journal of Enterostomal Therapy Nursing, 18*, 118–121.

Blazek, B., & McClellan, M. (1983). The effects of self-care instruction on locus of control in children. *Journal of School Health, 53*, 554–556.

Bliss-Holtz, V.J. (1988). Primiparas' prenatal concern for learning infant care. *Nursing Research, 37*, 20–24.

Bliss-Holtz, V.J. (1991). Developmental tasks of pregnancy and parental education. *International Journal of Childbirth Education, 6*(1), 29–31.

Bliss-Holtz, J., McLaughlin, K., & Taylor, S.G. (1990). Validating nursing theory for use within a computerized nursing information system. *Advances in Nursing Science, 13*(2), 46–52.

Bliss-Holtz, J., Taylor, S.G., & McLaughlin, K. (1992). Nursing theory as a base for a computerized nursing information system. *Nursing Science Quarterly, 5*, 124–128.

Bliss-Holtz, J., Taylor, S.G., McLaughlin, K., Sayers, P., & Nickle, L. (1992). Development of a computerized information system based on self-care deficit nursing theory. In J.M. Arnold & G.A. Pearson, *Computer applications in nursing education and practice* (pp. 87–93). New York: National League for Nursing.

Boon, E., & Graham, L. (1992). Hip arthroplasty for osteoarthritis. *British Journal of Nursing, 1*, 562–566.

Bracher, E. (1989). A model approach. *Nursing Times, 85*(43), 42–43.

Bramlett, M.H., Gueldner, S.H., & Sowell, R.L. (1990). Consumer-centric advocacy: Its connection to nursing frameworks. *Nursing Science Quarterly, 3*, 156–161.

Branch, M. (1985). Self-care: Black perspectives. In J. Riehl-Sisca, *The science and art of self-care* (pp. 181–188). Norwalk, CT: Appleton-Century-Crofts.

Brennan, M., & Duffy, M. (1992). Utilizing theory in practice to empower nursing. *Nursing Administration Quarterly, 16*(3), 32–33.

Brock, A.M., & O'Sullivan, P. (1985). A study to determine what variables predict institutionalization of elderly people. *Journal of Advanced Nursing, 10*, 533–537.

Buckley, H.B. (1990). Nurse practitioner intervention to improve postpartum appointment keeping in an outpatient family planning clinic. *Journal of the American Academy of Nurse Practitioners, 2*(1), 29–32.

Buckwalter, K.C., & Kerfoot, K.M. (1982). Teaching patients self care: A critical aspect of psychiatric discharge planning. *Journal of Psychiatric Nursing and Mental Health Services, 20*(5), 15–20.

Campbell, C. (1984). Orem's story. *Nursing Mirror, 159*(13), 28–30.

Campbell, J.C. (1986). Nursing assessment for risk of homicide with battered women. *Advances in Nursing Science, 8*(4), 36–51.

Campbell, J.C. (1989). A test of two explanatory models of women's responses to battering. *Nursing Research, 38*, 18–24.

Campuzano, M. (1982). Self-care following coronary artery bypass surgery. *Focus on Critical Care, 9*(2), 55–56.

Caradus, A. (1991). Nursing theory and operating suite nursing practice. *ACORN Journal, 4*(2), 29–30, 32.

Carlisle, J.B., Corser, N., Cull, V., DiMicco, W., Luther, L., McCaleb, A., Robuck, J., & Powell, K. (1993). Cardiovascular risk factors in young children. *Journal of Community Health Nursing, 10*, 1–9.

Chamorro, L.C. (1985). Self-care in the Puerto Rican community. In J. Riehl-Sisca, *The science and art of self-care* (pp. 189–195). Norwalk, CT: Appleton-Century-Crofts.

Chang, B., Uman, G., Linn, L., Ware, J., & Kane, R. (1984). The effect of systematically varying components of nursing care on satisfaction in elderly ambulatory women. *Western Journal of Nursing Research, 6*, 367–386.

Chang, B., Uman, G., Linn, L., Ware, J., & Kane, R. (1985). Adherence to health care regimens among elderly women. *Nursing Research, 34*, 27–31.

Chin, S. (1985). Can self-care theory be applied to families? In J. Riehl-Sisca, *The science and art of self-care* (pp. 56–62). Norwalk, CT: Appleton-Century-Crofts.

Clark, J., & Bishop, J. (1988). Model-making. *Nursing Times, 84*(27), 37–40.

Cleveland, S.A. (1989). Re: Perceived self-care agency: A LISREL factor analysis of Bickel and Hanson's Questionnaire [Letter to the editor]. *Nursing Research, 38*, 59.

Clinton, J.F., Denyes, M.J., Goodwin, J.O., & Koto, E.M. (1977). Developing criterion measures of nursing care: Case study of a process. *Journal of Nursing Administration, 7*(7), 41–45.

Compton, P. (1989). Drug abuse: A self-care deficit. *Journal of Psychosocial Nursing and Mental Health Services, 27*(3), 22–26.

Craig, C. (1989). Mr. Simpson's hip replacement, *Nursing (London), 3*(44), 12–19.

Cretain, G.K. (1989). Motivational factors in breast self-examination: Implications for nurses. *Cancer Nursing, 12*, 250–256.

Crews, J. (1972). Nurse-managed cardiac clinics. *Cardio-Vascular Nursing, 8*, 15–18.

Crockett, M.S. (1982). Self-reported coping histories of adult psychiatric and nonpsychiatric subjects and controls (Abstract). *Nursing Research, 31*, 122.

Davidhizar, R., & Cosgray, R. (1990). The use of Orem's model in psychiatric rehabilitation assessment. *Rehabilitation Nursing, 15*(1), 39–41.

Degenhart-Leskosky, S.M. (1989). Health education needs of adolescent and nonadolescent mothers. *Journal of Obstetric, Gynecologic, and Neonatal Nursing, 18*, 238–244.

Del Togno-Armanasco, V., Olivas, G.S., & Harter, S. (1989). Developing an integrated nursing care management model. *Nursing Management, 20*(10), 26–29.

Dennis, L.I. (1989). Soviet hospital nursing: A model for self-care. *Journal of Nursing Education, 28*, 76–77.

Denyes, M.J. (1982). Measurement of self-care agency in adolescents (Abstract). *Nursing Research, 31*, 63.

Denyes, M.J., Neuman, B.M., & Villarruel, A.M. (1991). Nursing actions to prevent and alleviate pain in hospitalized children. *Issues in Comprehensive Pediatric Nursing, 14*, 31–48.

Derstine, J.B. (1992). Theory-based advanced rehabilitation nursing: Is it a reality? *Holistic Nursing Practice, 6*(2), 1–6.

Dibner, L.A., & Murphy, J.S. (1991). Nurse entrepreneurs. *Journal of Psychosocial Nursing and Mental Health Services, 29*(5), 30–34.

Dier, K.A. (1987). A model for collaboration in nursing practice: Thailand and Canada. In K.J. Hannah, M. Reimer, W.C. Mills, & S. Letourneau (Eds.), *Clinical judgment and decision making: The future with nursing diagnosis* (pp. 323–327), New York: John Wiley & Sons.

Dodd, M.J. (1982). Assessing patient self-care for side effects of cancer chemotherapy— Part 1. *Cancer Nursing, 5*, 447–451.

Dodd, M.J. (1983). Self-care for side effects in cancer chemotherapy: An assessment of nursing interventions—Part 2. *Cancer Nursing, 6*, 63–67.

Dodd, M.J. (1984a). Measuring informational

intervention for chemotherapy knowledge and self-care behavior. *Research in Nursing and Health, 7,* 43–50.

Dodd, M.J. (1984b). Patterns of self-care in cancer patients receiving radiation therapy. *Oncology Nursing Forum, 11,* 23–27.

Dodd, M.J. (1987). Efficacy of proactive information on self-care in radiation therapy patients. *Heart and Lung, 16,* 538–544.

Dodd, M.J. (1988a). Efficacy of proactive information on self-care in chemotherapy patients. *Patient Education and Counseling, 11,* 215–225.

Dodd, M.J. (1988b). Patterns of self-care in patients with breast cancer. *Western Journal of Nursing Research, 10,* 7–24.

Doherty, S. (1992). Care plans—a personal view. *British Journal of Theatre Nursing, 2*(5), 4–5.

Dropkin, M.J. (1981). Development of a self-care teaching program for postoperative head and neck patients. *Cancer Nursing, 4,* 103–106.

Duffey, J., Miller, M.P., & Parlocha, P. (1993). Psychiatric home care: A framework for assessment and intervention. *Home Healthcare Nurse, 11*(2), 22–28.

Duman, L. (1992). [Nursing care based on Orem's theory.] *The Canadian Nurse, 88*(6), 36–39.

Duncan, S., & Murphy, F. (1988). Embracing a conceptual model. *The Canadian Nurse, 84*(4), 24–26.

Dunn, B. (1990). Alcohol dependency: Health promotion and Orem's model. *Nursing Standard, 4*(40), 34.

Dyer, S. (1990). Team work for personal patient care. *Nursing the Elderly, 3*(7), 28–30.

Ewing, G. (1989). The nursing preparation of stoma patients for self-care. *Journal of Advanced Nursing, 14,* 411–420.

Facteau, L.M. (1980). Self-care concepts and the care of the hospitalized child. *Nursing Clinics of North America, 15,* 145–155.

Fawcett, J., Archer, C.L., Becker, D., Brown, K.K., Gann, S., Wong, M.J., & Wurster, A.B. (1992). Guidelines for selecting a conceptual model of nursing: Focus on the individual patient. *Dimensions of Critical Care Nursing, 11,* 268–277.

Fawcett, J., Cariello, F.P., Davis, D.A., Farley, J., Zimmaro, D.M., & Watts, R.J. (1987). Conceptual models of nursing: Application to critical care nursing practice. *Dimensions of Critical Care Nursing, 6,* 202–213.

Feldsine, F. (1982). Options for transition into practice: Nursing process orientation program. *Journal of New York State Nurses' Association, 13,* 11–16.

Fenner, K. (1979). Developing a conceptual framework. *Nursing Outlook, 27,* 122–126.

Fernandez, R., Brennan, M.L., Alvarez, A.R., & Duffy, M.A. (1990). Theory-based practice: A model for nurse retention. *Nursing Administration Quarterly, 14*(4), 47–53.

Fernandez, R., & Wheeler, J.I. (1990). Organizing a nursing system through theory-based practice. In G.G. Mayer, M.J. Madden, & E. Lawrenz (Eds.), *Patient care delivery models* (pp. 63–83). Rockville, MD: Aspen.

Fields, L.M. (1987). A clinical application of the Orem nursing model in labor and delivery. *Emphasis: Nursing 2,* 102–108.

Finnegan, T. (1986). Self-care and the elderly. *New Zealand Nursing Journal, 79*(4), 10–13.

Fitch, M., Rogers, M., Ross E., Shea H., Smith, I., & Tucker, D. (1991). Developing a plan to evaluate the use of nursing conceptual frameworks. *Canadian Journal of Nursing Administration, 4*(1), 22–28.

Flanagan, M. (1991). Self-care for a leg ulcer. *Nursing Times, 87*(23), 67–68, 70, 72.

Flanagan, R. (1983). *Energy expenditure of normal females during three bathing techniques.* Unpublished thesis, University of Missouri, Columbia.

Foote, A., Holcombe, J., Piazza, D., & Wright, P. (1993). Orem's theory used as a guide for the nursing care of an eight-year-old child with leukemia. *Journal of Pediatric Oncology Nursing, 10*(1), 26–32.

Foster, P.C., & Janssens, N.P. (1985). Dorothea E. Orem. In Nursing Theories Conference Group, *Nursing theories: The base for professional nursing practice* (2nd ed., pp. 124–139). Englewood Cliffs, NJ: Prentice Hall.

Frederick, H.K., & Northam, E. (1938). *A textbook of nursing practice* (2nd ed.). New York: Macmillan.

Frey, M.A., & Fox, M.A. (1990). Assessing and teaching self-care to youths with diabetes mellitus. *Pediatric Nursing, 16,* 597–800.

Fukuda, N. (1990). Outcome standards for the client with chronic congestive heart failure. *Journal of Cardiovascular Nursing, 4*(3), 59–70.

Gallant, B.W., & McLane, A.M. (1979). Outcome criteria: A process for validation at the unit level. *Journal of Nursing Administration, 9*(1), 14–21.

Gammon, J. (1991). Coping with cancer: The role of self-care. *Nursing Practice, 4*(3), 11–15.

Gantz, S.B. (1980). A fourth-grade adventure in self-directed learning. *Topics in Clinical Nursing, 2*(2), 29–38.

Garvan, P., Lee, M., Lloyd K., & Sullivan, T.J. (1980). Self-care applied to the aged. *New Jersey Nurse, 10*(1), 3–5.

Gaut, D.A., & Kieckhefer, G.M. (1988). Assessment of self-care agency in chronically ill adolescents. *Journal of Adolescent Health Care, 9*, 55–60.

Geden, E.A. (1982). Effects of lifting techniques on energy expenditure: A preliminary investigation. *Nursing Research, 31*, 214–218.

Geden, E.A. (1985). The relationship between self-care theory and empirical research. In J. Riehl-Sisca, *The science and art of self-care* (pp. 265–270). Norwalk, CT: Appleton-Century-Crofts.

Germain, C.P., & Nemchik, R.M. (1989). Diabetes self-management and hospitalization. *Image: Journal of Nursing Scholarship, 20*, 74–78.

Goodwin, J.O. (1979). Programmed instruction for self-care following pulmonary surgery. *International Journal of Nursing Studies, 16*, 29–40.

Graff, B.M., Thomas, J.S., Hollingsworth, A.D., Cohen, S.M., & Rubin, M.M. (1992). Development of a postoperative self-assessment form. *Clinical Nurse Specialist, 6*, 47–50.

Gray, V.R., & Sergi, J.S. (1989). Family self-care. In P.J. Bomar (Ed.), *Nurses and family health promotion: Concepts, assessment, and interventions* (pp. 67–77). Baltimore: Williams & Wilkins.

Gulick, E.E. (1987). Parsimony and model confirmation of the ADL self-care scale for multiple sclerosis persons. *Nursing Research, 36*, 278–283.

Gulick, E.E. (1989). Model confirmation of the MS-related symptom checklist. *Nursing Research, 38*, 147–153.

Gulick, E.E. (1991). Self-assessed health and use of health services. *Western Journal of Nursing Research, 13*, 195–219.

Haas, D.L. (1990). Application of Orem's self-care deficit theory to the pediatric chronically ill population. *Issues in Comprehensive Pediatric Nursing, 13*, 253–264.

Hageman, P., & Ventura, M. (1981). Utilizing patient outcome criteria to measure the effects of a medication teaching regimen. *Western Journal of Nursing Research, 3*, 25–33.

Hagopian, G.A. (1991). The effects of a weekly radiation therapy newsletter on patients. *Oncology Nursing Forum, 18*, 1199–1203.

Hagopian, G.A., & Rubenstein, J.H. (1990). Effects of telephone call interventions on patients' well-being in a radiation therapy department. *Cancer Nursing, 13*, 339–344.

Hale, M., & Rhodes, G. (1985). *Care with a concept.* Chapel Hill, NC: Health Sciences Consortium. (Videotape).

Hamera, E.K., Peterson, K.A., Young, L.M., & Schaumloffel, M.M. (1992). Symptom monitoring in schizophrenia: Potential for enhancing self-care. *Archives of Psychiatric Nursing, 6*, 324–330.

Hamilton, L.W., & Creason, N.S. (1992). Mental status and functional abilities: Change in institutionalized elderly women. *Nursing Diagnosis, 3*, 81–86.

Hammonds, T.A. (1985). Self-care practices of Navajo Indians. In J. Riehl-Sisca, *The science and art of self-care* (pp. 171–180). Norwalk, CT: Appleton-Century-Crofts.

Hanchett, E.S. (1990). Nursing models and community as client. *Nursing Science Quarterly, 3*, 67–72.

Hanson, B.R., & Bickel, L. (1985). Development and testing of the questionnaire on perception of self-care agency. In J. Riehl-Sisca, *The science and art of self-care* (pp. 271–278). Norwalk, CT: Appleton-Century-Crofts.

Hanucharurnkul, S. (1989). Predictors of self-care in cancer patients receiving radiotherapy. *Cancer Nursing, 12*, 21–27.

Harman, L., Wabin, D., MacInnis, L., Baird, D., Mattiuzzi, D., & Savage, P. (1989). Developing clinical decision-making skills in staff nurses: An educational program. *Journal of Continuing Education in Nursing, 20*, 102–106.

Harper, D. (1984). Application of Orem's theoretical constructs to self-care medication behaviors in the elderly. *Advances in Nursing Science, 6*(3), 29–46.

Harrigan, J.F., Faro, B.Z., VanPutte, A., & Stoler, P. (1987). The application of locus of control to diabetes education in school-aged children. *Journal of Pediatric Nursing, 2*, 236–243.

Harris, J.K. (1980). Self-care is possible after cesarean delivery. *Nursing Clinics of North America, 15*, 191–204.

Harris, J.L., & Williams, L.K. (1991). Universal self-care requisites as identified by homeless elderly men. *Journal of Gerontological Nursing, 17*(6), 39–43.

Harrison, L.L., & Novak, D. (1988). Evaluation of a gerontological nursing continuing education programme: Effect on nurses' knowledge and attitudes and on patients' perceptions and satisfaction. *Journal of Advanced Nursing, 13,* 684–692.

Hartweg, D. (1993). Self-care actions of healthy middle-aged women to promote well-being. *Nursing Research, 42,* 221–227.

Hathaway, D.K., & Geden, E.A. (1983). Energy expenditure during leg exercise programs. *Nursing Research, 32,* 147–150.

Hathaway, D., & Strong, M. (1988). Theory, practice, and research in transplant nursing. *Journal of the American Nephrology Nurses Association, 15,* 9–12.

Hautman, M.A. (1987). Self-care responses to respiratory illnesses among Vietnamese. *Western Journal of Nursing Research, 9,* 223–243.

Hayward, M.B., Kish, J.P., Jr., Frey, G.M., Kirchner, J.M., Carr, L.S., & Wolfe, C.M. (1989). An instrument to identify stressors in renal transplant recipients. *Journal of the American Nephrology Nurses Association, 16,* 81–84.

Hedahl, K. (1983). Assisting the adolescent with physical disabilities through a college health program. *Nursing Clinics of North America, 18,* 257–274.

Henderson, V. (1955). *Textbook of the principles and practice of nursing* (5th ed.). New York: Macmillan.

Herrington, J., & Houston, S. (1984). Using Orem's theory: A plan for all seasons. *Nursing and Health Care, 5*(1), 45–47.

Hiromoto, B.M., & Dungan, J. (1991). Contract learning for self-care activities: A protocol study among chemotherapy outpatients. *Cancer Nursing, 14,* 148–154.

Hooten, S.L. (1992). Education of staff nurses to practice within a conceptual framework. *Nursing Administration Quarterly, 16*(3), 34–35.

Horn, B. (1978). Development of criterion measures of nursing care. (Abstract). In *Communicating nursing research. Vol 11:* New approaches to communicating nursing research (pp. 87–89). Boulder, CO: Western Interstate Commission for Higher Education.

Horn, B.J., & Swain, M.A. (1977). *Development of criterion measures of nursing care* (Vols. 1–2, NTIS Nos. PB-267 004 and PB-267 005). Ann Arbor, MI: University of Michigan.

Hughes, M.M. (1983). Nursing theories and emergency nursing. *Journal of Emergency Nursing, 9,* 95–97.

Humphreys, J. (1991). Children of battered women: Worries about their mothers. *Pediatric Nursing, 17,* 342–345, 354.

Hunter, L. (1992). Applying Orem to skin. *Nursing (London), 5*(4), 16–18.

Hurst, J.D., & Stullenbarger, B. (1986). Implementation of a self-care approach in a pediatric interdisciplinary phenylketonuria (PKU) clinic. *Journal of Pediatric Nursing, 1,* 159–163.

Huss, K., Salerno, M., & Huss, R.W. (1991). Computer-assisted reinforcement of instruction: Effects on adherence in adult atopic asthmatics. *Research in Nursing and Health, 14,* 259–267.

Husted, E., & Strzelecki, S. (1985). Orem: A foundation for nursing practice in a community hospital. In J. Riehl-Sisca, *The science and art of self-care* (pp. 199–207). Norwalk, CT: Appleton-Century-Crofts.

Jacobs, C.J. (1990). Orem's self-care model: Is it relevant to patients in intensive care? *Intensive Care Nursing, 6,* 100–103.

James, L.A. (1992). Nursing theory made practical. *Journal of Nursing Education, 31,* 42–44.

Jenny, J. (1988). Classification of nursing diagnosis: A self-care approach. In R.M. Carroll-Johnston (Ed.), *Classification of nursing diagnoses: Proceedings of the Eighth Conference: North American Nursing Diagnosis Association* (pp. 152–157). Philadelphia: JB Lippincott.

Jenny, J. (1989). Classifying nursing diagnoses: A self-care approach. *Nursing and Health Care, 10,* 83–88.

Jenny, J. (1991). Self-care deficit theory and nursing diagnosis: A test of conceptual fit. *Journal of Nursing Education, 30,* 227–232.

Jenny, J. (1992). Self-care taxonomy [Letter to the editor]. *Nursing Diagnosis, 3*(1), 44.

Johannsen, J.M. (1992). Self-care assessment: Key to teaching and discharge planning. *Dimensions of Critical Care Nursing, 11,* 48–56.

Jopp, M., Carroll, M.C., Waters, L. (1993). Using self-care theory to guide nursing management of the older adult after hospitalization. *Rehabilitation Nursing, 18,* 91–94.

Kam, B.W., & Werner, P.W. (1990). Self-care theory: Application to perioperative nursing. *Association of Operating Room Nurses Journal, 51,* 1365–1370.

Karl, C. (1982). The effect of an exercise program on self-care activities for the institutionalized elderly. *Journal of Gerontological Nursing, 8,* 282–285.

Kearney, B.Y., & Fleischer, B.J. (1979). Development of an instrument to measure exercise of self-care agency. *Research in Nursing and Health, 2,* 25–34.

Kerkstra, A., Castelein, E., & Philipsen, H. (1991). Preventive home visits to elderly people by community nurses in the Netherlands. *Journal of Advanced Nursing, 16,* 631–637.

Kirkpatrick, M.K., Brewer, J.A., & Stocks, B. (1990). Efficacy of self-care measures for premenstrual syndrome (PMS). *Journal of Advanced Nursing, 15,* 281–285.

Kitson, A.L. (1986). Indicators of quality in nursing care—an alternative approach. *Journal of Advanced Nursing, 11,* 133–144.

Komulainen, P. (1991). Occupational health nursing based on self-care theory. *American Association of Occupational Health Nursing Journal, 39,* 333–335.

Kotarbinski, T. (1965). *Praxiology: An introduction to the sciences of efficient action* (Trans. O. Wojtasiewicz). New York: Pergamon Press.

Kruger, S.F. (1988). The application of the self-care concept of nursing in the Wichita State University baccalaureate program. *Kansas Nurse, 63*(12), 6–7.

Kubricht, D. (1984). Therapeutic self-care demands expressed by outpatients receiving external radiation therapy. *Cancer Nursing, 7,* 43–52.

Kyle, B.A.S., & Pitzer, S.A. (1990). A self-care approach to today's challenges. *Nursing Management, 21*(3), 37–39.

Lacey, D. (1993). Using Orem's model in psychiatric nursing. *Nursing Standard, 7*(29), 28–30.

Lakin, J.A. (1988). Self-care, health locus of control, and health value among faculty women. *Public Health Nursing, 5,* 37–44.

Langland, R.M., & Farrah, S.J. (1990). Using a self-care framework for continuing education in gerontological nursing. *Journal of Continuing Education in Nursing, 21,* 267–270.

Langley, T. (1989). Please, deliver more incontinence pads. *Nursing Times, 85*(15), 73–75.

Laschinger, H.S. (1990). Helping students apply a nursing conceptual framework in the clinical setting. *Nurse Educator, 15*(3), 20–24.

Laurie-Shaw, B., & Ives, S.M. (1988a). Implementing Orem's self-care deficit theory: Part I—Selecting a framework and planning for implementation. *Canadian Journal of Nursing Administration, 1*(1), 9–12.

Laurie-Shaw, B., & Ives, S.M. (1988b). Part II: Implementing Orem's self-care deficit theory—Adopting a conceptual framework of nursing. *Canadian Journal of Nursing Administration, 1*(2), 16–19.

Leatt, P., Bay, K.S., & Stinson, S.M. (1981). An instrument for assessing and classifying patients by type of care. *Nursing Research, 30,* 145–150.

Lonergan, B.J.F. (1958). *Insight: A study of human understanding.* New York: Philosophical Library.

Lorensen, M., Holter, I.M., Evers, G.C., Isenberg, M.A., van Achterberg, T. (1993). Cross-cultural testing of the appraisal of self-care agency: ASA scale in Norway. *International Journal of Nursing Studies, 30,* 15–23.

Lott, T.F., Blazey, M.E., & West, M.G. (1992). Patient participation in health care: An underused resource. *Nursing Clinics of North America, 27,* 61–76.

MacDonald, G. (1991). Plans for a better future. *Nursing Times, 87*(31), 42–43.

Mack, C.H. (1992). Assessment of the autologous bone marrow transplant patient according to Orem's self-care model. *Cancer Nursing, 15,* 429–436.

MacLellan, M. (1989). Community care of a patient with multiple sclerosis. *Nursing (London), 3*(33), 28–32.

MacSweeny, J. (1992). A helpful assessment. *Nursing Times, 88*(29), 32–33.

Malik, U. (1992). Women's knowledge, beliefs and health practices about breast cancer and breast self-examination. *Nursing Journal of India, 83,* 186–190.

Marriner-Tomey, A. (1989). *Nursing theorists and their work* (2nd ed.). St. Louis: CV Mosby.

Mason, T., & Chandley, M. (1990). Nursing models in a special hospital: A critical analysis of efficacity. *Journal of Advanced Nursing, 15,* 667–673.

Maunz, E.R., & Woods, N.F. (1988). Self-care practices among young adult women: Influence of symptoms, employment, and sex-role orientation. *Health Care for Women International, 9,* 29–41.

McBride, S. (1987). Validation of an instrument to measure exercise of self-care agency. *Research in Nursing and Health, 10,* 311–316.

McCord, A.S. (1990). Teaching for tonsillectomies: Details mean better compliance. *Today's OR Nurse, 12*(6), 11–14.

McCoy, S. (1989). Teaching self-care in a market-oriented world. *Nursing Management, 20*(5), 22, 26.

McDermott, M.A.N. (1993). Learned helplessness as an interacting variable with self-care agency: Testing a theoretical model. *Nursing Science Quarterly*, 6, 28–38.

McFarland, S.M., Sasser, L., Boss, B.J., Dickerson, J.I., & Stelling, J.D. (1992). Self Care Assessment Tool for spinal cord injured persons. *SCI Nursing*, 9, 111–116.

McKeighen, R.J., Mehmert, P.A., & Dickel, C.A. (1991). Self-care deficit, bathing/hygiene: Defining characteristics and related factors utilized by staff nurses in an acute care setting. In R.M. Carroll-Johnston (Ed.), *Classification of nursing diagnosis: Proceedings of the Ninth Conference: North American Nursing Diagnosis Association* (pp. 247–248). Philadelphia: JB Lippincott.

McLaughlin, K., Taylor, S., Bliss-Holtz, J., Sayers, P., & Nickle, L. (1990). Shaping the future: The marriage of nursing theory and informatics. *Computers in Nursing*, 8, 174–179.

McVay, J. (1985). A beginning of service and caring. In J. Riehl-Sisca, *The science and art of self-care* (pp. 245–252). Norwalk, CT: Appleton-Century-Crofts.

McWilliams, B., Murphy, F., & Sobiski, A. (1988). Why self-care theory works for us. *The Canadian Nurse*, 84(9), 38–40.

Meeker, B.J., Rodriguez, L., & Johnson, J.M. (1992). A comprehensive analysis of preoperative patient education. *Today's OR Nurse*, 14(3), 11–18, 33–34.

Meleis, A.I. (1991). *Theoretical nursing: Development and progress* (2nd ed.). Philadelphia: JB Lippincott.

Meriney, D.K. (1990). Application of Orem's conceptual framework to patients with hypercalcemia related to breast cancer. *Cancer Nursing*, 13, 316–323.

Michael, M.M., & Sewall, K.S. (1980). Use of the adolescent peer group to increase the self-care agency of adolescent alcohol abusers. *Nursing Clinics of North America*, 15, 157–176.

Miller, J. (1989). DIY health care. *Nursing Standard*, 3(43), 35–37.

Miller, J.F. (1980). The dynamic focus of nursing: A challenge to nursing administration. *Journal of Nursing Administration*, 10(1), 13–18.

Miller, J.F. (1982). Categories of self-care needs of ambulatory patients with diabetes. *Journal of Advanced Nursing*, 7, 25–31.

Mitchell, P., & Irvin, N. (1977). Neurological examination: Nursing assessment for nursing purposes. *Journal of Neurosurgical Nursing*, 9(1), 23–28.

Monsen, R.B. (1992). Autonomy, coping, and

self-care agency in healthy adolescents and in adolescents with spina bifida. *Journal of Pediatric Nursing*, 7, 9–13.

Moore, J.B. (1987a). Determining the relationship of autonomy to self-care agency or locus of control in school-age children. *Maternal-Child Nursing Journal*, 16, 47–60.

Moore, J.B. (1987b). Effects of assertion training and first aid instruction on children's autonomy and self-care agency. *Research in Nursing and Health*, 10, 101–109.

Moore, J.B. (1993). Predictors of children's self-care performance: Testing the theory of self-care deficit. *Scholarly Inquiry for Nursing Practice*, 7, 199–212.

Moore, J.B., & Gaffney, K.F. (1989). Development of an instrument to measure mothers' performance of self-care activities for children. *Advances in Nursing Science*, 12(1), 76–83.

Moore, R. (1989). Diogenes syndrome. *Nursing Times*, 85(30), 46–48.

Morales-Mann, E.T., & Jiang, S.L. (1993). Applicability of Orem's conceptual framework: A cross-cultural point of view. *Journal of Advanced Nursing*, 18, 737–741.

Morse, W., & Werner, J.S. (1988). Individualization of patient care using Orem's theory. *Cancer Nursing*, 11, 195–202.

Moscovitz, A. (1984). Orem's theory as applied to psychiatric nursing. *Perspectives in Psychiatric Care*, 22(1), 36–38.

Mulkeen, H. (1989). Diabetes: Teaching the teaching of self-care. *Nursing Times*, 85(3), 63–65.

Mullin, V.I. (1980). Implementing the self-care concept in the acute care setting. *Nursing Clinics of North America*, 15, 177–190.

Mullin, V.I., & Weed, F. (1980, October). *Orem's self-care concept as a conceptual framework for a nursing curriculum*. Paper presented at Virginia Nurses' Association State Convention.

Munley, M.J., & Sayers, P.A. (1984). *Self-care deficit theory of nursing: A primer for application of the concepts*. North Brunswick, NJ: Personal and Family Health Associates.

Murphy, P.P. (1981). A hospice model and self-care theory. *Oncology Nursing Forum*, 8(2), 19–21.

Neil, R.M. (1984). Self care agency and spouses/companions of alcoholics. *Kansas Nurse*, 59(10), 3–4.

Norris, M.K.G. (1991). Applying Orem's theory to the long-term care of adolescent transplant recipients. *American Nephrol-*

ogy *Nurses' Association Journal, 18*, 45–47, 53.

Nowakowski, L. (1980). Health promotion/self-care programs for the community. *Topics in Clinical Nursing, 2*(2), 21–27.

Nunn, D., & Marriner-Tomey, A. (1989). Applying Orem's model in nursing administration. In B. Henry, C. Arndt, M. DiVincenti, & A. Marriner-Tomey (Eds.), *Dimensions of nursing administration: Theory, research, education, practice* (pp. 63–67). Boston: Blackwell Scientific Publications.

Nursing Development Conference Group. (1973). *Concept formalization in nursing: Process and product.* Boston: Little, Brown.

Nursing Development Conference Group. (1979). *Concept formalization in nursing: Process and product.* Boston: Little, Brown.

Oakley, D., Denyes, M.J., & O'Connor, N. (1989). Expanded nursing care for contraceptive use. *Applied Nursing Research, 2*, 121–127.

Oberst, M.T., Hughes, S.H., Chang, A.S., & McCubbin, M.A. (1991). Self-care burden, stress appraisal, and mood among persons receiving radiotherapy. *Cancer Nursing, 14*, 71–78.

O'Connor, C.T. (1990). Patient education with a purpose. *Journal of Nursing Staff Development, 6*, 145–147.

O'Donovan, S. (1990a). Nursing models: More of Orem. *Nursing the Elderly, 2*(3), 22–23.

O'Donovan, S. (1990b). Nursing models: More of Orem—Part 2. *Nursing the Elderly, 2*(4), 20–22.

Orem, D.E. (1956). *Hospital nursing service: An analysis.* Indianapolis: Division of Hospital and Institutional Services of the Indiana State Board of Health.

Orem, D.E. (1959). *Guides for developing curricula for the education of practical nurses.* Washington, DC: US Government Printing Office.

Orem, D.E. (1971). *Nursing: Concepts of practice.* New York: McGraw-Hill.

Orem, D.E. (1978, December). *A general theory of nursing.* Paper presented at the Second Annual Nurse Educator Conference, New York. (Cassette recording).

Orem, D.E. (1980). *Nursing: Concepts of practice* (2nd ed.). New York. McGraw-Hill.

Orem, D.E. (1983a). The family coping with a medical illness: Analysis and application of Orem's theory. In I.W. Clements & F.B. Roberts, *Family health: A theoretical*

approach to nursing care (pp. 385–386). New York: John Wiley & Sons.

Orem, D.E. (1983b). The family experiencing emotional crisis. Analysis and application of Orem's self-care deficit theory. In I.W. Clements & F.B. Roberts, *Family health: A theoretical approach to nursing care* (pp. 367–368). New York: John Wiley & Sons.

Orem, D.E. (1983c). The self-care deficit theory of nursing: A general theory. In I.W. Clements & F.B. Roberts, *Family health: A theoretical approach to nursing care* (pp. 205–217). New York: John Wiley & Sons.

Orem, D.E. (1984). Orem's conceptual model and community health nursing. In M.K. Asay & C.C. Ossler (Eds.), *Conceptual models of nursing: Applications in community health nursing. Proceedings of the Eighth Annual Community Health Nursing Conference* (pp. 35–50). Chapel Hill: Department of Public Health Nursing, School of Public Health, University of North Carolina.

Orem, D.E. (1985). *Nursing: Concepts of practice* (3rd ed.). New York: McGraw-Hill.

Orem, D.E. (1989). Theories and hypotheses for nursing administration. In B. Henry, M. DiVincenti, C. Arndt, & A. Marriner (Eds.), *Dimensions of nursing administration: Theory, research, education and practice* (pp. 55–62). Boston: Blackwell Scientific Publications.

Orem, D.E. (1990). A nursing practice theory in three parts, 1956–1989. In M.E. Parker (Ed.), *Nursing theories in practice* (pp. 47–60). New York: National League for Nursing.

Orem, D.E. (1991). *Nursing: Concepts of practice* (4th ed.). St. Louis: Mosby-Year Book.

Orem, D.E., & Taylor, S.G. (1986). Orem's general theory of nursing. In P. Winstead-Fry (Ed.), *Case studies in nursing theory* (pp. 37–71). New York: National League for Nursing.

Padilla, G.V., & Grant, M.M. (1982). Quality assurance programme for nursing. *Journal of Advanced Nursing, 7*, 135–145.

Palmer, P., & Meyers, F.J. (1990). An outpatient approach to the delivery of intensive consolidation chemotherapy to adults with acute lymphoblastic leukemia. *Oncology Nursing Forum, 17*, 553–558.

Palmer, S.J. (1993). Care of sick children by parents: A meaningful role. *Journal of Advanced Nursing, 18*, 185–191.

Park, P.B. (1989). Health care for the homeless: A self-care approach. *Clinical Nurse Specialist, 3*, 171–175.

Parsons, T. (1937). *The structure of social action.* New York: McGraw-Hill.

Parsons, T. (1951). *The social system.* New York: The Free Press.

Paternostro, I. (1992). Developing theory-based software for nurses, by nurses. *Nursing Administration Quarterly, 16*(3), 33–34.

Patterson, E., & Hale, E. (1985). Making sure: Integrating menstrual care practices into activities of daily living. *Advances in Nursing Science, 7*(3), 18–31.

Perras, S., & Zappacosta, A. (1982). The application of Orem's theory in promoting self-care in a peritoneal dialysis facility. *American Association of Nephrology Nurses and Technicians Journal, 9*(3), 37–39.

Petrlik, J.C. (1976). Diabetic peripheral neuropathy. *American Journal of Nursing, 76*, 1794–1797.

Phillips, J.R. (1977). Nursing systems and nursing models. *Image, 9*, 4–7.

Piemme, J.A., & Trainor, M.A. (1977). A first-year nursing course in a baccalaureate program. *Nursing Outlook, 25*, 184–187.

Porter, D., & Shamian, J. (1983). Self-care in theory and practice. *The Canadian Nurse, 79*(8), 21–23.

Porter, L., Youssef, M., Shaaban, I., & Ibrahim, W. (1992). Parenting enhancement among Egyptian mothers in a tertiary care setting. *Pediatric Nursing, 18*, 329–336, 386.

Priddy, J. (1989). Surgical care of the elderly. Home help. *Nursing Times, 85*(29), 30–32.

Raven, M. (1988–1989). Application of Orem's self-care model to nursing practice in developmental disability. *Australian Journal of Advanced Nursing, 6*(2), 16–23.

Raven, M. (1989). A conceptual model for care in developmental disability services. *Australian Journal of Advanced Nursing, 6*(4), 10–17.

Redfern, S. (1990). Care after a stroke. *Nursing (London), 4*(4), 7–11.

Rew, L. (1987). Children with asthma: The relationship between illness behaviors and health locus of control. *Western Journal of Nursing Research, 9*, 465–483.

Rew, L. (1990). Childhood sexual abuse: Toward a self-care framework for nursing intervention and research. *Archives of Psychiatric Nursing, 4*, 147–153.

Reid, B., Allen, A.F., Gauthier, T., & Campbell, H. (1989). Solving the Orem mystery:

An educational strategy. *Journal of Continuing Education in Nursing, 20*, 108–110.

Rhodes, V.A., Watson, P.M., & Hanson, B.M. (1988). Patients' descriptions of the influence of tiredness and weakness on self-care abilities. *Cancer Nursing, 11*, 186–194.

Richardson, A. (1991). Theories of self-care: Their relevance to chemotherapy-induced nausea and vomiting. *Journal of Advanced Nursing, 16*, 671–676.

Richeson, M., & Huch, M. (1988). Self-care and comfort: A framework for nursing practice. *New Zealand Nursing Journal, 81*(6), 26–27.

Riehl, J.P., & Roy, C. (1980). *Conceptual models for nursing practice* (2nd ed.). New York: Appleton-Century-Crofts.

Riehl-Sisca, J. (1985a). Determining criteria for graduate and undergraduate self-care curriculums. In J. Riehl-Sisca, *The science and art of self-care* (pp. 20–24). Norwalk, CT: Appleton-Century-Crofts.

Riehl-Sisca, J. (1985b). Epilogue: Future implications for the science and art of self-care. In J. Riehl-Sisca, *The science and art of self-care* (pp. 307–309). Norwalk, CT: Appleton-Century-Crofts.

Riehl-Sisca, J. (1985c). *The science and art of self-care.* Norwalk, CT: Appleton-Century-Crofts.

Riehl-Sisca, J.P. (1989). *Conceptual models for nursing practice* (3rd ed.). Norwalk, CT: Appleton & Lange.

Roach, K.G., & Woods, H.B. (1993). Implementing cooperative care on an acute care medical unit. *Clinical Nurse Specialist, 7*, 26–29.

Robichaud-Ekstrand, S. (1990). [Orem in medical-surgical nursing.] *The Canadian Nurse, 86*(5), 42–47.

Robinson, K.D., & Posner, J.D. (1992). Patterns of self-care needs and interventions related to biologic response modifier therapy: Fatigue as a model. *Seminars in Oncology Nursing, 8*(4, Suppl 1), 17–22.

Rosenthal, R. (1991). *Meta-analytic procedures for social research* (rev. ed.). Newbury Park, CA: Sage.

Rossow-Sebring, J., Carrieri, V., & Seward, H. (1992). Effect of Orem's model on nurse attitudes and charting behavior. *Journal of Nursing Staff Development, 8*, 207–212.

Rothlis, J. (1984). The effect of a self-help group on feelings of hopelessness and helplessness. *Western Journal of Nursing Research, 6*, 157–173.

Ruddick-Bracken, H., & Mackie, N. (1989).

Helping the workers help themselves. *Nursing Times*, 85(24), 75–76.

Sandman, P.O., Norberg, A., Adolfsson, R., Alexsson, K., & Hedley, V. (1986). Morning care of patients with Alzheimer-type dementia: A theoretical model based on direct observation. *Journal of Advanced Nursing*, 11, 369–378.

Schafer, S.L. (1989). An aggressive approach to promoting health responsibility. *Journal of Gerontological Nursing*, 15(4), 22–27.

Scherer, P. (1988). Hospitals that attract (and keep) nurses. *American Journal of Nursing*, 88, 34–40.

Seideman, R.Y. (1990). Effects of a premenstrual syndrome education program on premenstrual symptomatology. *Health Care for Women International*, 11, 491–501.

Siebert, K.D., Ganong, L.H., Hagemann, V., & Coleman, M. (1986). Nursing students' perceptions of a child: Influence of information on family structure. *Journal of Advanced Nursing*, 11, 333–337.

Smith, M.C. (1977). Self-care: A conceptual framework for rehabilitation nursing. *Rehabilitation Nursing*, 2(2), 8–10.

Smith, M.C. (1979). Proposed metaparadigm for nursing research and theory development: An analysis of Orem's self-care theory. *Image*, 11, 75–79.

Smith, M.J. (1987). A critique of Orem's theory. In R.R. Parse, *Nursing science: Major paradigms, theories, and critiques* (pp. 91–105). Philadelphia: WB Saunders.

Smith, J.M., & Sorrell, V. (1989). Developing wellness programs: A nurse-managed stay well center for senior citizens. *Clinical Nurse Specialist*, 3, 198–202.

Smits, J., & Kee, C.C. (1992). Correlates of self-care among the independent elderly: Self-concept affects well-being. *Journal of Gerontological Nursing*, 18(9), 13–18.

Snyder, M., Brugge-Wiger, P., Ahern, S., Connelly, S., De Pew, C., Kappas-Larson, P., Semmerling, E., & Wyble, S. (1991). Complex health problems: Clinically assessing self-management abilities. *Journal of Gerontological Nursing*, 17(4), 23–27.

Steele, N.F., & Sterling, Y.M. (1992). Application of the case study design: Nursing interventions for discharge readiness. *Clinical Nurse Specialist*, 6, 79–84.

Steele, S., Russell, F., Hansen, B., & Mills, B. (1989). Home management of URI in children with Down syndrome. *Pediatric Nursing*, 15, 484–488.

Storm, D.S., & Baumgartner, R.G. (1987). Achieving self-care in the ventilator-dependent patient: A critical analysis of a case study. *International Journal of Nursing Studies*, 24, 95–106.

Stockdale-Woolley, R. (1984). The effects of education on self-care agency. *Public Health Nursing*, 1, 97–106.

Story, E.L., & Ross, M.M. (1986). Family centered community health nursing and the Betty Neuman Systems Model. *Nursing Papers*, 18(2), 77–88.

Sullivan, T., & Monroe, D. (1986). A self-care practice theory of nursing the elderly. *Educational Gerontology*, 12, 13–26.

Swindale, J.E. (1989). The nurse's role in giving pre-operative information to reduce anxiety in patients admitted to hospital for elective minor surgery. *Journal of Advanced Nursing*, 14, 899–905.

Tadych, R. (1985). Nursing in multiperson units: The family. In J. Riehl-Sisca, *The science and art of self-care* (pp. 49–55). Norwalk, CT: Appleton-Century-Crofts.

Taira, F. (1991). Individualized medication sheets. *Nursing Economics*, 9, 56–58.

Taylor, S.G. (1985a). Curriculum development for preservice programs using Orem's theory of nursing. In J. Riehl-Sisca, *The science and art of self-care* (pp. 25–32). Norwalk, CT: Appleton-Century-Crofts.

Taylor, S.G. (1985b). Teaching self-care deficit theory to generic students. In J. Riehl-Sisca, *The science and art of self-care* (pp. 41–46). Norwalk, CT: Appleton-Century-Crofts.

Taylor, S.G. (1987). A model for nursing diagnosis and clinical decision making using Orem's self-care deficit theory of nursing. In K.J. Hannah, M. Reimer, W.C. Mills, & S. Letourneau (Eds.), *Clinical judgment and decision making: The future with nursing diagnosis* (pp. 84–86). New York: John Wiley & Sons.

Taylor, S.G. (1990). Practical applications of Orem's self-care deficit nursing theory. In M.E. Parker (Ed.), *Nursing theories in practice* (pp. 61–70). New York: National League for Nursing.

Taylor, S.G. (1991). The structure of nursing diagnoses from Orem's theory. *Nursing Science Quarterly*, 4, 24–32.

Taylor, S.G., & McLaughlin, K. (1991). Orem's general theory of nursing and community nursing. *Nursing Science Quarterly*, 4, 153–160.

Thomas, J.S., Graff, B.M., Hollingsworth, A.O., Cohen, S.M., & Rubin, M.M. (1992). Home visiting for a posthysterectomy population. *Home Healthcare Nurse*, 10(3), 47–52.

Titus, S., & Porter, P. (1989). Orem's theory applied to pediatric residential treatment. *Pediatric Nursing, 15,* 465–468, 556.

Tolentino, M.B. (1990). The use of Orem's self-care model in the neonatal intensive care unit. *Journal of Obstetric, Gynecologic, and Neonatal Nursing, 19,* 496–500.

Toth, J.C. (1980). Effect of structured preparation for transfer on patient anxiety on leaving coronary care unit. *Nursing Research, 29,* 28–34.

Turner, K. (1989). Orem's model and patient teaching. *Nursing Standard, 50*(3), 32–33.

Utz, S.W., & Ramos, M.C. (1993). Mitral value prolapse and its effects: A programme of inquiry within Orem's self-care deficit theory of nursing. *Journal of Advanced Nursing, 18,* 742–751.

van Achterberg, T., Lorensen, M., Isenberg, M.A., Evers, G.C.M., Levin, E., & Philipsen, H. (1991). The Norwegian, Danish and Dutch version of the Appraisal of Self-Care Agency Scale: Comparing reliability aspects. *Scandinavian Journal of Caring Sciences, 5,* 101–108.

Van Eron, M. (1985). Clinical application of self-care deficit theory. In J. Riehl-Sisca, *The science and art of self-care* (pp. 208–224). Norwalk, CT: Appleton-Century-Crofts.

Vasquez, M.A. (1992). From theory to practice: Orem's self-care nursing model and ambulatory care. *Journal of Post Anesthesia Nursing, 7,* 251–255.

Wagnild, G., Rodriguez, W., & Pritchett, P. (1987). Orem's self-care theory: A tool for education and practice. *Journal of Nursing Education, 26,* 343.

Walborn, K.A. (1980). A nursing model for the hospice: Primary and self-care nursing. *Nursing Clinics of North America, 15,* 205–217.

Walsh, M. (1989). Asthma: The Orem self-care nursing model approach. *Nursing (London), 3*(38), 19–21.

Weaver, M.T. (1987). Perceived self-care agency: A LISREL factor analysis of Bickel and Hanson's questionnaire. *Nursing Research, 36,* 381–387.

Weinrich, S.P. (1990). Predictors of older adults' participation in fecal occult blood screening. *Oncology Nursing Forum, 17,* 715–720.

Weintraub, F.N., & Hagopian, G.A. (1990). The effect of nursing consultation on anxiety, side effects, and self-care of patients receiving radiation therapy. *Oncology Nursing Forum, 17*(3, Suppl), 31–36.

Weis, A. (1988). Cooperative care: An application of Orem's self-care theory. *Patient Education and Counseling, 11,* 141–146.

Whenery-Tedder, M. (1991). Teaching acceptance. *Nursing Times, 87*(12), 36–39.

Whetstone, W.R. (1986). Social dramatics: Social skills development for the chronically mentally ill. *Journal of Advanced Nursing, 11,* 67–74.

Whetstone, W.R. (1987). Perceptions of self-care in East Germany: A cross-cultural empirical investigation. *Journal of Advanced Nursing, 12,* 167–176.

Whetstone, W.R., & Hansson, A.M.O. (1989). Perceptions of self-care in Sweden: A cross-cultural replication. *Journal of Advanced Nursing, 14,* 962–969.

Williams, P.D., Valderrama, D.M., Gloria, M.D., Pascoguin, L.G., Saavedra, L.D., De La Rama, D.T., Feny, T.C., Abaguin, C.M., & Zaldivar, S.B. (1988). Effects of preparation for mastectomy/hysterectomy on women's post-operative self-care behaviors. *International Journal of Nursing Studies, 25,* 191–206.

Woods, N.F. (1985). Self-care practices among young adult married women. *Research in Nursing and Health, 8,* 227–233.

Wollery, L. (1983). Self-care for the obstetrical patient. *Journal of Obstetric, Gynecologic, and Neonatal Nursing, 12,* 33–37.

Woolley, A.S., McLaughlin, J., & Durham, J.D. (1990). Linking diploma and bachelor's degree nursing education: An Illinois experiment. *Journal of Professional Nursing, 6,* 206–212.

Wright, J. (1988). Trolley full of trouble. *Nursing Times, 84*(9), 24–26.

Youssef, F.A. (1987). Discharge planning for psychiatric patients: The effects of a family-patient teaching programme. *Journal of Advanced Nursing, 12,* 611–616.

Zach, P. (1982). Self-care agency in diabetic ocular sequelae. *Journal of Ophthalmic Nursing Techniques, 1*(2), 21–31.

BIBLIOGRAPHY

PRIMARY SOURCES

Nursing Development Conference Group. (1973). *Concept formalization in nursing: Process and product.* Boston: Little, Brown.

Nursing Development Conference Group. (1979). *Concept formalization in nursing:*

Process and product. Boston: Little, Brown.

Orem, D.E. (1956). *Hospital nursing service: An analysis.* Indianapolis: Division of Hospital and Institutional Services of the Indiana State Board of Health.

Orem, D.E. (1959). *Guides for developing curricula for the education of practical nurses.* Washington, DC: US Government Printing Office.

Orem, D.E. (1971). *Nursing: Concepts of practice.* New York: McGraw-Hill.

Orem, D.E. (1980). *Nursing: Concepts of practice* (2nd ed.). New York: McGraw-Hill.

Orem, D.E. (1981). Nursing: A triad of action systems. In G.E. Lasker (Ed.), *Applied systems and cybernetics. Vol. IV. Systems research in health care, biocybernetics and ecology* (pp. 1729–1733). New York: Pergamon Press.

Orem, D.E. (1983). The family coping with a medical illness: Analysis and application of Orem's theory. In I.W. Clements & F.B. Roberts, *Family health: A theoretical approach to nursing care* (pp. 385–386). New York: John Wiley & Sons.

Orem, D.E. (1983). The family experiencing emotional crisis: Analysis and application of Orem's self-care deficit theory. In I.W. Clements & F.B. Roberts, *Family health: A theoretical approach to nursing care* (pp. 367–368). New York: John Wiley & Sons.

Orem, D.E. (1983). The self-care deficit theory of nursing: A general theory. In I.W. Clements & F.B. Roberts, *Family health: A theoretical approach to nursing care* (pp. 205–217). New York: John Wiley & Sons.

Orem, D.E. (1984). Orem's conceptual model and community health nursing. In M.K. Asay & C.C. Ossler (Eds.), *Conceptual models of nursing: Applications in community health nursing. Proceedings of the Eighth Annual Community Health Nursing Conference* (pp. 35–50). Chapel Hill: Department of Public Health Nursing, School of Public Health, University of North Carolina.

Orem, D.E. (1985). *Nursing: Concepts of practice* (3rd ed.). New York: McGraw-Hill.

Orem, D.E. (1987). Orem's general theory of nursing. In R.R. Parse, *Nursing science: Major paradigms, theories, and critiques* (pp. 67–89). Philadelphia: WB Saunders.

Orem, D.E. (1989). Theories and hypotheses for nursing administration. In B. Henry, M. DiVincenti, C. Arndt, & A. Marriner (Eds.), *Dimensions of nursing administra-*

tion: *Theory, research, education and practice* (pp. 55–62). Boston: Blackwell Scientific Publications.

Orem, D.E. (1990). A nursing practice theory in three parts, 1956–1989. In M.E. Parker (Ed.), *Nursing theories in practice* (pp. 47–60). New York: National League for Nursing.

Orem, D.E. (1991). *Nursing: Concepts of practice* (4th ed.). St. Louis: Mosby-Year Book.

Orem, D.E., & Parker, K.S. (Eds.) (1963). *Nurse education workshop proceedings.* Washington, DC: Catholic University of America.

Orem, D.E., & Taylor, S.G. (1986). Orem's general theory of nursing. In P. Winstead-Fry (Ed.), *Case studies in nursing theory* (pp. 37–71). New York: National League for Nursing.

COMMENTARY

Aggleton, P., & Chalmers, H. (1985). Orem's self-care model. *Nursing Times, 81*(1), 36–39.

Arrington, D.T., & Walborn, K.S. (1989). The comfort caregiver concept. *Caring, 8*(12), 24–27.

Bartle, J. (1991). Caring in relation to Orem's theory. *Nursing Standard, 5*(37), 33–36.

Biehler, B.A. (1992). Impact of role-sets on implementing self-care theory with children. *Pediatric Nursing, 18*, 30–34.

Biley, F., & Dennerley, M. (1990). Orem's model: A critical analysis. *Nursing (London), 4*(13), 19–22.

Bottorff, J.L. (1991). Nursing: A practice science of caring. *Advances in Nursing Science, 14*(1), 26–39.

Bramlett, M.H., Gueldner, S.H., & Sowell, R.L. (1990). Consumer-centric advocacy: Its connection to nursing frameworks. *Nursing Science Quarterly, 3*, 156–161.

Butterfield, S. (1983). In search of commonalities: An analysis of two theoretical frameworks. *International Journal of Nursing Studies, 20*, 15–22.

Cavanagh, S. (1991). Orem and the nursing process: New directions for the 1990s. *Nurse Practitioner, 4*(4), 26–28.

Chapman, P. (1984). Specifics and generalities: A critical examination of two nursing models. *Nurse Education Today, 4*, 141–144.

Chavasse, J.M. (1987). A comparison of three models of nursing. *Nurse Education Today, 7*(4), 177–186.

Clark, M.D. (1986). Application of Orem's theory of self-care: A case study. *Journal of Community Health Nursing, 3,* 127–135.

Davidhizar, R. (1988). Critique of Orem's self-care model. *Nursing Management, 19*(11), 78–79.

Davis, L.H., Dumas, R. Ferketich, S., Flaherty, M.J., Isenberg, M., Koerner, J.E., Lacey, B., Stern, P.N., Valente, S., & Meleis, A.I. (1992). AAN expert panel report: Culturally competent health care. *Nursing Outlook, 40,* 277–283.

Denyes, M.J. (1988). Orem's model used for health promotion: Directions from research. *Advances in Nursing Science, 11*(1), 13–21.

Eban, J.D., Gashti, N.N., Hayes, S.E., et al. (1994). Dorothea E. Orem: Self-care deficit theory of nursing. In A. Marriner-Tomey (Ed.): *Nursing theorists and their work* (3rd ed., pp. 181–198). St. Louis: Mosby-Year Book.

Eban, J.D., Gashti, N.N., Nation, M.J., Marriner-Tomey, A., & Nordmeyer, S.B. (1989). Dorothea E. Orem: Self-care deficit theory of nursing. In A. Marriner-Tomey, *Nursing theorists and their work* (2nd ed., pp. 118–132). St. Louis: CV Mosby.

Eban, J.D., Nation, M.J., Marriner, A., & Nordmeyer, S.B. (1986). Dorothea E. Orem: Self-care deficit theory of nursing. In A. Marriner, *Nursing theorists and their work* (pp. 117–130). St. Louis: CV Mosby.

Feathers, R.L. (1989). Orem's self-care nursing theory. In J.P. Riehl-Sisca, *Conceptual models for nursing practice* (3rd ed., pp. 369–375). Norwalk, CT: Appleton & Lange.

Fitzpatrick, J.J., Whall, A., Johnston, R., & Floyd, J. (1982). *Nursing models and their psychiatric mental health applications.* Bowie, MD: Brady.

Foster, P.C., & Janssens, N.P. (1980). Dorothea E. Orem. In Nursing Theories Conference Group, *Nursing theories: The base for professional nursing practice* (pp. 90–106). Englewood Cliffs, NJ: Prentice-Hall.

Foster, P.C., & Janssens, N.P. (1985). Dorothea E. Orem. In Nursing Theories Conference Group, *Nursing theories: The base for professional nursing practice* (2nd ed., pp. 124–139). Englewood Cliffs, NJ: Prentice-Hall.

Foster, P.C., & Janssens, N.P. (1990). Dorothea E. Orem. In J.B. George (Ed.), *Nursing theories: The base for professional nursing practice* (3rd ed., pp. 91–112). Norwalk, CT: Appleton & Lange.

Grypdonck, M. (1990). Theory development in nursing: Have the promises been fulfilled? A case study of Orem's theory. In *Proceedings of the 5th Conference of the Workgroup of European Nurse Researchers* (pp. 209–225). Budapest: The Workgroup.

Hanucharurnkul, S. (1989). Comparative analysis of Orem's and King's theories. *Journal of Advanced Nursing, 14,* 365–372.

Hartweg, D.L. (1990). Health promotion self-care within Orem's general theory of nursing. *Journal of Advanced Nursing, 15,* 35–41.

Hartweg, D.L. (1991). *Dorothea Orem: Self care deficit theory.* Newbury Park, CA: Sage.

Iveson-Iveson, J. (1982). Putting ideas into action. *Nursing Mirror, 155*(16), 49.

Johnston, R.L. (1983). Orem self-care model of nursing. In J.J. Fitzpatrick & A.L. Whall, *Conceptual models of nursing: Analysis and application* (pp. 137–155). Bowie, MD: Brady.

Johnston, R.L. (1989). Orem self-care model of nursing. In J.J. Fitzpatrick & A.L. Whall, *Conceptual models of nursing: Analysis and application* (2nd ed., pp. 165–184). Bowie, MD: Brady.

Keyser, P. (1985). Ethics of nurse-patient relationships in self-care model. In J. Riehl-Sisca, *The science and art of self-care* (pp. 14–19). Norwalk, CT: Appleton-Century-Crofts.

Kitson, A.L. (1987). A comparative analysis of lay-caring and professional (nursing) caring relationships. *International Journal of Nursing Studies, 24,* 155–165.

Leininger, M.M. (1992). Self-care ideology and cultural incongruities: Some critical issues. *Journal of Transcultural Nursing, 4*(1), 2–4.

Meleis, A.I. (1991). *Theoretical nursing: Development and progress* (2nd ed.). Philadelphia: JB Lippincott.

Melnyk, K. (1983). The process of theory analysis: An examination of the nursing theory of Dorothea E. Orem. *Nursing Research, 32,* 170–174.

Melnyk, K. (1983). Re: Nursing theory [Letter to the editor]. *Nursing Research, 32,* 318.

Melnyk, K. (1983). To the editor [Letter to the editor]. *Nursing Research, 32,* 383.

Allison, S. (1983). To the editor [Letter to the editor]. *Nursing Research, 32,* 381.

Burns, M., & Whelton, B. (1983). To the editor [Letter to the editor]. *Nursing Research, 32,* 381.

Geden, E. (1983). To the editor [Letter to the editor]. *Nursing Research, 32,* 381–382.

Orem, D. (1983). To the editor [Letter to the editor]. *Nursing Research, 32,* 382.

Pearson, B. (1983). To the editor [Letter to the editor]. *Nursing Research, 32,* 318.

Taylor, S. (1983). To the editor [Letter to the editor]. *Nursing Research, 32,* 382–383.

Morse, J.M., Solberg, S.M., Neander, W.L., Bottorff, J.L., & Johnson, J.L. (1990). Concepts of caring and caring as a concept. Advances in Nursing Science, 13(1), 1–14.

Munley, M.J., & Sayers, P.A. (1984). *Self-care deficit theory of nursing: A primer for application of the concepts.* North Brunswick, NJ: Personal and Family Health Associates.

Pace, J.C. (1985). An advocacy model for health care professionals. *Family and Community Health, 7*(4), 77–87.

Perry, P.D., & Sutcliffe, S.A. (1982). Conceptual frameworks for clinical practice. *Journal of Neurosurgical Nursing, 14,* 318–321.

Pesut, D.J. (1992). Self-regulation, self-management and self-care. *South Carolina Nurse, 7*(2), 22–23.

Purcell, C. (1993). Holistic care of a critically ill child. *Intensive Critical Care Nursing, 9,* 108–115.

Riehl-Sisca, J. (1985). Epilogue: Future implications for the science and art of self-care. In J. Riehl-Sisca, *The science and art of self-care* (pp. 307–309). Norwalk, CT: Appleton-Century-Crofts.

Riehl-Sisca, J.P. (1985). Orem's general theory of nursing: An interpretation. In J. Riehl-Sisca, *The science and art of self-care* (pp. 3–13). Norwalk, CT: Appleton-Century-Crofts.

Riehl-Sisca, J.P. (1989). Orem's general theory of nursing: An interpretation. In J.P. Riehl-Sisca, *Conceptual models for nursing practice* (3rd ed., pp. 359–368). Norwalk, CT: Appleton & Lange.

Rosenbaum, J. (1986). Comparison of two theorists on care: Orem and Leininger. *Journal of Advanced Nursing, 11,* 409–419.

Rosenbaum, J.N. (1989). Self-caring: Concept development for nursing. *Recent Advances in Nursing, 24,* 18–31.

Rourke, A.M. (1991). Self-care: Chore or challenge? *Journal of Advanced Nursing, 16,* 233–241.

Runtz, S.E., & Urtel, J.G. (1983). Evaluating your practice via a nursing model. *Nurse Practitioner, 8*(3), 30, 32, 37–40.

Simmons, S.J. (1990). The Health-Promoting Self-Care System Model: Directions for nursing research and practice. *Journal of Advanced Nursing, 15,* 1162–1166.

Smith, M.C. (1979). Proposed metaparadigm for nursing research and theory development: An analysis of Orem's self-care theory. *Image, 11,* 75–79.

Smith, M.J. (1987). A critique of Orem's theory. In R.R. Parse, *Nursing science: Major paradigms, theories, and critiques* (pp. 91–105). Philadelphia: WB Saunders.

Smith, S.R. (1981). Sound off! "Oremization," the curse of nursing. *RN, 44* (10), 83.

Spangler, Z.S., & Spangler, W.D. (1983). Self-care: A testable model. In P.L. Chinn (Ed.), *Advances in nursing theory development* (pp. 89–105). Rockville, MD: Aspen.

Steiger, N., & Lipson, J. (1985). *Self-care nursing: Theory and practice.* Bowie, MD: Brady.

Stern, P.N., & Harris, C.C. (1985). Women's health and the self-care paradox: A model to guide self-care readiness. *Health Care for Women International, 6,* 151–174.

Taylor, S. (1978, December/1979, January). The unique object and system of nursing. *Missouri Nurse,* 3–5.

Thibodeau, J.A. (1983). *Nursing models: Analysis and evaluation.* Monterey, CA: Wadsworth.

Underwood, P.R. (1990). Orem's self-care model: Principles and general applications (pp. 175–187). In D. Cormack & B. Reynolds (Eds.), *Psychiatric and mental health nursing.* London: Chapman and Hill.

Urbancic, J.C. (1992). Empowerment support with adult female survivors of childhood incest: Part I—Theories and research. *Archives of Psychiatric Nursing, 6,* 275–281.

Urbancic, J.C. (1992). Empowerment support with adult female survivors of childhood incest: Part II—Application of Orem's method of helping. *Archives of Psychiatric Nursing, 6,* 282–286.

Utz, S.W. (1990). Motivating self-care: A nursing approach. *Holistic Nursing Practice, 4*(2), 13–21.

Uys, L.R. (1987). Foundational studies in nursing. *Journal of Advanced Nursing, 12,* 275–280.

Walker, J.M., & Campbell, S.M. (1989). Pain assessment, nursing models, and the nursing process. *Recent Advances in Nursing, 24,* 47–61.

Walton, J. (1985). An overview: Orem's self-care deficit theory of nursing. *Focus on Critical Care, 12*(1), 54–58.

Whelen, E. (1984). Analysis and application of Dorothea Orem's self-care practice model. *Journal of Nursing Education, 23,* 342–345.

RESEARCH

Alexander, J.S., Younger, R.E., Cohen, R.M., & Crawford, L.V. (1988). Effectiveness of a nurse-managed program for children with chronic asthma. *Journal of Pediatric Nursing, 3,* 312–317.

Allen, J.D. (1988). Knowing what to weigh: Women's self-care activities related to weight. *Advances in Nursing Science, 11*(1), 47–60.

Allison, S.E. (1971). The meaning of rest: An exploratory nursing study. In *ANA clinical sessions* (pp. 191–205). New York: Appleton-Century-Crofts.

Arneson, S.W., & Triplett, J.L. (1990). Riding with Bucklebear: An automobile safety program for preschoolers. *Journal of Pediatric Nursing, 5,* 115–122.

Barron, M.L., Ganong, L.H., & Brown, M. (1987). An examination of preconception health teaching by nurse practitioners. *Journal of Advanced Nursing, 12,* 605–610.

Baulch, Y.S., Larson, P.J., Dodd, M.J., & Dietrich, C. (1992). The relationship of visual acuity, tactile sensitivity, and mobility of the upper extremities to proficient breast self-examination in women 65 and older. *Oncology Nursing Forum, 19* 1367–1372.

Belcher, D. (1992). The effect of a career awareness program on the success rate of the practical nursing student. (Abstract). *Kentucky Nurse, 40*(3), 18.

Bennett, J.A., DeMayo, M., & Saint Germain, M. (1993). Caring in the time of AIDS: The importance of empathy. *Nursing Administration Quarterly, 17*(2), 46–60.

Bidigare, S.A., & Oermann, M.H. (1991). Attitudes and knowledge of nurses regarding organ procurement. *Heart and Lung, 20,* 20–24.

Biggs, A.J. (1990). Family care-giver versus nursing assessments of elderly self-care abilities. *Journal of Gerontological Nursing, 16*(8), 11–16.

Bliss-Holtz, V.J. (1988). Primiparas' prenatal concern for learning infant care. *Nursing Research, 37,* 20—24.

Bliss-Holtz, V.J. (1991). Developmental tasks of pregnancy and parental education. *International Journal of Childbirth Education, 6*(1), 29–31.

Blazek, B., & McClellan, M. (1983). The effects of self-care instruction on locus of control in children. *Journal of School Health, 53,* 554–556.

Bottorff, J.L. (1988). Assessing an instrument in a pilot project: The self-care agency questionnaire. *Canadian Journal of Nursing Research, 20,* 7–16.

Brock, A.M., & O'Sullivan, P. (1985). A study to determine what variables predict institutionalization of elderly people. *Journal of Advanced Nursing, 10,* 533–537.

Buckley, H.B. (1990). Nurse practitioner intervention to improve postpartum appointment keeping in an outpatient family planning clinic. *Journal of the American Academy of Nurse Practitioners, 2*(1), 29–32.

Campbell, J.C. (1986). Nursing assessment for risk of homicide with battered women. *Advances in Nursing Science, 8*(4), 36–51.

Campbell, J.C. (1989). A test of two explanatory models of women's responses to battering. *Nursing Research, 38,* 18–24.

Carlisle, J.B., Corser, N., Cull, V., DiMicco, W., Luther, L., McCaleb, A., Robuck, J., & Powell, K. (1993). Cardiovascular risk factors in young children. *Journal of Community Health Nursing, 10,* 1–9.

Chang, B., Uman, G., Linn, L., Ware, J., & Kane, R. (1984). The effect of systematically varying components of nursing care on satisfaction in elderly ambulatory women. *Western Journal of Nursing Research, 6,* 367–386.

Chang, B., Uman, G., Linn, L., Ware, J., & Kane, R. (1985). Adherence to health care regimens among elderly women. *Nursing Research, 34,* 27–31.

Cleveland, S.A. (1989). Re: Perceived self-care agency: A LISREL factor analysis of Bickel and Hanson's Questionnaire [Letter to the editor]. *Nursing Research, 38,* 59.

Weaver, M.T. (1989). Response [Letter to the editor]. *Nursing Research, 38,* 59.

Conn, V. (1991). Self-care actions taken by older adults for influenza and colds. *Nursing Research, 40,* 176–181.

Conn, V.S., Taylor, S.G., & Kelley, S. (1991). Medication regimen complexity and adherence among older adults. *Image: Journal of Nursing Scholarship, 23,* 231–235.

Crockett, M.S. (1982). Self-reported coping histories of adult psychiatric and nonpsychiatric subjects and controls. (Abstract). *Nursing Research, 31,* 122.

Dashiff, C.J. (1992). Self-care capabilities in black girls in anticipation of menarche. *Health Care for Women International, 13,* 67–76.

Degenhart-Leskosky, S.M. (1989). Health education needs of adolescent and nonadolescent mothers. *Journal of Obstetric, Gynecologic, and Neonatal Nursing, 18,* 238–244.

Denyes, M.J. (1982). Measurement of self-care agency in adolescents. (Abstract). *Nursing Research, 31,* 63.

Denyes, M.J., Neuman, B.M., & Villarruel, A.M. (1991). Nursing actions to prevent and alleviate pain in hospitalized children. *Issues in Comprehensive Pediatric Nursing, 14,* 31–48.

Denyes, M.J., O'Connor, N.A., Oakley, D., & Ferguson, S. (1989). Integrating nursing theory, practice and research through collaborative practice. *Journal of Advanced Nursing, 14,* 141–145.

Dickson, G., & Lee-Villasenor, H. (1982). Nursing theory and practice: A self-care approach. *Advances in Nursing Science, 5*(1), 29–40.

Dodd, M.J. (1982). Assessing patient self-care for side effects of cancer chemotherapy — Part 1. *Cancer Nursing, 5,* 447–451.

Dodd, M.J. (1983). Self-care for side effects in cancer chemotherapy: An assessment of nursing interventions — Part 2. *Cancer Nursing, 6,* 63–67.

Dodd, M.J. (1984). Measuring informational intervention for chemotherapy knowledge and self-care behavior. *Research in Nursing and Health, 7,* 43–50.

Dodd, M.J. (1984). Patterns of self-care in cancer patients receiving radiation therapy. *Oncology Nursing Forum, 11,* 23–27.

Dodd, M.J. (1987). Efficacy of proactive information on self-care in radiation therapy patients. *Heart and Lung, 16,* 538–544.

Dodd, M.J. (1988). Efficacy of proactive information on self-care in chemotherapy patients. *Patient Education and Counseling, 11,* 215–225.

Dodd, M.J. (1988). Patterns of self-care in patients with breast cancer. *Western Journal of Nursing Research, 10,* 7–24.

Dodd, M.J., & Dibble, S.L. (1993). Predictors of self-care: A test of Orem's model. *Oncology Nursing Forum, 20,* 895–901.

Dowd, T.T. (1991). Discovering older women's experience of urinary incontinence. *Research in Nursing and Health, 14,* 179–186.

Edgar, L., Shamian, J., & Patterson, D. (1984). Factors affecting the nurse as a teacher and practicer of breast self-examination. *International Journal of Nursing Studies, 21,* 255–265.

Ewing, G. (1989). The nursing preparation of stoma patients for self-care. *Journal of Advanced Nursing, 14,* 411–420.

Fawcett, J., Ellis, V., Underwood, P., Naqvi, A., & Wilson, D. (1990). The effect of Orem's self-care model on nursing care in a nursing home setting. *Journal of Advanced Nursing, 15,* 659–666.

Frey, M.A., & Fox, M.A. (1990). Assessing and teaching self-care to youths with diabetes mellitus. *Pediatric Nursing, 16,* 597–800.

Gammon, J. (1991). Coping with cancer: The role of self-care. *Nursing Practice, 4*(3), 11–15.

Ganong, L.H., & Coleman, M. (1992). The effect of clients' family structure on nursing students' cognitive schemas and verbal behavior. *Research in Nursing and Health, 15,* 139–146.

Gast, H.L., Denyes, M.J., Campbell, J.C., Hartweg, D.L., Schott-Baer, D., & Isenberg, M. (1989). Self-care agency: Conceptualizations and operationalizations. *Advances in Nursing Science, 12*(1), 26–38.

Gaut, D.A., & Kieckhefer, G.M. (1988). Assessment of self-care agency in chronically ill adolescents. *Journal of Adolescent Health Care, 9,* 55–60.

Geden, E.A. (1982). Effects of lifting techniques on energy expenditure: A preliminary investigation. *Nursing Research, 31,* 214–218.

Geden, E.A. (1985). The relationship between self-care theory and empirical research. In J. Riehl-Sisca, *The science and art of self-care* (pp. 265–270). Norwalk, CT: Appleton-Century-Crofts.

Geden, E. (1989). The relationship between self-care theory and empirical research. In J.P. Riehl-Sisca, *Conceptual models for nursing practice* (3rd ed., pp. 377–382). Norwalk, CT: Appleton & Lange.

Geden, E., & Taylor, S. (1991). Construct and empirical validity of the self-as-carer inventory. *Nursing Research, 40,* 47–50.

Germain, C.P., & Nemchik, R.M. (1989). Diabetes self-management and hospitalization. *Image: Journal of Nursing Scholarship, 20,* 74–78.

Glanz, D., Ganong, L., & Coleman, M. (1989). Client gender, diagnosis, and family structure. *Western Journal of Nursing Research, 11,* 726–735.

Goodwin, J.O. (1979). Programmed instruction for self-care following pulmonary surgery. *International Journal of Nursing Studies, 16,* 29–40.

Gulick, E.E. (1987). Parsimony and model confirmation of the ADL self-care scale for multiple sclerosis persons. *Nursing Research, 36,* 278–283.

Gulick, E.E. (1988). The self-administered ADL scale for persons with multiple sclerosis. In C.F. Waltz, & O.L. Strickland (Eds.), *Measurement of Nursing Outcomes.* Vol. 1. *Measuring client outcomes* (pp. 128–159). New York: Springer.

Gulick, E.E. (1989). Model confirmation of

the MS-related symptom checklist. *Nursing Research, 38,* 147–153.

Gulick, E.E. (1989). Work performance by persons with multiple sclerosis: Conditions that impede or enable the performance of work. *International Journal of Nursing Studies, 26,* 301–311.

Gulick, E.E. (1991). Self-assessed health and use of health services. *Western Journal of Nursing Research, 13,* 195–219.

Hagopian, G. (1990). The measurement of self-care strategies of patients in radiation therapy. In O.L. Strickland & C.F. Waltz (Eds.), *Measurement of nursing outcomes.* Vol. *4. Measuring client self-care and coping skills* (pp. 475–570). New York: Springer.

Hagopian, G.A. (1991). The effects of a weekly radiation therapy newsletter on patients. *Oncology Nursing Forum, 18,* 1199–1203.

Hagopian, G.A., & Rubenstein, J.H. (1990). Effects of telephone call interventions on patients' well-being in a radiation therapy department. *Cancer Nursing, 13,* 339–344.

Hamera, E.K., Peterson, K.A., Young, L.M., & Schaumloffel, M.M. (1992). Symptom monitoring in schizophrenia: Potential for enhancing self-care. *Archives of Psychiatric Nursing, 6,* 324–330.

Hamilton, L.W., & Creason, N.S. (1992). Mental status and functional abilities: Change in institutionalized elderly women. *Nursing Diagnosis, 3,* 81–86.

Hanson, B.R., & Bickel, L. (1985). Development and testing of the questionnaire on perception of self-care agency. In J. Riehl-Sisca, *The science and art of self-care* (pp. 271–278). Norwalk, CT: Appleton-Century-Crofts.

Hanucharurnkul, S. (1989). Predictors of self-care in cancer patients receiving radiotherapy. *Cancer Nursing, 12,* 21–27.

Hanucharurnku[l], S., & Vinya-nguag, P. (1991). Effects of promoting patients' participation in self-care on postoperative recovery and satisfaction with care. *Nursing Science Quarterly, 4,* 14–20.

Harper, D. (1984). Application of Orem's theoretical constructs to self-care medication behaviors in the elderly. *Advances in Nursing Science, 6*(3), 29–46.

Harris, J.L., & Williams, L.K. (1991). Universal self-care requisites as identified by homeless elderly men. *Journal of Gerontological Nursing, 17*(6), 39–43.

Harrison, L.L., & Novak, D. (1988). Evaluation of a gerontological nursing continuing education programme: Effect on nurses' knowledge and attitudes and on

patients' perceptions and satisfaction. *Journal of Advanced Nursing, 13,* 684–692.

Hartley, L.A. (1988). Congruence between teaching and learning self-care: A pilot study. *Nursing Science Quarterly, 1,* 161–167.

Hartweg, D. (1993). Self-care actions of healthy middle-aged women to promote well-being. *Nursing Research, 42,* 221–227.

Hartweg, D., & Metcalfe, S. (1986). Self-care attitude changes of nursing students enrolled in a self-care curriculum — A longitudinal study. *Research in Nursing and Health, 9,* 347–353.

Hathaway, D.K., & Geden, E.A. (1983). Energy expenditure during leg exercise programs. *Nursing Research, 32,* 147–150.

Hautman, M.A. (1987). Self-care responses to respiratory illnesses among Vietnamese. *Western Journal of Nursing Research, 9,* 223–243.

Hayward, M.B., Kish, J.P., Jr., Frey, G.M., Kirchner, J.M., Carr, L.S., & Wolfe, C.M. (1989). An instrument to identify stressors in renal transplant recipients. *Journal of the American Nephrology Nurses Association, 16,* 81–84.

Hinojosa, R.J. (1992). Nursing interventions to prevent or relieve postoperative nausea and vomiting. *Journal of Post Anesthesia Nursing, 7,* 3–14.

Hiromoto, B.M., & Dungan, J. (1991). Contract learning for self-care activities: A protocol study among chemotherapy outpatients. *Cancer Nursing, 14,* 148–154.

Humphreys, J. (1991). Children of battered women: Worries about their mothers. *Pediatric Nursing, 17,* 342–345, 354.

Huss, K., Salerno, M., & Huss, R.W. (1991). Computer-assisted reinforcement of instruction: Effects on adherence in adult atopic asthmatics. *Research in Nursing and Health, 14,* 259–267.

jirovec, M.M., & Kasno, J. (1990). Self-care agency as a function of patient-environmental factors among nursing home residents. *Research in Nursing and Health, 13,* 303–309.

Jirovec, M.M., & Kasno, J. (1993). Predictors of self-care abilities among the institutionalized elderly. *Western Journal of Nursing Research, 15,* 314–326.

Jopp, M., Carroll, M.C., Waters, L. (1993). Using self-care theory to guide nursing management of the older adult after hospitalization. *Rehabilitation Nursing, 18,* 91–94.

Karl, C. (1982). The effect of an exercise program on self-care activities for the institutionalized elderly. *Journal of Gerontological Nursing, 8,* 282–285.

Kearney, B.Y., & Fleischer, B.J. (1979). Development of an instrument to measure exercise of self-care agency. *Research in Nursing and Health, 2,* 25–34.

Kerkstra, A., Castelein, E., & Philipsen, H. (1991). Preventive home visits to elderly people by community nurses in the Netherlands. *Journal of Advanced Nursing, 16,* 631–637.

Kirkpatrick, M.K., Brewer, J.A., & Stocks, B. (1990). Efficacy of self-care measures for perimenstrual syndrome (PMS). *Journal of Advanced Nursing, 15,* 281–285.

Klemm, L.W., & Creason, N.S. (1991). Self-care practices of women with urinary incontinence—A preliminary study. *Health Care for Women International, 12,* 199–209.

Krouse, H.J., & Roberts, S.J. (1989). Nurse-patient interactive styles: Power, control, and satisfaction. *Western Journal of Nursing Research, 11,* 717–725.

Kruger, S., Shawver, M., & Jones, L. (1980). Reactions of families to the child with cystic fibrosis. *Image, 12,* 67–72.

Kubricht, D. (1984). Therapeutic self-care demands expressed by outpatients receiving external radiation therapy. *Cancer Nursing, 7,* 43–52.

Lakin, J.A. (1988). Self-care, health locus of control, and health value among faculty women. *Public Health Nursing, 5,* 37–44.

Lorensen, M., Holter, I.M., Evers, G.C., Isenberg, M.A., van Achterberg, T. (1993). Cross-cultural testing of the appraisal of self-care agency: ASA scale in Norway. *International Journal of Nursing Studies, 30,* 15–23.

MacVicar, M.G., Winningham, M.L., & Nickel, J.L. (1989). Effects of aerobic interval training on cancer patients' functional capacity. *Nursing Research, 38,* 348–351.

Malik, U. (1992). Women's knowledge, beliefs and health practices about breast cancer and breast self-examination. *Nursing Journal of India, 83,* 186–190.

Massner, R.L., & Gardner, S.S. (1988). Specific outcomes of nurse-directed colorectal cancer screening. In C.F. Waltz, & O.L. Strickland (Eds.), *Measurement of nursing outcomes.* Vol. 1. *Measuring client outcomes* (pp. 443–456). New York: Springer.

Maunz, E.R., & Woods, N.F. (1988). Self-care practices among young adult women: Influence of symptoms, employment, and sex-role orientation. *Health Care for Women International, 9,* 29–41.

McBride, S. (1987). Validation of an instrument to measure exercise of self-care agency. *Research in Nursing and Health, 10,* 311–316.

McBride, S.H. (1991). Comparative analysis of three instruments designed to measure self-care agency. *Nursing Research, 40,* 12–16.

McCord, A.S. (1990). Teaching for tonsillectomies: Details mean better compliance. *Today's OR Nurse, 12*(6), 11–14.

McDermott, M.A.N. (1993). Learned helplessness as an interacting variable with self-care agency: Testing a theoretical model. *Nursing Science Quarterly, 6,* 28–38.

McElmurry, B.J., & Huddleston, D.S. (1991). Self-care and menopause: Critical review of research. *Health Care for Women International, 12,* 15–26.

McFarland, S.M., Sasser, L., Boss, B.J., Dickerson, J.L., & Stelling, J.D. (1992). Self-Care Assessment Tool for spinal cord injured persons, *SCI Nursing, 9,* 111–116.

Meeker, B.J., Sehrt Rodriquez, L., & Johnson, J.M. (1992). A comprehensive analysis of preoperative patient education. *Today's OR Nurse, 14*(3), 11–18, 33–34.

Miller, J.F. (1982). Categories of self-care needs of ambulatory patients with diabetes. *Journal of Advanced Nursing, 7,* 25–31.

Monsen, R.B. (1992). Autonomy, coping, and self-care agency in healthy adolescents and in adolescents with spina bifida. *Journal of Pediatric Nursing, 7,* 9–13.

Moore, J.B. (1987). Determining the relationship of autonomy to self-care agency or locus of control in school-age children. *Maternal-Child Nursing Journal, 16,* 47–60.

Moore, J.B. (1987). Effects of assertion training and first aid instruction on children's autonomy and self-care agency. *Research in Nursing and Health, 10,* 101–109.

Moore, J.B. (1993). Predictors of children's self-care performance: Testing the theory of self-care deficit. *Scholarly Inquiry for Nursing Practice, 7,* 199–212.

Denyes, M.J. (1993) Response to "Predictors of children's self-care performance: Testing the theory of self-care deficit." *Scholarly Inquiry for Nursing Practice, 7,* 213–217.

Moore, J.B., & Gaffney, K.F. (1989). Development of an instrument to measure mothers' performance of self-care activities for children. *Advances in Nursing Science, 12*(1), 76–83.

Murphy, E., & Freston, M.S. (1991). An analysis of theory-research linkages in published gerontologic nursing studies, 1983–1989. *Advances in Nursing Science, 13*(4), 1–13.

Neil, R.M. (1984). Self care agency and spouses/companions of alcoholics. *Kansas Nurse, 59*(10), 3–4.

Grant, M. (1990). Study critique. *Oncology Nursing Forum, 17*(3, Suppl), 36–38.

Oberst, M.T., Hugest, S.H., Chang, A.S., & McCubbin, M.A. (1991). Self-care burden, stress appraisal, and mood among persons receiving radiotherapy. *Cancer Nursing, 14*, 71–78.

Pallikkathayil, L., & Morgan, S.A. (1988). Emergency department nurses' encounters with suicide attempters: A qualitative investigation. *Scholarly Inquiry for Nursing Practice, 2*, 237–253.

Winstead-Fry, P. (1988). Response to "Emergency department nurses' encounters with suicide attempters: A qualitative investigation." *Scholarly Inquiry for Nursing Practice, 2*, 255–259.

Palmer, P., & Meyers, F.J. (1990). An outpatient approach to the delivery of intensive consolidation chemotherapy to adults with acute lymphoblastic leukemia. *Oncology Nursing Forum, 17*, 553–558.

Patterson, E., & Hale, E. (1985). Making sure: Integrating menstrual care practices into activities of daily living. *Advances in Nursing Science, 7*(3), 18–31.

Porter, L., Youssef, M., Shaaban, I., & Ibrahim, W. (1992). Parenting enhancement among Egyptian mothers in a tertiary care setting. *Pediatric Nursing, 18*, 329–336, 386.

Reed, P.G. (1989). Mental health of older adults. *Western Journal of Nursing Research, 11*, 143–163.

Rew, L. (1987). Children with asthma: The relationship between illness behaviors and health locus of control. *Western Journal of Nursing Research, 9*, 465–483.

Rew, L. (1987). The relationship between self-care behaviors and selected psychosocial variables in children with asthma. *Journal of Pediatric Nursing, 2*, 333–341.

Rhodes, V.A., Watson, P.M., & Hanson, B.M. (1988). Patients' descriptions of the influence of tiredness and weakness on self-care abilities. *Cancer Nursing, 11*, 186–194.

Richardson, A. (1992). Studies exploring self-care for the person coping with cancer treatment: A review. *International Journal of Nursing Studies, 29*, 191–204.

Riesch, S.K. (1988). Changes in the exercise of self-care agency. *Western Journal of Nursing Research, 10*, 257–273.

Riesch, S.K., & Hauck, M.R. (1988). The exercise of self-care agency: An analysis of construct and discriminant validity. *Research in Nursing and Health, 11*, 245–255.

Robinson, K.D., & Posner, J.D. (1992). Patterns of self-care needs and interventions related to biologic response modifier therapy: Fatigue as a model. *Seminars in Oncology Nursing, 8*(4, Suppl. 1), 17–22.

Rothert, M., Rovner, D., Holmes, M., et al. (1990). Women's use of information regarding hormone replacement therapy. *Research in Nursing and Health, 13*, 355–366.

Rothlis, J. (1984). The effect of a self-help group on feelings of hopelessness and helplessness. *Western Journal of Nursing Research, 6*, 157–173.

Sandman, P.O., Norberg, A., Adolfsson, R., Axelsson, K., & Hedley, V. (1986). Morning care of patients with Alzheimer-type dementia: A theoretical model based on direct observation. *Journal of Advanced Nursing, 11*, 369–378.

Saucier, C. (1984). Self concept and self-care management in school-age children with diabetes. *Pediatric Nursing, 10*, 135–138.

Schafer, S.L. (1989). An aggressive approach to promoting health responsibility. *Journal of Gerontological Nursing, 15*(4), 22–27.

Schott-Baer, D. (1993). Dependent care, caregiver burden, and self-care agency of spouse caregivers. *Cancer Nursing, 16*, 230–236.

Seideman, R.Y. (1990). Effects on a premenstrual syndrome education program on premenstrual symptomatology. *Health Care for Women International, 11*, 491–501.

Siebert, K.D., Ganong, L.H., Hagemann, V., & Coleman, M. (1986). Nursing students' perceptions of a child: Influence of information on family structure. *Journal of Advanced Nursing, 11*, 333–337.

Smits, J., & Kee, C.C. (1992). Correlates of self-care among the independent elderly: Self-concept affects well-being. *Journal of Gerontological Nursing, 18*(9), 13–18.

Steele, N.F., & Sterling, Y.M. (1992). Application of the case study design: Nursing interventions for discharge readiness. *Clinical Nurse Specialist, 6*, 79–84.

Stockdale-Woolley, R. (1984). The effects of education on self-care agency. *Public Health Nursing, 1*, 97–106.

Storm, D.S., & Baumgartner, R.G. (1987). Achieving self-care in the ventilator-dependent patient: A critical analysis of a case study. *International Journal of Nursing Studies, 24,* 95–106.

Sullivan, T.J. (1980). Self-care model for nursing. In *Directions for nursing in the 80s* (pp. 57–68). Kansas City: American Nurses Association.

Takahashi, J.J., & Bever, S.C. (1989). Preoperative nursing assessment: A research study. *Association of Operating Room Nurses Journal, 50,* 1022, 1024–1029, 1031–1032, 1034–1035.

Taylor, S.G. (1988). To the editor (Re: Lundh, Soder & Waerness article). *Image: Journal of Nursing Scholarship, 20,* 236.

Toth, J.C. (1980). Effect of structured preparation for transfer on patient anxiety on leaving coronary care unit. *Nursing Research, 29,* 28–34.

Utz, S.W., Hammer, J., Whitmire, V.M., & Grass, S. (1990). Perceptions of body image and health status in persons with mitral valve prolapse. *Image: Journal of Nursing Scholarship, 22,* 18–22.

Utz, S.W., & Ramos, M.C. (1993). Mitral value prolapse and its effects: A programme of inquiry within Orem's self-care deficit theory of nursing. *Journal of Advanced Nursing, 18,* 742–751.

Vallarruel, A.M., & Denyes, M.J. (1991). Pain assessment in children: Theoretical and empirical validity. *Advances in Nursing Science, 14*(2), 32–41.

van Achterberg, T., Lorensen, M., Isenberg, M.A., Evers, G.C.M., Levin, E., & Philipsen, H. (1991). The Norwegian, Danish and Dutch version of the Appraisal of Self-Care Agency Scale: Comparing reliability aspects. *Scandinavian Journal of Caring Sciences, 5,* 101–108.

Wagnild, G., Rodriguez, W., & Pritchett, P. (1987). Orem's self-care theory: A tool for education and practice. *Journal of Nursing Education, 26,* 343.

Wanich, C.K., Sullivan-Marx, E.M., Gottlieb, G.L., & Johnson, J.C. (1992). Functional status outcomes of a nursing intervention in hospitalized elderly. *Image: Journal of Nursing Scholarship, 24,* 201–207.

Weaver, M.T. (1987). Perceived self-care agency: A LISREL factor analysis of Bickel and Hanson's questionnaire. *Nursing Research, 36,* 381–387.

Webster, D., Leslie, L., McElmurry, B.J., Dan, A., Biordi, D., Boyer, D., Swider, S., Lipetz, M., & Newcomb, J. (1986). Re: Nursing practice in women's health— concept paper [Letter to the editor]. *Nursing Research, 35,* 143.

Weinrich, S.P. (1990). Predictors of older adults' participation in fecal occult blood screening. *Oncology Nursing Forum, 17,* 715–720.

Weintraub, F.N., & Hagopian, G.A. (1990). The effect of nursing consultation on anxiety, side effects, and self-care of patients receiving radiation therapy. *Oncology Nursing Forum, 17*(3, Suppl), 31–36.

Whetstone, W.R. (1986). Social dramatics: Social skills development for the chronically mentally ill. *Journal of Advanced Nursing, 11,* 67–74.

Whetstone, W.R. (1987). Perceptions of self-care in East Germany: A cross-cultural empirical investigation. *Journal of Advanced Nursing, 12,* 167–176.

Whetstone, W.R., & Hansson, A.M.O. (1989). Perceptions of self-care in Sweden: A cross-cultural replication. *Journal of Advanced Nursing, 14,* 962–969.

Williams, P.D., Valderrama, D.M., Gloria, M.D., Pascoguin, L.G., Saavedra, L.D., De La Rama, D.T., Ferry, T.C., Abaguin, C.M., & Zaldivar, S.B. (1988). Effects of preparation for mastectomy/hysterectomy on women's post-operative self-care behaviors. *International Journal of Nursing Studies, 25,* 191–206.

Woods, N.F. (1985). Self-care practices among young adult married women. *Research in Nursing and Health, 8,* 227–233.

Woods, N. (1989). Conceptualizations of self-care: Toward health-oriented models. *Advances in Nursing Science, 12*(1), 1–13.

Woods, N.F., Taylor, D., Mitchell, E.S., & Lentz, M.J. (1992). Perimenstrual symptoms and health-seeking behavior. *Western Journal of Nursing Research, 14,* 418–443.

Youssef, F.A. (1987). Discharge planning for psychiatric patients: The effects of a family-patient teaching programme. *Journal of Advanced Nursing, 12,* 611–616.

DOCTORAL DISSERTATIONS

Bach, C.A. (1989). The relationships among perceived control of activities of daily living, depression and life satisfaction in quadriplegic adults. *Dissertation Abstracts International, 49,* 2563B.

Baker, L.K. (1992). Predictors of self-care in adolescents with cystic fibrosis: A test and explication of Orem's theories of self-care and self-care deficit. *Dissertation Abstracts International, 53,* 1290B.

Banks, J. (1981). The effects of relaxation training and biofeedback on the weight of black, obese clients. *Dissertation Abstracts International, 42,* 965B.

Barkauskas, V.H. (1981). Effects of public health nursing interventions with primiparous mothers and their infants. *Dissertation Abstracts International*, *41*, 338B.

Beatty, E.R. (1992). Locus-of-control, self-actualization and self-care agency among registered nurses. *Dissertation Abstracts International*, *52*, 3523B.

Beauchesne, M.F. (1989). An investigation of the relationship between social support and the self care agency of mothers of developmentally disabled children. *Dissertation Abstracts International*, *50*, 121B.

Bliss-Holtz, V.J. (1986). Desire to learn infant care during the antepartal period: An exploratory study. *Dissertation Abstracts International*, *47*, 991B.

Brawn, J.W. (1987). Self care agency and adult health promotion. *Dissertation Abstracts International*, *48*, 1639B.

Brugge, P.A. (1982). The relationship between family as a social support system, health status, and exercise of self-care agency in the adult with a chronic illness. *Dissertation Abstracts International*, *42*, 4361B.

Budd, S.P. (1992). Women's health study: Self-efficacy and the rehabilitation experiences. *Dissertation Abstracts International*, *53*, 1291B.

Burkett, M.T.E. (1991). Relationships among reminiscence, self-esteem, and physical functioning in older African-American women. *Dissertation Abstracts International*, *51*, 3318B.

Burns, M.A. (1986). The use of self-care agency to meet the need for solitude and social interaction by chronically ill individuals. *Dissertation Abstracts International*, *47*, 992B–993B.

Clancy, M.T. (1984). Complementarity defined and measured as a specific component of the nursing care process in comparisons made between nurse-patient and physician-patient interactions. *Dissertation Abstracts International*, *44*, 3717B.

Cleveland, S.A. (1988). Assessment of self-care agency in patients with chronic obstructive pulmonary disease. *Dissertation Abstracts International*, *49*, 2124B.

Cofield, N.A. (1991). Effect of a health promotion program on self-care agency of children. *Dissertation Abstracts International*, *51*, 3777B.

Cunningham, G.D. (1990). Health promoting self-care behaviors in the community older adult. *Dissertation Abstracts International*, *50*, 4968B.

Davidson, J.D.U. (1989). Health embodiment: The relationship between self-care agency and health-promoting behaviors. *Dissertation Abstracts International*, *49*, 3102B.

Denyes, M.J. (1980). Development of an instrument to measure self-care agency in adolescents. *Dissertation Abstracts International*, *41*, 1716B.

Dodd, M.J. (1981). Enhancing self-care behaviors through informational interventions in patients with cancer who are receiving chemotherapy. *Dissertation Abstracts International*, *42*, 565B.

Eith, C.A. (1983). The nursing assessment of readiness for instruction of breast self-examination instrument (NAElB): Instrument development: *Dissertation Abstracts International*, *44*, 1780B.

Emerson, E.A. (1992). Playing for health: The process of play and self-expression in children who have experienced a sexual trauma. *Dissertation Abstracts International*, *53*, 2784B.

Evans, L.K. (1980). The relationship of needs awareness, locus of control, health state, and social support system to social interaction as a form of self-care behavior among elderly residents of public housing. *Dissertation Abstracts International*, *40*, 3662B–3663B.

Fernsler, J.L. (1984). A comparison of patient and nurse perceptions of patients' self-care deficits associated with cancer chemotherapy. *Dissertation Abstracts International*, *45*, 827B.

Folden, S.L. (1991). The effect of supportive-educative nursing interventions on post-stroke older adults' self-care perceptions. *Dissertation Abstracts International*, *52*, 159B.

Ford, D. (1988). Complications and referrals of patients with protein-calorie malnutrition. *Dissertation Abstracts International*, *49*, 1089B.

Fordham, P.N. (1990). A Q analysis of nursing behaviors which facilitate the grief work of parents with a premature infant in a neonatal intensive care unit. *Dissertation Abstracts International*, *51*, 661B.

Freeman, E.M. (1993). Self-care agency in gay men with HIV infection. *Dissertation Abstracts International*, *53*, 3400B.

Fuller, F.J. (1993). Health of elderly male dependent-care agents for a spouse with Alzheimer's disease. *Dissertation Abstracts International*, *53*, 4589B.

Garde, P.P. (1987). Orem's "self-care model" of nursing practice: Implications for program development in continuing education in nursing. *Dissertation Abstracts International*, 48, 284A.

Gast, H.L. (1984). The relationship between stages of ego development and developmental stages of health self care operations. *Dissertation Abstracts International*, 44, 3039B.

Good, M.P.L. (1992). Comparison of the effects of relaxation and music on postoperative pain. *Dissertation Abstracts International*, 53, 1783B.

Greenfield, P.H. (1990). A comparison of the self-care ability of employed women who have and have not maintained weight loss. *Dissertation Abstracts International*, 50, 3398B.

Haas, D.L. (1991). The relationship between coping dispositions and power components of dependent-care agency in parents of children with special health care needs. *Dissertation Abstracts International*, 52, 1351B.

Hanucharurnkul, S. (1989). Social support, self-care, and quality of life in cancer patients receiving radiotherapy in Thailand. *Dissertation Abstracts International*, 50, 494B.

Harris, J.L. (1990). Self-care actions of chronic schizophrenics associated with meeting solitude and social interaction self-care requisites. *Dissertation Abstracts International*, 50, 3920B.

Hartweg, D.L. (1992). Health promotion self-care actions of healthy, middle-aged women. *Dissertation Abstracts International*, 52, 6316B.

Harvey, B.L. (1987). Self-care practices of industrial workers to prevent low back pain. *Dissertation Abstracts International*, 48, 89B.

Hehn, D.M. (1986). Hospice care: Critical role behaviors related to self-care and role supplementation. *Dissertation Abstracts International*, 46, 2623B.

Humphreys, J.C. (1990). Dependent-care directed toward the prevention of hazards to life, health, and well-being in mothers and children who experience family violence. *Dissertation Abstracts International*, 51, 1744B.

Hurst, J.D. (1991). The relationship among self-care agency, risk-taking, and health risks in adolescents. *Dissertation Abstracts International*, 52, 1352B.

James, K.S. (1991). Factors related to self-care agency and self-care practices of obese adolescents. *Dissertation Abstracts International*, 52, 1955B.

Kain, C.D. (1986). Dorothea E. Orem's Self-Care Model of Nursing: Implications for program development in associate degree nursing education. *Dissertation Abstracts International*, 47, 994B.

Kennedy, L.M. (1991). The effectiveness of a self-care medication education protocol on the home medication behaviors of recently hospitalized elderly. *Dissertation Abstracts International*, 51, 3779B.

Lantz, J.M. (1982). Self-actualization: An indicator of self-care practices among adults 65 years and over. *Dissertation Abstracts International*, 42, 4017B.

Laurin, J. (1979). Development of a nursing process-outcome model based on Orem's concepts of nursing practice for quality nursing care evaluation. *Dissertation Abstracts International*, 40, 1122B.

Marten, M.L.C. (1983). The relationship of level of depression to perceived decision making capabilities of institutionalized elderly women. *Dissertation Abstracts International*, 43, 2855B–2856B.

Marz, MS. (1989). Effect of differentiated practice, conditioning factors and nursing agency on performance and strain of nurses in hospital settings. *Dissertation Abstracts International*, 50, 1856B.

McCaleb, K.A. (1992). Self-concept and self-care practices of healthy adolescents. *Dissertation Abstracts International*, 52, 3529B.

McDermott, M.A.N. (1990). The relationship between learned helplessness and self-care agency in adults as a function of gender and age. *Dissertation Abstracts International*, 50, 3403B.

Michaels, C.L. (1986). Development of a self-care assessment tool for hospitalized chronic obstructive pulmonary disease patients: A methodological study. *Dissertation Abstracts International*, 46, 3783B.

Monsen, R.B. (1989). Autonomy, coping, and self-care agency in healthy adolescents and in adolescents with spina bifida. *Dissertation Abstracts International*, 50, 2340B.

Musci, E.C. (1984). Relationship between family coping strategies and self-care during cancer chemotherapy treatments. *Dissertation Abstracts International*, 44, 3712B.

Neves, E.P. (1980). The relationship of hospitalized individuals' cognitive structure regarding health to their health self-care behaviors. *Dissertation Abstracts International*, 41, 522B.

Nicholas, P.K. (1991). Hardiness, self-care practices, and perceived health status in the elderly. *Dissertation Abstracts International*, 52, 1957B.

Olson, G.P. (1986). Perceived opportunity for and preference in decision-making of hospitalized men and women. *Dissertation Abstracts International, 47,* 572B–573B.

Parker, M.E. (1983). The use of Orem's self-care concept of nursing in curricula of selected baccalaureate programs of nursing education. *Dissertation Abstracts International, 43,* 2224A.

Passfro, V.A. (1989). Parental perceptions of neonatal intensive care unit discharge teaching. *Dissertation Abstracts International, 49,* 2569B.

Pinkerton, M. (1983). Self-care and burn-out in the professional nurse. *Dissertation Abstracts International, 44,* 1783B.

Pulliam, L.W. (1986). Relationship between social support and the nutritional status of patients receiving radiation therapy for cancer. *Dissertation Abstracts International, 46,* 262D.

Raven, M.C. (1990). Forging a new helping profession: The practice of Kinlein—1971–1986. *Dissertation Abstracts International, 50,* 1847B.

Rieder, K.A. (1982). The relationship among attitudinal, perceptual, and behavioral factors as indicators of hospitalized patients' participation in care. *Dissertation Abstracts International, 43,* 1044B.

Riley, C.P. (1989). Effects of a pulmonary rehabilitation program on dyspnea, self care, and pulmonary function of patients with chronic obstructive pulmonary disease. *Dissertation Abstracts International, 49,* 5231B.

Rowles, C.J. (1993). The relationship of selected personal and organizational variables and the tenure of directors of nursing in nursing homes. *Dissertation Abstracts International, 53,* 4593B.

Rozmus, C.L. (1991). A description of the maternal decision-making process regarding circumcision. *Dissertation Abstracts International, 51,* 3787B.

St. Onge, J.L. (1990). The relationship of self-care agency to health-seeking behaviors in caucasian and black U.S. veterans. *Dissertation Abstracts International, 50,* 3926B.

Scheetz, S.L. (1986). The relationship of social network characteristics to the performance of self-care by the chronically mentally ill adult in the community. *Dissertation Abstracts International, 47,* 2377B.

Schlatter, B.L. (1991). Control and satisfaction with the birth experience. *Dissertation Abstracts International, 52,* 164B.

Schorfheide, A.M. (1986). The relationship of reported self-care practice, parental motivation for self-care, and health locus of control with insulin dependent diabetic children and their families. *Dissertation Abstracts International, 46,* 3008B–3009B.

Schott-Baer, D. (1991). Family culture, family resources, dependent care, caregiver burden and self-care agency of spouses of cancer patients. *Dissertation Abstracts International, 51,* 3327B.

Scott, D.L. (1990). The relationship of knowledge and health locus-of-control of early adolescent males to the use of smokeless tobacco. *Dissertation Abstracts International, 50,* 4987B.

Simmons, S.J. (1990). Self-care agency and health-promoting behavior of a military population. *Dissertation Abstracts International, 51,* 2290B.

Sirles, A.T. (1986). The effect of a self-care health education program on parents' self-care knowledge, health locus of control and children's medical utilization rate. *Dissertation Abstracts International, 46,* 2628B.

Smith, C.T. (1990). The lived experience of staying healthy in rural black families. *Dissertation Abstracts International, 50,* 3925B.

Spezia, M.A. (1991). Family responses and self-care activities in school-age children with diabetes. *Dissertation Abstracts International, 52,* 2997B.

Stashinko, E. (1987). The relationship between self-perceptions of competence and self-care behaviors in third-grade children. *Dissertation Abstracts International, 48,* 1644D.

Stullenbarger, N.E. (1985). A Q-analysis of the self-care abilities of young, schoolaged children. *Dissertation Abstracts International, 45,* 2872B–2873B.

Underwood, P.R. (1979). Nursing care as a determinant in the development of self-care behavior by hospitalized adult schizophrenics. *Dissertation Abstracts International, 40,* 679B.

Vannoy, B.E. (1990). Relationships among basic conditioning factors, motivational dispositions, and the power element of self-care agency in people beginning a weight loss program. *Dissertation Abstracts International, 51,* 1197B.

Wells-Biggs, A.J. (1986). Hermeneutic interpretation of the work of Dorothea E. Orem: A nursing metaphor. *Dissertation Abstracts International, 47,* 576B.

Willard, G.A. (1990). Development of an instrument to measure the functional status of hospitalized patients. *Dissertation Abstracts International, 51,* 2823B.

MASTER'S THESES

Alvey, C.J. (1989). The relationship between perceived social support and health promotive self-care behaviors in older adults. *Master's Abstracts International, 27,* 41.

Baldwin, B.S. (1992). Female caregivers of elderly relatives with dementia: Implications for day center intervention. *Master's Abstracts International, 30,* 92.

Barbel, L.L. (1989). Perceived learning needs of cardiac patients. *Master's Abstracts International, 27,* 90.

Belcher, D.H. (1991). The effect of a career awareness program on the success rate of the practical nurse student. *Master's Abstracts International, 29,* 638.

Cipolla, R.M. (1993). Retrospective record review of lost work days and a cumulative trauma disorders abatement program in a clothing manufacturer: Implications for nursing. *Master's Abstracts International, 31,* 268.

Coker, C. (1989). An impact evaluation of a therapeutic touch continuing education activity. *Master's Abstracts International, 27,* 251.

Daniels, A.E., & McMahan, T.A. (1993). Self-care burden in women with human immunodeficiency virus. *Master's Abstracts International, 31,* 269.

Davidson, J.D.U. (1988). Historical perspective of self-care agency among elderly Mennonites at the turn of the twentieth century. *Master's Abstracts International, 26,* 418.

Desmond, A.M. (1989). The relationship between loneliness and social interaction in women prisoners. *Master's Abstracts International, 27,* 93.

Drake Wilke, C.B. (1989). Health behavior and patterns of solvent use of recreational woodcrafters. *Master's Abstracts International, 17,* 270.

Edwards, C.J. (1988). Self-care agency and job satisfaction in patients recovering from a myocardial infarction. *Master's Abstracts International, 26,* 236.

Feigenbaum, J. (1993). Palliative care volunteers' descriptions of the stressors experienced in their relationship with clients coping with terminal illness at home. *Master's Abstracts International, 31,* 301.

Fillingame, M. (1991). Preoperative self-care agency and postoperative self-care outcomes in ambulatory surgical patients. *Master's Abstracts International, 29,* 91.

French, E.D. (1988). Relationship between perceptions of social support and maternal perceptions of infants. *Master's Abstracts International, 26,* 157.

Galbreath, C. (1990). The relationships of community health nurses' health beliefs, their practice of the self-care requisite of breast self-examination, and the influence on client teaching. *Master's Abstracts International, 28,* 408.

Gaslin, T.C. (1993). Client perception of antepartal education information. *Master's Abstracts International, 31,* 272.

Giermek, C. (1990). The relationship of the locus-of-control and self-care practices in the patient with basal cell skin cancer. *Master's Abstracts International, 28,* 575.

Grachek, M.K. (1988). The relationship between loneliness and self-care practices of elderly residents of a senior housing complex. *Master's Abstracts International, 26,* 105.

Gustek, E.D. (1992). Barriers to self-care health practices in the single female patient. *Master's Abstracts International, 30,* 708.

Guswiler, K.A. (1991). Cancer patients' responses to chemotherapy teaching on side effect management. *Master's Abstracts International, 29,* 642.

Halleron, P. (1989). Health promotion/disease prevention in health services: Towards the development of a self-care model. *Master's Abstracts International, 27,* 500.

Harmer, M.A. (1993). Perceptions of public health nurses and principals of adolescents' self-care deficits. *Master's Abstracts International, 31,* 299.

Harper, B. (1993). Nurses' beliefs about social support and the effect of nursing care on cardiac clients attitudes in reducing cardiac risk factors. *Master's Abstracts International, 31,* 273.

Harter, J.W. (1989). Self-care action demands identified by female myocardial infarction patients. *Master's Abstracts International, 27,* 254.

Haynes, L.A. (1988). The relationship between perceived exercise of self-care agency of diabetics and reported compliance to the diabetic regimen. *Master's Abstracts International, 26,* 106.

Ho, G-F. (1990). Self-help practice in persons with rheumatoid arthritis. *Master's Abstracts International, 28,* 410.

Hollstein, M.S. (1989). The relationship between self-care practice and social support in frail elderly community residents. *Master's Abstracts International, 27,* 96.

Jackson, L.E. (1989). Self-care agency and limitations with respect to contraceptive behavior of Mexican-American women. *Master's Abstracts International, 27,* 97.

Jacobi, D.A. (1990). Effectiveness of cerebral palsy discharge planning instruction using scripted role playing for undergraduate nursing students. *Master's Abstracts International, 28,* 576.

Jaster, S.E. (1992). Self-care burden with radiotherapy for head and neck cancer. *Master's Abstracts International, 30,* 95.

Jayroe, L.S. (1990). The effect of competency-based interviews upon the outcome of graduate nurses' orientation. *Master's Abstracts International, 28,* 273.

Jefferies, M.A. (1991). Testicular self-examination: The effectiveness of an educational program for professional men. *Master's Abstracts International, 29,* 93.

Keesler, C.A. (1992). The study of the characteristics of health beliefs, value placed on health, and locus of control of adults participant in a cancer screening program. *Master's Abstracts International, 30,* 1292.

Kiplinger, M.S. (1989). A study of self-care agency of adolescents with asthma and their self-care practices. *Master's Abstracts International, 27,* 377.

Kohlmeier, C.M. (1989). Impact of the chronically ill child on maternal locus-of-control. *Master's Abstracts International, 27,* 491.

Lawton, L.L. (1992). Patient's perceptions of being prepared for self-care following discharge from an acute care setting. *Master's Abstracts International, 30,* 711.

Lyons, E.M. (1993). Relationship between literacy and compliance in middle-aged adults with essential hypertension. *Master's Abstracts International, 31,* 2778.

Marciniak, C.J. (1989). A comparison of self-care agency in prepared and unprepared women who have had caesarean deliveries. *Master's Abstracts International, 27,* 257.

Martinez, R.H. (1991). A study of caregivers of elderly veterans. *Master's Abstracts International, 29,* 96.

Masiulaniec, B.A.S. (1990). Self-care practices of a selected homeless population. *Master's Abstracts International, 28,* 63.

McNamara, N.T. (1993). Older healthy Hispanic women's beliefs about breast cancer. *Master's Abstracts International, 31,* 278.

Molde, J. (1990). Self-care agency: Relationship to nurses' attitudes toward urinary incontinence. *Master's Abstracts International, 28,* 414.

Myers, T.C. (1988). An examination of the relationship between self-esteem, the perceived social support systems, and the self-care nutritional practices of adult working women. *Master's Abstracts International, 26,* 422.

Panczykowski, C.A. (1991). The chronically ill adolescent's perception of the effects of primary nursing on self-care abilities. *Master's Abstracts International, 29,* 649.

Price, H.J. (1988). Variables influencing burden in spousal and adult child primary caregivers of persons with Alzheimer's disease in the home setting. *Master's Abstracts International, 26,* 244.

Ragan, C.A. (1988). Self-care practices of the homeless. *Master's Abstracts International, 26,* 110.

Reynolds, S.K. (1990). Exercise of self-care agency and patient satisfaction with nursing care. *Master's Abstracts International, 28,* 114.

Riley, S. (1990). A study of the relationship between an AIDS health education curriculum and self-care agency of middle school students. *Master's Abstracts International, 28,* 582.

Schumann, C.A. (1988). The relationship between absenteeism and job satisfaction in staff nurses. *Master's Abstracts International, 26,* 111.

Seymour, S.F. (1991). Preoperative self-care agency and postoperative self-care outcomes in ambulatory surgical patients. *Master's Abstracts International, 29,* 91.

Smith, C.I. (1991). Comparison of diet and exercise versus diet alone in relapse of obesity. *Master's Abstracts International, 29,* 268.

Sturt, M.K. (1992). Self-care practices of women who experience nausea and vomiting during pregnancy. *Master's Abstracts International, 30,* 1301.

Thrasher, C. (1992). The effect of an educational program on handwashing behaviors of registered nurses in a home health care agency. *Master's Abstracts International, 30,* 100.

Valone, J.D. (1992). Aerobic exercise self-care agency and the prevention of the health deviation of a second cardiovascular event. *Master's Abstracts International, 30,* 302.

Verostko-Harty, M.A. (1990). Self-care, locus-of-control and the prevention of decubitus ulcers. *Master's Abstracts International, 28,* 116.

Wambach, K.A. (1990). The effect of lactation consultant contact on early breastfeeding problems. *Master's Abstracts International, 28,* 116.

Ward, S.T. (1991). Physical restraint use on the confused elderly patient in an acute care setting: A retrospective study. *Master's Abstracts International, 29,* 653.

Webb, R.J. (1989). A comparison between hemodialysis and CAPD as a function of locus-of-control. *Master's Abstracts International, 28,* 117.

Wetmore, D.E. (1989). Expressed concerns of individuals with HIV positive antibody reaction. *Master's Abstracts International, 27,* 106.

Witman, M.A.M. (1992). Effects of videotaped basic cancer information on self-reported state anxiety of newly-diagnosed cancer patients. *Master's Abstracts International, 30,* 719.

Witherspoon, B.B. (1989). Post-hospitalization management of acute postoperative pain with a self-directed relaxation technique. *Master's Abstracts International, 27,* 383.

EDUCATION

Berbiglia, V.A. (1991). A case study: Perspectives on a self-care deficit nursing theory-based curriculum. *Journal of Advanced Nursing, 16,* 1158–1163.

Farnham, S., & Fowler, M. (1985). Demedicalization, bilingualization, and reconceptualization: Teaching Orem's self-care model to the RN-BSN student. In J. Riehl-Sisca, *The science and art of self-care* (pp. 35–40). Norwalk, CT: Appleton-Century-Crofts.

Fenner, K. (1979). Developing a conceptual framework. *Nursing Outlook, 27,* 122–126.

Goodwin, J.O. (1980). A cross-cultural approach to integrating nursing theory and practice. *Nurse Educator, 5(6),* 15–20.

Herrington, J., & Houston, S. (1984). Using Orem's theory: A plan for all seasons. *Nursing and Health Care 5(1),* 45–47.

Kruger, S.F. (1988). The application of the self-care concept of nursing in the Wichita State University baccalaureate program. *Kansas Nurse, 63(12),* 6–7.

Langland, R.M., & Farrah, S.J. (1990). Using a self-care framework for continuing education in gerontological nursing. *Journal of Continuing Education in Nursing, 21,* 267–270.

Laschinger, H.S. (1990). Helping students apply a nursing conceptual framework in the clinical setting. *Nurse Educator, 15(3),* 20–24.

Mulkeen, H. (1989). Diabetes: Teaching the teaching of self-care. *Nursing Times, 85(3),* 63–65.

Piemme, J.A., & Trainor, M.A. (1977). A first-year nursing course in a baccalaureate program. *Nursing Outlook, 25,* 184–187.

Richeson, M., & Huch, M. (1988). Self-care and comfort: A framework for nursing practice. *New Zealand Nursing Journal, 81(6),* 26–27.

Riehl-Sisca, J. (1985). Determining criteria for graduate and undergraduate self-care curriculums. In J. Riehl-Sisca, *The science and art of self-care* (pp. 20–24). Norwalk, CT: Appleton-Century-Crofts.

Taylor, S.G. (1985). Curriculum development for preservice programs using Orem's theory of nursing. In J. Riehl-Sisca, *The science and art of self-care* (pp. 25–32). Norwalk, CT: Appleton-Century-Crofts.

Taylor, S.G. (1985). Teaching self-care deficit theory to generic students. In J. Riehl-Sisca, *The science and art of self-care* (pp. 41–46). Norwalk, CT: Appleton-Century-Crofts.

Woolley, A.S., McLaughlin, J., & Durham, J.D. (1990). Linking diploma and bachelor's degree nursing education: An Illinois experiment. *Journal of Professional Nursing, 6,* 206–212.

ADMINISTRATION

Allison, S.E. (1973). A framework for nursing action in a nurse-conducted diabetic management clinic. *Journal of Nursing Administration, 3(4),* 53–60.

Allison, S.E. (1985). Structuring nursing practice based on Orem's theory of nursing: A nurse administrator's perspective. In J. Riehl-Sisca, *The science and art of self-care* (pp. 225–235). Norwalk, CT: Appleton-Century-Crofts.

Allison, S.E., McLaughlin, K., & Walker, D. (1991). Nursing theory: A tool to put nursing back into nursing administration. *Nursing Administration Quarterly, 15(3),* 72–78.

Angeles, D.M. (1991). An Orem-based NICU orientation checklist. *Neonatal Network, 9(7),* 43–48.

Aukamp, V. (1988). Defining characteristics of knowledge deficit in the third trimester. In R.M. Carroll-Johnston (Ed.), *Classification of nursing diagnosis: Proceedings of the Eighth Conference: North American Nursing Diagnosis Association* (pp. 299–306). Philadelphia: JB Lippincott.

Avery, P. (1992). Self-care in the hospital setting: The Prince Henry Hospital experience. *Lamp, 49*(2), 26–28.

Backscheider, J.E. (1974). Self-care requirements, self-care capabilities and nursing systems in the diabetic nurse management clinic. *American Journal of Public Health, 64*, 1138–1146.

Baldwin, J., & Davis, L.L. (1989). Assessing parents as health educators. *Pediatric Nursing, 15*, 453–457.

Barnes, L.P. (1991). Teaching self-care to children. *American Journal of Maternal Child Nursing, 16*, 101.

Bliss-Holtz, J., McLaughlin, K., & Taylor, S.G. (1990). Validating nursing theory for use within a computerized nursing information system. *Advances in Nursing Science, 13*(2), 46–52.

Bliss-Holtz, J., Taylor, S.G., & McLaughlin, K. (1992). Nursing theory as a base for a computerized nursing information system. *Nursing Science Quarterly, 5*, 124–128.

Bliss-Holtz, J., Taylor, S.G., McLaughlin, K., Sayers, P., & Nickle, L. (1992). Development of a computerized information system based on self-care deficit nursing theory. In J.M. Arnold & G.A. Pearson, *Computer applications in nursing education and practice* (pp. 87–93). New York: National League for Nursing.

Brennan, M., & Duffy, M. (1992). Utilizing theory in practice to empower nursing. *Nursing Administration Quarterly, 16*(3), 32–33.

Campbell, C. (1984). Orem's story. *Nursing Mirror, 159*(13), 28–30.

Chang, B.L. (1980). Evaluation of health care professionals in facilitating self-care: Review of the literature and a conceptual model. *Advances in Nursing Science, 3*(1), 43–58.

Clark, J., & Bishop, J. (1988). Model-making. *Nursing Times, 84*(27), 37–40.

Clinton, J.F., Denyes, M.J., Goodwin, J.O., & Koto, E.M. (1977). Developing criterion measures of nursing care: Case study of a process. *Journal of Nursing Administration, 7*(7), 41–45.

Coleman, L.J. (1980). Orem's self-care concept of nursing. In J.P. Riehl & C. Roy, *Conceptual models for nursing practice* (2nd ed., pp. 315–328). New York: Appleton-Century-Crofts.

Crews, J. (1972). Nurse-managed cardiac clinics. *Cardio-Vascular Nursing, 8*, 15–18.

Del Togno-Armanasco, V., Olivas, G.S., & Harter, S. (1989). Developing an integrated nursing care management model. *Nursing Management, 20*(10), 26–29.

Dennis, L.I. (1989). Soviet hospital nursing: A model for self-care. *Journal of Nursing Education, 28*, 76–77.

Derstine, J.B. (1992). Theory-based advanced rehabilitation nursing: Is it a reality? *Holistic Nursing Practice, 6*(2), 1–6.

Dibner, L.A., Murphy, J.S. (1991). Nurse entrepreneurs. *Journal of Psychosocial Nursing and Mental Health Services, 29*(5), 30–34.

Dier, K.A. (1987). A model for collaboration in nursing practice: Thailand and Canada. In K.J. Hannah, M. Reimer, W.C. Mills, & S. Letourneau (Eds.), *Clinical judgment and decision making: The future with nursing diagnosis* (pp. 323–327). New York: John Wiley & Sons.

Doherty, S. (1992). Care plans—a personal view. *British Journal of Theatre Nursing, 2*(5), 4–5.

Duncan, S., & Murphy, F. (1988). Embracing a conceptual model. *The Canadian Nurse, 84*(4), 24–26.

Dyer, S. (1990). Team work for personal patient care. *Nursing the Elderly, 3*(7), 28–30.

Estes, S.D., & Hart, M. (1993). A model for the development of the CNS role in adolescent health promotion self-care. *Clinical Nurse Specialist, 7*, 111–115.

Feldsine, F. (1982). Options for transition into practice: Nursing process orientation program. *Journal of New York State Nurses' Association, 13*, 11–16.

Fernandez, R., Brennan, M.L., Alvarez, A.R., & Duffy, M.A. (1990). Theory-based practice: A model for nurse retention. *Nursing Administration Quarterly, 14*(4), 47–53.

Fernandez, R., & Wheeler, J.I. (1990). Organizing a nursing system through theory-based practice. In G.G. Mayer, M.J. Madden, & E. Lawrenz (Eds.), *Patient care delivery models* (pp. 63–83). Rockville, MD: Aspen.

Fondiller, S. (1991). The new look in nursing documentation. *American Journal of Nursing, 91*, 65–67, 70–71, 73–74, 75.

Fridgen, R., & Nelson, S. (1992). Teaching tool for renal transplant recipients using Orem's self-care model. *CANNT Journal, 2*(3), 18–26.

Fukuda, N. (1990). Outcome standards for the client with chronic congestive heart failure. *Journal of Cardiovascular Nursing, 4*(3), 59–70.

Gallant, B.W., & McLane, A.M. (1979). Outcome criteria: A process for validation at the unit level. *Journal of Nursing Administration, 9*(1), 14–21.

Graff, B.M., Thomas, J.S., Hollingsworth, A.D., Cohen, S.M., & Rubin, M.M. (1992). Development of a postoperative self-assessment form. *Clinical Nurse Specialist, 6*, 47–50.

Hageman, P., & Ventura, M. (1981). Utilizing patient outcome criteria to measure the effects of a medication teaching regimen. *Western Journal of Nursing Research, 3*, 25–33.

Harman, L., Wabin, D., MacInnis, L., Baird, D., Mattiuzzi, D., & Savage, P. (1989). Developing clinical decision-making skills in staff nurses: An educational program. *Journal of Continuing Education in Nursing, 20*, 102–106.

Hathaway, D., & Strong, M. (1988). Theory, practice, and research in transplant nursing. *Journal of the American Nephrology Nurses Association, 15*, 9–12.

Holzemer, W.L. (1992). Linking primary health care and self-care through case management. *International Nursing Review, 39*, 83–89.

Hooten, S.L. (1992). Education of staff nurses to practice within a conceptual framework. *Nursing Administration Quarterly, 16*(3), 34–35.

Horn, B. (1978). Development of criterion measures of nursing care. (Abstract). In *Communicating nursing research. Vol 11: New approaches to communicating nursing research* (pp 87–89). Boulder, CO: Western Interstate Commission for Higher Education.

Horn, B.J., & Swain, M.A. (1976). An approach to development of criterion measures for quality patient care. In *Issues in evaluation research* (pp. 74–82). Kansas City: American Nurses Association.

Horn, B.J., & Swain, M.A. (1977). Development of criterion measures of nursing care (Vols. 1–2, NTIS Nos. PB-267 004 and PB-267 005). Ann Arbor, MI: University of Michigan.

Hunter, L. (1992). Applying Orem to skin. *Nursing (London), 5*(4), 16–18.

Husted, E., & Strzelecki, S. (1985). Orem: A foundation for nursing practice in a community hospital. In J. Riehl-Sisca, *The science and art of self-care* (pp. 199–207). Norwalk, CT: Appleton-Century-Crofts.

Isenberg, M.A. (1991). Insights from Orem's nursing theory on differentiating nursing practice: In I.E. Goertzen (Ed.), *Differentiating nursing practice: Into the twenty-first century* (pp. 45–49). Kansas City, MO: American Academy of Nursing.

Jenny, J. (1991). Self-care deficit theory and nursing diagnosis: A test of conceptual fit. *Journal of Nursing Education, 30*, 227–232.

Johannsen, J.M. (1992). Self-care assessment: Key to teaching and discharge planning. *Dimensions of Critical Care Nursing, 11*, 48–56.

Kappeli, S. (1987). The influence of nursing models on clinical decision making I. In K.J. Hannah, M. Reimer, W.C. Mills, & S. Letourneau (Eds.), *Clinical judgment and decision making: The future with nursing diagnosis* (pp. 33–41). New York: John Wiley & Sons.

Kitson, A.L. (1986). Indicators of quality in nursing care—an alternative approach. *Journal of Advanced Nursing, 11*, 133–144.

Laurie-Shaw, B., & Ives, S.M. (1988). Implementing Orem's self-care deficit theory. Part I—Selecting a framework and planning for implementation. *Canadian Journal of Nursing Administration, 1*(1), 9–12.

Laurie-Shaw, B., & Ives, S.M. (1988). Part II. Implementing Orem's self-care deficit theory: Adopting a conceptual framework of nursing. *Canadian Journal of Nursing Administration, 1*(2), 16–19.

Leatt, P., Bay, K.S., & Stinson, S.M. (1981). An instrument for assessing and classifying patients by type of care. *Nursing Research, 30*, 145–150.

Lott, T.F., Blazey, M.E., & West, M.G. (1992). Patient participation in health care: An underused resource. *Nursing Clinics of North America, 27*, 61–76.

Loveland-Cherry, C., Whall, A., Griswold, E., Bronneville, R., & Page, G. (1985). A nursing protocol based on Orem's self-care model: Application with aftercare clients. In J. Riehl-Sisca, *The science and art of self-care* (pp. 285–297). Norwalk, CT: Appleton-Century-Crofts.

Mason, T., & Chandley, M. (1990). Nursing models in a special hospital: A critical analysis of efficacity. *Journal of Advanced Nursing, 15*, 667–673.

MacLeod, J.A., & Sella, S. (1992). One year later: Using role theory to evaluate a new delivery system. *Nursing Forum, 27*(2), 20–28.

McCoy, S. (1989). Teaching self-care in a market-oriented world. *Nursing Management, 20*(5), 22, 26.

McKeighen, R.J., Mehmert, P.A., & Dickel, C.A. (1991). Self-care deficit, bathing/hygiene: Defining characteristics and related factors utilized by staff nurses in an acute care setting. In R.M. Carroll-Johnston

(Ed.), *Classification of nursing diagnosis: Proceedings of the Ninth Conference: North American Nursing Diagnosis Association* (pp. 247–248). Philadelphia: JB Lippincott.

McLaughlin, K., Taylor, S., Bliss-Holtz, J., Sayers, P., & Nickle, L. (1990). Shaping the future: The marriage of nursing theory and informatics. *Computers in Nursing, 8,* 174–179.

McVay, J. (1985). A beginning of service and caring. In J. Riehl-Sisca, *The science and art of self-care* (pp. 245–252). Norwalk, CT: Appleton-Century-Crofts.

McWilliams, B., Murphy, F., & Sobiski, A. (1988). Why self-care theory works for us. *The Canadian Nurse, 84*(9), 38–40.

Mehta, S.M. (1993). Applying Orem's self-care framework. *Geriatric Nursing, 14,* 182–185.

Michaels, C. (1985). Clinical specialist consultation to assess self-care agency among hospitalized COPD patients. In J. Riehl-Sisca, *The science and art of self-care* (pp. 279–284). Norwalk, CT: Appleton-Century-Crofts.

Miller, J.F. (1980). The dynamic focus of nursing: A challenge to nursing administration. *Journal of Nursing Administration, 10*(1), 13–18.

Nunn, D., & Marriner-Tomey, A. (1989). Applying Orem's model in nursing administration. In B. Henry, C. Arndt, M. Di-Vincenti, & A. Marriner-Tomey (Eds.), *Dimensions of nursing administration: Theory, research, education, practice* (pp. 63–67). Boston: Blackwell Scientific Publications.

O'Connor, C.T. (1990). Patient education with a purpose. *Journal of Nursing Staff Development, 6,* 145–147.

Padilla, G.V., & Grant, M.M. (1982). Quality assurance programme for nursing. *Journal of Advanced Nursing, 7,* 135–145.

Paternostro, I. (1992). Developing theory-based software for nurses, by nurses. *Nursing Administration Quarterly, 16*(3), 33–34.

Porter, D., & Shamian, J. (1983). Self-care in theory and practice. *The Canadian Nurse, 79*(8), 21–23.

Reid, B., Allen, A.F., Gauthier, T., & Campbell, H. (1989). Solving the Orem mystery: An educational strategy. *Journal of Continuing Education in Nursing, 20,* 108–110.

Roach, K.G., & Woods, H.B. (1993). Implementing cooperative care on an acute care medical unit. *Clinical Nurse Specialist, 7,* 26–29.

Romine, S. (1986). Applying Orem's theory of self-care to staff development. *Journal of Nursing Staff Development, 2*(2), 77–79.

Rossow-Sebring, J., Carrieri, V., & Seward, H. (1992). Effect of Orem's model on nurse attitudes and charting behavior. *Journal of Nursing Staff Development, 8,* 207–212.

Scherer, P. (1988). Hospitals that attract (and keep) nurses. *American Journal of Nursing, 88,* 34–40.

Sella, S., & MacLeod, J.A. (1991). One year later: Evaluating a changing delivery system. *Nursing Forum, 26*(2), 5–11.

Smith, J.M., & Sorrell, V. (1989). Developing wellness programs: A nurse-managed stay well center for senior citizens. *Clinical Nurse Specialist, 3,* 198–202.

Snyder, M., Brugge-Wiger, P., Ahern, S., Connelly, S., DePew, C., Kappas-Larson, P., Semmerling, E., & Wyble, S. (1991). Complex health problems: Clinically assessing self-management abilities. *Journal of Gerontological Nursing, 17*(4), 23–27.

Taira, F. (1991). Individualized medication sheets. *Nursing Economics, 9,* 56–58.

Taylor, S.G. (1987). A model for nursing diagnosis and clinical decision making using Orem's self-care deficit theory of nursing. In K.J. Hannah, M. Reimer, W.C. Mills, & S. Letourneau (Eds.), *Clinical judgment and decision making: The future with nursing diagnosis* (pp. 84–86). New York: John Wiley & Sons.

Taylor, S.G. (1991). The structure of nursing diagnoses from Orem's theory. *Nursing Science Quarterly, 4,* 24–32.

Van Eron, M. (1985). Clinical application of self-care deficit theory. In J. Riehl-Sisca, *The science and art of self-care* (pp. 208–224). Norwalk, CT: Appleton-Century-Crofts.

Watson, S. (1989). The graduate experience: A professional development program for college health nurses based on a conceptual model of nursing. *Mid-Atlantic College Health Association News,* Winter, 10.

Weis, A. (1988). Cooperative care: An application of Orem's self-care theory. *Patient Education and Counseling, 11,* 141–146.

PRACTICE

Alford, D.M. (1985). Self-care practices in ambulatory nursing clinics for older adults. In J. Riehl-Sisca, *The science and art of self-care* (pp. 253–261). Norwalk, CT: Appleton-Century-Crofts.

Anderson, S.B. (1992). Guillain-Barré syndrome: Giving the patient control. *Journal of Neuroscience Nursing, 24,* 158–162.

Anna, D.J., Christensen, D.G., Hohon, S.A., Ord, L., & Wells, S.R. (1978). Implementing Orem's conceptual framework. *Journal of Nursing Administration, 8*(11), 8–11.

Atkins, F.D. (1992). An uncertain future: Children of mentally ill parents. *Journal of Psychosocial Nursing and Mental Health Services, 30*(8), 13–16.

Beckmann, C.A. (1987). Maternal-child health in Brazil. *Journal of Obstetric, Gynecologic, and Neonatal Nursing, 16,* 238–241.

Beed, P. (1991). Sight restored. *Nursing Times, 87*(30), 46–48.

Behi, R. (1986). Look after yourself. *Nursing Times, 82*(37), 35–37.

Bilitski, J.S. (1981). Nursing science and the laws of health: The test of substance as a step in the process of theory development. *Advances in Nursing Science, 4*(1), 15–29.

Blaylock, B. (1991). Enhancing self-care of the elderly client: Practical teaching tips for ostomy care. *Journal of Enterostomal Therapy Nursing, 18,* 118–121.

Bracher, E. (1989). A model approach. *Nursing Times, 85*(43), 42–43.

Bromley, B. (1980). Applying Orem's self-care theory in enterostomal therapy. *American Journal of Nursing, 80,* 245–249.

Buckwalter, K.C., & Kerfoot, K.M. (1982). Teaching patients self care: A critical aspect of psychiatric discharge planning. *Journal of Psychiatric Nursing and Mental Health Services, 20*(5), 15–20.

Bunting, S.M. (1989). Stress on caregivers of the elderly. *Advances in Nursing Science, 11*(2), 63–73.

Burnside, I. (1988). *Nursing and the aged: A self-care approach* (3rd ed.). New York: McGraw-Hill.

Calley, J.M., Dirksen, M., Engalla, M., & Hennrich, M.L. (1980). The Orem self-care nursing model. In J.P. Riehl & C. Roy, *Conceptual models for nursing practice* (2nd ed., pp. 302–314). New York: Appleton-Century-Crofts.

Campuzano, M. (1982). Self-care following coronary artery bypass surgery. *Focus on Critical Care, 9*(2), 55–56.

Caradus, A. (1991). Nursing theory and operating suite nursing practice. *ACORN Journal, 4*(2), 29–30, 32.

Catanese, M.L. (1987). Vaginal birth after cesarean: Recommendations, risks, realities, and the client's right to know. *Holistic Nursing Practice, 2*(1), 35–43.

Chamorro, L.C. (1985). Self-care in the Puerto Rican community. In J. Riehl-Sisca, *The science and art of self-care* (pp. 189–195). Norwalk, CT; Appleton-Century-Crofts.

Chin, S. (1985). Can self-care theory be applied to families? In J. Riehl-Sisca, *The science and art of self-care* (pp. 56–62). Norwalk, CT: Appleton-Century-Crofts.

Clark, A.P. (1985). Self-care by the person with diabetes mellitus. In J. Riehl-Sisca, *The science and art of self-care* (pp. 126–131). Norwalk, CT: Appleton-Century-Crofts.

Clang, E.D. (1985). Nursing system design for a young married diabetic. In J. Riehl-Sisca, *The science and art of self-care* (pp. 113–125). Norwalk, CT: Appleton-Century-Crofts.

Cohen, R. (1985). Sexual and self-care practices of adults. In J. Riehl-Sisca, *The science and art of self-care* (pp. 298–306). Norwalk, CT: Appleton-Century-Crofts.

Comptom, P. (1989). Drug abuse: A self-care deficit. *Journal of Psychosocial Nursing and Mental Health Services, 27*(3), 22–26.

Connelly, C.E. (1987). Self-care and the chronically ill patient. *Nursing Clinics of North America, 22,* 621–629.

Craig, C. (1989). Mr. Simpson's hip replacement. *Nursing (London), 3*(44), 12–19.

Cretain, G.K. (1989). Motivational factors in breast self-examination: Implications for nurses. *Cancer Nursing, 12,* 250–256.

delaCruz, L.A.D. (1988). In search of psychiatric nursing theory: An exploration of Orem's self-care model's applicability. *Canadian Journal of Psychiatric Nursing, 29*(3), 10–16.

Dashiff, C.J. (1988). Theory development in psychiatric-mental health nursing: An analysis of Orem's theory. *Archives of Psychiatric Nursing, 2,* 366–372.

Davidhizar, R., & Cosgray, R. (1990). The use of Orem's model in psychiatric rehabilitation assessment. *Rehabilitation Nursing, 15*(1), 39–41.

Dear, M.R., & Keen, M.F. (1982). Promotion of self-care in the employee with rheumatoid arthritis. *Occupational Health Nursing, 30*(1), 32–34.

Dropkin, M.J. (1981). Development of a self-care teaching program for postoperative head and neck patients. *Cancer Nursing, 4,* 103–106.

Duffey, J., Miller, M.P., & Parlocha, P. (1993). Psychiatric home care: A framework for assessment and intervention. *Home Healthcare Nurse, 11*(2), 22–28.

Dumas, L. (1992). (Nursing care based on Orem's theory.) *The Canadian Nurse, 88*(6), 36–39.

Dunn, B. (1990). Alcohol dependency: Health promotion and Orem's model. *Nursing Standard, 4*(40), 34.

Dunphy, J., & Jackson, E. (1985). Planning nursing care for the postpartum mother and her newborn. In J. Riehl-Sisca, *The science and art of self-care* (pp. 63–90). Norwalk, CT: Appleton-Century-Crofts.

Eichelberger, K.M., Kaufman, D.N., Rundahl, M.E., & Schwartz, N.E. (1980). Self-care nursing plan: Helping children to help themselves. *Pediatric Nursing, 6*(3), 9–13.

Eliopoulos, C. (1984). A self care model for gerontological nursing. *Geriatric Nursing, 4*, 366–369.

Facteau, L.M. (1980). Self-care concepts and the care of the hospitalized child. *Nursing Clinics of North America, 15*, 145–155.

Fawcett, J., Archer, C.L., Becker, D., Brown, K.K., Gann, S., Wong, M.J., & Wurster, A.B. (1992). Guidelines for selecting a conceptual model of nursing: Focus on the individual patient. *Dimensions of Critical Care Nursing, 11*, 268–277.

Fawcett, J., Cariello, F.P., Davis, D.A., Farley, J., Zimmaro, D.M., & Watts, R.J. (1987). Conceptual models of nursing: Application to critical care nursing practice. *Dimensions of Critical Care Nursing, 6*, 202–213.

Fields, L.M. (1987). A clinical application of the Orem nursing model in labor and delivery. *Emphasis: Nursing, 2*, 102–108.

Finnegan, T. (1986). Self-care and the elderly. *New Zealand Nursing Journal, 79*(4), 10–13.

Fitzgerald, S. (1980). Utilizing Orem's self-care nursing model in designing an educational program for the diabetic. *Topics in Clinical Nursing, 2*(2), 57–65.

Flanagan, M. (1991). Self-care for a leg ulcer. *Nursing Times, 87*(23), 67–68, 70, 72.

Foote, A., Holcombe, J., Piazza, D., & Wright, P. (1993). Orem's theory used as a guide for the nursing care of an eight-year-old child with leukemia. *Journal of Pediatric Oncology Nursing, 10*(1), 26–32.

Frey, M.A., & Denyes, M.J. (1989). Health and illness self-care in adolescents with IDDM: A test of Orem's theory. *Advances in Nursing Science, 12*(1), 67–75.

Fridgen, R., & Nelson, S. (1992). Teaching tool for renal transplant recipients using Orem's self-care model. *CANNT, 2*(3), 18–26.

Gantz, S.B. (1980). A fourth-grade adventure in self-directed learning. *Topics in Clinical Nursing, 2*(2), 29–38.

Garrett, A.P. (1985). A nursing system design for a patient with myocardial infarction. In J. Riehl-Sisca, *The science and art of self-care* (pp. 142–160). Norwalk, CT: Appleton-Century-Crofts.

Garvan, P., Lee, M., Lloyd K., & Sullivan, T.J. (1980). Self-care applied to the aged. *New Jersey Nurse, 10*(1), 3–5.

Geyer, E. (1990). Self-care issues for the elderly. *Dimensions in Oncology Nursing, 4*(2), 33–35.

Gibson, K.T. (1980). The type A personality: Implications for nursing practice. *Cardio-Vascular Nursing, 16*(5), 25–28.

Goldstein, N., Zink, M., Stevenson, L., Anderson, M., Wollery, L., & DePompolo, T. (1983). Self-care: A framework for the future. In P.L. Chinn (Ed.), *Advances in nursing theory development* (pp. 107–121). Rockville, MD: Aspen.

Gray, V.R., & Sergi, J.S. (1989). Family self-care. In P.J. Bomar (Ed.), *Nurses and family health promotion: Concepts, assessment, and interventions* (pp. 67–77). Baltimore: Williams & Wilkins.

Haas, D.L. (1990). Application of Orem's self-care deficit theory to the pediatric chronically ill population. *Issues in Comprehensive Pediatric Nursing, 13*, 253–264.

Hammonds, T.A. (1985). Self-care practices of Navajo Indians. In J. Riehl-Sisca, *The science and art of self-care* (pp. 171–180). Norwalk, CT: Appleton-Century-Crofts.

Hanchett, E.S. (1988). *Nursing frameworks and community as client: Bridging the gap.* Norwalk, CT: Appleton & Lange.

Hanchett, E.S. (1990). Nursing models and community as client. *Nursing Science Quarterly, 3*, 67–72.

Harrigan, J.F., Faro, B.Z., VanPutte, A., & Stoler, P. (1987). The application of locus of control to diabetes education in school-aged children. *Journal of Pediatric Nursing, 2*, 236–243.

Harris, J.K. (1980). Self-care is possible after cesarean delivery. *Nursing Clinics of North America, 15*, 191–204.

Hedahl, K. (1983). Assisting the adolescent with physical disabilities through a college health program. *Nursing Clinics of North America, 18*, 257–274.

Hewes, C.J., & Hannigan, E.P. (1985). Self-care model and the geriatric patient. In J. Riehl-Sisca, *The science and art of self-care* (pp. 161–167). Norwalk, CT: Appleton-Century-Crofts.

Hurst, J.D., & Stullenbarger, B. (1986). Implementation of a self-care approach in a pediatric interdisciplinary phenylketonuria

(PKU) clinic. *Journal of Pediatric Nursing, 1*, 159–163.

Hughes, M.M. (1983). Nursing theories and emergency nursing. *Journal of Emergency Nursing, 9*, 95–97.

Jacobs, C.J. (1990). Orem's self-care model: Is it relevant to patients in intensive care? *Intensive Care Nursing, 6*, 100–103.

James, L.A. (1992). Nursing theory made practical. *Journal of Nursing Education, 31*, 42–44.

Joseph, L.S. (1980). Self-care and the nursing process. *Nursing Clinics of North America, 15*, 131–143.

Kam, B.W., & Werner, P.W. (1990). Self-care theory: Application to perioperative nursing. *Association of Operating Room Nurses Journal, 51*, 1365–1370.

Keohane, N.S., & Lacey, L.A. (1991). Preparing the woman with gestational diabetes for self-care: Use of a structured teaching plan by nursing staff. *Journal of Obstetric, Gynecologic, and Neonatal Nursing, 20*, 189–193.

Kerr, J.A.C. (1985). A case of adolescent turmoil: Use of the self-care model. In J. Riehl-Sisca, *The science and art of self-care* (pp. 105–112). Norwalk, CT: Appleton-Century-Crofts.

Komulainen, P. (1991). Occupational health nursing based on self-care theory. *American Association of Occupational Health Nursing Journal, 39*, 333–335.

Kyle, B.A.S., & Pitzer, S.A. (1990). A self-care approach to today's challenges. *Nursing Management, 21*(3), 37–39.

Lacey, D. (1993). Using Orem's model in psychiatric nursing. *Nursing Standard, 7*(29), 28–30.

Langley, T. (1989). Please, deliver more incontinence pads. *Nursing times, 85*(15), 73–75.

MacDonald, G. (1991). Plans for a better future. *Nursing Times, 87*(31), 42–43.

Mack, C.H. (1992). Assessment of the autologous bone marrow transplant patient according to Orem's self-care model. *Cancer Nursing, 15*, 429–436.

MacLellan, M. (1989). Community care of a patient with multiple sclerosis. *Nursing (London), 3*(33), 28–32.

MacSweeny, J. (1992). A helpful assessment. *Nursing Times, 88*(29), 32–33.

Marten, L. (1978). Self-care nursing model for patients experiencing radical change in body image. *Journal of Obstetric, Gynecologic, and Neonatal Nursing, 7*(6), 9–13.

Matteson, M.A., & McConnell, E.S. (1988). *Gerontological nursing: Concepts and practice.* Philadelphia: WB Saunders.

McConnell, E.S. (1988). A conceptual framework for gerontological nursing practice. In M.A. Matteson & E.S. McConnell (Eds.), *Gerontological nursing: Concepts and practice* (pp. 6–55). Philadelphia: WB Saunders.

McCracken, M.J. (1985). A self-care approach to pediatric chronic illness. In J. Riehl-Sisca, *The science and art of self-care* (pp. 91–104). Norwalk, CT: Appleton-Century-Crofts.

McIntyre, K. (1980). The Perry model as a framework for self-care. *Nurse Practitioner, 5*(6), 34–38.

Meriney, D.K. (1990). Application of Orem's conceptual framework to patients with hypercalcemia related to breast cancer. *Cancer Nursing, 13*, 316–323.

Michael, M.M., & Sewall, K.S. (1980). Use of the adolescent peer group to increase the self-care agency of adolescent alcohol abusers. *Nursing Clinics of North America, 15*, 157–176.

Miller, J. (1989). DIY health care. *Nursing Standard, 3*(43), 35–37.

Mitchell, P., & Irvin, N. (1977). Neurological examination: Nursing assessment for nursing purposes. *Journal of Neurosurgical Nursing, 9*(1), 23–28.

Moore, R. (1989). Diogenes syndrome. *Nursing Times, 85*(30), 46–48.

Morales-Mann, E.T., & Jiang, S.L. (1993). Applicability of Orem's conceptual framework: A cross-cultural point of view. *Journal of Advanced Nursing, 18*, 737–741.

Morse, W., & Werner, J.S. (1988). Individualization of patient care using Orem's theory. *Cancer Nursing, 11*, 195–202.

Moscovitz, A. (1984). Orem's theory as applied to psychiatric nursing. *Perspectives in Psychiatric Care, 22*(1), 36–38.

Mullin, V.I. (1980). Implementing the self-care concept in the acute care setting. *Nursing Clinics of North America, 15*, 177–190.

Murphy, P.P. (1981). A hospice model and self-care theory. *Oncology Nursing Forum, 8*(2), 19–21.

Nickle-Gallagher, L. (1985). Structuring nursing practice based on Orem's general theory: A practitioner's perspective. In J. Riehl-Sisca, *The science and art of self-care* (pp. 236–244). Norwalk, CT: Appleton-Century-Crofts.

Norris, M.K.G. (1991). Applying Orem's theory to the long-term care of adolescent transplant recipients. *American Nephrology Nurses' Association Journal, 18*, 45–47, 53.

Nowakowski, L. (1980). Health promotion/

self-care programs for the community. *Topics in Clinical Nursing*, 2(2), 21–27.

Oakley, D., Denyes, M.J., & O'Connor, N. (1989). Expanded nursing care for contraceptive use. *Applied Nursing Research*, 2, 121–127.

O'Donovan, S. (1990). Nursing models: More of Orem. *Nursing the Elderly*, 2(3), 22–23.

O'Donovan, S. (1990). Nursing models: More of Orem—Part 2. *Nursing the Elderly*, 2(4), 20–22.

O'Donovan, S. (1992). Simon's nursing assessment. *Nursing Times*, 88(2), 30–33.

Padula, C.A. (1992). Self-care and the elderly: Review and implications. *Public Health Nursing*, 9, 22–28.

Palmer, S.J. (1993). Care of sick children by parents: A meaningful role. *Journal of Advanced Nursing*, 18, 185–191.

Park, P.B. (1989). Health care for the homeless: A self-care approach. *Clinical Nurse Specialist*, 3, 171–175.

Perras, S., & Zappacosta, A. (1982). The application of Orem's theory in promoting self-care in a peritoneal dialysis facility. *American Association of Nephrology Nurses and Technicians Journal*, 9(3), 37–39.

Petrlik, J.C. (1976). Diabetic peripheral neuropathy. *American Journal of nursing*, 76, 1794–1797.

Pletcher, M.S. (1985). Nutrition self-care: An adaptation and component of the therapeutic regimen. In J. Riehl-Sisca, *The science and art of self-care* (pp. 132–141). Norwalk, CT: Appleton-Century-Crofts.

Priddy, J. (1989). Surgical care of the elderly. Home help. *Nursing Times*, 85(29), 30–32.

Raven, M. (1988–1989). Application of Orem's self-care model to nursing practice in developmental disability. *Australian Journal of Advanced Nursing*, 6(2), 16–23.

Raven, M. (1989). A conceptual model for care in developmental disability services. *Australian Journal of Advanced Nursing*, 6(4), 10–17.

Redfern, S. (1990). Care after a stroke. *Nursing (London)*, 4(4), 7–11.

Rew, L. (1990). Childhood sexual abuse: Toward a self-care framework for nursing intervention and research. *Archives of Psychiatric Nursing*, 4, 147–153.

Richardson, A. (1991). Theories of self-care: Their relevance to chemotherapy-induced nausea and vomiting. *Journal of Advanced Nursing*, 16, 671–676.

Robichaud-Ekstrand, S. (1990). [Orem in medical-surgical nursing.] *The Canadian Nurse*, 86(5), 42–47.

Roper, J.M., Shapira, J., & Chang, B. (1991). Agitation in the demented patient. A framework for management. *Journal of Gerontological Nursing*, 17(3), 17–21.

Ruddick-Bracken, H., & Mackie, N. (1989). Helping the workers help themselves. *Nursing Times*, 85(24), 75–76.

Smith, M.C. (1977). Self-care: A conceptual framework for rehabilitation nursing. *Rehabilitation Nursing*, 2(2), 8–10.

Smith, M.C. (1989). An application of Orem's theory in nursing practice. *Nursing Science Quarterly*, 2, 159–161.

Steele, S., Russell, F., Hansen, B., & Mills, B. (1989). Home management of URI in children with Down syndrome. *Pediatric Nursing*, 15, 484–488.

Sullivan, T., & Monroe, D. (1986). A self-care practice theory of nursing the elderly. *Educational Gerontology*, 12, 13–26.

Sullivan, T., & Monroe, D. (1987). Self-care model for long term care. *California Nurse*, 83(6), 6–7.

Swindale, J.E. (1989). The nurse's role in giving pre-operative information to reduce anxiety in patients admitted to hospital for elective minor surgery. *Journal of Advanced Nursing*, 14, 899–905.

Tadych, R. (1985). Nursing in multiperson units: The family. In J. Riehl-Sisca, *The science and art of self-care* (pp. 49–55). Norwalk, CT: Appleton-Century-Crofts.

Taylor, S.G. (1988). Nursing theory and nursing process: Orem's theory in practice. *Nursing Science Quarterly*, 1, 111–119.

Taylor, S.G. (1989). An interpretation of family within Orem's general theory of nursing. *Nursing Science Quarterly*, 1, 131–137.

Taylor, S.G. (1990). Practical applications of Orem's self-care deficit nursing theory. In M.E. Parker (Ed.) *Nursing theories in practicer* (pp. 61–70). New York: National League for Nursing.

Taylor, S.G., & McLaughlin, K. (1991). Orem's general theory of nursing and community nursing. *Nursing Science Quarterly*, 4, 153–160.

Thomas, J.S., Graff, B.M., Hollingsworth, A.O., Cohen, S.M., & Rubin, M.M. (1992). Home visiting for a posthysterectomy population. *Home Healthcare Nurse*, 10(3), 47–52.

Titus, S., & Porter, P. (1989). Orem's theory applied to pediatric residential treatment. *Pediatric Nursing*, 15, 465–468, 556.

Tolentino, M.B. (1990). The use of Orem's self-care model in the neonatal intensive care unit. *Journal of Obstetric, Gynecologic, and Neonatal Nursing, 19*, 496–500.

Turner, K. (1989). Orem's model and patient teaching. *Nursing Standard, 50*(3), 32–33.

Underwood, P.R. (1980). Facilitating self-care. In Pothier, P. (Ed.), *Psychiatric nursing: A basic text* (pp. 115–132). Boston: Little, Brown.

Vasquez, M.A. (1992). From theory to practice: Orem's self-care nursing model and ambulatory care. *Journal of Post Anesthesia Nursing, 7*, 251–255.

Walborn, K.A. (1980). A nursing model for the hospice: Primary and self-care nursing. *Nursing Clinics of North America, 15*, 205–217.

Walsh, M. (1989). Asthma: The Orem self-care nursing model approach. *Nursing (London), 3*(38), 19–21.

Walsh, M., & Judd, M. (1989). Long term immobility and self care: The Orem nursing approach. *Nursing Standard, 3*(41), 34–36.

Welsh, M.D., & Clochesy, J.M. (Eds.). (1990). *Case studies in cardiovascular critical care nursing.* Rockville, MD: Aspen.

Whenery-Tedder, M. (1991). Teaching acceptance. *Nursing Times, 87*(12), 36–39.

Wollery, L. (1983). Self-care for the obstetrical patient. *Journal of Obstetric, Gynecologic, and Neonatal Nursing, 12*, 33–37.

Wright, J. (1988). Trolley full of trouble. *Nursing Times, 84*(9), 24–26.

Zach, P. (1982). Self-care agency in diabetic ocular sequelae. *Journal of Ophthalmic Nursing Techniques, 1*(2), 21–31.

CHAPTER 8

Rogers' Science of Unitary Human Beings*

This chapter presents an analysis and evaluation of Martha E. Rogers' conceptual model of nursing, which is referred to as the Science of Unitary Human Beings. Rogers (personal communication, June 17, 1987) regards her work as an abstract conceptual system that "is not of the same order as the other conceptual models, nor does it derive from the same world view. Rather, it derives from a different world view and deals with a different phenomenon." The Science of Unitary Human Beings does, however, fit the definition of a conceptual model used in this book.

The concepts of the Science of Unitary Human Beings and their dimensions are listed below. Each concept and its dimensions are defined and described later in this chapter.

KEY CONCEPTS

ENERGY FIELDS
Human
Environmental
OPENNESS
PATTERN
PANDIMENSIONALITY
PRINCIPLES OF HOMEODYNAMICS
Resonancy
Helicy
Integrality
HEALTH
An Expression of the Life Process
NURSING

A Learned Profession
A Science and an Art
GOAL OF NURSING
Promotion of Health and Well-Being
NURSING PROCESS
Pattern Manifestation Appraisal
Deliberative Mutual Patterning
THEORY OF ACCELERATING
  EVOLUTION
THEORY OF RHYTHMICAL
  CORRELATES OF CHANGE
THEORY OF PARANORMAL
  PHENOMENA

*Martha E. Rogers died March 13, 1994.

ANALYSIS OF ROGERS' SCIENCE
OF UNITARY HUMAN BEINGS

This section presents an analysis of the Science of Unitary Human Beings. The analysis draws from several of Rogers' publications, including her 1970 book, *An Introduction to the Theoretical Basis of Nursing;* her 1989 book chapter, "Nursing: A science of unitary man"; her 1990a book chapter, "Nursing: Science of unitary, irreducible human beings: Update 1990"; and her 1992b journal article, "Nursing science and the space age."

Origins of the Model

Historical Evolution and Motivation

Rogers first presented what has come to be known as the Science of Unitary Human Beings in her 1970 book, *An Introduction to the Theoretical Basis of Nursing.* Further development and refinement of the conceptual system was presented by Rogers (1978a) at the Second Annual Nurse Educator Conference. This presentation, with additional refinements, was later published in Riehl and Roy's (1980) book, *Conceptual Models for Nursing Practice* (Rogers, 1980a). The latter two papers also introduced theoretical formulations derived from the conceptual system. An expanded explanation of the conceptual system, as well as a comprehensive discussion of the theories derived from it, were presented in a series of video and audio tapes in 1980 (Rogers, 1980b – g). Further refinements of the conceptual system were published in Malinski's (1986a) book, *Explorations on Martha Rogers' Science of Unitary Human Beings* (Rogers, 1986). Still further refinements were published in Barrett's (1990d) book, *Visions of Rogers' Science-Based Nursing* (Rogers, 1990a), and in Rogers' 1992b journal article. The revisions and refinements in the Science of Unitary Human Beings are a reflection of Rogers' concern with language and the insights she has gained over the years from new knowledge. She commented:

> The development of a science of unitary human beings is a never-ending process. This abstract system first presented some years ago has continued to gain substance. Concomitantly, early errors have undergone correction, definitions have been revised for greater clarity and accuracy, and updating of content is ongoing. (Rogers, 1992b, p. 28)

Several changes have been made in the conceptual system. The notion of development, per se, has been dropped because it "implies certain kinds of linearity" (Rogers, cited in Malinski, 1986b, p. 11). The term for the person evolved from man (Rogers, 1970) to unitary man (Rogers, 1980a) and finally to unitary human beings (Rogers, 1986).

The basic concepts or building blocks of the Rogerian conceptual system evolved from energy field, wholeness, openness, unidirectional, pattern and organization, and sentience and thought (Rogers, 1970) to energy field, openness, pattern, and four-dimensional (Rogers, 1980a) to energy field, openness, pattern, and multidimensional (Rogers, 1990a) and now to energy field, openness, pattern, and pandimensional (Rogers, 1992b).

Rogers eliminated the term unidirectional because it led to the false interpretation of human development as linear. Multidimensional replaced four-dimensional in an effort "to select words best suited to portray one's thought . . . Multidimensional provides for an infinite domain without limit" (Rogers, 1990a, p. 7). Pandimensional replaced multidimensional for the same reason. Rogers (1992b) explained that despite the term name changes, its definition has remained the same.

The principles of homeodynamics evolved from reciprocy, synchrony, helicy, and resonancy (Rogers, 1970) to helicy, resonancy, and complementarity (Rogers, 1980a) to helicy, resonancy, and integrality (Rogers, 1986). The principles of reciprocy and synchrony were eliminated and the principle of complementarity was replaced by the principle of integrality because the terms reciprocy, synchrony, and complementarity lead to the false interpretation of separation between the human and environmental energy fields. Furthermore, the notion of mutual and simultaneous interaction, with its false connotation of separate human and environmental fields, evolved into the principle of complementarity and then to the principle of integrality. A recent change has been in the definition of the principle of helicy. In this case, probabilistic was replaced by unpredictable because "the literature now points up that unpredictability transcends probability" (Rogers, 1990a, p. 7).

Rogers (1978b) stated that she deliberately set out to develop a conceptual system when she realized that "there had to be a body of knowledge that was specific to and unique to nursing, or there was no need for higher education in nursing at all." Rogers' recognition of the need for an organized body of nursing knowledge was evident in her early writings on nursing education, especially in the books, *Educational Revolution in Nursing* (Rogers, 1961) and *Reveille in Nursing* (Rogers, 1964).

Rogers is a pioneer in the development of unique nursing knowledge. She is one of the first modern nurse scholars to explicitly identify man as the central phenomenon of interest to the discipline of nursing (Newman, 1972). Moreover, she focused attention on the environment as an equally important phenomenon for study. Rogers (1978a, 1992a) traced the dual concern with people and their environments to Nightingale. She explained, "Rogerian science of irreducible human beings provides a framework rooted in a new reality and directed toward moving us from what might be called a prescientific era to a scientific era. Certainly Nightingale laid a firm foundation for this kind of an approach to nursing knowledge and its use" (1992a, p. 61).

Philosophical Claims

Rogers (1978a) stated that she directed her efforts "to evolve a conceptual system that would give identity to nursing as a knowledgeable endeavor." The following assumptions provided the foundation for the Science of Unitary Human Beings:

1. Nursing is a learned profession.

2. The explication of an organized body of abstract knowledge specific to nursing is indispensable to nursing's transition from prescience to science.

3. Nursing is both an empirical science and an art.

4. Nursing science is an organized body of abstract knowledge arrived at by scientific research and logical analysis.

5. The art of nursing is the utilization of scientific nursing knowledge for the betterment of people.

6. People need knowledgeable nursing.

7. The practice of nursing is the use of nursing knowledge in human service.

8. The descriptive, explanatory, and predictive principles that direct nursing practice are derived from a conceptual system.

9. Nursing's long-established concern is with people and their worlds.

10. People have the capacity to participate knowingly and probabilistically in the process of change. (Rogers, 1970, 1978a, 1978b, 1980a, 1986, 1992b)

Central to the Science of Unitary Human Beings is Rogers' (1980a, 1992b) rejection of the notion of causality. She has stated, "The appearance of causality is an illusion, a mirage" (1980a, p. 334) and "In a universe of open systems, causality is not an option" (1992b, p. 30).

Rogers (1992b) believes in "a humane and optimistic view of life's potentials [that] grows as a new reality appears" (p. 28). She also believes that nursing is a basic, open-ended science that builds and refines as "new knowledge brings new insights" (p. 28).

Furthermore, Rogers (1992b) believes that energy fields "constitute the fundamental unit of both the living and the nonliving." (p. 30). Energy fields, Rogers (1992b) believes, "are not biological fields, physical fields, social fields, or psychological fields. Nor are human and environmental fields a summation of biological, physical, social, and psychological fields" (p. 30).

Moreover, Rogers (1992b) believes in a "new vision of a world encompassing far more than planet earth . . . [and a future] of growing diversity, of accelerating evolution, and of nonrepeating rhythmicities" (p. 33).

Strategies for Knowledge Development

Rogers (1992b) used a deductive approach to develop her conceptual system that yielded "a creative synthesis of facts and ideas . . . an emergent, a new product" (p. 28). She explained that the Science of Unitary Human Beings

> has not derived from one or more of the basic sciences. Neither has it come out of a vacuum. It flows instead in novel ways from a multiplicity of knowledge, from many sources, to create a kaleidoscope of potentialities. In turn, fundamental concepts are identified and significant terms are defined congruent with the evolving system. . . . Neither does it derive from . . . applied sciences, nor is it a summation of knowledge drawn from other fields. Nursing, instead, consists of its own unique irreducible mix. (p. 28)

Influences from Other Scholars

Rogers has always emphasized the uniqueness of nursing knowledge in general and the Science of Unitary Human Beings in particular. She has, however, clearly stated that the new product that is her conceptual system was synthesized from the work of many scholars in adjunctive disciplines. Indeed, Rogers has cited many notable philosophers and scientists, including Bertalanffy (1960), Bohm (1980), Burr and Northrop (1935), Capra (1982), Chardin (1961), Einstein (1961), Fuller (1981), Goldstein (1939), Herrick (1956), Lewin (1964), Polanyi (1958), Russell (1953), Sheldrake (1981), and Stewart (1989), among others.

Rogers (1985c) implied that system theory and knowledge gleaned from the exploration of space have been especially influential in the development and refinement of the Science of Unitary Human Beings when she stated:

> The introduction of systems theories several decades ago set in motion new ways of perceiving people and their world. Science and technology escalated. Space exploration revised old views. New knowledge merged with new ways of thinking. The second industrial revolution was born—far more dramatic in its implications and potentials than the first. A pressing need to study people in ways that would enhance their humanness coordinate with accelerating technological advances forced a search for new models. (p. 16)

World View

Rogers (1992b) claimed that a new world view, "compatible with the most progressive knowledge available . . . has become a necessary prelude to studying human health and to determining modalities for its promotion both on this planet and in outer space. The [Science of Unitary Human Beings] is rooted in this new world view, a pandimensional view of people and their world" (pp. 27–28). In addition, Rogers (1990b) commented, "My own work focuses on developing a holistic world view by proposing a science of unitary, irreducible beings that is coordinate with a world view that includes outer space. . . . A holistically oriented space-age paradigm is the substance of nursing's science of unitary, irreducible human beings" (pp. 106–107).

Sellers (1991) maintained that the Science of Unitary Human Beings "is an eclectic synthesis of idealism, progressivism, and humanism that moves away from rationalism and scientific realism" (p. 147). Sarter (1988) pointed out that the major philosophical threads of the Science of Unitary Human Beings are "holism, process, [pan]dimensionality, evolution, energy fields, openness, noncausality, and pattern" (p. 54). Hanchett (1992) pointed out the similarities between certain concepts of the Science of Unitary Human Beings and the Madhyamika-Prasangika school of Tibetan Buddhism. She commented that "The activity and awareness of the energy field of Rogers' science bear relationships to the Buddhist concept[s] of karma . . . [and] direct perception. Rogers' denial of parts as constituting the person is similar to the Buddhist argument that the aggregates do not constitute the person" (p. 170). In addition, Hanchett noted that the Rogerian notion of unique pattern within the integral human and environmental energy fields "is similar to the functioning of recognizable, conventional persons and phenomena within the interconnected web of dependent arising in the middle way consequence school of Tibetan Buddhist philosophy" (p. 170). The new world view reflected by the Science of Unitary Human Beings, and the world view that incorporates the philosophical positions identified by Sellers (1991), Sarter (1988), and Hanchett (1992) is *simultaneous action.*

In keeping with the simultaneous action world view, the Science of Unitary Human Beings clearly reflects a holistic view of the person and environment. In fact, the person and the environment are clearly conceptualized as irreducible, indivisible wholes.

Although the Science of Unitary Human Beings reflects a holistic view of the world, Rogers (1992b) does not use the term holistic because of its ambiguous and varied meanings. She pointed out, "The use of the term unitary human beings is not to be confused with current popular usage of the term holistic, generally signifying a summation of parts, whether few or many. The unitary nature of environment is equally irreducible. The concept of a field provides a means of perceiving people and their respective environments as irreducible wholes" (p. 29).

The human energy field is regarded as an active organism who is integral with the environmental energy field. Rogers (1992b) stated, "People's capacity to participate knowingly in the process of change is postulated" (p. 28).

Moreover, human and environmental energy fields change continuously. Change is, therefore, regarded as natural and desirable. In fact, "Change just is" (Rogers, Doyle, Racolin, & Walsh, 1990, p. 377). Change is creative and innovative, always in the direction of increasing diversity.

Thus, the person is always progressing, always reaching toward his or her potential. Indeed, "Change is continuous, relative, and innovative. The increasing diversity of field patterning characterizes this process of change. Individual differences serve only to point up the significance of this relative diversity" (Rogers, 1992b, p. 31).

Rogers (1970) explicitly rejected the reaction world view tenet of reductionism, with its focus on parts, stating, "Reductionism, representative of an atomistic world view in which complex things are built up of simple elements, is contrary to a perception of wholeness" (p. 87). She also stated that her conceptual system "is humanistic, not mechanistic. Moreover, this is an optimistic model though not a utopian one" (Rogers, 1987d, p. 141). She also explicitly rejected mechanistic causality, stating, "In a universe of open systems, causality is not an option. Acausality had come in with quantum theory. . . . Causality is invalid" (Rogers, 1986, p. 5). Furthermore, Rogers (1970) rejected the reaction world view of the person as reacting to environmental stimuli. She commented, "The all-too-common perception of man predominantly subjected to multiple negative environmental influences with pathological outcomes denies man's unity with nature and his evolutionary becoming" (p. 85).

Unique Focus of the Model

The Science of Unitary Human Beings is concerned with " people and their worlds in a pandimensional universe" (Rogers, 1992b, p. 29). The distinction between nursing and other disciplines and the uniqueness of nursing, according to Rogers (1990b), lie in the phenomenon of central interest to each, in what is known rather than what is done in practice. From the perspective of the Science of Unitary Human Beings, the phenomenon of central concern is "the study of unitary, irreducible human beings and their respective environments" (p. 108). Elaborating, Rogers (1992b) stated:

> The uniqueness of nursing, like that of other sciences, lies in the phenomenon central to its focus. For nurses, that focus consists of a long-established concern with people and the world they live in. It is the natural forerunner of an organized, abstract system encompassing people and their environments. The irreducible nature of individuals is different from the sum of their parts. Furthermore, the integrality of people and their environments coordinates with a pandimensional universe of open systems, points to a new paradigm, and initiates the identity of nursing as a science. (p. 28)

The human and environmental energy fields, then, are the special areas of concern. More specifically, the Rogerian conceptual system is concerned with those patterns of the human and environmental energy fields that are associated with maximum well-being, as well-being is defined by the society in which the human being is located. Rogers

(1987c) has underscored the point that the Science of Unitary Human Beings does not deal with health problems, but rather is concerned with the "evolution of change in the direction of wherever human beings think they are going."

Riehl and Roy (1974, 1980) classified the Science of Unitary Human Beings as a systems model. Riehl-Sisca (1989) classified it as a developmental model. Careful review of the content of the Rogerian conceptual system indicates that it reflects characteristics of both systems and developmental models.

The basic characteristic of systems model, integration of parts, was addressed in Rogers' (1992b) statements that unitary human beings and their environments are irreducible and indivisible energy fields that "have their own identity and are not to be confused with parts" (p. 30); unitary human beings are regarded as "irreducible wholes [and] a whole cannot be understood when it is reduced to its particulars" (p. 29); and "the irreducible nature of individuals is different from the sum of their parts" (p. 28). The characteristic, system, was addressed in the discussion of the human and environmental energy fields as open systems. Rogers (1992b) pointed out that from her perspective, this means that the energy fields are always open — "not a little bit or sometimes, but continuously" (p. 30). The characteristic of environment was addressed explicitly and was defined as a pandimensional energy field that is integral with the human pandimensional energy field (Rogers, 1992b).

Boundary was not addressed explicitly in the recent versions of the Science of Unitary Human Beings. The lack of boundaries is evident in Rogers' (1986) statement that the "human and environmental fields are infinite and integral with one another" (p. 5). The characteristic of tension, stress, strain, and conflict also was not addressed in the Science of Unitary Human Beings. Rogers clearly rejected the idea that any external force impinges on the human field. Rather, the human and environmental fields are integral.

Rogers (1992b) regarded the characteristics of equilibrium and steady state as obsolete. Instead, she presented an innovative view of the relationship between human beings and their environments that goes beyond general system thinking. For Rogers, there is no fixed equilibrium point or even a dynamic equilibrium nor is there any feedback process of input and output. Rather, the principle of integrality postulates that the human and environmental energy fields engage in the continuous mutual process of change. "The continuous change," Rogers (1992b) noted, "emerges out of nonequilibrium and exhibits punctualism not gradualism. In addition, change is accelerating" (p. 32).

Although Rogers addressed the characteristics of systems models, she placed major emphasis on human development in the form of evolutionary changes in human field pattern. Rogers (cited in Malinski, 1986b), however, no longer uses the term human development "because development implies certain kinds of linearity" (p. 11).

The developmental model characteristics of growth, development, maturation, change, and direction of change are addressed by the principles of helicy and resonancy. These principles postulate that field pattern is characterized by continuous change that is innovative, unpredictable, and increasing in diversity. The direction of change is always toward increasing diversity, from lower frequency to higher frequency wave patterns (Rogers, 1992b).

Identifiable state is addressed by the concept of pattern. According to Rogers (1992b), pattern is "the distinguishing characteristic of an energy field perceived as a single wave . . . it gives identity to the field" (p. 30).

The form of progression most clearly reflected by the Rogerian conceptual system is the differentiated type. The principle of helicy postulates that human and environmental field patterns increase in diversity and are characterized by nonrepeating rhythmicities. Although the term helicy might imply a spiral, Chin's (1980) definition of that form as returning to former problems but dealing with them at a higher level is at odds with Rogers' (1980a) contention that "there is no going back, no repetition" (p. 333).

The developmental model characteristic of forces is not addressed. In fact, such an idea is rejected by Rogers. Rather, she posits that the nature of the energy field is to evolve. No special forces are required for this. Thus, the potentiality for development is overt.

Meleis (1991) regarded the Science of Unitary Human Beings as a prominent example of the outcomes category of models and also classified it within her person-environment interaction category. Marriner-Tomey (1989) placed Rogers' work in the energy fields category. Barnum (1994) relegated Rogers' work to her enhancement category.

Content of the Model: Concepts

Person and Environment

Rogers (1986) identified unitary human beings and their environments as the central focus of her conceptual system. The relationship between unitary human beings and their environments is such that they must be discussed together and within the context of the four basic concepts of the Science of Unitary Human Beings—**energy fields, openness, pattern,** and **pandimensionality**. Rogers (1992b) pointed out that the concept of **energy field** represents "a means of perceiving people and their respective environments as irreducible wholes" (p. 29). She went on to explain that "Field . . . is a unifying concept and energy signifies the dynamic nature of the field. Energy fields are infinite and pandimensional; they are in continuous motion" (p. 30).

Rogers (1992b) identified two energy fields—the *human energy field* and the *environmental energy field*. Unitary human beings and the environment, then, are energy fields. The unitary human being is defined as "an irreducible, indivisible, pandimensional energy field identified by pattern and manifesting characteristics that are specific to the whole and which cannot be predicted from knowledge of the parts" (p. 29). The environment is defined as "an irreducible, [indivisible] pandimensional energy field identified by pattern and integral with the human field" (p. 29).

Rogers (1992b) pointed out that "human beings and the environment *are* energy fields; they do not *have* energy fields" (p. 30). Consequently, the possessive cannot be used when referring to a human or an environmental energy field.

Human and environmental energy fields are **open**. Rogers (1992b) maintained that there is no variance in the openness of the human and environmental energy fields, explaining that "energy fields are open, not a little bit or sometimes, but continuously" (p. 30).

Energy fields have **pattern**. Rogers (1992b) defined pattern as "the distinguishing characteristic of an energy field perceived as a single wave" (p. 30). Elaborating on that concept, Rogers stated, "Pattern is an abstraction, its nature changes continuously, and it gives identity to the field. . . . each human field pattern is unique and is integral with its own unique environmental field pattern" (p. 30).

The pattern of an energy field is conceptualized as a wave phenomenon. Rogers (1970) noted, "A multiplicity of waves characterizes the universe. Light waves, sound waves, thermal waves, atomic waves, gravity waves flow in rhythmic patterns" (p. 101).

Energy field patterns change continuously. The change, according to Rogers (1992b), is continuous, relative, innovative, increasingly diverse, and unpredictable. This means that there is no repetition in human life, no regression to former states or stages. Rather, the human and environmental field patterns change constantly, always evolving into other novel, innovative forms (Rogers, 1970). Although the direction of changes is invariant, the rate of change may vary for an individual over the course of life. Change also varies among individuals. Indeed, "individual differences . . . point up the significance of this relative diversity" (Rogers, 1992b, p. 31).

Energy field patterns are not, according to Rogers (1992b), directly observable. Rather, "manifestations of field patterning are observable events in the real world. They are postulated to emerge out of the human-environmental field mutual process" (p. 31). Manifestations of energy field pattern range from the physical body to such rhythmical phenomena as diversity in the experiences of time passing, the speed of motion, and sleep-wake cycles. With regard to the body, Rogers stated, "I consider physical bodies to be manifestations of field [pattern]" (Rogers et al., 1990, p. 377). The diversity in rhythmical phenomena is elaborated in Table 8–1. In referring to that table, Rogers (1990a) explained, "The evolution of life and non-life is a dynamic, irreducible, nonlinear process

TABLE 8-1. **MANIFESTATIONS OF RELATIVE DIVERSITY IN FIELD PATTERNING**

Less diverse	More diverse	
Longer rhythms	Shorter rhythms	Seem continuous
Slower motion	Faster motion	Seem continuous
Lower frequency	Higher frequency	Seem continuous
Time experienced as slower	Time experienced as faster	Timelessness
Pragmatic	Imaginative	Visionary
Sleeping	Waking	Beyond waking

Adapted from Rogers, M.E. (1990). Nursing: Science of unitary, irreducible, human beings: Update 1990. In E.A.M. Barrett (Ed.), *Visions of Rogers' science-based nursing* (p. 9). New York: National League for Nursing, with permission.

characterized by increasing complexification of energy field patterning. The nature of change is unpredictable and increasingly diverse" (p. 8).

Rogers (1992b) described human and environmental energy fields as **pandimensional**. She defined pandimensionality as "a nonlinear domain without spatial or temporal attributes" (p. 29). Rogers claims that pandimensional "best expresses the idea of a unitary whole" (p. 31). Furthermore, she noted that "one does not move into or become pandimensional. Rather, this is a way of perceiving reality" (p. 31). Thus, all reality for Rogers is pandimensional and in such a pandimensional world, "the relative nature of change becomes explicit" (p. 31).

Rogers (1992b) has extended the notion of the human energy field to groups. She commented that the Science of Unitary Human Beings "is equally as applicable to groups as it is to individuals. The group energy field to be considered is identified. It may be a family, a social group, or a community, a crowd or some other combination" (p. 30). Group energy fields have the same characteristics as individual energy fields—they are continuously open and integral with their own environmental fields, they are pandimensional, and they have pattern that changes continuously.

Rogers (1992b) formulated three mutually exclusive **principles of homeodynamics** to explicitly and concisely state her ideas about human and environmental energy field patterns. The principles are equally applicable to individual and group fields.

The *principle of resonancy* delineates the direction of evolutionary change in energy field pattern. Resonancy is the "continuous change from lower to higher frequency wave patterns in human and environmental fields" (Rogers, 1990a, p. 8).

The *principle of helicy* speaks to the continuous change that characterizes human and environmental field patterns. Helicy is the "continuous, innovative, unpredictable, increasing diversity of human and environmental field patterns" (Rogers, 1990a, p. 8).

The *principle of integrality* emphasizes the nature of the relationship between the human and environmental fields. Integrality is the "continuous mutual human field and environmental field process" (Rogers, 1990a, p. 8).

Health

Rogers (1970) defined **health** as *an expression of the life process.* She referred to health and illness, ease and dis-ease, normal and pathological processes, and maximum well-being and sickness. Such dichotomous notions, Rogers (1970) maintained, "are arbitrarily defined, culturally infused, and value laden" (p. 85). She went on to explain,

> Health and sickness, however defined, are expressions of the process of life. Whatever meaning they may have is derived out of an understanding of the life process in its totality. Life's deviant course demands that it be viewed in all of its dimensions if valid explanations of its varied manifestations are to emerge. (p. 85)

Wellness and illness, then, are not differentiated within the context of the Science of Unitary Human Beings. Rather, they are considered value terms imposed by society. As such, "manifestations of human and environmental field pattern deemed to have high value are labeled wellness by the society, and those deemed to have low value are labeled illness" (Rogers, 1980f). Similarly, "Well being is a value, it is not an absolute" (Rogers et al., 1990, p. 378) and "Disease and pathology are value terms applied when the human field manifests characteristics that may be deemed undesirable" (Rogers, 1992b, p. 33). More specifically, within the Science of Unitary Human Beings,

> There are no absolute norms for health. There are patterns that emerge from the human process that may cause pain, happiness, illness, or any behavior. Society labels some of these behaviors "sick." What behaviors a society accepts as sick or well varies with culture and history. Families also have their own definitions of sick or well. . . . So there are no absolutes about what constitutes sickness or wellness. (Madrid & Winstead-Fry, 1986, p. 91)

In keeping with the Science of Unitary Human Beings, Madrid and Winstead-Fry then defined health as "participation in the life process by choosing and executing behaviors that lead to the maximum fulfillment of a person's potential" (p. 91).

Despite her lack of differentiation of wellness and illness, Rogers (1970) viewed those health states in the form of a continuum. She explained:

> Health and illness are part of the same continuum. They are not dichotomous conditions. The multiple events taking place along life's axis denote the extent to which man is achieving his maximum health potential and vary in their expressions from greatest health to those conditions which are incompatible with maintaining life processes. (p. 125)

However, Rogers (1970) indicated that she thinks society views wellness and illness as dichotomous, discrete entities.

Nursing

Rogers (1992b) regards **nursing** as *a learned profession that is both a science and an art.* The *science of* nursing is "an organized body of abstract knowledge arrived at by scientific research and logical analysis" (p. 28). Rogers went on to say, "Historically, the term 'nursing' most often has been used as a verb signifying 'to do,' rather than as a noun meaning 'to know.' When nursing is identified as a science the term 'nursing' becomes a noun signifying 'a body of abstract knowledge'" (pp. 28–29).

The *art of* nursing "is the creative use of the science of nursing for human betterment" (Rogers, 1992b, p. 28). The combination of nursing as art and science is evident in Rogers' (1992c) description of nursing as "compassionate concern for human beings. It is the heart that understands and the hand that soothes. It is the intellect that synthesizes many learnings into meaningful ministrations" (p. 1339).

Rogers (1970, 1992c) described nursing's mission as social, stating,

Nursing exists to serve people. Its direct and over-riding responsibility is to society . . . the safe practice of nursing depends on the nature and amount of scientific nursing knowledge the individual brings to practice and the imaginative, intellectual judgment with which such knowledge is made explicit in service to mankind. (1970, p. 122)

Nursing's abstract system is the outgrowth of concern for human health and welfare. The science of nursing aims to provide a growing body of theoretical knowledge whereby nursing practice can achieve new levels of meaningful service to man. (1970, p. 88)

Nursing's story is a magnificent epic of service to mankind. It is about people: how they are born, and live and die; in health and in sickness; in joy and in sorrow. Its mission is the translation of knowledge into human service. . . . [Nursing is] a field long dedicated to serving the health needs of people. (1992c, p. 1339)

The social mission of nursing is also evident in Rogers' (1970) statement concerning the scope of nursing's service to people:

The arenas of nursing's services extend into all areas where there are people: at home, at school, at work, at play; in hospital, nursing home, and clinic; on this planet and now moving into outer space. (p. 86)

The **goal of nursing** identified by Rogers is predicated on a view of the practitioner as "an environmental component for the individual receiving services" (Rogers, 1970, pp. 124–125). The following quotes indicate that the goal of nursing focuses on the *promotion of health and well-being* and on the integral relationship between the human and environmental energy fields:

The primary focus of nursing is to promote health. (Rogers, 1992a, p. 61)
The purpose of nurses is to promote health and well-being for all persons wherever they are. (Rogers, 1992b, p. 28)
The purpose of nursing is to promote human betterment wherever people are, on planet earth or in outer space. (Rogers, 1992b, p. 33)
Nurses participate in the process of change, to help people move toward what is deemed better health. (Rogers, 1980g)

Nursing is appropriate in all areas of health care, as is evident in the following statement: "Nursing is engaged in maintenance and promotion of health and rehabilitation of the sick and disabled from conception through dying" (Rogers, 1978a). Although Rogers mentioned prevention of disease in her 1970 book, she later pointed out that prevention is a negative concept that is contradicted by the tenets of the Science of Unitary Human Beings (Rogers, 1980g). She also pointed out that promotion of health is a more positive, optimistic concept and, therefore, is consistent with the Science of Unitary Human Beings.

The **nursing process**, according to Rogers (1970), follows from the science of nursing. She explained:

Broad principles are put together in novel ways to help explain a wide range of events and multiplicity of individual differences. Action, based on predictions arising out of intellectual skill in the merging of scientific principles, becomes underwritten by intellectual judgments. (pp. 87–88)

Rogers (1978b) regarded the nursing process as a modality for implementation of nursing knowledge but lacking in any substance of its own. She did not specify a particular nursing process format but did mention assessment, diagnosis, goal setting, intervention, and evaluation in her 1970 book. Although Rogers' recent publications and presentations do not address nursing process, some elements can be extracted from those and related works.

Rogers (1970) maintained that the nursing process must focus on the person as a unified whole. Moreover, Rogers (1980f, 1980g, 1992b) has continuously emphasized the need for individualized nursing care. She noted that as the diversity of energy field pattern increases, "so too will individualization of [nursing] services" (1992b, p. 33). She maintained that the individualization of nursing services is necessary to help people achieve their maximum potential in a positive fashion. The nurse must look at each individual and determine the range of behaviors that are normal for him or her. Diversity among individuals always must be taken into account, for it has distinct implications for what will be done and how it will be done.

The diversity of human and environment energy field pattern manifestations is apprehended through what Rogers (1990a, 1992b) has referred to as synthesis and pattern seeing. Elaborating, Barrett (1988) identified *pattern manifestation appraisal* as the first phase of the Rogerian practice methodology. She defined pattern manifestation appraisal as "the continuous process of identifying manifestations of the human and environmental fields that relate to current health events" (p. 50). Cowling (1990b) explained that human field pattern is appraised "through manifestations of the pattern in the form of experience, perception, and expressions" (p. 52). He referred to experience in its broadest sense, not just sensory experience. Experiences of pattern manifestation are accompanied by perception and are expressed in such diverse forms as verbal responses, responses to questionnaires, and personal ways of living and relating. Relevant pattern information includes sensations, thoughts, feelings, awareness, imagination, memory, introspective insights, intuitive apprehensions, recurring themes and issues that pervade one's life, metaphors, visualizations, images, nutrition, work and play, exercise, substance use, sleep/wake cycles, safety, decelerated/accelerated field rhythms, space-time shifts, interpersonal networks, and professional health care access and use (Barrett, 1990b; Cowling, 1990b).

The diversity of field pattern manifestations within an individual and between individuals mandates novel nursing intervention. The novelty of nursing intervention is explained by Rogers (1970) in the following quotation:

> Judicious and wise identification of interventive measures consonant with the diagnostic pattern and the purposes to be achieved in any given situation requires the imaginative pulling together of nursing knowledges in new ways according to the particular needs of the individual or group. (p. 125)

Rogers (1970) acknowledged the importance of technological tools and personal procedural activities as nursing interventions, but pointed out that "it must be thoroughly understood that tools and procedures are adjuncts to practice and are safe and meaningful only to the extent that knowledgeable nursing judgments underwrite their selection and the ways in which they may be used" (p. 126). The Science of Unitary Human Beings, Rogers (1990a) pointed out, "sparks new interventive modalities —that evolve as life evolves from earth to space and beyond" (p. 10). Many of the new modalities are noninvasive. In fact, Rogers (1990a) maintains that "the practice of nursing will be characterized primarily by noninvasive modalities" (p. 10) and has for several years cited the potential benefits of noninvasive modalities in relation to health and well being. She regards such noninvasive modalities as therapeutic touch, imagery, meditation, relaxation, unconditional love, attitudes of hope, humor, upbeat moods, and the use of sound, color, and motion as particularly consistent with the Science of Unitary Human Beings (Rogers, 1985c, 1987b, 1990a, 1992b; Rogers et al., 1990).

Other appropriate noninvasive modalities are health education, wellness counseling, nutrition counseling, meaningful presence, meaningful dialogue, affirmations (expressions of intentionality), bibliotherapy, journal keeping, and esthetic experiences of art, poetry, and nature (Barrett, 1990b). A potential modality is virtual reality, which is a "computer-generated reality that creates the illusion that the physical body is manifesting in a place where the physical body is not located" (Barrett, 1993, p. 11). Virtual reality may be regarded as "a form of power, i.e., a specific way whereby the capacity to participate knowingly in change is enhanced. In this form of power, one participates in dramatically changing the experience of our mutual process with the environment" (Barrett, 1993, p. 15).

Nursing interventions are implemented in the second phase of the Rogerian practice methodology, *deliberative mutual patterning*. Barrett (1988) defined deliberative mutual patterning as "the continuous process whereby the nurse with the client patterns the environmental field to promote harmony related to the health events" (p. 50). In this phase of the Rogerian practice methodology, "the nurse facilitates the client's actualization of potentials for health and well being. . . . The nurse does not attempt to change anyone to conform to arbitrary health ideals. Rather, nursing care enhances the client's efforts to actualize health potentials from his or her point of view. The nurse helps [to] create an environment where healing conditions are optimal and invites clients to heal themselves as they participate in various modalities used in deliberative mutual patterning" (Barrett, 1990c, pp. 34, 36).

The outcomes of nursing intervention are evaluated by means of a return to pattern manifestation appraisal. Cowling (1990b) explained, "Evaluation requires a return to the original appraisal format after monitoring and collecting additional pattern information as it unfolds during the implementation of nursing intervention strategies. The pattern information is considered in the context of continually emerging health patterning goals affirmed by the client" (p. 61).

Content of the Model: Propositions

Rogers repeatedly linked the metaparadigm concepts person and environment. This linkage is most evident in the principle of integrality: "[The] continuous mutual human field and environmental field process" (Rogers, 1990a, p. 8).

Person, environment, and nursing are linked in this statement: "For nurses, that focus consists of a long-established concern with people and the world they live in. It is the natural forerunner of an organized, abstract system encompassing people and their environments" (Rogers, 1992b, p. 28).

Person, health, and nursing are linked in this statement: "Nurses participate in the process of change, to help people move toward what is deemed better health" (Rogers, 1980g).

The linkage of all four metaparadigm concepts—person, environment, health, and nursing—is evident in the following statements:

The purpose of nurses is to promote health and well-being for all persons wherever they are. (Rogers, 1992b, p. 28)

The purpose of nursing is to promote human betterment wherever people are, on planet earth or in outer space. (Rogers, 1992b, p. 33)

EVALUATION OF ROGERS' SCIENCE OF UNITARY HUMAN BEINGS

This section presents an evaluation of the Science of Unitary Human Beings. The evaluation is based on the results of the analysis as well as on publications by others who have used or commented on the Rogerian conceptual system.

Explication of Origins

The origins of the Science of Unitary Human Beings are evident. Rogers identified various refinements in the conceptual system and explained the reasons for changes in terminology. She also explained why she decided to develop a conceptual system and explicitly identified many of the assumptions undergirding the Science of Unitary Human Beings. Other philosophical claims, in the forms of beliefs held by Rogers about people, their environments, health, and nursing, were easily extracted from her publications. These assumptions and beliefs indicate that Rogers views nursing as a legitimate science and an art that must base its practice on a body of knowledge that has been validated by empirical research. The assumptions also indicate that Rogers values a unitary view of the person and the environment. Rogers pointed out that that perspective of the person identifies nursing as a unique discipline.

Rogers emphasized her view that health is socially defined, which suggests that she expects specific goals for nursing intervention to be based on the values of society, not those of the nurse alone. Moreover, Rogers' discussion of nursing intervention indicates that she values individualized care for each person. In fact, individualized care is mandated by the Science of Unitary Human Beings due to the uniqueness and diversity of each human energy field.

Rogers explained how she drew from the knowledge of various sciences in developing the Science of Unitary Human Beings, and she cited the works of several scholars from adjunctive disciplines. Refinements in the Science of Unitary Human Beings can clearly be traced to new knowledge in nursing and adjunctive disciplines. For example, in explaining the word change in the principle of helicy from probabilistic to unpredictable, Rogers (1990a, 1992b) cited publications about chaos theory.

Comprehensiveness of Content

The Science of Unitary Human Beings is sufficiently comprehensive with regard to depth of content. The many revisions and refinements in the conceptual system attest to Rogers' concern for precision in language. Rogers defined and described the four metaparadigm concepts—person, environment, health, nursing—sufficiently for a conceptual model. Person and environment were clearly defined, and the relationship between unitary human beings and their environments was explicitly identified. Health was defined through its relation to the life process, and determination of wellness and illness was considered a social value.

Furthermore, nursing was defined, and emphasis was placed on its characteristics as a noun. The goal of nursing was clearly delineated. A nursing process, in the form of the Rogerian practice methodology, was extracted from Rogers' publications and from publications by two of the main proponents of the Science of Unitary Human Beings.

The Science of Unitary Human Beings is consistent with scientific findings. This is particularly evident in Rogers' insistence that nursing actions must stem from an organized and valid knowledge base. Indeed, Rogers repeatedly emphasized that nursing is an empirical science, such that any and all judgments must be based on scientific knowledge. She commented, "The education of nurses gains its identity by the transmission of nursing's body of theoretical knowledge. The practice of nurses, therefore, is the creative use of this knowledge in human service" (Rogers, 1992b, p. 29).

In fact, Rogers (1970, 1987a) has always maintained that nursing practice must be theory-based. Indeed, she stated that "Nursing practice must be flexible and creative, individualized and socially oriented, compassionate and skillful. Professional practitioners in nursing must be continuously translating theoretical knowledge into human service. . . . Nursing's conceptual system provides the foundation for nursing practice" (1970, p. 128).

She also stated, "For nurses to fulfill their social and professional responsibilities in the days ahead demands that their practice be based upon a substantive theoretical base specific to nursing. . . . The practice of nurses is the use of this knowledge in service to people" (1987a, pp. 121–122). Furthermore, Rogers (1980a) commented, "Broad principles to guide practice must replace rule-of-thumb" (p. 337).

The dynamic nature of nursing is evident in the following statement: "The dynamic nature of life signifies continuous revision of the nature and meaning of diagnostic data and concomitant revision of interventional measures" (Rogers, 1970, p. 125). In addition, the dynamic nature of the practice methodology is evident in the phase of deliberative mutual patterning as nurse and client are in continuous mutual process, and is also evident in the return to pattern manifestation appraisal for evaluation of intervention outcomes.

The Science of Unitary Human Beings is compatible with ethical standards for nursing practice. Rogers (1992b) noted that "continued emphasis on human rights, client decision-making, and noncompliance with the traditional rules of thumb are . . . necessary dimensions of the new science and art of nursing" (p. 33).

Rogers clearly linked the metaparadigm concepts person and environment and also linked these concepts with health and with nursing. The linkage among all four metaparadigm concepts was concisely stated in two statements regarding the purpose of nursing.

The Science of Unitary Human Beings is comprehensive in breadth of content. The Rogerian conceptual system can be used in diverse settings, ranging from community-based health services to hospitals to the "human advent into outer space" (Rogers, 1992b, p. 27), and with people experiencing virtually any health-related condition from birth through death, "in health and in sickness, in joy and in sorrow" (Rogers, 1992c, p. 1339). Furthermore, the Science of Human Beings is equally applicable to individuals and groups, including families, social groups, communities, and crowds (Rogers, 1992b).

The breadth of the Science of Unitary Human Beings is further supported by the direction it provides for nursing research, education, administration, and practice. Rules for each area are being formulated.

Rules for nursing research are developing. Rogers noted, "Science is never finished. It is always open ended" (Rogers et al., 1990, p. 380). Rogers (1987a) also noted, "The future of research in nursing is based on a commitment to nursing as a science in its own right. The science of nursing is identified as the science of unitary human beings" (p. 123). Consequently, research is crucial for the continued refinement of the Science of Unitary Human Beings.

The phenomena to be studied are unitary human beings and their environments. "The study of nursing as a science," Rogers (1990b) maintained, "is the study of the phenomena central to nursing: unitary, irreducible, human beings and their environments. It is not the study of other fields or theories deriving from other fields. . . . The study of nurses and what they do is not the study of nursing anymore than the study of biologists and what they do is the study of biology" (p. 111).

The problems to be studied are the manifestations of human and environmental field patterns, especially pattern profiles, which are clusters of related pattern manifestations (Phillips, 1989, 1991). The purpose of Science of Unitary Human Beings-based research is to develop theoretical knowledge about "unitary, irreducible, indivisible human and environmental fields: people and their world" (Rogers, 1992b, p. 29).

Given Rogers' emphasis on nursing as a service to all people, wherever they may be, virtually any setting and any person or group would be appropriate for study, with the proviso that both person or group and environment are taken into account. Both basic and applied research are needed to continue to develop nursing knowledge. Basic research, according to Rogers (1992b), "provides new knowledge" (p. 28). In particular, "the focus and goal of basic research in nursing science . . . [is] pattern seeing" (Reeder, 1984, p. 22). In contrast, applied research "tests the new knowledge already available" in practical situations (Rogers, 1992b, p. 28). Rogers (1987a) maintained that "Applied research should replace the use of the phrase 'clinical research.' According to dictionaries the term clinical means 'investigation of a disease in the living subject by observation as distinguished from controlled study, something done at the bedside.' These definitions are inappropriate and inadequate for the scope and purposes of nursing" (p. 22).

Rogers (1992b) advocates the use of a variety of qualitative and quantitative research methods, including philosophical and descriptive approaches. Reeder (1986) maintained that Husserlian phenomenology is an appropriate approach to Science of Unitary Human Beings-based basic research. Cowling (1986b) added existentialism, ecological thinking, dialectical thinking, and historical inquiries, as well as methods that focus on the uniqueness of each person, such as imagery, direct questioning, personal structural analysis, and the Q-sort to the list of appropriate methodologies. Furthermore, case studies and longitudinal research designs that focus on the identification of human and environmental field patterns are more appropriate than cross-sectional designs, given Rogers' emphasis on the uniqueness of the unitary human being (Fawcett, 1994).

Cowling (1986b) pointed out that although descriptive and correlational designs are consistent with the Science of Unitary Human Beings, strict experimental designs are of "questionable value," given the fact that "the unitary system is a noncausal model of reality" (p. 73). Cowling's (1986b) recommendation of correlational designs is supported by Rogers' statements that "There is no causality, but there are relationships" (Rogers et al., 1990, p. 380) and "Association does not mean causality" (Rogers, 1992b, p. 30). Cowling (1986b) went on to say, however, that quasi-experimental and experimental designs "may be appropriate to specific theoretical propositions because they provide a mechanism for testing probabilistic change manifested from human environmental process" (p. 73).

Rogers (1987a) pointed out that "there are incongruities and contradictions between holistic directions in nursing and the forms of inquiry used by nurses. . . . There is a critical need for new tools of measurement appropriate to new paradigms" (p. 122). In fact, a few instruments have been directly derived from the Science of Unitary Human Beings. These instruments are discussed in the social utility section on nursing research later in this chapter.

Data analysis techniques must take the unitary nature of human beings and the integrality of the human and environmental energy fields into account. Consequently, "the use of standard data analysis techniques that employ the components of variance model of statistics [is precluded], for this statistical model is logically inconsistent with the assumption of holism stating that the whole is greater than the sum of parts" (Fawcett & Downs, 1986, p. 87). Cowling (1986b) indicated that "multivariate analysis procedures, particularly canonical correlation, can be useful methods for generating a constellation of variables representing human field pattern properties" (p. 73). The problem here, however, is that canonical correlation is a component of variance procedure, as are all parametric correlational techniques.

Reeder (1984) maintained that ongoing testing of the Science of Unitary Human Beings "cannot be done through the logical empiricist criterion of meaning, testing the hypodeductive system for consistency, and then testing correspondence to the world (mind/body dualism). But rather, the [conceptual] system can be continuously tested through the manifestation of the integral evidence of human and environmental fields and through the relationships between phenomena, which arise from integral evidence" (p. 22).

The emphasis in the Rogerian conceptual system on the integrality of human and environmental energy fields indicates that research conducted within the context of the Science of Unitary Human Beings will enhance understanding of the continuous mutual process of human and environmental energy fields and manifestations of changes in energy field patterns. Ultimately, Science of Unitary Human Beings-based research will yield "a body of knowledge specific to nursing" (Rogers, 1992b, p. 29).

Most of the rules for nursing education have been formulated. Rogers (1985a) recognizes both professional and technical nursing education. She differentiated the two types of programs and the two types of practice on the basis of the nature and amount of knowledge that underwrites the two separate career paths. The focus of the curriculum and the purposes of professional nursing education are identified in the following quotations:

> The education of professional practitioners in nursing requires the transmission of a body of scientific knowledge specific to nursing. This body of knowledge determines the safety and scope of nursing practice. The imaginative and creative use of knowledge for the betterment of man finds expression in the art of nursing. Education opens the doorway to developing the art of practice. The purpose of professional education is to provide the knowledge and tools whereby an individual may become an artist in his field. (Rogers, 1970, p. 88)

> The education of nurses has identity in transmission of nursing's body of theoretical knowledge. (Rogers, 1987a, p. 121)

> The primary purpose of the educational program is to transmit a body of scholarly knowledge in nursing. (Rogers, 1985a, p. 382)

Rogers (cited in Takahashi, 1992) claims that the study of nursing "should be rooted in the study of humankind" (p. 89). More specifically, Rogers (1990b) maintained that the study of the Science of Unitary

Human Beings must be "central to the education of nurses" (p. 111). The content of nursing programs should include courses that will provide a sound general education that is perhaps more far-reaching than typical. Indeed, Rogers (1987a) maintained that "the liberal arts and sciences including extraterrestrial matters" should be part of the content of technical, professional, and advanced nursing education programs (p. 121).

Specific courses in the adjunctive disciplines that are appropriate as a background for the study of the Science of Unitary Human Beings include written and spoken English, foreign language, mathematics, and history (Rogers, 1961), as well as astronomy, modern physics, Eastern philosophy, logic, ethics, cultural anthropology, economics, political science, and computer science (Barrett, 1990a). The level of required content is implied in Rogers' (1987a) discussion of the focus of baccalaureate, master's, and doctoral education. She explained, "Baccalaureate degree graduates in nursing properly possess beginning tools of inquiry and are able to exploit knowledge for the improvement of practice. Master's degree graduates in nursing possess more sophisticated tools of study, identify more complex problems, and design and implement applied research. Basic research requires doctoral study in nursing with a high level of scholarly sophistication and the ability to push back frontiers of knowledge" (p. 122).

Young (1985) indicated that the principles of resonancy, helicy, and integrality are the "major integrating concepts of the curriculum" (p. 60) and outlined a sequence of content at one school of nursing. She explained that the principles are introduced in the first course in the nursing major and are then considered at more advanced levels of understanding and application in subsequent courses. The stages of the human life process, from conception through aging and in stages of terminal illness and dying, can provide the organizational theme for the sequence of didactic content and practicum experiences (Mathwig, Young, & Pepper, 1990; Young, 1985).

Rogers' discussions of nursing education indicate that education for professional nursing occurs at the baccalaureate, master's, and doctoral levels in senior college and university settings. Students must meet the requirements for matriculation in professional nursing programs in those settings. Moreover, Rogers (1985a) noted that "The quality of professional education does not exceed the quality of the faculty. Preparation for full college and university teaching is at the doctoral level" (p. 382).

The rule dealing with teaching-learning strategies is not yet fully formulated. Young (1985) commented that "teaching-learning is a complex, interactive process of growth and development. As faculty and students explore together the meaning of Rogerian concepts, they continue to develop new insights and creative applications for the practice of nursing" (p. 68). Barrett (1990a) emphasized the need to use "processes that teach students how to learn, how to think critically, how to see patterns, find meanings, and gain scholarly insights" (p. 312). Mathwig et al. (1990) maintained that "the development of the student's awareness of self as an aspect of the client's environmental energy field and the dynamic role the nurse's energy field pattern has on the client" needs to be emphasized (p. 320). Rogers (1990b) added that "In the educational process we do not need to teach students how to do everything. Rather we need to teach them how to figure out how to do everything" (p. 111).

On a more pragmatic note, Rogers (1985a) maintained that teaching-learning strategies should include didactic content and laboratory experiences encompassing "maintenance and promotion of health, [as well as] care and rehabilitation of the sick and disabled" (p. 382). She went on to say that laboratory study is "a necessary adjunct [to didactic content] whereby students have the opportunity to demonstrate their capacity to translate theory into practice. . . . Laboratory study is directed toward the healthy and the sick of all ages and conditions. Laboratory settings include homes, schools, industrial settings, clinics, hospitals, and other places where people may be" (p. 382).

Rules for nursing administration can be extracted from publications by Rogers and those proponents of the Science of Unitary Human Beings who have begun to discuss the application of the conceptual system to structures for the delivery of nursing services. Within the context of the Science of Unitary Human Beings, nursing services are regarded as energy fields that "must be seen as more than employees and staffing schedules, more than a body count of functionaires required to staff a shift. All shifts and all nurses should be viewed as interdependent" (Caroselli-Dervan, 1990, p. 154). Gueldner (1989) added that the "administrative system consists of all human and environmental fields integral to the system, and is potentially so complex as to extend to infinity" (p. 114).

The distinctive focus of Science of Unitary Human Beings–based nursing practice is to use nursing knowledge in a creative manner. The purpose to be fulfilled by nursing services is health promotion.

The practitioners of professional nursing should hold valid baccalaureate or higher degrees in nursing. Indeed, Rogers (1992b) maintained that "Autonomous nursing practice directed by nurses holding valid baccalaureate and higher degrees with an upper division major in nursing science is central to the future" (p. 33). Furthermore, professional practitioners should be licensed as such. In fact, Rogers (1985b) has claimed that "Licensure for professional practice in nursing is long overdue. In its absence, human health is jeopardized, fraudulence in recruitment practices continues, and placement of a high value on ignorance is pervasive. Licensing laws for professional practice must be written and professional examinations must be developed. People are at stake" (p. 384).

Nursing services are delivered in many different settings. Rogers (1992b) advocates "Broad community-based health promotion services [that] provide the umbrella" for all health services (p. 33). She maintained that community-based health services should take precedence over hospital-based sick services and should extend to "multiple extra-terrestrial centers" (p. 33). Rogers (1990a, 1990b) regards hospitals and nursing homes as supplemental or satellite services that are pathology- and disease-oriented. She predicts that "As health promotion takes over, fewer and fewer people will need sick services as they currently exist" (1990a, p. 10).

Caroselli-Dervan (1990) noted that the leaders of nursing services must be visionary and willing to embrace innovative and creative change. Alligood (1989) pointed out that "a major function of the administrator is identifying ways of patterning fields to assure integrated behaviors for clients and employees" (p. 109). Gueldner (1989) maintained that "the goal of all nurse administrators is to increase the capacity of each individual in a system to participate knowingly in change. All administrative energy, therefore, should be directed to changes in the environment that will enhance harmonious, symphonic human-environmental field interactions" (p. 115). Gueldner went on to say that "all management energy should be directed to . . . the well-being of each client" (p. 117).

Gueldner (1989) noted that management strategies should be designed "to enhance positive field interactions between staff members and their respective environments. . . . [Moreover,] the administrative climate should be open and supportive; the administrative model should be designed to enhance the self-esteem, actualization, confidence, available options, freedom of choice, and opportunities for individual and group development" (p. 117).

Caroselli-Dervan (1990) and Rizzo (1990) view the strategy of participatory management, operationalized in the form of power sharing, as consistent with the Science of Unitary Human Beings. More specifically, participatory management with power sharing is operationalized as the situation in which "the primary nurse is able to make autonomous decisions and involve his or her primary patients and their significant others" (Rizzo, 1990, p. 161).

Gueldner (1989) noted that administrative policies should include provision for staff development, continuing educational opportunities, and appropriate systems of communication. Staff development should focus on helping "each nurse [to] use him- or herself as a therapeutic agent and mobilize other resources needed to increase awareness, capacity, and choice" (p. 117). A high priority should be based on continuing education, inasmuch as "knowing participation in change is based on being informed" (p. 117). Communication systems should "reflect a positive view of the contributions of each individual within a system" (p. 117).

Rules for nursing practice may be extracted from publications by Rogers and those proponents of the Science of Unitary Human Beings who have begun to describe a specific Rogerian practice methodology. "The practice of nursing," Rogers (1992b) claimed, "is the creative use of [nursing's body of theoretical] knowledge in human service" (p. 29). The purpose of nursing "is to promote health and well-being for all persons wherever they are" (Rogers, 1992b, p. 28). Clinical problems of interest are those manifestations of human and environmental field patterning that nursing as a discipline and society as a whole deem relevant for nursing. Nursing may be practiced in any setting in which nurses encounter people, ranging from the community to hospitals to outer space. All people of all ages, both as individual human energy fields and as group energy fields, are legitimate recipients of nursing care.

The Rogerian practice methodology, described by Barrett (1988, 1990b) and Cowling (1990b), focuses on the human and environmental energy fields. The two phases of pattern manifestation appraisal and deliberative mutual patterning represent "concern [with] human life patterning and reflect the wholeness of the unitary person in continuous innovative change with the universe" (Barrett, 1990b, p. 35). Emphasis is placed on the need to individualize nursing services as intraindividual and interindividual energy field pattern manifestations become increasingly diverse. Nursing interventions emphasize diverse noninvasive modalities.

Science of Unitary Human Beings–based nursing practice contributes to human betterment, however that might be defined by a society. Moreover, nursing practice guided by the Science of Unitary Human Beings can assist both patient and nurse "to become aware of their own rhythms and to make choices among a range of options congruent with their perceptions of well-being" (Malinski, 1986c, p. 29). Nursing guided by the Science of Unitary Human Beings also leads to acceptance of diversity as the norm and of the integral connectedness of human beings and their environments, as well as to viewing change as positive (Malinski, 1986c).

Logical Congruence

There is no evidence of logical incompatibility in the content of the Science of Unitary Human Beings. The content of the Rogerian conceptual system flows directly from Rogers' philosophical claims, and the distinctive view of the person and the environment is carried throughout all components of the Rogerian conceptual system. Furthermore, the characteristics of systems and developmental models that are reflected in the content of the Science of Unitary Human Beings are addressed in a logically congruent manner.

Generation of Theory

Rogers (1980a, 1986, 1992b) derived three rudimentary theories from the Science of Unitary Human Beings. The **Theory of Accelerating Evo-**

lution posits that evolutionary change is speeding up and that the range of diversity of life processes is widening. More specifically, the theory postulates that change proceeds "in the direction of higher wave frequency field pattern . . . characterized by growing diversity" (1980a, p. 334). "The higher frequency wave patterns manifesting growing diversity," Rogers explained, "portend new norms to coordinate with this accelerating change" (1992b, p. 32). Examples of new norms offered by Rogers are higher blood pressure readings in all age groups compared with readings from a few decades ago and increased length of the average waking period. Moreover, the theory provides a novel explanation for hyperactivity in children, regarding that pattern manifestation as accelerating evolution of the human energy field. Rogers (1992b) commented, "interestingly, gifted children and the so-called hyperactive [children] not uncommonly manifest similar behaviors. It would seem more reasonable, then, to hypothesize that hyperactivity was accelerating evolution, rather than to denigrate rhythmicities that diverge from outdated norms and erroneous expectations" (p. 32).

The **Theory of Rhythmical Correlates of Change** focuses on human and environmental energy field rhythms, which "are not to be confused with biologic rhythms or psychologic rhythms or similar particulate phenomena" (Rogers, 1980a, p. 335). "Manifestations of the speeding up of human field rhythms," Rogers (1992b) explained, "are coordinate with higher frequency environmental field patterns. Humans and their environments evolve and change together" (p. 32). The theory proposes that the accelerating evolution and increasing diversity of human field patterns are integral with accelerating evolution and increasing diversity in environmental field patterns. Evidence for the theory includes the population explosion and increased longevity along with quickened environmental motion, growing atmospheric and cosmological complexity, escalating levels of science and technology, and development of space communities.

The **Theory of Paranormal Phenomena** provides explanations for precognition, déjà vu, clairvoyance, and telepathy. Rogers (1980a) pointed out that within the Science of Unitary Human Beings "such occurrences become 'normal' rather than 'paranormal'" (p. 335). This is because in a pandimensional world, there is neither linear time nor any separation of human and environmental fields, so that the present is relative to the person. The theory also provides an explanation for the efficacy of such alternative methods of healing as meditation, imagery, and therapeutic touch. Rogers (1992b) commented, "Meditative modalities, for example, bespeak 'beyond waking' [pattern] manifestations" (p. 32).

Krieger (1975) introduced the alternative, noninvasive healing method of therapeutic touch into the nursing literature. Miller (1979) placed therapeutic touch within the context of the Science of Unitary Human beings, stating that "The . . . science of unitary [human beings] as formulated by Rogers, may be used to account for the phenomenon of the therapeutic touch in healing, a phenomenon that other theories have failed to explain" (p. 279). Within the Science of Unitary Human Beings, therapeutic touch is viewed as a noninvasive modality that involves both pattern manifestation appraisal and deliberative human/environmental energy field patterning. Thus, therapeutic touch reflects the principles of resonancy and integrality (Quinn & Strelkauskas, 1993). Boguslawski (1979) noted that therapeutic touch is thought to involve a transfer of energy from nurse to patient, with resultant change in the energy field pattern. More specifically, therapeutic touch is conceptualized as "knowledgeable and purposive patterning of nurse-environmental/patient-environmental energy field process (Meehan, 1993, p. 73).

Rogers (1980a, 1986) cited several examples of changes in human life that she claimed as support for her theories. For example, she noted that Toffler's (1970, 1980) work provides evidence of the increasing rate of change in many aspects of life. She also noted that sleep/wake patterns are changing, such that people of all ages sleep less now. More definitive empirical evidence supporting her theory of rhythmic correlates comes from work by Johnston, Fitzpatrick, and Donovan (1982), who found that developmental stage is related to past and future time orientation.

Other theories have been derived from the Rogerian conceptual system. Newman (1986) has constructed a grand theory of health—the Theory of Health as Expanding Consciousness—from the concepts of time, space, movement, consciousness, and pattern. The central thesis of the theory is that health is the expansion of consciousness. According to Newman (1986), the meaning of life and health are found in the evolving process of expanding consciousness. More specifically, the theory asserts that "every person in every situation, no matter how disordered and hopeless it may seem, is part of the universal process of expanding consciousness" (Newman, 1992, p. 650).

Parse (1981, 1992) formulated a grand theory, now called the Theory of Human Becoming, that "synthesizes Martha E. Rogers's principles and concepts about man with major tenets and concepts from existential-phenomenological thought" (1981, p. 4). In particular, Parse based her theory on Rogers' principles of helicy, complementarity (now integrality), and resonancy; and her concepts of energy field, openness, pattern and organization, and four-dimensionality (now pandimensionality); as well as on the existential phenomenological tenets of human subjectivity and intentionality and the concepts of co-constitution, coexistence, and situated freedom. The central thesis of the Theory of Human Becoming is that "humans participate with the universe in the cocreation of health" (1992, p. 37). Parse (cited in Takahashi, 1992) explained that "Human becoming refers to the human being structuring meaning multidimensionally while cocreating rhythmical patterns of relating and cotranscending with possibles" (p. 86).

Fitzpatrick (1983, 1989) derived the Life Perspective Rhythm Model, which could be considered a grand theory, from the Rogerian conceptual system and from the findings of research by Fitzpatrick (1980), Fitzpatrick and Donovan (1978), and Fitzpatrick, Donovan, and Johnston (1980). The life perspective rhythm model, according to Fitzpatrick (1989), "is a developmental model which proposes that the process of human development is characterized by rhythms. Human development occurs within the context of continuous person-environment interaction. Basic human rhythms that describe the development of persons include the identified indices of holistic human functioning, that is, temporal patterns, motion patterns, consciousness patterns, and perceptual patterns. The rhythmic correlates developed by Rogers are consistent with this life perspective rhythm model" (p. 405).

Barrett (1986) derived a middle-range theory of power—the Theory of Knowing Participation in Change—from the principle of helicy. Power is defined as "the capacity to participate knowingly in the nature of change characterizing the continuous repatterning of the human and environmental fields" (p. 174). Elaborating, Barrett (1986) explained that knowing participation "is being aware of what one is choosing to do, feeling free to do it, and doing it intentionally. Awareness and freedom to act intentionally guide participation in choices and involvement in creating changes" (p. 175).

Ference (1986b, 1989b) derived the middle-range Theory of Human Field Motion from the principle of resonancy. The theory proposes that "as a human field engages in ever-higher levels of human field motion, the pattern evolves toward greater complexity, diversity, and differentiation" (1989b, p. 123). Ference (1989b) cited empirical evidence of the correlates of human field motion, stating that "Human field motion expands with increased physical motion, with meditation, with risk-taking, and with higher levels of participation in change" (p. 123).

Reed (1991) reformulated knowledge about self-transcendence from various life span theories within the context of the Science of Unitary Human Beings. "Self transcendence," she explained, "was identified as a particular pattern of expansion of conceptual boundaries" (p. 72). The reformulated theory proposes that "expansion of conceptual boundaries through intrapersonal, interpersonal, and temporal experiences [is] developmentally appropriate in individuals confronted with end-of-own-life issues [and that] expansion of self-boundaries [is] positively related to indicators of well-being in these individuals" (p. 72).

Leddy (1993) has reconceptualized the principle of integrality through an extensive review of the literature from many adjunctive disciplines. Her work led to the development of the Human Energy Systems (HES) Model, three middle-range theories, and two instruments. The middle-range descriptive theories of well-being, health, and nursing were directly derived from the HES model. The Well-Being Index was designed to measure well-being, defined as "a dynamic state characterized by perceived purpose and power to influence change" (Leddy, 1993, p. 57). The Synchrony Scale was designed to measure ease and expansion of synchrony, which is defined as concomitant patterning of human/environment participation (Leddy, personal communication, September 4, 1993).

Credibility

Social Utility

The social utility of the Science of Unitary Human Beings is well-documented by its use as a guide for nursing research, education, administration, and practice. National Rogerian Conferences, sponsored by New York University Division of Nursing, the Division of Nursing Alumni Association, and Upsilon Chapter of Sigma Theta Tau International, have been held in New York City every 2 to 3 years since 1983. Malinski's (1986a) edited book, *Explorations on Martha Rogers' Science of Unitary Human Beings*, and Barrett's (1990d) edited book, *Visions of Rogers' Science-Based Nursing*, are devoted exclusively to reports of and issues related to research and practice derived from the Science of Unitary Human Beings. Two other books, *Martha E. Rogers: Eighty Years of Excellence*, and *Martha E. Rogers: Her Life and Her Work*, both edited by Barrett and Malinski, were published in 1994. Still another book, *Rogers' Scientific Art of Nursing Practice*, which is edited by Madrid and Barrett and contains the papers presented at the Fourth Rogerian Conference, was also published in 1994. In addition, a journal entitled *Visions: The Journal of Rogerian Nursing Science* premiered in 1993.

The use of the Science of Unitary Human Beings requires considerable background and ongoing study. Rogers (1990b) maintained that the implementation of nursing practice based on the Science of Unitary Human Beings requires a commitment to life-long learning and the use of what nurses know as well as what they can imagine. Implementation also requires creativity and compassion. The new reality represented by the Science of Unitary Human Beings requires "new ways of thinking, new questions, new interpretations" (Rogers, 1990b, p. 111). In particular, nurses "should learn to think through what it is they are dealing with and then practice will always be new and innovative" (Rogers, cited in Takahashi, 1992, p. 89).

Rogers' conception of the person as a unitary human being and the presentation of the Science of Unitary Human Beings in just four concepts and three principles might be considered elegant in its simplicity, yet as Newman (1972) noted, "Many a graduate student will attest to the difficulty of reorganizing one's thinking about [the person] in order to consider [him or her] a unified being and not as a composite of organs and systems and various psychosocial components" (pp. 451–452). Although the same thing might be said about any conceptual model that puts forth a holistic view of the person, some nurses find it especially difficult for the Science of Unitary Human Beings.

The difficulty may be due to the fact that viewing the world from the perspective of the Science of Unitary Human Beings "requires a new synthesis, a creative leap and inculcation of new attitudes and values" (Rogers, 1989, p. 188) or it may be due to the fact that the Science of Unitary Human Beings is made up of terms and ideas that are unfamiliar to some people. However, Rogers (1970, 1978a, 1980b, 1986, 1990a, 1992b) has repeatedly defended her terminology, pointing out that she selected terms that are in the general language and initially defined those terms according to the dictionary. As the conceptual system evolved, Rogers recognized the need for more specific definitions to facilitate uniformity of usage and precision. She noted that that procedure is common in all sciences. Nevertheless, use of the Science of Unitary Human Beings must be preceded by mastery of a vocabulary that may be new to many nurses. This task can be facilitated by use of the glossary of terms that is included in several of Rogers' (1986, 1990a, 1992b) recent publications.

The application of the Science of Unitary Human Beings in nursing practice is feasible. Ference (1989b) outlined a 12-month plan for introducing the Rogerian conceptual system into a nursing service setting that provides an overview of the human and material resources required. The first level, which takes approximately 6 months and consists of five phases, involves introducing the Rogerian conceptual system to the administrators and staff.

The first phase, awareness, requires approximately 10 hours spread over 4 to 6 weeks and focuses on learning. Planned discussions between a "faculty expert" and the nursing staff are supplemented with readings and annotated references.

During the second phase, testing, the staff becomes acclimated to the Rogerian conceptual system through such activities as patient care conferences that focus on integrating the Rogerian conceptual system into everyday clinical situations.

During the third phase, readiness, the staff begins to write care plans, which they use to explain the Rogerian conceptual system to their peers. In addition, the staff begins to implement the care plans "with much sharing of new modalities of care as [they] integrate the [Science of Unitary Human Beings] into their traditional practice" (p. 124).

The fourth phase, expert reinforcement, typically occurs after about 30 hours of formal instruction. In this phase, feedback is provided to the staff from an expert in the Rogerian conceptual system. Ference (1989b) noted that role modeling is a particularly effective strategy during the fourth phase, especially for staff who may be skeptical or those who have difficulty understanding the content of and nursing modalities associated with the Science of Unitary Human Beings.

The expert reinforcement phase evolves into the fifth phase, peer reinforcement, as the staff becomes more proficient with implementation. The fifth phase also involves evaluation by means of a nursing process audit tool that can be used by peers to critique adherence of practice to the Rogerian conceptual system. In addition, conferences and direct observation are used by peers and by the expert to evaluate the extent to which practice reflects the Science of Unitary Human Beings.

The second level focuses on administrative and policy matters and requires another 6 months for completion. During that time, the nursing philosophy, nursing standards of care, nursing documentation system, and quality assurance program are revised in accord with the Science of Unitary Human Beings.

Mason and Patterson (1990) noted that although Science of Unitary Human Beings-based nursing practice certainly is feasible and is associated with beneficial patient outcomes, its proper use may be limited "in the secure environment of a special hospital" for mentally handicapped people (p. 141). In addition, Mason and Chandley (1990) commented that the application of the conceptual system in special hospitals for the criminally insane "remains unsuccessful, not least of all because of its highly complex philosophical nature, but also because it cannot influence the politico-legal components" (p. 671).

NURSING RESEARCH. The utility of the Science of Unitary Human Beings for nursing research is well documented. Ference (1986a) traced the evolution of research that has been guided by the Rogerian conceptual system. She noted that the early studies, all of which were conducted as doctoral dissertations at New York University, "were based upon some guiding assumptions and a philosophy that the nurse cares for the whole person" (p. 37). Her retrospective analysis of these studies yielded groupings of research. In the mid-1960s, studies focused on human development, such as Porter's (1968) research, and on man-environment interaction, exemplified by Mathwig's (1968) research. Research conducted from the late 1960s to the late 1970s focused on body image, exemplified by Fawcett's (1977) and Chodil's (1979) studies. Several studies completed in the early to mid-1970s focused on the variable of time, such as the research by Newman (1971) and Fitzpatrick (1976). Studies conducted during the early 1970s also focused on locus of control, field independence, and differentiation, exemplified by research conducted by Barnard (1973), Miller (1974), and Swanson (1976).

Ference (1986a) pointed out that much of the early research only mentioned Rogers' work and used theories borrowed from other disciplines as a basis for hypotheses. Research conducted during the late 1970s and into the 1980s used the Rogerian conceptual system in a more comprehensive manner, often identifying a particular principle of homeodynamics as the focus of study. One of the first studies that reflected that focus was conducted by Ference (1980) herself. All Science of Unitary Human Beings–based doctoral dissertations and master's theses that could be retrieved from *Dissertation Abstracts International* and *Master's Abstracts International* are listed in the bibliography at the end of this chapter.

A review of the published full reports of Science of Unitary Human Beings–based research revealed some instrument development studies, a few descriptive studies, many correlational studies, and several experimental studies. Ference (1986b) developed the Human Field Motion Test to measure the person's perception of the frequency of energy field motion. Barrett (1986) developed the Power as Knowing Participation in Change Test to measure the person's capacity to participate knowingly in change, that is, the person's awareness of what he or she is choosing to do, feeling free to do it, and doing it intentionally. Paletta (1990) designed the Temporal Experience Scales (TES) to measure "the continuous mutual process of the human field with the movement of events in the environmental field" (p. 240). Three independent scales comprise the TES—the Time Dragging Scale, the Time Racing Scale, and the Timelessness Scale. Wright's (1991) Human Energy Field Assessment Form was developed "to record findings related to the human energy field assessment as it is practiced in therapeutic touch" (1991, p. 635). The form permits recording of the location and intensity of energy field disturbances as well as the strength of the overall energy field. Carboni (1992) developed the Mutual Exploration of the Healing Human Field–Environmental Field Relationship instrument "to capture the changing configurations of energy field patterns of the healing human field-environmental field relationship in order to provide data useful for identifying and understanding this relationship" (p. 137). One form of the instrument can be used by the nurse and the individual client, and another form can be used by the nurse and two or more individuals as the client. Johnston (1993) designed the Human Field Image Metaphor Scale as a measure of human field image, which is "an individual awareness of the infinite wholeness of the human field" (personal communication from Rogers, 1991, cited in Johnston, 1993, p. 55) and a manifestation of the human and environmental field mutual process (Phillips, 1990).

Banonis (1989) described the experience of recovering from addiction within the context of the Rogerian conceptual system and Parse's (1981) theory of man-living-health. Malinski (1991) described the experiences of older couples with laughing at oneself. She proposed that laughing at oneself is a form of knowing participation in the process of health patterning. Reeder (1991) described the meaning of laughing at oneself. Gulick and Bugg (1992) described the multidimensional health patterning, in the form of symptoms and activities of daily living, of people with multiple sclerosis. Using qualitative methods, Heidt (1990) and Samarel (1992) described the beneficial effects of therapeutic touch.

Correlational research derived from the Rogerian conceptual system has examined the relationships between such variables as creativity, actualization, and empathy (Alligood 1986, 1991); mystical experience, differentiation, and creativity (Cowling, 1986a); the experience of dying, the experience of paranormal events, and creativity (McEvoy, 1990); diverse environmental conditions, temporal experience, and perception of restfulness (Smith, 1984, 1986); temporal experience and human time, defined as boundarylessness, openness, continuous change, creativity, and innovation (Paletta, 1990); perception of the speed of time and the process of dying (Rawnsley, 1986); time experience, creativity, differentiation and human field motion (Ference, 1986b); human field motion, human field rhythms, creativity, diversity of sensory phenomena, perception of time moving fast, and waking periods (Yarcheski & Mahon, 1991); imposed motion and human field motion (Gueldner, 1986); human field motion and power (Barrett, 1986); human field motion and preferred visible wavelengths (Benedict & Burge, 1990); visible lightwaves and the experience of pain (McDonald, 1986); and hyperactivity and perception of short wavelength light (Malinski, 1986d).

Other relationships that have been investigated include gender role identity, femininity, and self-concept during pregnancy and the postpartum (Brouse, 1985); self-actualization, conception of health, and choices about health practices (Laffrey, 1985); perceived body size, conversational distance, body weight, and self-actualization (Clarke, 1986); and body temperature, activation, and well-being (Mason, 1988).

Several experimental Science of Unitary Human Beings–based studies have focused on the effects of noninvasive modalities, including therapeutic touch and guided imagery. The efficacy of therapeutic touch has been investigated with regard to hemoglobin level (Krieger, 1974); anxiety (Quinn, 1984, 1989); anxiety, mood, time perception, perception of therapeutic touch effectiveness, and immune function (Quinn & Strelkauskas, 1993); time distortion (Quinn, 1992); tension headache pain (Keller & Bzdek, 1986); and postoperative pain (Meehan, 1993). The studies of the effects of guided imagery have focused on the experience of time and human field motion (Butcher & Parker, 1988, 1990).

In addition, Goldberg and Fitzpatrick (1980) studied the effect of movement therapy on morale and self-esteem. Gil and Atwood (1981) studied the effects of epidermal growth factor on wound healing. Meehan (1992) studied the effect of budgetary knowledge on staff nurses' attitudes toward administration and cost containment. Floyd (1983, 1984) studied the sleep-wake cycles of rotating shift workers and the interactions between individual circadian rhythms of sleep and wakefulness and the rest-activity schedule in a psychiatric hospital. Gaydos and Farnham (1988) explored the differences in individuals' heart rate and blood pressure when petting a dog with whom they had a companion bond, when petting an unknown dog, and when reading quietly.

The investigation of family-related phenomena is evident in some studies derived from the Rogerian conceptual system. Schodt (1989) studied the pattern of relationships among father-fetus attachment, mother-fetus attachment, and couvade. Boyd (1990) investigated mother-daughter identification through examination of the relationships between attachment, conflict, and mother and daughter identities. Sanchez (1989) examined the relationships between empathy, diversity, and telepathy in mother-daughter dyads. The extension of the Rogerian conceptual system to the family is also evident in Fawcett's (1989) summary of the findings from a program of research designed to examine similarities in wives' and husbands' pregnancy-related experiences, including body image changes and physical and psychological symptoms.

Other published research reports have cited Rogers' work but present no evidence that the studies were directly derived from the Rogerian conceptual system. Lum et al. (1978) used Rogers' (1970) definition of nursing in their study of the effects of nursing activities on outcomes for oncology patients receiving chemotherapy. Reed (1987) noted that her study of the relationship between spirituality and well-being in terminally ill persons is within the context of the concept of transcendence, which she regarded as an aspect of various models, including Rogers'. Tompkins (1980) referred to Rogers' work, as well as to other conceptual models, in her discussion of her study findings. Smith (1983) noted that the view of family used in her study of family development when a teenage mother and her infant are incorporated into the household was consistent with Rogers' work.

NURSING EDUCATION. The utility of the Science of Unitary Human Beings for nursing education is documented. Rogers (cited in Safier, 1977) commented, "I know that many schools are using my book [*An Introduction to the Theoretical Basis of Nursing*], and also that many students are being oriented to this sort of thinking" (p. 328). Riehl's (1980) finding that Rogers' model was "being taught, practiced by students, and implemented by faculty" (p. 398) provided empirical evidence to support that statement. Riehl did not, however, provide the names of schools using the Rogerian conceptual system.

More specific evidence of the use of the Science of Unitary Human Beings as a curriculum guide is available. The Rogerian conceptual system has been used to guide the development of the curriculum for the baccalaureate, master's, and doctoral programs at New York University Division of Nursing in New York City. Rogers (1978b) outlined the sequence of nursing courses in the baccalaureate program, which is structured according to stages of human development in a chronological fashion starting with the neonate. Mathwig et al. (1990) presented additional discussion of the baccalaureate nursing curriculum at New York University. Young (1985) and later Mathwig et al. (1990) presented a detailed discussion of use of the Science of Unitary Human Beings in the baccalaureate program at Washburn University School of Nursing in Topeka, Kansas. Mathwig et al. (1990) also presented a detailed discussion of the

Science of Unitary Human Beings–based baccalaureate curriculum for registered nurses at Mercy College in Dobbs Ferry, New York.

NURSING ADMINISTRATION. The utility of the Science of Unitary Human Beings for nursing administration is beginning to be documented in the literature. Nursing practice is guided by the Science of Unitary Human Beings at the Veterans Administration Medical Center in San Diego, California (Garon, 1991; Kodiath, 1991), the University of Michigan Surgical Intensive Care Unit in Ann Arbor (Smith, Kupferschmid, Dawson, & Briones, 1991), an inpatient/outpatient interdisciplinary Pain Management Clinic located within an acute care hospital (Joseph, 1990), and in private nursing practices (Barrett, 1990a, 1992; Hill & Oliver, 1993; Forker & Billings, 1989).

Garon (1991) presented a Science of Unitary Human Beings–based format for the holistic assessment of patients in the home setting who experience chronic pain. Tettero, Jackson, and Wilson (1993) described a Science of Unitary Human Beings–based nursing assessment tool for use in various clinical situations. Madrid and Winstead-Fry (1986) described a format for assessment based on the correlates of patterning.

Falco and Lobo (1985) presented a detailed nursing process format based on the principles of homeodynamics that can be used to develop nursing care plans for patients with various health problems. Smith et al. (1991) described a Science of Unitary Human Beings–based nursing process format for use in a family-centered surgical intensive care unit. They listed relevant questions to ask to elicit information for the assessment, diagnosis, implementation, and evaluation phases of the nursing process, within the context of the principles of helicy, resonancy, and complementarity (now integrality).

Decker (1989) devised a Science of Unitary Human Beings–based nursing practice model for use at an outpatient geriatric assessment center. The model encompasses observation of behavior, assessment of the person and environment, diagnosis of total person function, establishment of congruent goals, implementation of interventions, guidance of patterning, and evaluation of total person function. She pointed out that "the role of the clinical nurse specialist as a member of the geriatric assessment team is clarified when nursing actions are based [on the principles of helicy, resonancy, and integrality]" (p. 28).

Hanchett (1979) developed several assessment tools based on the Rogerian conceptual system and general system theory. Those tools were designed specifically for assessment of the energy, individuality, and pattern and organization of communities.

NURSING PRACTICE. Rogers (1987a) maintained that "the practical implications [of the Science of Unitary Human Beings] for human health and well-being are already demonstrable" (p. 123). Indeed, the utility of the Science of Unitary Human Beings for creative nursing care of individuals of various ages and with diverse medical conditions is documented in the literature. Blair (1979) and Rogers (1986) discussed care of the hyperactive child. Katch (1983), Rogers (1986), Alligood (1990), and Cowling (1990a) discussed the utility of the Rogerian conceptual system for nursing care of the aged.

Levine (1976) derived a theoretical explanation of the experience of pregnancy and implications for practice from an early version of the Rogerian conceptual system. She stated, "Pregnancy illustrates how needs arising within the female's field cause an inner-directed, contracted field experience that persists and intensifies throughout the 9 months, diminishes severely during labor and delivery, and reexpands around lactation. Implications for family and health personnel during these stages are knowledge, acceptance, and support of the female. . . . It becomes important to minimize environmental factors that could present or arrest the female's field contraction and expansion at the various states of pregnancy" (p. 15).

Rogers (1986) discussed the utility of her conceptual system for nursing care of persons with hypertension and for the dying person. Madrid and Winstead-Fry (1986) used their Science of Unitary Human Beings–based assessment format to determine the energy field pattern for a 35-year-old man with a cerebral aneurysm and then described the planning, intervention, and evaluation phases of the nursing process for this patient. Whelton (1979) combined the Rogerian conceptual system with a nursing process format and knowledge from physiology, psychology, and sociology to outline nursing care plans for patients with decreased cardiac output and those with impaired neurological function. She then applied the resultant conceptual-theoretical system to the care of a noncompliant patient with decreased cardiac output and a history of diabetes and hypertension, and a patient with total disability due to recurrent meningioma.

Kodiath (1991) interpreted the nursing care of a 51-year-old woman with chronic pain within the context of the Science of Unitary Human Beings. Buczny, Speirs, and Howard (1989) and Ference (1989a) applied the Rogerian conceptual system to the care of terminally ill patients.

Tuyn (1992) described nursing practice that combines the Science of Unitary Human Beings with brief, solution-oriented therapy. Thompson (1990) discussed the psychodynamics and nursing care of a client with a borderline personality disorder within the context of the Science of Unitary Human Beings.

Meehan (1990) described the use of therapeutic touch with a patient experiencing pain from metastatic cancer. Newshan (1989) described the use of therapeutic touch for the control of respiratory and gastrointestinal symptoms, fever, pain, and anxiety in a 29-year-old man with AIDS. Madrid (1990) used therapeutic touch, along with environmental patterning, in the care of a 30-year-old man with AIDS. Payne (1989) applied therapeutic touch with patients at a rehabilitation center. Hill and Oliver

(1993) explained how they use therapeutic touch in a mental health nursing practice.

Barrett (1990b) described the use of health patterning in her private nursing practice. She regards health patterning as "a nursing science alternative to psychotherapy" (p. 105), defining it as "the process of assisting clients with their knowing participation in change" (Barrett, 1990c, p. 38). Health patterning is accomplished through a variety of modalities, one of which is power enhancement. "Power," Barrett (1990c) explained, "is the avenue whereby humans participate in creating their own reality by actualizing some potentials for change rather than others" (p. 38). In a later publication, Barrett (1992) described the use of innovative imagery, a health-patterning modality that enhances power by assisting clients with their knowing participation in change.

Other publications have addressed the application of the Science of Unitary Human Beings to the family. Whall (1981) constructed a logically congruent conceptual-theoretical system of nursing knowledge from the Rogerian conceptual system, Fawcett's (1975) extension of the conceptual system to the family system, and theories of family functioning. She then developed a guide for assessment of families, organized according to individual subsystem considerations, interactional patterns, unique characteristics of the whole family system, and environmental interface synchrony. Rogers (1983a, 1983b) extended the conceptual system to the family system and presented a discussion of the use of the extension of her conceptual system in specific family situations. Johnston (1986) and Reed (1986) derived family therapy protocols from the Rogerian conceptual system.

Hanchett (1990) explained how the Science of Unitary Human Beings can be extended for use in the community, with the community as the client. Forker and Billings (1989) discussed the application of the Rogerian conceptual system in the community in the form of a clinical group encounter with an aging population.

Social Congruence

Implementation of the Science of Unitary Human Beings carries with it the understanding that "Nursing, as a learned profession, has no dependent functions. Like all other professions, nursing has many collaborative functions, which are indispensable to providing society with a higher order of service than any one profession can offer. Moreover, no profession has the knowledge, competence, or prerogative to delegate anything to another profession. Each profession is responsible for determining its own boundaries within the context of social need" (Rogers, 1985a, p. 381). Consequently, "professionally educated nurses are independent practitioners prepared to knowledgeably provide health services to individuals, families, groups, and communities. They are accountable for their own acts and liable to the public they serve. They are peer participants in collaborative judgments made with professional personnel in other fields" (Rogers 1985a, p. 382).

Rogers' view of professional practice, coupled with her focus on health promotion and noninvasive modalities of nursing intervention directed to all people, wherever they are, may exceed the expectations of some consumers of health care, some nurses, and some other health care team members. In fact, the Science of Unitary Human Beings reflects a view of people and their environments that requires a new way of thinking that not all people are willing or interested in undertaking. Indeed, the Science of Unitary Human Beings "will not be accepted if a nurse cannot perceive [energy] fields and resonating waves as the 'real world' of nursing" (Barnum, 1990, p. 43).

However, as more consumers recognize the value, cost-effectiveness, and benefits of health promotion and noninvasive modalities, and as health care reform requires new views of what constitutes appropriate care, the nursing activities guided by the Science of Unitary Human Beings should be more fully accepted and even anticipated.

The Science of Unitary Human Beings is congruent with societal expectations that individuals should participate actively in decisions about their health care. In fact, Rogers (cited in Randell, 1992) noted, "Our job is better health, and people do better making their own choices. The best prognosis is for the individual who is non-compliant" (p. 181). Bramlet, Gueldner, and Sowell (1990) pointed out that Rogers' position reflects consumer-centric advocacy.

Proponents, of course, find Science of Unitary Human Beings–based nursing practice congruent with their views of nursing. In fact, for many of its proponents, the Rogerian conceptual system and its related theories and research comprise the nursing science. For example, Blair (1979) commented, "Nursing science as conceptualized by Rogers provides a sound basis for achieving the goal of nursing—to serve man throughout the life process" (p. 302).

Rogers (1987c) has pointed out that her perspective of nursing is humanistic and optimistic but not utopian. Rogers' humanistic and scholarly approach to nursing has been cited as "a model for emulation" by Hugh R.K. Barber (1987, p. 12), a physician. He pointed out that "the new orientation of the nursing profession is achieving in a more sophisticated manner what physicians have been striving to achieve. However, while nursing is drawing closer to this goal, physicians seem to be slowly moving in the opposite direction" (p. 15).

Social Significance

Rogers (1992b) maintained that the purpose of Science of Unitary Human Beings–based nursing practice is "to promote health and well-

being for all persons wherever they are" (p. 28). Whelton (1979) specu-
lated that use of the Rogerian conceptual system could make differences
in clients' health status. She stated, "By entering into a scientifically
based therapeutic relationship with the patient, the nurse can make the
difference between the patient continuing a life of inadvertent self-
destruction or reaching for his optimum health potential" (p. 19). Miller
(1979) noted, "If Rogers' [conceptual system] is followed, then perhaps
nursing approaches would take into account a wider range of behavioral
variability among individuals" (p. 286).

The evidence supporting the social significance of Science of Unitary
Human Beings–based nursing practice is mixed, with evaluation focused
primarily on the effects of the use of therapeutic touch. Anecdotal evidence comes from practitioners, who claim that therapeutic touch elicits
a profound relaxation response, promotes a positive mood state, and reduces anxiety, pain, and the need for pain medication (Jurgens, Meehan,
& Wilson, 1987; Newshan, 1989).

Empirical evidence provides some support for the anecdotal claims.
Qualitative and quantitative studies have systemically documented the
beneficial effects of therapeutic touch, including increased relaxation,
reduced pain and anxiety, and increased positive mood (Heidt, 1990;
Meehan, 1993; Samarel, 1992). Experimental research has, however,
yielded mixed results. In one study, Quinn (1984) found that therapeutic
touch resulted in a reduction in state anxiety, but that finding was not
replicated in her later investigation (1989). More carefully controlled
studies are warranted.

Contributions to the Discipline of Nursing

Rogers was one of the first nurse scholars to explicitly identify the
person as the central phenomenon of nursing's concern. Summarizing the
significance of that contribution to nursing knowledge, Newman (1972)
stated, "Much of the confusion about what we should be studying was
eliminated, in my opinion, when Rogers identified the phenomenon
which is the center of nursing's purpose: MAN. . . . The clear-cut delineation of man as the focus of nursing gave direction for the development
of theory that is not just relevant to nursing, but basic to nursing" (pp.
451–452).

Although other conceptual models consider the person in a holistic
manner, Rogers' view of the person as a unitary human being is distinctive in that no parts or components or subsystems of the person are
delineated—the person is a unified whole. Furthermore, although other
conceptual models consider the environment and its relationship with the
person, Rogers' view of person and environment as integral energy fields
is unique and visionary.

Commenting on the contributions of her model, Rogers (cited in

Safier, 1977) stated, "The conceptual system . . . provides for a substantive body of knowledge in nursing that will have relevance for all workers concerned with people, but with special relevance for nurses, not because it matters to nurses per se, but because it matters to human beings, and consequently to nurses" (p. 320). Moreover, Rogers (1986) pointed out that "the Science of Unitary Human Beings identifies nursing's uniqueness and signifies the potential of nurses to fulfill their social responsibility in human service" (p. 8).

Whall (1987) noted that the Rogerian conceptual system has advanced the discipline of nursing through the many debates it has sparked. She pointed out that the conceptual system "has generated lively debates and seems to have raised more questions than it answers. It has explained disparate views while engendering debate regarding techniques that may be used to measure concepts and relationships. The debates engendered by [Rogers'] model have in a sense forced nursing to move on. In a sense, it forced nurse scholars to question and seek answers again and again. If this . . . is in essence the value of a [conceptual model], Rogers' framework will stand as a milestone" (p. 158).

Rogers, along with most other authors of nursing models, has continued to refine her conceptual system. Speaking to the need for continued evolution of her model, Rogers (1970) stated, "The emergence of a science of nursing demands a clear, unequivocal conceptual frame of reference. This is not to propose that nursing's conceptual system is either static or inflexible. Quite the contrary. In its evolution it is properly subject to reformulation and change as empirical knowledge grows, as conceptual data achieve greater clarity, and as the interconnectedness between ideas takes on new dimensions" (p. 84).

Rogers has been largely successful in her commitment to advancing the discipline of nursing through development of a unique and substantive body of knowledge. She commented, "The future of nursing is based on a commitment to nursing as a science in its own right. The science of nursing is identified as the science of unitary human beings. The research potentials of nursing's abstract system are multiple. It is logically and scientifically tenable, it is flexible and open-ended. The practice implications for human health and well-being are already demonstrable" (Rogers, 1987a, p. 123).

Potential users of the Rogerian conceptual system are urged to consider its strengths and its limitations and work to systematically evaluate the credibility of relevant conceptual-theoretical-empirical structures as guides for the plethora of nursing activities for which it was developed. The advancement, continued refinement, and evaluation of the credibility of the Science of Unitary Human Beings should be ensured by the scholarly work of the members of the Society of Rogerian Scholars, which was founded in 1986. The Society is committed "to fostering the development of the Science of Unitary Human Beings by providing a formal, organized structure for the stimulation, development, and exchange of ideas" (Society of Rogerian Scholars, 1993). The Society publishes the quarterly newsletter, *Rogerian Nursing Science News*, and the annual journal, *Visions: The Journal of Rogerian Nursing Science.*

In conclusion, Martha Rogers has made a substantial contribution to the discipline of nursing by proposing a visionary paradigm that should be an appropriate guide for nursing activities as human beings continue to evolve and as we move farther into the space age. As Rogers (1990b) stated,

> As a holistic reality revolutionizes our thinking and as space exploration and space living provide spin-off from space that can be helpful on planet Earth, nursing will change, as will other fields. We are on the threshold of a fantastic and unimagined future. Our potential for human service is greater than it has ever been. (p. 112)

REFERENCES

Alligood, M.R. (1986). The relationship of creativity, actualization, and empathy in unitary human development. In V.M. Malinski (Ed.), *Explorations on Martha Rogers' Science of Unitary Human Beings* (pp. 145–160). Norwalk, CT: Appleton-Century-Crofts.

Alligood, M.R. (1989). Applying Rogers' model to nursing administration: Emphasis on environment, health. In B. Henry, C. Arndt, M. DiVincenti, & A. Marriner-Tomey (Eds.), *Dimensions of nursing administration: Theory, research, education, and practice.* (pp. 105–111). Boston: Blackwell Scientific Publications.

Alligood, M.R. (1990). Nursing care of the elderly: Futuristic projections. In E.A.M. Barrett (Ed.), *Visions of Rogers' science based nursing* (pp. 129–142). New York: National League for Nursing.

Alligood, M.R. (1991). Testing Rogers' theory of accelerating change. The relationships among creativity, actualization, and empathy in persons 18 to 92 years of age. *Western Journal of Nursing Research, 13,* 84–96.

Banonis, B.C. (1989). The lived experience of recovering from addiction: A phenomenological study. *Nursing Science Quarterly, 2,* 37–43.

Barber, H.R.K. (1987). Editorial: Trends in nursing: A model for emulation. *The Female Patient, 12*(3), 12, 14.

Barnard, R.M. (1973). Field independence-dependence and selected motor abilities. *Dissertation Abstracts International, 34,* 2737B.

Barnum, B.J.S. (1990). *Nursing theory: Analysis, application, evaluation* (3rd ed). Glenview, IL: Scott, Foresman/Little, Brown Higher Education.

Barnum, B.J.S. (1994). *Nursing theory: Analysis, application, evaluation* (4th ed). Philadelphia: JB Lippincott.

Barrett, E.A.M. (1986). Investigation of the principle of helicy: The relationship of human field motion and power. In V.M. Malinski (Ed.), *Explorations on Martha Rogers' Science of Unitary Human Beings* (pp. 173–188). Norwalk, CT: Appleton-Century-Crofts.

Barrett, E.A.M. (1988). Using Rogers' science of unitary human beings in nursing practice. *Nursing Science Quarterly, 1,* 50–51.

Barrett, E.A.M. (1990a). The continuing revolution of Rogers' science-based nursing education. In E.A.M. Barrett (Ed.), *Visions of Rogers' science-based nursing* (pp. 303–317). New York: National League for Nursing.

Barrett, E.A.M. (1990b). Health patterning with clients in a private practice environment. In E.A.M. Barrett (Ed.), *Visions of Rogers' science-based nursing* (pp. 105–115). New York: National League for Nursing.

Barrett, E.A.M. (1990c). Rogers' science-based nursing practice. In E.A.M. Barrett (Ed.), *Visions of Rogers' science-based nursing* (pp. 31–44). New York: National League for Nursing.

Barrett, E.A.M. (Ed.). (1990d). *Visions of Rogers' science-based nursing.* New York: National League for Nursing.

Barrett, E.A.M. (1992). Innovative imagery: A health-patterning modality for nursing practice. *Journal of Holistic Nursing, 10,* 154–166.

Barrett, E.A.M. (1993). Virtual reality: A health patterning modality for nursing in space. *Visions: The Journal of Rogerian Nursing Science, 1,* 10–21.

Barrett, E.A.M., & Malinski, V.M. (Eds.). (1994a). *Martha E. Rogers: Eighty years of excellence.* New York: Society of Rogerian Scholars.

Barrett, E.A.M., & Malinski, V.M. (Eds.). (1994b). *Martha E. Rogers: Her life and her work.* Philadelphia: FA Davis.

Benedict, S.C., & Burge, J.M. (1990). The relationship between human field motion and preferred visible wavelengths. *Nursing Science Quarterly, 3,* 73–80.

Bertalanffy, L. (1960). *Problems of life.* New York: Harper Torchbooks.

Blair, C. (1979). Hyperactivity in children: Viewed within the framework of synergistic man. *Nursing Forum, 18,* 293–303.

Boguslawski, M. (1979). The use of therapeutic touch in nursing. *Journal of Continuing Education in Nursing, 10*(4), 9–15.

Bohm, D. (1980). *Wholeness and the implicate order.* Boston: Routledge & Kegan Paul.

Boyd, C. (1990). Testing a model of mother-daughter identification. *Western Journal of Nursing Research, 12,* 448–468.

Bramlett, M.H., Gueldner, S.H., & Sowell, R.L. (1990). Consumer-centric advocacy: Its connection to nursing frameworks. *Nursing Science Quarterly, 3,* 156–161.

Brouse, S.H. (1985). Effect of gender role identity on patterns of feminine and self-concept scores from late pregnancy to early postpartum. *Advances in Nursing Science, 7*(3), 32–40.

Buczny, B., Speirs, J., & Howard, J.R. (1989). Nursing care of a terminally ill client. Applying Martha Rogers' conceptual framework. *Home Healthcare Nurse, 7*(4), 13–18.

Burr, H.S., & Northrop, F.S.C. (1935). The electro-dynamic theory of life. *Quarterly Review of Biology, 10,* 322–333.

Butcher, H.K., & Parker, N.I. (1988). Guided imagery within Rogers' Science of Unitary Human Beings. An experimental study. *Nursing Science Quarterly, 1,* 103–110.

Butcher, H.K., & Parker, N.I. (1990). Guided imagery within Rogers' Science of Unitary Human Beings: An experimental study. In E.A.M. Barrett (Ed.), *Visions of Rogers' science based nursing* (pp. 269–286). New York: National League for Nursing.

Capra, F. (1982). *The turning point.* New York; Simon & Schuster.

Carboni, J.T. (1992). Instrument development and the measurement of unitary constructs. *Nursing Science Quarterly, 5,* 134–142.

Caroselli-Dervan, C. (1990). Visionary opportunities for knowledge development in nursing administration. In E.A.M. Barrett (Ed.), *Visions of Rogers' science based nursing* (pp. 151–158). New York: National League for Nursing.

Chardin, P.T. (1961). *The phenomenon of man.* New York: Harper Torchbooks.

Chin, R. (1980). The utility of systems models and developmental models for practitioners. In J.P. Riehl & C. Roy, *Conceptual models for nursing practice* (2nd ed., pp. 21–37). New York: Appleton-Century-Crofts.

Chodil, J.J. (1979). An investigation of the relation between perceived body space, actual body space, body image boundary, and self-esteem. *Dissertation Abstracts International, 39,* 3760B.

Clarke, P.N. (1986). Theoretical and measurement issues in the study of field phenomena. *Advances in Nursing Science, 9*(1), 29–39.

Cowling, W.R. III. (1986a). The relationship of mystical experience, differentiation, and creativity in college students. In V.M. Malinski (Ed.), *Explorations on Martha Rogers' Science of Unitary Human Beings* (pp. 131–143). Norwalk, CT: Appleton-Century-Crofts.

Cowling, W.R. III. (1986b). The science of unitary human beings: Theoretical issues, methodological challenges, and research realities. In V.M. Malinski (Ed.), *Explorations on Martha Rogers' Science of Unitary Human Beings* (pp. 65–77). Norwalk, CT: Appleton-Century-Crofts.

Cowling, W.R. III. (1990a). Chronological age as an anomalie of evolution. In E.A.M. Barrett (Ed.), *Visions of Rogers' science based nursing* (pp. 143–150). New York: National League for Nursing.

Cowling, W.R. III (1990b). A template for unitary pattern-based nursing practice. In E.A.M. Barrett (Ed.), *Visions of Rogers' science-based nursing* (pp. 45–65). New York: National League for Nursing.

Decker, K. (1989). Theory in action. The geriatric assessment team. *Journal of Gerontological Nursing, 15*(10), 25–28.

Einstein, A. (1961). *Relativity.* New York: Crown.

Falco, S.M., & Lobo, M.L. (1985). Martha E. Rogers. In *Nursing Theories Conference*

Group, nursing theories: The base for professional nursing practice (2nd ed., pp. 214–234). Englewood Cliffs, NJ: Prentice-Hall.

Fawcett, J. (1975). The family as a living open system: An emerging conceptual framework for nursing. *International Nursing Review, 22,* 113–116.

Fawcett, J. (1977). The relationship between spouses' strength of identification and their patterns of change in perceived body space and articulation of body concept during and after pregnancy. *Dissertation Abstracts International, 37,* 4396B.

Fawcett, J. (1989). Spouses' experiences during pregnancy and the postpartum: A program of research and theory development. *Image: Journal of Nursing Scholarship, 21,* 149–152.

Fawcett, J. (1994). Theory development using quantitative methods within the science of unitary human beings. In M. Madrid & E.A.M. Barrett (Eds.), *Rogers' scientific art of nursing practice.* New York: National League for Nursing.

Fawcett, J., & Downs, F.S. (1986). *The relationship of theory and research.* Norwalk, CT: Appleton-Century-Crofts.

Ference, H.M. (1980). The relationship of time experience, creativity traits, differentiation and human field motion: An empirical investigation of Rogers' correlates of synergistic human development. *Dissertation Abstracts International, 40,* 5206B.

Ference, H.M. (1986a). Foundations of a nursing science and its evolution: A perspective. In V.M. Malinski (Ed.), *Explorations on Martha Rogers' Science of Unitary Human Beings* (pp. 25–32). Norwalk, CT: Appleton-Century-Crofts.

Ference, H.M. (1986b). The relationship of time experience, creativity traits, differentiation, and human field motion. In V.M. Malinski (Ed.), *Explorations on Martha Rogers' Science of Unitary Human Beings* (pp. 95–106). Norwalk, CT: Appleton-Century-Crofts.

Ference, H.M. (1989a). Comforting the dying: Nursing practice according to the Rogerian model. In J.P. Riehl-Sisca, *Conceptual models for nursing practice* (3rd ed., pp. 197–205). Norwalk, CT: Appleton & Lange.

Ference, H.M. (1989b). Nursing science theories and administration. In B. Henry, C. Arndt, M. DiVincenti, & A. Marriner-Tomey (Eds.), *Dimensions of nursing administration: Theory, research, education,*

and practice (pp. 121–131). Boston: Blackwell Scientific Publications.

Fitzpatrick, J.J. (1976). An investigation of the relationship between temporal orientation, temporal extension, and time perception. *Dissertation Abstracts International, 36,* 3310B.

Fitzpatrick, J.J. (1980). Patients' perceptions of time: Current research. *International Nursing Review, 27,* 148–153, 160.

Fitzpatrick, J.J. (1983). Life perspective rhythm model. In J.J. Fitzpatrick & A.L. Whall, *Conceptual models of nursing: Analysis and application* (pp. 295–302). Bowie, MD: Brady.

Fitzpatrick, J.J. (1989). A life perspective rhythm model. In J.J. Fitzpatrick & A.L. Whall, *Conceptual models of nursing: Analysis and application* (2nd ed., pp. 401–407). Norwalk, CT: Appleton & Lange.

Fitzpatrick, J.J., & Donovan, M.J. (1978). Temporal experience and motor behavior among the aging. *Research in Nursing and Health, 1,* 60–68.

Fitzpatrick, J.J., Donovan, M.J., & Johnston, R.L. (1980). Experience of time during the crisis of cancer. *Cancer Nursing, 3,* 191–194.

Floyd, J.A. (1983). Research using Rogers's conceptual system: Development of a testable theorem. *Advances in Nursing Science, 5*(2), 37–48.

Floyd, J.A. (1984). Interaction between personal sleep-wake rhythms and psychiatric hospital rest-activity schedule. *Nursing Research, 33,* 255–259.

Forker, J.E., & Billings, C.V. (1989). Nursing therapeutics in a group encounter. *Archives of Psychiatric Nursing, 3,* 108–112.

Fuller, R.B. (1981). *Critical path.* New York: St. Martin's Press.

Garon, M. (1991). Assessment and management of pain in the home care setting: Application of Rogers' Science of Unitary Human Beings. *Holistic Nursing Practice, 6*(1), 47–57.

Gaydos, L.S., & Farnham, R. (1988). Human-animal relationships within the context of Rogers' principle of integrality. *Advances in Nursing Science, 10*(4), 72–80.

Gill, B.P., & Atwood, J.R. (1981). Reciprocy and helicy used to relate mEFG and wound healing. *Nursing Research, 30,* 68–72.

Goldberg, W.G., & Fitzpatrick, J.J. (1980). Movement therapy with the aged. *Nursing Research, 29,* 339–346.

Goldstein, K. (1939). *The organism.* New York: American Book Company.

Gueldner, S.H. (1986). The relationship between imposed motion and human field motion in elderly individuals living in nursing homes. In V.M. Malinski (Ed.), *Explorations on Martha Rogers' Science of Unitary Human Beings* (pp. 161–172). Norwalk, CT: Appleton-Century-Crofts.

Gueldner, S.H. (1989). Applying Rogers' model to nursing administration: Emphasis on client and nursing. In B. Henry, C. Arndt, M. DiVincenti, & A. Marriner-Tomey (Eds.), *Dimensions of nursing administration: Theory, research, education, and practice* (pp. 113–119). Boston: Blackwell Scientific Publications.

Gulick, E.E., & Bugg, A. (1992). Holistic health patterning in multiple sclerosis. *Research in Nursing and Health, 15,* 175–185.

Hanchett, E.S. (1979). *Community health assessment: A conceptual tool kit.* New York: John Wiley & Sons.

Hanchett, E.S. (1990). Nursing models and community as client. *Nursing Science Quarterly, 3,* 67–72.

Hanchett, E.S. (1992). Concepts from eastern philosophy and Rogers' Science of Unitary Human Beings. *Nursing Science Quarterly, 5,* 164–170.

Heidt, P.R. (1990). Openness: A qualitative analysis of nurses' and patients' experiences of therapeutic touch. *Image: Journal of Nursing Scholarship, 22,* 180–186.

Herrick, J. (1956). *The evolution of human nature.* Austin: University of Texas Press.

Hill, L., & Oliver, N. (1993). Technique integration: Therapeutic touch and theory-based mental health nursing. *Journal of Psychosocial Nursing and Mental Health Services, 31*(2), 19–22.

Johnston, L.W. (1993). The development of the human field image metaphor scale. *Visions: The Journal of Rogerian Nursing Science, 1,* 55–56.

Johnston, R.L. (1986). Approaching family intervention through Rogers' conceptual model. In A.L. Whall, *Family therapy theory for nursing: Four approaches* (pp. 11–32). Norwalk, CT: Appleton-Century-Crofts.

Johnston, R.L., Fitzpatrick, J.J., & Donovan, M.J. (1982). Developmental stage: Relationship to temporal dimensions. (Abstract). *Nursing Research, 31,* 120.

Joseph, L. (1990). Practical application of Rogers' theoretical framework for nursing. In M.E. Parker (Ed.), *Nursing theories in practice* (pp. 115–125). New York: National League for Nursing.

Jurgens, A., Meehan, T.C., Wilson, H.L.

(1987). Therapeutic touch as a nursing intevention. *Holistic Nursing Practice, 2*(1), 1–13.

Katch, M.P. (1983). A negentropic view of the aged. *Journal of Gerontological Nursing, 9,* 656–660.

Keller, E., & Bzdek, V.M. (1986). Effects of therapeutic touch on tension headache pain. *Nursing Research, 35,* 101–106.

Kodiath, M.F. (1991). A new view of the chronic pain client. *Holistic Nursing Practice, 6*(1), 41–46.

Krieger, D. (1974). The relationship of touch, in intent to help or heal to subjects' in vivo hemoglobin values: A study in personalized interaction. In American Nurses' Association, *Ninth Nursing Research Conference* (pp. 39–58). Kansas City, MO: American Nurses' Association.

Krieger, D. (1975). Therapeutic touch: The imprimatur of nursing. *American Journal of Nursing, 75,* 784–787.

Laffrey, S.C. (1985). Health behavior choice as related to self-actualization and health conception. *Western Journal of Nursing Research, 7,* 279–295.

Leddy, S.K. (1993). Controversies column: Commentary and critique. *Visions: The Journal of Rogerian Nursing Science, 1,* 56–57.

Levine, N.H. (1976). A conceptual model for obstetric nursing. *Journal of Obstetric, Gynecologic, and Neonatal Nursing, 5*(2), 9–15.

Lewin, K. (1964). *Field theory in the social sciences.* (D. Cartwright, Ed.) New York: Harper Torchbooks.

Lum, J.J., Chase, M., Cole, S.M., Johnson, A., Johnson, J.A., & Link, M.R. (1978). Nursing care of oncology patients receiving chemotherapy. *Nursing Research, 27,* 340–346.

Madrid, M. (1990). The participating process of human field patterning in an acute-care environment. In E.A.M. Barrett (Ed.), *Visions of Rogers science based nursing* (pp. 93–104). New York: National League for Nursing.

Madrid, M., & Barrett, E.A.M. (1994). *Rogers' scientific art of nursing practice.* New York: National League for Nursing.

Madrid, M., & Winstead-Fry, P. (1986). Rogers's conceptual model. In P. Winstead-Fry (Ed.), *Case studies in nursing theory* (pp. 73–102). New York: National League for Nursing.

Malinski, V.M. (Ed.). (1986a). *Explorations on Martha Rogers' Science of Unitary Human Beings.* Norwalk, CT: Appleton-Century-Crofts.

Malinski, V.M. (1986b). Further ideas from Martha Rogers. In V.M. Malinski (Ed.), *Explorations on Martha Rogers' Science of Unitary Human Beings* (pp. 9–14). Norwalk, CT: Appleton-Century-Crofts.

Malinski, V.M. (1986c). Nursing practice within the science of unitary human beings. In V.M. Malinski (Ed.), *Explorations on Martha Rogers' Science of Unitary Human Beings* (pp. 25–32). Norwalk, CT: Appleton-Century-Crofts.

Malinski, V.M. (1986d). The relationship between hyperactivity in children and perception of short wavelength light. In V.M. Malinski (Ed.), *Explorations on Martha Rogers' Science of Unitary Human Beings* (pp. 107–118). Norwalk, CT: Appleton-Century-Crofts.

Malinski, V.M. (1991). The experience of laughing at oneself in older couples. *Nursing Science Quarterly, 4,* 69–75.

Marriner-Tomey, A. (1989). *Nursing theorists and their work* (2nd ed.). St. Louis: CV Mosby.

Mason, D.J. (1988). Circadian rhythms of body temperature and activation and the well-being of older women. *Nursing Research, 37,* 276–281.

Mason, T., & Chandley, M. (1990). Nursing models in a special hospital: A critical analysis of efficacity. *Journal of Advanced Nursing, 15,* 667–673.

Mason, T., & Patterson, R. (1990). A critical review of the use of Rogers' model within a special hospital: A single case study. *Journal of Advanced Nursing, 15,* 130–141.

Mathwig, G.M. (1968). Living open systems, reciprocal adaptations and the life process. *Dissertation Abstracts International, 29,* 666B.

Mathwig, G.M., Young, A.A., & Pepper, J.M. (1990). Using Rogerian science in undergraduate and graduate nursing education. In E.A.M. Barrett (Ed.), *Visions of Rogers' science based nursing* (pp. 319–334). New York: National League for Nursing.

McDonald, S.F. (1986). The relationship between visible lightwaves and the experience of pain. In V.M. Malinski (Ed.), *Explorations on Martha Rogers' Science of Unitary Human Beings* (pp. 119–130). Norwalk, CT: Appleton-Century-Crofts.

McEvoy, M.D. (1990). The relationships among the experience of dying, the experience of paranormal events, and creativity in adults. In E.A.M. Barrett (Ed.), *Visions of Rogers' science based nursing* (pp. 209–228). New York: National League for Nursing.

Meehan, D.B. (1992). Effects of budgetary knowledge on staff nurses attitudes toward administration and cost containment. (Abstract). *Kentucky Nurse, 40*(2), 12.

Meehan, T.C. (1990). The science of unitary human beings and theory-based practice: Therapeutic touch. In E.A.M. Barrett (Ed.), *Visions of Rogers' science based nursing* (pp. 67–82). New York: National League for Nursing.

Meehan, T.C. (1993). Therapeutic touch and postoperative pain: A Rogerian research study. *Nursing Science Quarterly, 6,* 69–78.

Meleis, A.I. (1991). *Theoretical nursing: Development and progress* (2nd ed.). Philadelphia: JB Lippincott.

Miller, L.A. (1979). An explanation of therapeutic touch using the science of unitary man. *Nursing Forum, 18,* 278–287.

Miller, S.R. (1974). An investigation of the relationship between mothers' general fearfulness, their daughters' locus of control, and general fearfulness in the daughter. *Dissertation Abstracts International, 35,* 2281B.

Newman, M.A. (1971). An investigation of the relationship between gait tempo and time perception. *Dissertation Abstracts International, 32,* 2821B.

Newman, M.A. (1972). Nursing's theoretical evolution. *Nursing Outlook, 20,* 449–453.

Newman, M.A. (1986). *Health as expanding consciousness.* St. Louis: CV Mosby.

Newman, M.A. (1992). Window on health as expanding consciousness. In M. O'Toole (Ed.), *Miller-Keane encyclopedia and dictionary of medicine, nursing, and allied health* (5th ed., p. 650). Philadelphia: WB Saunders.

Newshan, G. (1989). Therapeutic touch for symptom control in persons with AIDS. *Holistic Nursing Practice, 3*(4), 45–51.

Paletta, J.R. (1990). The relationship of temporal experience to human time. In E.A.M. Barrett (Ed.), *Visions of Rogers' science based nursing* (pp. 239–254). New York: National League for Nursing.

Parse, R.R. (1981). *Man-Living-Health: A theory of nursing.* New York: John Wiley & Sons. Reprinted 1989. Albany, NY: Delmar.

Parse, R.R. (1992). Human becoming: Parse's theory of nursing. *Nursing Science Quarterly, 5,* 35–42.

Payne, M.B. (1989). The use of therapeutic touch with rehabilitation clients. *Rehabilitation Nursing, 14*(2), 69–72.

Phillips, J.R. (1989). Science of Unitary

Human Beings: Changing research perspectives. *Nursing Science Quarterly, 2,* 57-60.

Phillips, J.R. (1990). Changing human potentials and future visions of nursing: A human field image perspective. In E.A.M. Barrett (Ed.), *Visions of Rogers' science based nursing* (pp. 13-25). New York: National League for Nursing.

Phillips, J.R. (1991). Human field research. *Nursing Science Quarterly, 4,* 142-143.

Polanyi, M. (1958). *Personal knowledge.* Chicago: University of Chicago Press.

Porter, L. (1968). Physical-physiological activity and infants' growth and development. *Dissertation Abstracts International, 28,* 4829B.

Quinn, J.F. (1984). Therapeutic touch as energy exchange: Testing the theory. *Advances in Nursing Science, 6*(2), 42-49.

Quinn, J.F. (1989). Therapeutic touch as energy exchange: Replication and extension. *Nursing Science Quarterly, 2,* 79-87.

Quinn, J.F. (1992). Holding sacred space: The nurse as healing environment. *Holistic Nursing Practice, 6*(4), 26-36.

Quinn, J.F., & Strelkauskas, A.J. (1993). Psychoimmunologic effects of Therapeutic Touch on practitioners and recently bereaved recipients: A pilot study. *Advances in Nursing Science, 15*(4), 13-26.

Randell, B.P. (1992). Nursing theory: The 21st century. *Nursing Science Quarterly, 5,* 176-184.

Rawnsley, M.M. (1986). The relationship between the perception of the speed of time and the process of dying. In V.M. Malinski (Ed), *Explorations on Martha Rogers' Science of Unitary Human Beings* (pp. 79-93). Norwalk, CT: Appleton-Century- Crofts.

Reed, P.G. (1986). The developmental conceptual framework: Nursing reformulations and applications for family therapy. In A.L. Whall, *Family therapy for nursing: Four approaches* (pp. 69-91). Norwalk, CT: Appleton-Century-Crofts.

Reed, P.G. (1987). Spirituality and well-being in terminally ill hospitalized adults. *Research in Nursing and Health, 10,* 335-344.

Reed, P.G. (1991). Toward a nursing theory of self-transcendence: Deductive reformulation using developmental theories. *Advances in Nursing Science, 13*(4), 64-77.

Reeder, F. (1984). Philosophical issues in the Rogerian science of unitary human beings. *Advances in Nursing Science, 6*(2), 14-23.

Reeder, F. (1986). Basic theoretical research in the conceptual system of unitary human beings. In V.M. Malinski (Ed.), *Explorations on Martha Rogers' Science of Unitary Human Beings* (pp. 45-64). Norwalk, CT: Appleton-Century-Crofts.

Reeder, F. (1991). The importance of knowing what to care about: A phenomenological inquiry using laughing at oneself as a clue. In P.L. Chinn (Ed.), *Anthology on caring* (pp. 259-279). New York: National League for Nursing.

Riehl, J.P. (1980). Nursing models in current use. In J.P. Riehl & C. Roy, *Conceptual models for nursing practice* (2nd ed., pp. 393-398). New York: Appleton-Century-Crofts.

Riehl, J.P., & Roy, C. (1974). *Conceptual models for nursing practice.* New York: Appleton-Century-Crofts.

Riehl, J.P., & Roy, C. (1980). *Conceptual models for nursing practice* (2nd ed). New York: Appleton-Century-Crofts.

Riehl-Sisca, J.P. (1989). Conceptual models for nursing practice (3rd ed.). Norwalk, CT: Appleton & Lange.

Rizzo, J.A. (1990). Nursing service as an energy field: A response to "Visionary opportunities for knowledge development in nursing administration." In E.A.M. Barrett (Ed.), *Visions of Rogers science based nursing* (pp. 159-164). New York: National League for Nursing.

Rogers, M.E. (1961). *Educational revolution in nursing.* New York: Macmillan.

Rogers, M.E. (1964). *Reveille in nursing.* Philadelphia: FA Davis.

Rogers, M.E. (1970). *An introduction to the theoretical basis of nursing.* Philadelphia: FA Davis.

Rogers, M.E. (1978a, December). *Nursing science: A science of unitary man.* Paper presented at Second Annual Nurse Educator Conference, New York. (Cassette recording).

Rogers, M.E. (1978b, December). *Application of theory in education and service.* Paper presented at Second Annual Nurse Educator Conference, New York. (Cassette recording).

Rogers, M.E. (1980a). Nursing: A science of unitary man. In J.P. Riehl & C. Roy, *Conceptual models for nursing practice* (2nd ed., pp. 329-337). New York: Appleton-Century-Crofts.

Rogers, M.E. (1980b). *Science of unitary man. Tape I: Unitary man and his world: A paradigm for nursing.* New York: Media for Nursing. (Cassette recording).

Rogers, M.E. (1980c). *Science of unitary*

man. *Tape II: Developing an organized abstract system: Synthesis of facts and ideas for a new product.* New York: Media for Nursing. (Cassette recording).

Rogers, M.E. (1980d). *Science of unitary man. Tape III: Principles and theories: Directions for description, explanation and prediction.* New York: Media for Nursing. (Cassette recording).

Rogers, M.E. (1980e). *Science of unitary man. Tape IV: Theories of accelerating evolution, paranormal phenomena and other events.* New York: Media for Nursing. (Cassette recording).

Rogers, M.E. (1980f). *Science of unitary man. Tape V: Health and illness: New perspectives.* New York: Media for Nursing. (Cassette recording).

Rogers, M.E. (1980g). *Science of unitary man. Tape VI: Interventive modalities: Translating theories into practice.* New York: Media for Nursing. (Cassette recording).

Rogers, M.E. (1983a). The family coping with a surgical crisis: Analysis and application of Rogers' theory of nursing. In I.W. Clements & F.B. Roberts, *Family health: A theoretical approach to nursing care* (pp. 390–391). New York: John Wiley & Sons.

Rogers, M.E. (1983b). Science of unitary human beings: A paradigm for nursing. In I.W. Clements and F.B. Roberts, *Family health: A theoretical approach to nursing care* (pp. 219–227). New York: John Wiley & Sons.

Rogers, M.E. (1985a). The nature and characteristics of professional education for nursing. *Journal of Professional Nursing, 1*, 381–383.

Rogers, M.E. (1985b). The need for legislation for licensure to practice professional nursing. *Journal of Professional Nursing, 1*, 384.

Rogers, M.E. (1985c). A paradigm for nursing. In R. Wood & J. Kekahbah (Eds.), *Examining the cultural implications of Martha E. Rogers' Science of Unitary Human Beings* (pp. 13–23). Lecompton, KS: Wood-Kekahbah Associates.

Rogers, M.E. (1986). Science of unitary human beings. In V.M. Malinski (Ed.), *Explorations on Martha Rogers' Science of Unitary Human Beings* (pp. 3–8). Norwalk, CT: Appleton-Century-Crofts.

Rogers, M.E. (1987a). Nursing research in the future. In J. Roode (Ed.), *Changing patterns in nursing education* (pp. 121–123). New York: National League for Nursing.

Rogers, M.E. (1987b, May). Rogers' framework. Paper presented at Nurse Theorist Conference, Pittsburgh, PA. (Cassette recording).

Rogers, M.E. (1987c, May). *Small group D.* Discussion at Nurse Theorist Conference, Pittsburgh PA. (Cassette recording).

Rogers, M.E. (1987d). Rogers' Science of Unitary Human Beings. In R.R. Parse, Nursing science: Major paradigms, theories, and critiques (pp. 139–146). Philadelphia: WB Saunders.

Rogers, M.E. (1989). Nursing: A science of unitary human beings. In J.P. Riehl-Sisca, *Conceptual models for nursing practice* (3rd ed., pp. 181–188). Norwalk, CT: Appleton & Lange.

Rogers, M.E. (1990a). Nursing: Science of unitary, irreducible, human beings: Update 1990. In E.A.M. Barrett (Ed.), *Visions of Rogers' science-based nursing* (pp. 5–11). New York: National League for Nursing.

Rogers, M.E. (1990b). Space-age paradigm for new frontiers in nursing. In M.E. Parker (Ed.), *Nursing theories in practice* (pp. 105–113). New York: National League for Nursing.

Rogers, M.E. (1992a). Nightingale's notes on nursing: Prelude to the 21st century. In F.N. Nightingale, *Notes on nursing: What it is, and what it is not* (commemorative edition, pp. 58–62). Philadelphia: JB Lippincott.

Rogers, M.E. (1992b). Nursing science and the space age. *Nursing Science Quarterly, 5*, 27–34.

Rogers, M.E. (1992c). Window on science of unitary human beings. In M. O'Toole (Ed.), *Miller-Keane encyclopedia and dictionary of medicine, nursing, and allied health* (p. 1339). Philadelphia: WB Saunders.

Rogers, M.E., Doyle, M.B., Racolin, A., & Walsh, P.C. (1990). A conversation with Martha Rogers on nursing in space. In E.A.M. Barrett (Ed.), *Visions of Rogers' science based nursing* (pp. 375–386). New York: National League for Nursing.

Russell, B. (1953). On the notion of cause, with applications to the free-will problem. In H. Feigl & M. Brodbeck (Eds.), *Readings in the philosophy of science* (pp. 387–407). New York: Appleton-Century-Crofts.

Safier, G. (1977). *Contemporary American leaders: An oral history.* New York: McGraw-Hill.

Samarel, N. (1992). The experience of receiving therapeutic touch. *Journal of Advanced Nursing, 17*, 651–657.

Sanchez, R. (1989). Empathy, diversity, and telepathy in mother-daughter dyads: An empirical investigation utilizing Rogers' conceptual framework. *Scholarly Inquiry for Nursing Practice, 3,* 29–44.

Sarter, B. (1988). Philosophical sources of nursing theory. *Nursing Science Quarterly, 1,* 52–59.

Schodt, C.M. (1989). Parental-fetal attachment and couvade: A study of patterns of human-environment integrality. *Nursing Science Quarterly, 2,* 88–97.

Sellers, S.C. (1991). A philosophical analysis of conceptual models of nursing. *Dissertation Abstracts International, 52,* 1937B. (University Microfilms No. AAC9126248).

Sheldrake, R. (1981). *A new science of life.* Los Angeles: Jeremy Tarcher.

Smith, K., Kupferschmid, B.J., Dawson, C., & Briones, T.L. (1991). A family-centered critical care unit. *AACN Clinical Issues, 2,* 258–268.

Smith, L. (1983). A conceptual model of families incorporating an adolescent mother and child into the household. *Advances in Nursing Science, 6*(1), 45–60.

Smith, M.J. (1984). Temporal experience and bed rest: Replication and refinement. *Nursing Research, 33,* 298–302.

Smith, M.J. (1986). Human-environment process: A test of Rogers' principle of integrality. *Advances in Nursing Science, 9*(1), 21–28.

Society of Rogerian Scholars. (1993). *Membership brochure.* Pensacola, FL: The Society.

Stewart, I. (1989). *Does God play dice? The mathematics of chaos.* Cambridge, MA: Brasil Blackwell.

Swanson, A. (1976). An investigation of the relationship between a child's general fearfulness and the child's mother's anxiety, self differentiation, and accuracy of perception of her child's general fearfulness. *Dissertation Abstracts International, 36,* 3313B.

Takahashi, T. (1992). Perspectives on nursing knowledge. *Nursing Science Quarterly, 5,* 86–91.

Tettero, I., Jackson, S., & Wilson, S. (1993). Theory to practice: Developing a Rogerian-based assessment tool. *Journal of Advanced Nursing, 18,* 776–782.

Tompkins, E.S. (1980). Effect of restricted mobility and dominance on perceived duration. *Nursing Research, 29,* 333–338.

Thompson, J.E. (1990). Finding the borderline's border: Can Martha Rogers help? *Perspectives in Psychiatric Care, 26*(4), 7–10.

Toffler, A. (1970). *Future shock.* New York: Random House.

Toffler, A. (1980). *The third wave.* New York: William Morrow.

Tuyn, L.K. (1992). Solution-oriented therapy and Rogerian nursing science: An integrated approach. *Archives of Psychiatric Nursing, 6,* 83–89.

Whall, A.L. (1981). Nursing theory and the assessment of families. *Journal of Psychiatric Nursing and Mental Health Services, 19*(1), 30–36.

Whall, A.L. (1987). A critique of Rogers's framework. In R.R. Parse, *Nursing science: Major paradigms, theories, and critiques* (pp. 147–158). Philadelphia: WB Saunders.

Whelton, B.J. (1979). An operationalization of Martha Rogers' theory throughout the nursing process. *International Journal of Nursing Studies, 16,* 7–20.

Wright, S.M. (1991). Validity of the human energy field assessment form. *Western Journal of Nursing Research, 13,* 635–647.

Yarcheski, A., & Mahon, N.E. (1991). An empirical test of Rogers' original and revised theory of correlates in adolescents. *Research in Nursing and Health, 14,* 447–455.

Young, A.A. (1985). The Rogerian conceptual system: A framework for nursing education and service. In R. Wood & J. Kekahbah (Eds.), *Examining the cultural implications of Martha E. Rogers' Science of Unitary Human Beings* (pp. 53–69). Lecompton, KS: Wood-Kekahbah Associates.

BIBLIOGRAPHY

PRIMARY SOURCES

Barrett, E.A.M., & Malinski, V.M. (Eds.). (1994). *Martha E. Rogers: Eighty years of excellence.* New York: Society of Rogerian Scholars.

Barrett, E.A.M., & Malinski, V.M. (Eds.). (1994). *Martha E. Rogers: Her life and her work.* Philadelphia: FA Davis.

Malinski, V.M. (1986). Further ideas from Martha Rogers. In V.M. Malinski (Ed.), *Explorations on Martha Rogers' Science of*

Unitary Human Beings (pp. 9-14). Norwalk, CT: Appleton-Century-Crofts.

Randell, B.P. (1992). Nursing theory: The 21st century. *Nursing Science Quarterly, 5,* 176-184.

Rogers, M.E. (1961). *Educational revolution in nursing.* New York: Macmillan.

Rogers, M.E. (1963). Some comments on the theoretical basis of nursing practice. *Nursing Science, 1*(1), 11-13, 60-61.

Rogers, M.E. (1964). *Reveille in nursing.* Philadelphia: FA Davis.

Rogers, M.E. (1970). *An introduction to the theoretical basis of nursing.* Philadelphia: FA Davis.

Rogers, M.E. (1980). Nursing: A science of unitary man. In J.P. Riehl & C. Roy, *Conceptual models for nursing practice* (2nd ed., pp. 329-337). New York: Appleton-Century-Crofts.

Rogers, M.E. (1980). *Science of unitary man. Tape I: Unitary man and his world: A paradigm for nursing.* New York: Media for Nursing. (Cassette recording).

Rogers, M.E. (1980). *Science of unitary man. Tape II. Developing an organized abstract system: Synthesis of facts and ideas for a new product.* New York: Media for Nursing. (Cassette recording).

Rogers, M.E. (1980). *Science of unitary man. Tape III: Principles and theories: Directions for description, explanation and prediction.* New York: Media for Nursing. (Cassette recording).

Rogers, M.E. (1980). *Science of unitary man. Tape IV: Theories of accelerating evolution, paranormal phenomena and other events.* New York: Media for Nursing. (Cassette recording).

Rogers, M.E. (1980). *Science of unitary man. Tape V: Health and illness: New perspectives.* New York: Media for Nursing. (Cassette recording).

Rogers, M.E. (1980). *Science of unitary man. Tape VI: Interventive modalities: Translating theories into practice.* New York: Media for Nursing. (Cassette recording).

Rogers, M.E. (1981). Science of unitary man. A paradigm for nursing. In G.E. Lasker (Ed.), *Applied systems and cybernetics: Vol. 4. Systems research in health care, biocybernetics and ecology* (pp. 1719-1722). New York: Pergamon Press.

Rogers, M.E. (1983). The family coping with a surgical crisis. Analysis and application of Rogers' theory of nursing. In I.W. Clements & F.B. Roberts, *Family health: A theoretical approach to nursing care* (pp. 390-391). New York: John Wiley & Sons.

Rogers, M.E. (1983). Science of unitary human beings: A paradigm for nursing. In I.W. Clements and F.B. Roberts, *Family health: A theoretical approach to nursing care* (pp. 219-227). New York: John Wiley & Sons.

Rogers, M.E. (1985). A paradigm for nursing. In R. Wood & J. Kekahbah (Eds.), *Examining the cultural implications of Martha E. Rogers' Science of Unitary Human Beings* (pp. 13-23). Lecompton, KS: Wood-Kekahbah Associates.

Rogers, M.E. (1986). Science of unitary human beings. In V.M. Malinski (Ed.), *Explorations on Martha Rogers' Science of Unitary Human Beings* (pp. 3-8). Norwalk, CT: Appleton-Century-Crofts.

Rogers, M.E. (1987). Nursing research in the future. In J. Roode (Ed.), *Changing patterns in nursing education* (pp. 121-123). New York: National League for Nursing.

Rogers, M.E. (1987). Rogers' Science of Unitary Human Beings. In R.R. Parse, *Nursing science: Major paradigms, theories, and critiques* (pp. 139-146). Philadelphia: WB Saunders.

Rogers, M.E. (1988). Nursing science and art: A prospective. *Nursing Science Quarterly, 1,* 99-102.

Rogers, M.E. (1989). Nursing: A science of unitary human beings. In J.P. Riehl-Sisca, *Conceptual models for nursing practice* (3rd ed., pp. 181-188). Norwalk, CT: Appleton & Lange.

Rogers, M.E. (1990). Nursing: Science of unitary, irreducible, human beings: Update 1990. In E.A.M. Barrett (Ed.), *Visions of Rogers' science-based nursing* (pp. 5-11). New York: National League for Nursing.

Rogers, M.E. (1990). Space-age paradigm for new frontiers in nursing. In M.E. Parker (Ed.), *Nursing theories in practice* (pp. 105-113). New York: National League for Nursing.

Rogers, M.E. (1992). Nightingale's notes on nursing: Prelude to the 21st century. In F.N. Nightingale, *Notes on nursing: What it is, and what it is not* (commemorative edition, pp. 58-62). Philadelphia: JB Lippincott.

Rogers, M.E. (1992). Nursing science and the space age. *Nursing Science Quarterly, 5,* 27-34.

Rogers, M.E. (1992). Window on science of unitary human beings. In M. O'Toole (Ed.), *Miller-Keane encyclopedia and dictionary of medicine, nursing, and allied health* (p. 1339). Philadelphia: WB Saunders.

Rogers, M.E., Doyle, M.B., Racolin, A., & Walsh, P.C. (1990). A conversation with

Martha Rogers on nursing in space. In E.A.M. Barrett (Ed.), *Visions of Rogers' science based nursing* (pp. 375–386). New York: National League for Nursing.

Safier, G. (1977). *Contemporary American leaders: An oral history*. New York: McGraw-Hill.

Takahashi, T. (1992). Perspectives on nursing knowledge. *Nursing Science Quarterly*, 5, 86–91.

COMMENTARY

Aggleton, P., & Chalmers, H. (1984). Rogers' unitary field model. *Nursing Times*, 80(50), 35–39.

Allanach, E.J. (1988). Perceived supportive behaviors and nursing occupational stress: An evolution of consciousness. *Advances in Nursing Science*, 10(2), 73–82.

Andersen, M.D., & Smereck, G.A.D. (1989). Personalized nursing LIGHT model. *Nursing Science Quarterly*, 2, 120–130.

Andersen, M.D., & Smereck, G.A.D. (1992). The consciousness rainbow: An explication of Rogerian field pattern manifestations. *Nursing Science Quarterly*, 5, 72–79.

Barber, H.R.K. (1987). Editorial: Trends in nursing: A model for emulation. *The Female Patient* 12(3), 12, 14.

Barrett, E.A.M. (1989). A nursing theory of power for nursing practice: Derivation from Rogers' paradigm. In J.P. Riehl-Sisca, *Conceptual models for nursing practice* (3rd ed., pp. 207–217). Norwalk, CT: Appleton & Lange.

Barrett, E.A.M. (Ed.) (1990). *Visions of Rogers' science based nursing*. New York: National League for Nursing.

Barrett, E.A.M. (1990). Visions of Rogerian science in the future of humankind. In E.A.M. Barrett (Ed.), *Visions of Rogers science based nursing* (pp. 357–362). New York: National League for Nursing.

Barrett, E.A.M. (1991). Space nursing. *Cutis*, 48, 299–303.

Biley, F. (1990). Rogers' model: An analysis. *Nursing (London)*, 4(15), 31–33.

Biley, F. (1992). The perception of time as a factor in Rogers' science of unitary human beings: A literature review. *Journal of Advanced Nursing*, 17, 1141–1145.

Black, G., & Haight, B.K. (1992). Integrality as a holistic framework for the life-review process. *Holistic Nursing Practice*, 7(1), 7–15.

Blair, C. (1979). Hyperactivity in children: Viewed within the framework of synergistic man. *Nursing Forum*, 18, 293–303.

Boyd, C. (1985). Toward an understanding of mother-daughter identification using concept analysis. *Advances in Nursing Science*, 7(3), 78–86.

Bradley, D.B. (1987). Energy fields: Implications for nurses. *Journal of Holistic Nursing*, 5(1), 32–35.

Bramlett, M.H., Gueldner, S.H., & Boettcher, J.H. (1993). Reflections on the science of unitary human beings in terms of Kuhn's requirement for explanatory power. *Visions: The Journal of Rogerian Nursing Science*, 1, 22–35.

Bramlett, M.H., Gueldner, S.H., & Sowell, R.L. (1990). Consumer-centric advocacy: Its connection to nursing frameworks. *Nursing Science Quarterly*, 3, 156–161.

Buenting, J.A. (1993). Human energy field and birth: Implications for research and practice. *Advances in Nursing Science*, 15(4), 53–59.

Butcher, H.K., & Forchuk, C. (1992). The overview effect: The impact of space exploration on the evolution of nursing science. *Nursing Science Quarterly*, 5, 118–123.

Butterfield, S.E. (1983). In search of commonalities: An analysis of two theoretical frameworks. *International Journal of Nursing Studies*, 20, 15–22.

Caggins, R.P. (1991). The Caggins synergy nursing model. *The ABNF Journal*, 2(1), 15–18.

Carboni, J.T. (1991). A Rogerian theoretical tapestry. *Nursing Science Quarterly*, 4, 130–136.

Cerilli, K., & Burd, S. (1989). An analysis of Martha Rogers' nursing as a science of unitary human beings. In J.P. Riehl-Sisca, *Conceptual models for nursing practice* (3rd ed., pp. 189–195). Norwalk, CT: Appleton & Lange.

Cody, W.K. (1991). Multidimensionality: Its meaning and significance. *Nursing Science Quarterly*, 4, 140–141.

Compton, M.A. (1989). A Rogerian view of drug abuse: Implications for nursing. *Nursing Science Quarterly*, 2, 98–105.

Crawford, G. (1982). The concept of pattern in nursing: Conceptual development and measurement. *Advances in Nursing Science*, 5(1), 1–6.

Daily, I.S., Maupin, J.S., Murray, C.A., et al. (1994). Unitary human beings. In A. Marriner-Tomey, *Nursing theorists and their work* (3rd ed., pp. 211–230). St. Louis: Mosby-Year Book.

Daily, I.S., Maupin, J.S., & Satterly, M.C. (1986). Martha E. Rogers. Unitary human beings. In A. Marriner, *Nursing theorists* and their work (pp. 345–360). St. Louis: CV Mosby.

Daily, I.S., Maupin, J.S., Satterly, M.C., Schnell, D.L., & Wallace, T.L. (1989). Martha E. Rogers: Unitary human beings. In A. Marriner-Tomey, Nursing theorists and their work (2nd ed., pp. 402–419). St. Louis: CV Mosby.

Davidson, A.W., & Ray, M.A. (1991). Studying the human-environment phenomenon using the science of complexity. Advances in Nursing Science, 14(2), 73–87.

DeFeo, D.J. (1990). Change: A central concern of nursing. Nursing Science Quarterly, 3, 88–94.

Falco, S.M., & Lobo, M.L. (1980). Martha E. Rogers. In Nursing Theories Conference Group, Nursing theories: The base for professional nursing practice (pp. 164–183). Englewood Cliffs, NJ: Prentice-Hall.

Falco, S.M., & Lobo, M.L. (1985). Martha E. Rogers. In Nursing Theories Conference Group, Nursing theories: The base for professional nursing practice (2nd ed., pp. 214–234). Englewood Cliffs, NJ: Prentice-Hall.

Falco, S.M., & Lobo, M.L. (1990). Martha E. Rogers. In J.B. George (Ed.), Nursing theories: The base for professional nursing practice (3rd ed., pp. 211–230). Norwalk, CT: Appleton & Lange.

Fawcett, J. (1975). The family as a living open system: An emerging conceptual framework for nursing. International Nursing Review, 22, 113–116.

Fisher, L.R., & Reichenbach, M.A. (1987/1988). From Tinkerbell to Rogers. (How a fairy tale facilitated an understanding of Rogers' theory of unitary being.) Nursing Forum, 23, 5–9.

Fitzpatrick, J.J. (1983). Life perspective rhythm model. In J.J. Fitzpatrick & A.L. Whall, Conceptual models of nursing: Analysis and evaluation (pp. 295–302). Bowie, MD: Brady.

Fitzpatrick, J.J. (1988). Theory based on Rogers' conceptual model. Journal of Gerontological Nursing, 14(9), 14–19.

Fitzpatrick, J.J. (1989). A life perspective rhythm model. In J.J. Fitzpatrick & A.L. Whall, Conceptual models of nursing: Analysis and application (2nd ed., pp. 401–407). Norwalk, CT: Appleton & Lange.

Fitzpatrick, J.J., Whall, A.L., Johnston, R.L., & Floyd, J.A. (1982). Nursing models and their psychiatric mental health applications. Bowie, MD: Brady.

Freda, M.C. (1989). A role model of leadership in and advocacy for nursing. Nursing Forum, 24(3–4), 9–13.

Garon, M. (1992). Contributions of Martha Rogers to the development of nursing knowledge. Nursing Outlook, 40, 67–72.

Gioiella, E. (1989). Professionalizing nursing: A Rogers legacy. Nursing Science Quarterly, 2, 61–62.

Greiner, D.S. (1991). Rhythmicities. Nursing Science Quarterly, 4, 21–23.

Hanchett, E.S. (1992). Concepts from Eastern philosophy and Rogers' Science of Unitary Human Beings. Nursing Science Quarterly, 5, 164–170.

Hardin, S. (1990). A caring community. In M. Leininger & J. Watson (Eds.). The caring imperative in education (pp. 217–225). New York: National League for Nursing.

Hektor, L.M. (1989). Martha E. Rogers: A life history. Nursing Science Quarterly, 2, 63–73.

Huch, M.H. (1991). Perspectives on health. Nursing Science Quarterly, 4, 33–40.

Iveson-Iveson, J. (1982). The four dimensional nurse. Nursing Mirror, 155(22), 52.

Joseph, L. (1991). The energetics of conscious caring for the compassionate healer. In D.A. Gaut & M.M. Leininger, Caring: The compassionate healer (pp. 51–60). New York: National League for Nursing.

Katch, M.P. (1983). A negentropic view of the aged. Journal of Gerontological Nursing, 9, 656–660.

Leddy, S.K. (1993). Controversies column: Commentary and critique. Visions: The Journal of Rogerian Nursing Science, 1, 56–57.

Levine, N.H. (1976). A conceptual model for obstetric nursing. Journal of Obstetric, Gynecologic, and Neonatal Nursing, 5(2), 9–15.

Lutjens, L.R.J. (1991). Martha Rogers: The Science of Unitary Human Beings. Newbury Park, CA: Sage.

Malinski, V.M. (1986). Afterword. In V.M. Malinski (Ed.), Explorations on Martha Rogers' Science of Unitary Human Beings (pp. 189–191). Norwalk, CT: Appleton-Century-Crofts.

Malinski, V.M. (1986). Contemporary science and nursing: Parallels with Rogers. In V.M. Malinski (Ed.), Explorations on Martha Rogers' Science of Unitary Human Beings (pp. 15–23). Norwalk, CT: Appleton-Century-Crofts.

Malinski, V.M. (Ed.). (1986). Explorations on Martha Rogers' Science of Unitary

Human Beings. Norwalk, CT: Appleton-Century-Crofts.

Malinski, V.M. (1990). The meaning of a progressive world view in nursing: Rogers's Science of Unitary Human Beings. In N.L. Chaska (Ed.), The nursing profession: Turning points (pp. 237–244). St. Louis: CV Mosby.

Malinski, V.M. (1990). The Rogerian science of unitary human beings as a knowledge base for nursing in space. In E.A.M. Barrett (Ed.), Visions of Rogers science based nursing (pp. 363–374). New York: National League for Nursing.

Malinski, V.M. (1993). Therapeutic touch: The view from Rogerian nursing science. Visions: The Journal of Rogerian Nursing Science, 1, 45–54.

Martin, M-L., Forchuk, C., Santopinto, M., & Butcher, H.K. (1992). Alternative approaches to nursing practice: Application of Peplau, Rogers, and Parse. Nursing Science Quarterly, 5, 80–85.

Meleis, A.I. (1991). Theoretical nursing: Development and progress (2nd ed.). Philadelphia: JB Lippincott.

Miller, L.A. (1979). An explanation of therapeutic touch using the science of unitary man. Nursing Forum, 18, 278–287.

Newman, M.A. (1972). Nursing's theoretical evolution. Nursing Outlook, 20, 449–453.

Newman, M.A. (1979). Theory development in nursing. Philadelphia: FA Davis.

Newman, M.A. (1986). Health as expanding consciousness. St. Louis: CV Mosby.

Newman, M.A. (1990). Newman's theory of health as praxis. Nursing Science Quarterly, 3, 37–41.

Parse, R.R. (1981). Man-Living-Health: A theory of nursing. New York: John Wiley & Sons. Reprinted 1989. Albany, NY: Delmar.

Parse, R.R. (1989). Martha E. Rogers: A birthday celebration. (Editorial). Nursing Science Quarterly, 2, 55.

Parse, R.R. (1992). Human becoming: Parse's theory of nursing. Nursing Science Quarterly, 5, 35–42.

Phillips, J.R. (1990). Changing human potentials and future visions of nursing: A human field image perspective. In E.A.M. Barrett (Ed.), Visions of Rogers' science based nursing (pp. 13–25). New York: National League for Nursing.

Quillin, S.I.M., & Runk, J.A. (1983). Martha Rogers' model. In J.J. Fitzpatrick & A.L. Whall, Conceptual models of nursing: Analysis and application (pp. 245–261). Bowie, MD: Brady.

Quillin, S.I.M., & Runk, J.A. (1989). Martha

Rogers' unitary person model. In J.J. Fitzpatrick & A.L. Whall, Conceptual models of nursing: Analysis and application (2nd ed., pp. 285–300). Bowie, MD: Brady.

Rapacz, K.M. (1993). Imagination column: From pragmatic to imaginative to visionary. Visions: The Journal of Rogerian Nursing Science, 1, 58–59.

Rawnsley, M. (1985). H-E-A-L-T-H: A Rogerian perspective. Journal of Holistic Nursing, 3(1), 26.

Reed, P.G. (1991). Toward a nursing theory of self-transcendence: Deductive reformulation using developmental theories. Advances in Nursing Science, 13(4), 64–77.

Reeder, F. (1984). Philosophical issues in the Rogerian science of unitary human beings. Advances in Nursing Science, 6(2), 14–23.

Reeder, F. (1993). The science of unitary human beings and interpretive human science. Nursing Science Quarterly, 6, 13–24.

Rigley, A. (1980). Martha Rogers — Challenging ideas for nursing. The Lamp, 37(2), 20–22.

Rogers, M.E. (1985). The need for legislation for licensure to practice professional nursing. Journal of Professional Nursing, 1, 384.

Roy, C. (1974). Rogers' theoretical basis of nursing. In J.P. Riehl & C. Roy, Conceptual models for nursing practice (pp. 96–99). New York: Appleton-Century-Crofts.

Sarter, B. (1987). Evolutionary idealism: A philosophical foundation for holistic nursing theory. Advances in Nursing Science, 9(2), 1–9.

Sarter, B. (1988). Philosophical sources of nursing theory. Nursing Science Quarterly, 1, 52–59.

Sarter, B. (1988). The stream of becoming: A study of Martha Rogers's theory. New York: National League for Nursing.

Sarter, B. (1989). Some critical philosophical issues in the science of unitary human beings. Nursing Science Quarterly, 2, 74–78.

Schorr, J.A. Manifestations of consciousness and the developmental phenomenon of death. Advances in Nursing Science, 6(1), 26–35.

Schroeder, C., & Smith, M.C. (1991). Nursing conceptual frameworks arising from field theory: A critique of the body as manifestation of underlying field. Commentary: Disembodiment or "Where's the body in field theory?" [Schroeder]. Response: Affirming the unitary perspective

[Smith]. *Nursing Science Quarterly, 4*, 146–152.

Smith, M.C. (1988). Testing propositions derived from Rogers' conceptual system. *Nursing Science Quarterly, 1*, 60–67.

Smith, M.C. (1990). Pattern in nursing practice. *Nursing Science Quarterly, 3*, 57–59.

Smith, M.J. (1988). Perspectives on nursing science. *Nursing Science Quarterly, 1*, 80–85.

Smith, M.J. (1989). Four dimensionality: Where to go with it. *Nursing Science Quarterly, 2*, 56.

Uys, L.R. (1987). Foundational studies in nursing. *Journal of Advanced Nursing, 12*, 275–280.

Whall, A.L. (1987). A critique of Rogers's framework. In R.R. Parse, *Nursing science: Major paradigms, theories, and critiques* (pp. 147–158). Philadelphia: WB Saunders.

Wheeler, K. (1988). A nursing science approach to understanding empathy. *Archives of Psychiatric Nursing, 2*, 95–102.

Wilson, L.M., & Fitzpatrick, J.J. (1984). Dialectic thinking as a means of understanding systems-in-development: Relevance to Rogers's principles. *Advances in Nursing Science, 6*(2), 24–41.

Moccia, P. (1985). A further investigation of "Dialectical thinking as a means of understanding systems-in-development: Relevance to Rogers's principles." *Advances in Nursing Science, 7*(4): 33–38.

RESEARCH

Alligood, M.R. (1986). The relationship of creativity, actualization, and empathy in unitary human development. In V.M. Malinski (Ed.), *Explorations on Martha Rogers' Science of Unitary Human Beings* (pp. 145–160). Norwalk, CT: Appleton-Century-Crofts.

Alligood, M.R. (1991). Testing Rogers' theory of accelerating change: The relationships among creativity, actualization, and empathy in persons 18 to 92 years of age. *Western Journal of Nursing Research, 13*, 84–96.

Artinian, N.T. (1992). Spouse adaptation to mate's CABG surgery: 1-year follow-up. *American Journal of Critical Care, 1*, 36–42.

Banonis, B.C. (1989). The lived experience of recovering from addiction: A phenomenological study. *Nursing Science Quarterly, 2*, 37–43.

Barrett, E.A.M. (1986). Investigation of the principle of helicy: The relationship of human field motion and power. In V.M. Malinski (Ed.), *Explorations on Martha Rogers' Science of Unitary Human Beings* (pp. 173–188). Norwalk, CT: Appleton-Century-Crofts.

Barrett, E.A.M. (1990). Rogerian patterns of scientific inquiry. In E.A.M. Barrett (Ed.), *Visions of Rogers' science based nursing* (pp. 169–188). New York: National League for Nursing.

Benedict, S.C., & Burge, J.M. (1990). The relationship between human field motion and preferred visible wavelengths. *Nursing Science Quarterly, 3*, 73–80.

Boyd, C. (1990). Testing a model of mother-daughter identification. *Western Journal of Nursing Research, 12*, 448–468.

Brouse, S.H. (1985). Effect of gender role identity on patterns of feminine and self-concept scores from late pregnancy to early postpartum. *Advances in Nursing Science, 7*(3), 32–40.

Butcher, H.K., & Parker, N.I. (1988). Guided imagery within Rogers' Science of Unitary Human Beings: An experimental study. *Nursing Science Quarterly, 1*, 103–110.

Butcher, H.K., & Parker, N.I. (1990). Guided imagery within Rogers' Science of Unitary Human Beings: An experimental study. In E.A.M. Barrett (Ed.), *Visions of Rogers' science based nursing* (pp. 269–286). New York: National League for Nursing.

Rapacz, K.E. (1990). The patterning of time experience and human field motion during the experience of pleasant guided imagery: A discussion. In E.A.M. Barrett (Ed.), *Visions of Rogers' science based nursing* (pp. 287–294). New York: National League for Nursing.

Butcher, H.K., & Parker, N.I. (1990). Response to "Discussion of a study of pleasant guided imagery." In E.A.M. Barrett (Ed.), *Visions of Rogers' science based nursing* (pp. 295–297). New York: National League for Nursing.

Carboni, J.T. (1992). Instrument development and the measurement of unitary constructs. *Nursing Science Quarterly, 5*, 134–152.

Clarke, P.N. (1986). Theoretical and measurement issues in the study of field phenomena. *Advances in Nursing Science, 9*(1), 29–39.

Cowling, W.R., III. (1986). The relationship of mystical experience, differentiation, and creativity in college students. In V.M. Malinski (Ed.), *Explorations on Martha Rogers' Science of Unitary Human Beings* (pp. 131–143). Norwalk, CT: Appleton-Century-Crofts.

Cowling, W.R., III. (1986). The science of unitary human beings: Theoretical issues, methodological challenges, and research realities. In V.M. Malinski (Ed.), *Explorations on Martha Rogers' Science of Unitary Human Beings* (pp. 65–77). Norwalk, CT: Appleton-Century-Crofts.

Crawford, G. (1985). A theoretical model of support network conflict experienced by new mothers. *Nursing Research, 34,* 100–102.

Drake, M.L., Verhulst, D., Fawcett, J., & Barger, D.F. (1988). Spouses' body image changes during and after pregnancy: A replication in Canada. *Image: The Journal of Nursing Scholarship, 20,* 88–92.

Drake, M.L., Verhulst, D., & Fawcett, J. (1988). Physical and psychological symptoms experienced by Canadian women and their husbands during pregnancy and the postpartum. *Journal of Advanced Nursing, 13,* 436–440.

Fawcett, J. (1977). The relationship between identification and patterns of change in spouses' body images during and after pregnancy. *International Journal of Nursing Studies, 14,* 199–213.

Fawcett, J. (1978). Body image and the pregnant couple. *American Journal of Maternal Child Nursing, 3,* 227–233.

Fawcett, J. (1989). Spouses' experiences during pregnancy and the postpartum (brief report). *Applied Nursing Research, 2,* 49–50.

Fawcett, J. (1989). Spouses' experiences during pregnancy and the postpartum: A program of research and theory development. *Image: Journal of Nursing Scholarship, 21,* 149–152.

Eberhard, S.H. (1990). Letter to the editor. *Image: Journal of Nursing Scholarship, 22,* 197.

Fawcett, J. (1990). Response to Letter to the editor. *Image: Journal of Nursing Scholarship, 22,* 197.

Fawcett, J., Bliss-Holtz, V.J., Haas, M.B., Leventhal, M., & Rubin, M. (1986). Spouses body image changes during and after pregnancy: A replication and extension. *Nursing Research, 35,* 220–243.

Fawcett, J., & York, R. (1986). Spouses' physical and psychological symptoms during pregnancy and the postpartum. *Nursing Research, 35,* 144–148.

Fawcett, J., & York, R. (1987). Spouses' strength of identification and reports of symptoms during pregnancy and the postpartum. *Florida Nursing Review, 2*(2), 1–10.

Ference, H.M. (1986). Foundations of a nursing science and its evolution: A perspective. In V.M. Malinski (Ed.), *Explorations on Martha Rogers' Science of Unitary Human Beings* (pp. 25–32). Norwalk, CT: Appleton-Century-Crofts.

Ference, H.M. (1986). The relationship of time experience, creativity traits, differentiation, and human field motion. In V.M. Malinski (Ed.), *Explorations on Martha Rogers' Science of Unitary Human Beings* (pp. 95–106). Norwalk, CT: Appleton-Century-Crofts.

Fitzpatrick, J.J. (1980). Patients' perceptions of time: Current research. *International Nursing Review, 27,* 148–153, 160.

Floyd, J.A. (1983). Research using Rogers's conceptual system: Development of a testable theorem. *Advances in Nursing Science, 5*(2), 37–48.

Floyd, J.A. (1984). Interaction between personal sleep-wake rhythms and psychiatric hospital rest-activity schedule. *Nursing Research, 33,* 255–259.

Gaydos, L.S., & Farnham, R. (1988). Human-animal relationships within the context of Rogers' principle of integrality. *Advances in Nursing Science, 10*(4), 72–80.

Gill, B.P., & Atwood, J.R. (1981). Reciprocy and helicy used to relate mEFG and wound healing. *Nursing Research, 30,* 68–72.

Kim, H.S. (1983). Use of Rogers' conceptual system in research: Comments. *Nursing Research, 32,* 89–91.

Atwood, J.R., & Gill-Rogers, B. (1984). Metatheory methodology and practicality: Issues in research uses of Rogers' science of unitary man. *Nursing Research, 33,* 88–91.

Girardin, B.W. (1992). Lightwave frequency and sleep wake frequency in well, full-term neonates. *Holistic Nursing Practice, 6*(4), 57–66.

Goldberg, W.G., & Fitzpatrick, J.J. (1980). Movement therapy with the aged. *Nursing Research, 29,* 339–346.

Gueldner, S.H. (1986). The relationship between imposed motion and human field motion in elderly individuals living in nursing homes. In V.M. Malinski (Ed.), *Explorations on Martha Rogers' Science of Unitary Human Beings* (pp. 161–172). Norwalk, CT: Appleton-Century-Crofts.

Gulick, E.E., & Bugg, A. (1992). Holistic health patterning in multiple sclerosis. *Research in Nursing and Health, 15,* 175–185.

Heidt, P.R. (1990). Openness: A qualitative analysis of nurses' and patients' experiences of therapeutic touch. *Image: Journal of Nursing Scholarship, 22,* 180–186.

Johnston, L.W. (1993). The development of the human field image metaphor scale. *Visions: The Journal of Rogerian Nursing Science, 1,* 55–56.

Keller, E., & Bzdek, V.M. (1986). Effects of therapeutic touch on tension headache pain. *Nursing Research, 35,* 101–106.

Krieger, D. (1974). The relationship of touch, in intent to help or heal to subjects' in vivo hemoglobin values: A study in personalized interaction. In *American Nurses' Association, Ninth Nursing Research Conference* (pp. 39–58). Kansas City, MO: American Nurses' Association.

Laffrey, S.C. (1985). Health behavior choice as related to self-actualization and health conception. *Western Journal of Nursing Research, 7,* 279–295.

Malinski, V.M. (1986). The relationship between hyperactivity in children and perception of short wavelength light. In V.M. Malinski (Ed.), *Explorations on Martha Rogers' Science of Unitary Human Beings* (pp. 107–118). Norwalk, CT: Appleton-Century-Crofts.

Malinski, V.M. (1991). The experience of laughing at oneself in older couples. *Nursing Science Quarterly, 4,* 69–75.

Mason, D.J. (1988). Circadian rhythms of body temperature and activation and the well-being of older women. *Nursing Research, 37,* 276–281.

McDonald, S.F. (1986). The relationship between visible lightwaves and the experience of pain. In V.M. Malinski (Ed.), *Explorations on Martha Rogers' Science of Unitary Human Beings* (pp. 119–130). Norwalk, CT: Appleton-Century-Crofts.

McEvoy, M.D. (1990). The relationships among the experience of dying, the experience of paranormal events, and creativity in adults. In E.A.M. Barrett (Ed.), *Visions of Rogers' science based nursing* (pp. 209–228). New York: National League for Nursing.

Winstead-Fry, P. (1990). Reflections on death as a process: A response to a study of the experience of dying. In E.A.M. Barrett (Ed.), *Visions of Rogers' science based nursing* (pp. 229–236). New York: National League for Nursing.

McEvoy, M.D. (1990). Response to "Reflections on death as a process." In E.A.M. Barrett (Ed.), *Visions of Rogers' science based nursing* (pp. 237–238). New York: National League for Nursing.

Meehan, D.B. (1992). Effects of budgetary knowledge on staff nurses' attitudes toward administration and cost containment. (Abstract). *Kentucky Nurse, 40*(2), 12.

Meehan, T.C. (1990). Theory development. In E.A.M. Barrett (Ed.), *Visions of Rogers' science based nursing* (pp. 197–208). New York: National League for Nursing.

Meehan, T.C. (1993). Therapeutic touch and postoperative pain: A Rogerian research study. *Nursing Science Quarterly, 6,* 69–78.

Paletta, J.R. (1990). The relationship of temporal experience to human time. In E.A.M. Barrett (Ed.), *Visions of Rogers' science based nursing* (pp. 239–254). New York: National League for Nursing.

Rawnsley, M.M. (1990). What time is it? A response to a study of temporal experience. In E.A.M. Barrett (Ed.), *Visions of Rogers' science based nursing* (pp. 255–264). New York: National League for Nursing.

Paletta, J.R. (1990). Response to "What time is it?" In E.A.M. Barrett (Ed.), *Visions of Rogers' science based nursing* (pp. 265–268). New York: National League for Nursing.

Phillips, J.R. (1989). Science of unitary human beings: Changing research perspectives. *Nursing Science Quarterly, 2,* 57–60.

Phillips, J.R. (1991). Human field research. *Nursing Science Quarterly, 4,* 142–143.

Porter, L.S. (1972). The impact of physical-physiological activity on infants' growth and development. *Nursing Research, 21,* 210–219.

Porter, L.S. (1972). Physical-physiological activity and infants' growth and development. In American Nurses' Association, *Seventh Nursing Research Conference* (pp. 1–43). New York: American Nurses' Association.

Quinn, J.F. (1984). Therapeutic touch as energy exchange: Testing the theory. *Advances in Nursing Science, 6*(2), 42–49.

Quinn, J.F. (1989). Therapeutic touch as energy exchange: Replication and extension. *Nursing Science Quarterly, 2,* 79–87.

Quinn, J.F. (1992). Holding sacred space: The nurse as healing environment. *Holistic Nursing Practice, 6*(4), 26–36.

Quinn, J.F., & Strelkauskas, A.J. (1993). Psychoimmunologic effects of Therapeutic Touch on practitioners and recently bereaved recipients: A pilot study. *Advances in Nursing Science, 15*(4), 13–26.

Rawnsley, M.M. (1986). The relationship between the perception of the speed of time and the process of dying. In V.M. Malinski

(Ed.), *Explorations on Martha Rogers' Science of Unitary Human Beings* (pp. 79–93). Norwalk, CT: Appleton-Century-Crofts.

Rawnsley, M.M. (1990). Structuring the gap from conceptual system to research design within a Rogerian world view. In E.A.M. Barrett (Ed.), *Visions of Rogers' science based nursing* (pp. 189–197). New York: National League for Nursing.

Reed, P.G. (1989). Mental health of older adults. *Western Journal of Nursing Research, 11*, 143–163.

Reeder, F. (1986). Basic theoretical research in the conceptual system of unitary human beings. In V.M. Malinski (Ed.), *Explorations on Martha Rogers' Science of Unitary Human Beings* (pp. 45–64). Norwalk, CT: Appleton-Century-Crofts.

Reeder, F. (1991). The importance of knowing what to care about: A phenomenological inquiry using laughing at oneself as a clue. In P.L. Chinn (Ed.), *Anthology on caring* (pp. 259–279). New York: National League for Nursing.

Rogers, M.E. (1987). Nursing research in the future. In J. Roode (Ed.), *Changing patterns in nursing education* (pp. 121–123). New York: National League for Nursing.

Samarel, N. (1992). The experience of receiving therapeutic touch. *Journal of Advanced Nursing, 17*, 651–657.

Sanchez, R. (1989). Empathy, diversity, and telepathy in mother-daughter dyads: An empirical investigation utilizing Rogers' conceptual framework. *Scholarly Inquiry for Nursing Practice, 3*, 29–44.

Rawnsley, M.M. (1989). Response to "Empathy, diversity, and telepathy in mother-daughter dyads: An empirical investigation utilizing Rogers' conceptual framework." *Scholarly Inquiry for Nursing Practice, 3*, 45–51.

Schodt, C.M. (1989). Parental-fetal attachment and couvade: A study of patterns of human-environment integrality. *Nursing Science Quarterly, 2*, 88–97.

Smith, M.J. (1975). Changes in judgment of duration with different patterns of auditory information for individuals confined to bed. *Nursing Research, 24*, 93–98.

Smith, M.J. (1979). Duration experience for bed-confined subjects: A replication and refinement. *Nursing Research, 28*, 139–144.

Smith, M.J. (1984). Temporal experience and bed rest: Replication and refinement. *Nursing Research, 33*, 298–302.

Smith, M.J. (1986). Human-environment process: A test of Rogers' principle of inte-grality. *Advances in Nursing Science, 9*(1), 21–28.

Wright, S.M. (1991). Validity of the human energy field assessment form. *Western Journal of Nursing Research, 13*, 635–647.

Yarcheski, A., & Mahon, N.E. (1991). An empirical test of Rogers' original and revised theory of correlates in adolescents. *Research in Nursing and Health, 14*, 447–455.

DOCTORAL DISSERTATIONS

Allen, V.L.R. (1989). The relationship among time experience, human field motion, and clairvoyance: An investigation in the Rogerian conceptual system. *Dissertation Abstracts International, 50*, 121B.

Barnard, R.M. (1973). Field independence-dependence and selected motor abilities. *Dissertation Abstracts International, 34*, 2737B.

Barrett, E.A.M. (1984). An empirical investigation of Martha E. Rogers' principle of helicy: The relationship of human field motion and power. *Dissertation Abstracts International, 45*, 615A.

Bilitski, J.S. (1986). Assessment of adult day care program and client health characteristics in U.S. Region III. *Dissertation Abstracts International, 46*, 3460A.

Bramlett, M.H. (1991). Power, creativity and reminiscence in the elderly. *Dissertation Abstracts International, 51*, 3317B.

Branum, Q.K. (1986). Power as knowing participation in change: A model for nursing intervention. *Dissertation Abstracts International, 46*, 3780B.

Bray, J.D. (1990). The relationships of creativity, time experience and mystical experience. *Dissertation Abstracts International, 50*, 3394B.

Brouse, S.H. (1984). Patterns of feminine and self concept scores of pregnant women from the third trimester to six weeks postpartum. *Dissertation Abstracts International, 45*, 827B.

Brown, P.W. (1993). Sibling relationship qualities following the crisis of divorce. *Dissertation Abstracts International, 53*, 5639B.

Caroselli-Dervan, C. (1991). The relationship of power and feminism in female nurse executives in acute care hospitals. *Dissertation Abstracts International, 52*, 2990B.

Chandler, G.E. (1987). The relationship of nursing work environment to empowerment and powerlessness. *Dissertation Abstracts International, 47*, 4822B.

Chodil, J.J. (1979). An investigation of the relation between perceived body space, actual body space, body image boundary, and self-esteem. *Dissertation Abstracts International, 39,* 3760B.

Conner, G.K. (1986). The manifestations of human field motion, creativity, and time experience patterns of female and male parents. *Dissertation Abstracts International, 47,* 1926B.

Cora, V.L. (1986). Family life process of intergenerational families with functionally dependent elders. *Dissertation Abstracts International, 47,* 568B.

Cowling, W.R. III. (1984). The relationship of mystical experience, differentiation, and creativity in college students: An empirical investigation of the principle of helicy in Rogers' Science of Unitary Man. *Dissertation Abstracts International, 45,* 458A.

Daffron, J.M. (1989). Patterns of human field motion and human health. *Dissertation Abstracts International, 49,* 4229B.

DeSevo, M.R. (1991). Temporal experience and the preference for musical sequence complexity: A study based on Martha Rogers' conceptual system. *Dissertation Abstracts International, 52,* 2992B.

Dzurec, L.C. (1987). The nature of power experienced by individuals manifesting patterning labeled schizophrenic: An investigation of the principle of helicy. *Dissertation Abstracts International, 47,* 4467B.

Edwards, J.V. (1991). The relationship of contrasting selections of music and human field motion. *Dissertation Abstracts International, 52,* 2992B.

Evans, B.A. (1991). The relationship among a pattern of influence in the organizational environment, power of the nurse, and the nurse's empathic attributes: A manifestation of integrality. *Dissertation Abstracts International, 51,* 5244B.

Fawcett, J. (1977). The relationship between spouses' strength of identification and their patterns of change in perceived body space and articulation of body concept during and after pregnancy. *Dissertation Abstracts International, 37,* 4396B.

Feigenbaum, J.C. (1988). Historical trends in the role expectations of faculty in collegiate programs of professional nursing, 1901–1970. *Dissertation Abstracts International, 49,* 2125B.

Ference, H.M. (1980). The relationship of time experience, creativity traits, differentiation and human field motion: An empirical investigation of Rogers' correlates of synergistic human development. *Dissertation Abstracts International, 40,* 5206B.

Fitzpatrick, J.J. (1976). An investigation of the relationship between temporal orientation, temporal extension, and time perception. *Dissertation Abstracts International, 36,* 3310D.

Flatt, M.M. (1992). Life history of men with Alzheimer's disease and their spousal caregivers: Relevance for grounded theory of family care. *Dissertation Abstracts International, 53,* 315A.

Floyd, J.A. (1983). Hospitalization, sleep-wake patterns, and circadian type of psychiatric patients. *Dissertation Abstracts International, 43,* 3535B–3536B.

Fry, J.E. (1985). Reciprocity in mother-child interaction, correlates of attachment, and family environment in three-year-old children with congenital heart disease. *Dissertation Abstracts International, 46,* 113B.

Girardin, B.W. (1991). The relationship of lightwave frequency to sleep-wakefulness frequency in well, full-term hispanic neonates. *Dissertation Abstracts International, 52,* 748B.

Gueldner, S.H. (1983). A study of the relationship between imposed motion and human field motion in elderly individuals living in nursing homes. *Dissertation Abstracts International, 44,* 1411B.

Guthrie, B.J. (1988). The relationships of tolerance of ambiguity, preference for processing information in the mixed mode to differentiation in female college students: An empirical investigation of the homeodynamic principle of helicy. *Dissertation Abstracts International, 49,* 74B.

Hastings-Tolsma, M.T. (1993). The relationship of diversity of human field pattern to risk-taking and time experience: An investigation of Rogers' principles of homeodynamics. *Dissertation Abstracts International, 53,* 4029B.

Hektor, L.M. Nursing, science, and gender: Florence Nightingale and Martha E. Rogers. *Dissertation Abstracts International, 53,* 4590B.

Johnston, R.L. (1981). Temporality as a measure of unidirectionality with the Rogerian conceptual framework of nursing science. *Dissertation Abstracts International, 41,* 3740B.

Krause, D.A.B. (1992). The impact of an individually tailored nursing intervention on human field patterning in clients who experience dyspnea. *Dissertation Abstracts International, 53,* 1293B.

Kutlenios, R.M. (1986). A comparison of holistic, mental and physical health nursing interventions with the elderly. *Dissertation Abstracts International, 47,* 995B.

Lothian, J.A. (1990). Continuing to breastfeed. *Dissertation Abstracts International, 51,* 665B.

Ludomirski-Kalmanson, B. (1985). The relationship between the environmental energy wave frequency pattern manifest in red light and blue light and human field motion in adult individuals with visual sensory perception and those with total blindness. *Dissertation Abstracts International, 45,* 2094B.

MacDonald, G.C. (1992). Adolescent mother-infant dyads: Enhancing interactive reciprocy. *Dissertation Abstracts International, 52,* 5192B.

Macrae, J.A. (1983). A comparison between meditating subjects and non-meditating subjects on time experience and human field motion. Dissertation Abstracts International, 43, 3537B.

Malinski, V.M. (1981). The relationship between hyperactivity in children and perception of short wavelength light: An investigation into the conceptual system proposed by Dr. Martha E. Rogers. *Dissertation Abstracts International, 41,* 4459B.

Mathwig, G.M. (1968). Living open systems, reciprocal adaptations and the life process. *Dissertation Abstracts International, 29,* 666B.

McCanse, R.L. (1988). Healthy death readiness: Development of a measurement instrument. *Dissertation Abstracts International, 48,* 2606B.

McDonald, S.F. (1981). A study of the relationship between visible lightwaves and the experience of pain. *Dissertation Abstracts International, 42,* 569B.

McEvoy, M.D. (1988). The relationship among the experience of dying, the experience of paranormal events, and creativity in adults. *Dissertation Abstracts International, 48,* 2264B.

Miller, F.A. (1985). The relationship of sleep, wakefulness, and beyond waking experiences: A descriptive study of M. Rogers' concept of sleep-wake rhythm. *Dissertation Abstracts International, 46,* 116B.

Miller, S.R. (1974). An investigation of the relationship between mothers' general fearfulness, their daughters' locus of control, and general fearfulness in the daughter. *Dissertation Abstracts International, 35,* 2281B.

Moccia, P. (1980). A study of the theory-practice dialectic: Towards a critique of the science of man. *Dissertation Abstracts International, 41,* 2560B.

Moore, G. (1982). Perceptual complexity, memory and human duration experience. *Dissertation Abstracts International, 42,* 4363B.

Morris, D.L. (1992). An exploration of elder's perceptions of power and well-being. *Dissertation Abstracts International, 52,* 4125B.

Newman, M.A. (1971). An investigation of the relationship between gait tempo and time perception. *Dissertation Abstracts International, 32,* 2821B.

Oliver, N.R. (1988). Processing unacceptable behaviors of coworkers: A naturalistic study of nurses at work. *Dissertation Abstracts International, 49,* 75B.

Paletta, J.L. (1988). The relationship of temporal experience to human time. *Dissertation Abstracts International, 49,* 1621B–1622B.

Pohl, J.M. (1993). Mother-daughter relationships and adult daughters' commitment to caregiving for their aging disabled mothers. *Dissertation Abstracts International, 53,* 6225B.

Porter, L. (1968). Physical-physiological activity and infants' growth and development. *Dissertation Abstracts International, 28,* 4829B.

Quillin, S.I.M. (1984). Growth and development of infant and mother and mother-infant synchrony. *Dissertation Abstracts International, 44,* 3718B.

Quinn, A.A. (1989). Integrating a changing me: A grounded theory of the process of menopause for perimenopausal women. *Dissertation Abstracts International, 50,* 126B.

Quinn, J.F. (1982). An investigation of the effects of therapeutic touch done without physical contact on state anxiety of hospitalized cardiovascular patients. *Dissertation Abstracts International, 43,* 1797B.

Raile, M.M. (1983). The relationship of creativity, actualization and empathy in unitary human development: A descriptive study of M. Rogers' principle of helicy. *Dissertation Abstracts International, 44,* 449B.

Rankin, M.K. (1985). Effect of sound wave repatterning on symptoms of menopausal women. *Dissertation Abstracts International, 46,* 796B–797B.

Rapacz, K.E. (1992). Human patterning and chronic pain. *Dissertation Abstracts International, 52,* 4670B.

Rasch, R.F.R. (1988). The development of a taxonomy for the nursing process: A deductive approach based on an analysis of the discipline of nursing and application of set theory. *Dissertation Abstracts International, 49*, 2132B.

Rawnsley, M.M. (1977). Perceptions of the speed of time in aging and in dying: An empirical investigation of the holistic theory of nursing proposed by Martha Rogers. *Dissertation Abstracts International, 38*, 1652B.

Reeder, F. (1985). Nursing research, holism and philosophies of science: Points of congruence between E. Husserl and M.E. Rogers. *Dissertation Abstracts International, 44*, 2498B–2499B.

Rizzo, J.A. (1991). An investigation of the relationahips of life satisfaction, purpose in life, and power in individuals sixty-five years and older. *Dissertation Abstracts International, 51*, 4280B.

Sanchez, R.O. (1987). The relationship of empathy, diversity, and telepathy in mother-daughter dyads. *Dissertation Abstracts International, 47*, 3297B.

Sarter, B. (1985). The stream of becoming: A metaphysical analysis of Rogers' Model of Unitary Man. *Dissertation Abstracts International, 45*, 2106B.

Schodt, C.M. (1990). Patterns of parent-fetus attachment and the couvade syndrome: An application of human-environment integrality as postulated in the Science of Unitary Human Beings. *Dissertation Abstracts International, 50*, 4455B.

Sellers, S.C. (1991). A philosophical analysis of conceptual models of nursing. *Dissertation Abstracts International, 52*, 1937B.

Smith, C.T. (1991). The lived experience of staying healthy in rural black families. *Dissertation Abstracts International, 50*, 3925B.

Smith, M.C. (1987). An investigation of the effects of different sound frequencies on vividness and creativity of imagery. *Dissertation Abstracts International, 47*, 3708B.

Straneva, J.A.E. (1993). Therapeutic touch and in vitro erythropoiesis. *Dissertation Abstracts International, 54*, 1338B.

Swanson, A. (1976). An investigation of the relationship between a child's general fearfulness and the child's mother's anxiety, self differentiation, and accuracy of perception of her child's general fearfulness. *Dissertation Abstracts International, 36*, 3313B.

Thomas, D.J. (1993). The lived experience of people with liver transplants. *Dissertation Abstracts International, 54*, 747B.

Trangenstein, P.A. (1989). Relationships of power and job diversity to job satisfaction and job involvement: An empirical investigation of Rogers' principle of integrality. *Dissertation Abstracts International, 49*, 3110B–3111B.

Wright, S.M. (1989). Development and construct validity of the energy field assessment form. *Dissertation Abstracts International, 49*, 3113B.

Yaros, P.S. (1986). The relationship of maternal rhythmic behavior and infant interactional attention. *Dissertation Abstracts International, 47*, 136B.

MASTER'S THESES

Black, P.A. (1990). Powerlessness: A common experience shared by clients with an acute myocardial infarction. *Master's Abstracts International, 28*, 270.

Bryan, M.A. (1990). The effects of guided imagery on axiety levels of clients undergoing magnetic resonance imaging. *Master's Abstracts International, 28*, 570.

Butcher, H.K. (1987). Repatterning of time experience and human field motion during the experience of pleasant guided imagery: An experimental investigation within Rogers' Science of Unitary Human Beings. *Master's Abstracts International, 25*, 282.

Draus, C.A. (1988). The relationship of locus of control to decision-making behaviors in the first-line nurse manager. *Master's Abstracts International, 26*, 103.

Emmett, P.R. (1990). Nurse's knowledge, attitudes, and willingness to interact with clients with acquired immune deficiency syndrome. *Master's Abstracts International, 28*, 407.

Meskimen, K.L. (1993). The relationship of patterned environmental sound on restfulness of adult ICU patients. *Masters Abstracts International, 31*, 767.

Ziolkowski, I.H. (1990). Happiness and its relationship to rhythmic patterns of physiological processes in the elderly female residing in adult care facilities. *Master's Abstracts International, 28*, 585.

EDUCATION

Barrett, E.A.M. (1990). The continuing revolution of Rogers' science-based nursing education. In E.A.M. Barrett (Ed.), *Visions of Rogers' science based nursing* (pp. 303–318). New York: National League for Nursing.

Hanley, M.A. (1990). Concept-integration: A board game as a learning tool. In E.A.M.

Barrett (Ed.), *Visions of Rogers' science based nursing* (pp. 335–344). New York: National League for Nursing.

Mathwig, G.M., Young, A.A., & Pepper, J.M. (1990). Using Rogerian science in undergraduate and graduate nursing education. In E.A.M. Barrett (Ed.), *Visions of Rogers' science based nursing* (pp. 319–334). New York: National League for Nursing.

Rogers, M.E. (1961). *Educational revolution in nursing.* New York: Macmillan.

Rogers, M.E. (1963). Building a strong educational foundation. *American Journal of Nursing, 63*(6), 94–95.

Rogers, M.E. (1964). *Reveille in nursing.* Philadelphia: FA Davis.

Rogers, M.E. (1985). The nature and characteristics of professional education for nursing. *Journal of Professional Nursing, 1*, 381–383.

Rogers, M.E. (1985). Nursing education: Preparation for the future. In *Patterns in education: The unfolding of nursing* (pp. 11–14). New York: National League for Nursing.

Swanson, A.R. (1990). Issues in dissertation proposal development. In E.A.M. Barrett (Ed.), *Visions of Rogers' science based nursing* (pp. 345–351). New York: National League for Nursing.

Wood, R., & Kekahbah, J. (Eds.). (1985). *Examining the cultural implications of Martha E. Rogers's Science of Unitary Human Beings.* Lecompton, KS: Wood-Kekahbah Associates.

ADMINISTRATION

Alligood, M.R. (1989). Applying Rogers' model to nursing administration: Emphasis on environment, health. In B. Henry, C. Arndt, M. DiVincenti, & A. Marriner-Tomey (Eds.), *Dimensions of nursing administration: Theory, research, education, and practice.* (pp. 105–111). Boston: Blackwell Scientific Publications.

Caroselli-Dervan, C. (1990). Visionary opportunities for knowledge development in nursing administration. In E.A.M. Barrett (Ed.), *Visions of Rogers' science based nursing* (pp. 151–158). New York: National League for Nursing.

Rizzo, J.A. (1990). Nursing service as an energy field: A response to "Visionary opportunities for knowledge development in nursing administration." In E.A.M. Barrett (Ed.), *Visions of Rogers' science based nursing* (pp. 159–164). New York: National League for Nursing.

Decker, K. (1989). Theory in action: The geriatric assessment team. *Journal of Gerontological Nursing, 15*(10), 25–28.

Ference, H.M. (1989). Nursing science theories and administration. In B. Henry, C. Arndt, M. DiVincenti, & A. Marriner-Tomey (Eds.), *Dimensions of nursing administration: Theory, research, education, and practice* (pp. 121–131). Boston: Blackwell Scientific Publications.

Garon, M. (1991). Assessment and management of pain in the home care setting: Application of Rogers' Science of Unitary Human Beings. *Holistic Nursing Practice, 6*(1), 47–57.

Gueldner, S.H. (1989). Applying Rogers' model to nursing administration: Emphasis on client and nursing. In B. Henry, C. Arndt, M. DiVincenti, & A. Marriner-Tomey (Eds.), *Dimensions of nursing administration: Theory, research, education, and practice* (pp. 113–119). Boston: Blackwell Scientific Publications.

Hanchett, E.S. (1979). *Community health assessment: A conceptual tool kit.* New York: John Wiley & Sons.

Mason, T., & Chandley, M. (1990). Nursing models in a special hospital: A critical analysis of efficacity. *Journal of Advanced Nursing, 15*, 667–673.

Mason, T., & Patterson, R. (1990). A critical review of the use of Rogers' model within a special hospital: A single case study. *Journal of Advanced Nursing, 15*, 130–141.

Smith, K., Kupferschmid, B.J., Dawson, C., & Briones, T.L. (1991). A family-centered critical care unit. *AACN Clinical Issues, 2*, 258–268.

Tettero, I., Jackson, S., & Wilson, S. (1993). Theory to practice: Developing a Rogerian-based assessment tool. *Journal of Advanced Nursing, 18*, 776–782.

PRACTICE

Alligood, M.R. (1990). Nursing care of the elderly: Futuristic projections. In E.A.M. Barrett (Ed.), *Visions of Rogers' science based nursing* (pp. 129–142). New York: National League for Nursing.

Barrett, E.A.M. (1988). Using Rogers' science of unitary human beings in nursing practice. *Nursing Science Quarterly, 1*, 50–51.

Barrett, E.A.M. (1990). Health patterning in clients in a private practice. In E.A.M. Barrett (Ed.), *Visions of Rogers' science based nursing* (pp. 105–116). New York: National League for Nursing.

Barrett, E.A.M. (1990). Rogers' science-based nursing practice. In E.A.M. Barrett (Ed.), *Visions of Rogers' science based nursing* (pp. 31–44). New York: National League for Nursing.

Barrett, E.A.M. (1992). Innovative imagery: A health-patterning modality for nursing practice. *Journal of Holistic Nursing, 10,* 154–166.

Barrett, E.A.M. (1993). Virtual reality: A health patterning modality for nursing in space. *Visions: The Journal of Rogerian Nursing Science, 1,* 10–21.

Black, G., & Haight, B.K. (1992). Integrality as a holistic framework for the life-review process. *Holistic Nursing Practice, 7*(1), 7–15.

Boguslawski, M. (1979). The use of therapeutic touch in nursing. *Journal of Continuing Education in Nursing, 10*(4), 9–15.

Boguslawski, M. (1990). Unitary human field practice modalities. In E.A.M. Barrett (Ed.), *Visions of Rogers' science based nursing* (pp. 83–92). New York: National League for Nursing.

Buczny, B., Speirs, J., & Howard, J.R. (1989). Nursing care of a terminally ill client: Applying Martha Rogers' conceptual framework. *Home Healthcare Nurse, 7*(4), 13–18.

Christensen, P., Sowell, R., & Gueldner, S.H. (1993). Nursing in space: Theoretical foundations and potential practice applications within Rogerian science. *Visions: The Journal of Rogerian Nursing Science, 1,* 36–44.

Cowling, W.R. III. (1990). Chronological age as an anomalie of evolution. In E.A.M. Barrett (Ed.), *Visions of Rogers' science based nursing* (pp. 143–150). New York: National League for Nursing.

Cowling, W.R. III. (1990). A template for unitary pattern-based nursing practice. In E.A.M. Barrett (Ed.), *Visions of Rogers' science based nursing* (pp. 45–66). New York: National League for Nursing.

Ference, H.M. (1989). Comforting the dying: Nursing practice according to the Rogerian model. In J.P. Riehl-Sisca, *Conceptual models for nursing practice* (3rd ed., pp. 197–205). Norwalk, CT: Appleton & Lange.

Forker, J.E., & Billings, C.V. (1989). Nursing therapeutics in a group encounter. *Archives of Psychiatric Nursing, 3,* 108–112.

Hanchett, E.S. (1988). *Nursing frameworks and community as client: Bridging the gap.* Norwalk, CT: Appleton & Lange.

Hanchett, E.S. (1990). Nursing models and community as client. *Nursing Science Quarterly, 3,* 67–72.

Heggie, J.R., Schoenmehl, P.A., Chang, M.K., & Crieco, C. (1989). Selection and implementation of Dr. Martha Rogers' nursing conceptual model in an acute care setting. *Clinical Nurse Specialist, 3,* 143–147.

Hill, L., & Oliver, N. (1993). Technique integration: Therapeutic touch and theory-based mental health nursing. *Journal of Psychosocial Nursing and Mental Health Services, 31*(2), 19–22.

Johnston, R.L. (1986). Approaching family intervention through Rogers' conceptual model. In A.L. Whall, *Family therapy theory for nursing: Four approaches* (pp. 11–32). Norwalk, CT: Appleton-Century-Crofts.

Jones, D.A., Dunbar, C.F., & Jirovec, M.M. (1982). *Medical-surgical nursing: A conceptual approach.* New York: McGraw-Hill.

Joseph, L. (1990). Practical application of Rogers' theoretical framework for nursing. In M.E. Parker (Ed.), *Nursing theories in practice* (pp. 115–125). New York: National League for Nursing.

Jurgens, A., Meehan, T.C., Wilson, H.L. (1987). Therapeutic touch as a nursing intervention. *Holistic Nursing Practice, 2*(1), 1–13.

Kodiath, M.F. (1991). A new view of the chronic pain client. *Holistic Nursing Practice, 6*(1), 41–46.

Madrid, M. (1990). The participating process of human field patterning in an acute-care environment. In E.A.M. Barrett (Ed.), *Visions of Rogers' science based nursing* (pp. 93–104). New York: National League for Nursing.

Madrid, M., & Barrett, E.A.M. (1994). *Rogers' scientific art of nursing practice.* New York: National League for Nursing.

Madrid, M., & Winstead-Fry, P. (1986). Rogers's conceptual model. In P. Winstead-Fry (Ed.), *Case studies in nursing theory* (pp. 73–102). New York: National League for Nursing.

Magan, S.J., Gibbon, E.J., & Mrozek, R. (1990). Nursing theory applications: A practice model. *Issues in Mental Health Nursing, 11,* 297–312.

Malinski, V.M. (1986). Nursing practice within the science of unitary human beings. In V.M. Malinski (Ed.), *Explorations on Martha Rogers' Science of Unitary Human Beings* (pp. 25–32). Norwalk, CT: Appleton-Century-Crofts.

Meehan, T.C. (1990). The science of unitary

human beings and theory-based practice: Therapeutic touch. In E.A.M. Barrett (Ed.), *Visions of Rogers' science based nursing* (pp. 67–82). New York: National League for Nursing.

Newshan, G. (1989). Therapeutic touch for symptom control in persons with AIDS. *Holistic Nursing Practice, 3*(4), 45–51.

Payne, M.B. (1989). The use of therapeutic touch with rehabilitation clients. *Rehabilitation Nursing, 14*(2), 69–72.

Quinn, J.F. (1979). One nurse's evolution as a healer. *American Journal of Nursing, 79,* 662–664.

Reed, P.G. (1986). The developmental conceptual framework: Nursing reformulations and applications for family therapy. In A.L. Whall, *Family therapy for nursing: Four approaches* (pp. 69–91). Norwalk, CT: Appleton-Century-Crofts.

Thomas, S.D. (1990). Intentionality in the human-environment encounter in an ambulatory care environment. In E.A.M. Barrett (Ed.), *Visions of Rogers' science based nursing* (pp. 117–128). New York: National League for Nursing.

Thompson, J.E. (1990). Finding the borderline's border: Can Martha Rogers help? *Perspectives in Psychiatric Care, 26*(4), 7–10.

Tuyn, L.K. (1992). Solution-oriented therapy and Rogerian nursing science: An integrated approach. *Archives of Psychiatric Nursing, 6,* 83–89.

Webb, J. (1992). A new lease on life. *Nursing Times, 88*(11), 30–32.

Whall, A.L. (1981). Nursing theory and the assessment of families. *Journal of Psychiatric Nursing and Mental Health Services, 19*(1), 30–36.

Whelton, B.J. (1979). An operationalization of Martha Rogers' theory throughout the nursing process. *International Journal of Nursing Studies, 16,* 7–20.

Roy's Adaptation Model

This chapter presents an analysis and evaluation of Sister Callista Roy's Adaptation Model of Nursing. Roy's work clearly fits the definition of conceptual model used in this book. In fact, Roy has always referred to her work as a conceptual model.

The concepts of the Roy Adaptation Model and their dimensions are listed below. Each concept and its dimension are defined and described later in this chapter.

KEY CONCEPTS

ADAPTIVE SYSTEM
Regulator Subsystem
Cognator Subsystem
ADAPTIVE MODES
Physiological
  Basic Physiological Needs
  Regulator Process
Self-Concept
  Physical Self
  Personal Self
Role Function
  Primary Role
  Secondary Roles
  Tertiary Roles
Interdependence
  Significant Others
  Support Systems
ENVIRONMENT
Focal Stimulus
Contextual Stimuli
Residual Stimuli
ADAPTATION LEVEL
ADAPTIVE RESPONSES

INEFFECTIVE RESPONSES
GOAL OF NURSING
To Promote Adaptation
NURSING PROCESS
Assessment of Behavior
Assessment of Stimuli
Nursing Diagnosis
Goal Setting
Intervention
Evaluation
THEORY OF THE PERSON AS AN
  ADAPTIVE SYSTEM
THEORY OF THE PHYSIOLOGICAL
  MODE
THEORY OF THE SELF-CONCEPT
  MODE
THEORY OF THE ROLE FUNCTION
  MODE
THEORY OF THE
  INTERDEPENDENCE MODE
NURSING MODEL OF COGNITIVE
  PROCESSING

ANALYSIS OF ROY'S ADAPTATION MODEL

This section presents an analysis of the Roy Adaptation Model. The analysis draws heavily from the latest major book about the model, *The Roy Adaptation Model: The Definitive Statement* (Roy & Andrews, 1991).

Origins of the Model

Historical Evolution and Motivation

Roy first published the basic ideas that make up her conceptual model in 1970 in an article entitled, "Adaptation: A conceptual framework for nursing." She went on to publish additional elements of the model and implications for practice and education in 1971 and 1973. The model was explicated more fully in a chapter of the 1974 edition of the Riehl and Roy book, *Conceptual Models for Nursing Practice* (Roy, 1974). A major expansion of the model was presented in Roy's 1976b text, *Introduction to Nursing: An Adaptation Model*. Refinements of the model then were presented in Roy's 1978a speech at the Second Annual Nurse Educator Conference, in the 1980 edition of Riehl and Roy's book (Roy, 1980), and in Roy and Roberts's 1981 text, *Theory Construction in Nursing: An Adaptation Model*. Further refinements in the model were published in the second edition of Roy's (1984a) text, *Introduction to Nursing: An Adaptation Model*, in the Andrews and Roy (1986) book, *Essentials of the Roy Adaptation Model*, and in a chapter (Roy, 1989) of the third edition of *Conceptual Models for Nursing Practice* (Riehl-Sisca, 1989).

Roy articulated her philosophical claims in the 1988b journal article, "An explication of the philosophical assumptions of the Roy Adaptation Model," and she elaborated on her definitions of adaptation and health in the 1990 journal article, "Strengthening the Roy adaptation model through conceptual clarification: Commentary and response" (Artinian & Roy, 1990). The 1991 text, *The Roy Adaptation Model: The Definitive Statement* (Roy & Andrews, 1991) contains still further refinements in the model. The authors explicitly stated that the purpose of that book was "to assume the role of the definitive text on the model" (Roy & Andrews, 1991, p. xvii). A recent book chapter, "The Roy Adaptation Model: Theoretical update and knowledge for practice" (Roy & Corliss, 1993), presented additional refinements.

In tracing the historical development of her conceptual model, Roy (1989) stated:

> The Roy model had its beginning in 1964 when the author was challenged to develop a conceptual model for nursing in a seminar with Dorothy E. Johnson, at the University of California, Los Angeles. The adaptation concept, presented in a psychology class, had impressed the author as an appropriate conceptual framework for nursing. The work on adaptation by the physiologic psychologist, Harry Helson, was added to the beginning concept and the model's present form began to take shape. In subsequent years the model was developed as a framework for

nursing practice, research, and education. In 1968 work began on operationalizing the model in the baccalaureate nursing curriculum at Mount
Saint Mary's College in Los Angeles. The first class of students to study
with the model began their nursing major in the spring of 1970 and were
graduated in June, 1972. Use of the model in nursing practice led to
further clarification and refinement. In the summer of 1971 a pilot
research study was conducted and in 1976 to 1977 a survey research
study was done that led to some tentative confirmations of the model.
(p. 105)

Development of the model continued during the 1970s, according to Andrews and Roy (1991a), as "more than 1500 faculty and students at Mount
St. Mary's College in Los Angeles helped to clarify, refine, and extend the
basic concepts of the Roy Adaptation Model for nursing" (p. 4).

By accepting Johnson's challenge to develop a conceptual model, Roy
joined the group of nurse scholars who recognized the need to explicate a
body of nursing knowledge. Indeed, she stated:

> As nursing education moves more and more into institutions of
> higher learning, the nurse educator needs a basis for developing a body
> of nursing knowledge. And as the general public becomes more sophis-
> ticated in knowing the meaning of good health, it expects the nurse to
> provide care based on scientific knowledge. It is from the theoretical
> conceptual framework of any discipline that its area of practice, its body
> of knowledge, and its scientific basis are developed. (Roy, 1970, p. 42)

Philosophical Claims

Roy (1987c, 1988b, 1989) has presented the philosophical claims undergirding the Roy Adaptation Model in the form of scientific and philosophical assumptions and values about nursing. She commented, "These
assumptions have constituted the basis for and are evident in the specific
description of the following major concepts of the Roy Adaptation Model
—the person, the environment, health, and nursing" (Andrews & Roy,
1991a, p. 6).

Roy (1992) explained that the Roy Adaptation Model "assumes the
universal importance of promoting adaptation in states of health and
illness" (p. 66). She further explained that the Roy Adaptation Model is
based on scientific and philosophical assumptions reflecting "holism,
mutuality, control processes, activity, creativity, purpose, and value" (Roy,
1987c, p. 43).

The scientific assumptions were drawn from general system theory
(Bertalanffy, 1968) and Helson's (1964) adaptation level theory. Elaborating, Roy (1987c) stated:

> The [general system] theory assumptions focus primarily on holism,
> interdependence, control processes, information feedback, and, most
> importantly, the highly complex nature of living systems. Helson fo-
> cused on all behavior as adaptive. He believed that this behavior is the
> function of both the stimulus coming in, how light or dark it is, how hot

the room is, and the adaptation level. The process of responding positively as well as very actively is also significant from Helson's view. (p. 37)

The following specific scientific assumptions were explicated by Roy (1989):

1. The person is a bio-psycho-social being.

2. The person is in constant interaction with a changing environment.

3. To cope with a changing world, the person uses both innate and acquired mechanisms, which are biologic, psychologic, and social in origin.

4. Health and illness are one inevitable dimension of the person's life.

5. To respond positively to environmental changes, the person must adapt.

6. Adaptation is a function of the stimulus a person is exposed to and his or her adaptation level.

7. The person's adaptation level is such that it comprises a zone indicating the range of stimulation that will lead to a positive response.

8. The person is conceptualized as having four modes of adaptation: physiologic needs, self-concept, role function, and interdependence relations. (pp. 106–108)

Roy and Corliss (1993) revised and restated the scientific assumptions. They identified the assumptions from general system theory as:

1. Holism — a system is a set of units so related or connected as to form a unity or whole.

2. Interdependence — a system is a whole that functions as a whole by virtue of the interdependence of its parts.

3. Control Processes — a system has inputs, outputs, and control and feedback processes.

4. Information Feedback — input, in the form of a standard or feedback, often is referred to as information.

5. Complexity of Living Systems — living systems are almost infinitely more complex than mechanical systems and have standards and feedback to direct their functioning as a whole. (pp. 216–217)

Roy and Corliss (1993) drew from Helson's (1964) adaptation level theory for the following scientific assumptions:

1. Behavior as Adaptive — human behavior represents adaptation to environmental and organismic forces.

2. Adaptation as a Function of Stimuli and Adaptation Level — adaptive behavior is a function of the stimulus and adaptation level, that is, the pooled effect of the focal, contextual, and residual stimuli.

3. Individual, Dynamic Adaptation Levels — adaptation is a process of responding positively to environmental changes; this positive response decreases the responses necessary to cope with the stimuli and increases sensitivity to respond to other stimuli.

4. Positive and Active Processes of Responding — responses reflect the state of the organism as well as the properties of stimuli and hence are regarded as active processes. (Roy & Corliss, 1993, p. 217)

The philosophical assumptions on which the Roy Adaptation Model was based encompass several values and beliefs associated with the general principles of humanism and veritivity. Humanism, according to Roy (1988b), refers to "a broad movement in philosophy and psychology that recognizes the person and subjective dimensions of human experience as central to knowing and valuing" (p. 29). The tenets of humanism that are relevant to the Roy Adaptation Model are creative power, purposefulness, holism, subjectivity, and interpersonal relationships. In particular, Roy (1988b) believes that the individual "(a) shares in creative power, (b) behaves purposefully, not in a sequence of cause and effect, (c) possesses intrinsic holism, and (d) strives to maintain integrity and to realize the need for relationships" (p. 32).

Roy (1984a) pointed out that nursing has always "been concerned about the value of the human person" (p. 36). She then described the linkage between humanism and her conceptual model. She stated:

> As humanistic nurses, we believe in the person's own creative power. Roy places emphasis on the person's own coping abilities. Nurses see processes moving purposefully and not merely as chains of cause and effect. Roy views adaptation as an ongoing purposive process. Nursing's holistic approach is rooted in humanism. Roy's theoretical work is attempting to describe persons' functioning holistically and to point out holistic approaches to nursing care of persons. Nursing accepts the humanistic approach to valuing other persons' opinions and viewpoints . . . Nursing has long recognized the significance of interpersonal relationships. This humanistic value also is basic to the Roy Adaptation Model's nursing process. (p. 36)

Veritivity is a philosophical premise that asserts that "there is an absolute truth" (Roy, 1988b, p. 29). Roy (1987c) explained:

> On a more global level, the primacy of the notion of integration reflecting on holism, mutuality and control processes of the system, leads to the principle of "verativity," [sic] a term coined recently when speaking of values for science. It comes from the Latin word veritas, meaning truth. In the adaptive person, verativity [sic] reflects activity, creativity, unity, purpose, and value. (p. 45)

As a principle of human nature, veritivity "affirms a common purposefulness of human existence" (Roy, 1988b, p. 30). More specifically, Roy (1988b) believes that "the individual in society is viewed in the context of the (a) purposefulness of human existence, (b) unity of purpose of humankind, (c) activity and creativity for the common good, and (d) value and meaning of life" (p. 32).

Roy and Corliss (1993) reaffirmed the principles of humanism and veritivity as the source of the philosophical assumptions undergirding the Roy Adaptation Model. They explained that the assumptions from humanism are:

1. Creativity—person's own creative power.

2. Purposefulness—person's behavior is purposeful and not merely a chain of cause and effect.

3. Holism—person is holistic.

4. Interpersonal process—the interpersonal relationship is significant. (pp. 217–218)

The following assumptions from veritivity, according to Roy and Corliss (1993), are derived from "the Teilhardian [Chardin, 1959, 1965] view of the universe and the orthogenesis of humankind" (p. 218):

1. Purposefulness of human existence.

2. Unity of purpose

3. Activity [and] creativity.

4. Value and meaning of life. (p. 218)

Roy (1989) identified four values that undergird the goal of nursing. She pointed out, "These values are not proven within the model, but are assumed to be truths that made the overall goal of nursing worthwhile" (p. 109). Following are the values:

1. Nursing's concern with the person as a total being in the areas of health and illness is a socially significant activity.

2. The nursing goal of supporting and promoting patient adaptation is important for patient welfare.

3. Promoting the process of adaptation is assumed to conserve patient energy; thus nursing makes an important contribution to the overall goal of the health team by making energy available for the healing process.

4. Nursing is unique because it focuses on the patient as a person adapting to those stimuli present as a result of his or her position on the health-illness continuum. (p. 109)

Strategies for Knowledge Development

The Roy Adaptation Model evolved from a combination of inductive and deductive thinking. Roy (1992) explained, "As a young staff nurse I was immediately impressed with the resilience of children in the recovery process, both from disease and from the many changes of hospitalization, with even a small amount of well-timed nursing care. Thus, my original insights into viewing the person as having innate and acquired abilities to deal with a changing environment were developed. Later I articulated this belief by using the concept of adaptation" (p. 64).

Deduction was clearly the approach used by Roy to develop her conceptualization of adaptation and the factors that influence the level of adaptation. In fact, she drew heavily from Helson's (1964) work on adaptation of the retina of the eye to environmental changes. Moreover, her conceptualization of the person as an adaptive system was deduced from general system theory.

Roy used an inductive approach to identify the four modes of adaptation. This was accomplished through classification of "about 500 samples of behavior of patients collected by nursing students over a period of several months in all clinical settings" (Roy, 1971, p. 255). The classification was based in part on Strickler and LaSor's (1970) work on threats in crisis situations. The modes were then compared with the typologies developed by Abdellah, Beland, Martin, and Matheney (1960) and McCain (1965).

Influences from Other Scholars

Roy (1988c) noted that her personal and professional life has been shaped by "my family, my religious commitment, my teachers, and my mentors" (p. 292). She is the second child and first daughter in a large nuclear family. She joined the religious community of the Sisters of Saint Joseph of Carondelet when she completed high school. She completed her undergraduate nursing studies at Mount St. Mary's College in Los Angeles and went on to graduate study at the University of California, Los Angeles.

Andrews and Roy (1991a) explained that "The roots of the [Roy Adaptation] Model lie in Roy's own personal and professional background . . . Under the mentorship of Dorothy E. Johnson, Roy became convinced of the importance of defining nursing. She was influenced also by studies in the social sciences, and clinical practice in pediatric nursing provided experience with the resiliency of the human body and spirit" (p. 4).

In addition to acknowledging the contributions to her thinking made by her mentor, Dorothy Johnson, Roy (1978a) acknowledged her colleagues at Mount St. Mary's College, nursing students across the country, and other nurse theorists. In particular, she cited the influences of Dorothy Johnson's focus on behavior, Martha Rogers' concern with holistic man, and Dorothea Orem's notion of self-care. Roy (1988c) also acknowledged the contributions of Dr. Burton Meyer, who "gave me a firm grounding in both inductive and deductive processes for developing a framework, as well as in the meticulous steps of design, data collection, and analysis" during her graduate study at the University of California, Los Angeles (p. 293); and Dr. Connie Robinson, who provided mentorship in "the world of basic and clinical neurosciences" during her Robert Wood Johnson Clinical Nurse Scholars postdoctoral fellowship at the University of California, San Francisco (p. 296).

Roy (1970; Andrews & Roy, 1991a; Roy & Corliss, 1993) stated that the scientific foundation for the Roy Adaptation Model comes from the work of Helson (1964) and Bertalanffy (1968). Roy's notions of coping are tied to the work of Coelho, Hamburg, and Adams (1974) and Lazarus, Averill, and Opton (1974). She also drew from Levine (1966) and compared the concepts of her model with ideas put forth by Henderson (1960), Nightingale (1859), and Peplau (1952). Elaborating on influences from Nightingale, Roy (1992) noted that her own work is congruent with Nightingale's beliefs about "how to promote 'health existences' and the proper use of the environment to aid the natural reparative processes" (p. 64).

In addition, Roy (1988b) acknowledged the influence of several philosophers on the development of her philosophical assumptions. Among those whose works were cited are Chardin (1956, 1959, 1965), Ewing (1951), Kant (Boas, 1957), Popper (Popper & Eccles, 1981), and Rush (1981). Elaborating, Roy and Corliss (1993) explained that the philosophical assumptions

> . . . stem from Roy's lifelong study, conviction, and living of a theologically-based religious faith. In addition, Roy built upon both undergraduate and graduate studies in philosophy, especially related to the nature of person and the place of persons in a cosmos set in motion by a loving Creator. Early on she studied the philosophies of Aristotle and Thomas Aquinas, as well as the philosophical roots and historical methods of hermeneutical exegesis of biblical texts. Later the works of Freud, Jung, Adler, de Chardin, Kant, Hegel, Marx, and Freire were added. A strong basis in sociology, social psychology, and anthropology opened doors into structural analysis, empirical deductive knowledge strategies, interactionist theory, and phenomenology. Current teaching of the epistemology of nursing has allowed Roy to study the philosophy of science movements affecting nursing over the past few decades and the thinking of current nurse philosophers. (p. 218)

World View

The Roy Adaptation Model reflects the *reciprocal interaction* world view. Roy repeatedly emphasized the need to view the person as a holistic adaptive system that "functions as a whole and is more than the mere sum of its parts. . . . The person functions in a holistic manner with each aspect [of the Roy Adaptation Model] related to and affected by the others" (Andrews & Roy, 1991a, pp. 6–7, 21).

Roy also emphasized the active nature of the person. This is evident in the description of adaptive as meaning that "the human system has the capacity to adjust effectively to changes in the environment and, in turn, affects the environment" (Andrews & Roy, 1991a, p. 7). The active nature of the person is also evident in the description of the person's active participation in the nursing process, as noted in the following comment:

> According to this nursing model, the person is to be respected as an active participant in his care. It is the information that the patient shares with the nurse that forms the assessment. The goal arrived at is one of mutual agreement between nurse and patient. Interventions are the options that the nurse provides for the patient. (Roy & Roberts, 1981, p. 47)

The Roy Adaptation Model emphasizes continuous change. In fact, Roy (1978a) emphatically denied that the model promotes the status quo or is a static view. She stated, "Coping means the person continually raises his adaptation level." It may be inferred, then, that change is a natural and desirable condition for the person. The continuous nature of change was addressed explicitly in the description of life and the environment as constantly changing. Change is also reflected in the definition of adaptive responses as those that promote growth, and is further demonstrated in Roy's (1978a) assumption that "the person as a totality has great potential for self-actualization."

Unique Focus of the Model

The Roy Adaptation Model focuses on the responses of the adaptive system to a constantly changing environment. Adaptation is the central feature and a core concept of the model. Problems in adaptation arise when the adaptive system is unable to cope with or respond to constantly changing stimuli from the internal and external environments in a manner that maintains the integrity of the system (Andrews & Roy, 1991b; Roy, 1989). A typology of the indicators of positive adaptation and commonly recurring problems in adaptation is given in Table 9-1.

Roy (1989) maintained that the Roy Adaptation Model "can be viewed primarily as a systems model, although it also contains interactionist levels of analysis " (p. 105). Examination of the content of the model revealed that that is an accurate classification.

The systems model characteristic of system is addressed in the designation of the person as an open adaptive system. Andrews and Roy (1991a) explained, "In order to understand persons as adaptive systems, it is important to grasp the meaning of the term system. Broadly defined, a system is a set of parts connected to function as a whole for some purpose, and it does so by virtue of the interdependence of its parts" (p. 7). The subsystems are the regulator and cognator mechanisms, which are linked through the process of perception (Roy & Roberts, 1981).

Environment is described as "the world around and within" the adaptive system (Andrews & Roy, 1991a, p. 8). More specifically, the environment, both internal and external, is made up of focal, contextual, and residual stimuli. The relationship between the adaptive system and its environment is described in terms of the influences of the environment on the adaptive system and the system's capacity to alter the environment. "The nurse soon learns that the person never acts in isolation, but is influenced by the environment and in turn affects the environment" (Andrews & Roy, 1991a, p. 8).

The systems model characteristic of boundary is not addressed explicitly in the Roy Adaptation Model. The characteristic of tension, stress, strain, and conflict is addressed in the form of internal and external environmental strains. Roy (1989) explained, "Increased force, or tension, comes from strains within the [adaptive] system or from the environment that impinges on the system" (p. 105). More specifically, the tension is created by the focal, contextual, and residual stimuli from the internal and external environments.

TABLE 9–1. A TYPOLOGY OF INDICATORS OF POSITIVE ADAPTATION AND ADAPTATION PROBLEMS

Indicators of Positive Adaptation	Commonly Recurring Adaptation Problems
Physiological Mode: Oxygenation	Physiological Mode: Oxygenation
Stable processes of ventilation	Hypoxia/shock
Stable pattern of gas exchange	Ventilatory impairment
Adequate transport of gases	Inadequate gas exchange or transport
Adequate processes of compensation	Altered tissue perfusion
	Poor recruitment of compensatory processes for changing oxygen need
Physiological Mode: Nutrition	Physiological Mode: Nutrition
Stable digestive processes	Weight 20–25% above/below average
Adequate nutrition pattern for body requirements	Nutrition more/less than body requirements
Metabolic and other nutritive needs met during altered means of ingestion	Anorexia
	Nausea and vomiting
	Ineffective coping strategies for altered means of ingestion
Physiological Mode: Elimination	Physiological Mode: Elimination
Effective homeostatic bowel processes	Diarrhea
Stable pattern of bowel elimination	Bowel/bladder incontinence
Effective processes of urine formation	Constipation
Stable pattern of urine elimination	Urinary retention
Effective coping strategies for altered elimination	Flatulence
	Ineffective strategies for altered elimination
Physiological Mode: Activity and Rest	Physiological Mode: Activity and Rest
Integrated processes of mobility	Inadequate pattern of activity and rest
Adequate recruitment of compensatory movement processes during inactivity	Restricted mobility, gait, and/or coordination
Effective pattern of activity and rest	Activity intolerance
Effective sleep pattern	Immobility
Effective environmental changes for altered sleep conditions	Disuse consequences
	Potential for sleep pattern disturbance
	Fatigue
	Sleep deprivation
Physiological Mode: Protection	Physiological Mode: Protection
Intact skin	Disrupted skin integrity
Effective processes of immunity	Pressure sores
Effective healing response	Itching

Adequate secondary protection for changes in skin integrity and immune status

Physiological Mode: Senses
Effective processes of sensation
Effective integration of sensory input into information
Stable patterns of perception, i.e., interpretation and appreciation of input
Effective coping strategies for altered sensation

Physiological Mode: Fluids and Electrolytes
Stable processes of water balance
Stability of salts in body fluids
Balance of acid/base status
Effective chemical buffer regulation

Physiological Mode: Neurological Function
Effective processes of arousal/attention; sensation/perception; coding, concept formation, memory, language; planning; motor responses
Integrated thinking and feeling processes
Plasticity and functional effectiveness of developing, aging, and altered nervous system

Physiological Mode: Endocrine Function
Effective hormonal regulation of metabolic and body processes
Effective hormonal regulation of reproductive development
Stable patterns of closed loop negative feedback hormone systems
Stable patterns of cyclical hormone rhythms
Effective coping strategies for stress

Delayed wound healing
Infection
Potential for ineffective coping with allergic reaction
Ineffective coping with changes in immune status

Physiological Mode: Senses
Impairment of a primary sense
Potential for injury/loss of self-care abilities
Potential for distorted communication
Stigma
Sensory monotony/distortion
Sensory overload/deprivation
Acute pain
Chronic pain
Perceptual impairment
Ineffective coping strategies for sensory impairment

Physiological Mode: Fluids and Electrolytes
Dehydration
Edema
Intracellular water retention
Shock
Hyper or hypo calcemia, kalemia, or natremia
Acid/base imbalance
Ineffective buffer regulation for changing pH

Physiological Mode: Neurological Function
Decreased level of consciousness
Defective cognitive processing
Memory deficits
Instability of behavior and mood
Ineffective compensation for cognitive deficit
Potential for secondary brain damage

Physiological Mode: Endocrine Function
Ineffective hormone regulation, reflected in fatigue, irritability, heat intolerance
Ineffective reproductive development
Instability of hormone system loops
Instability of internal cyclical rhythms
Stress

(Continued)

TABLE 9–1. **A TYPOLOGY OF INDICATORS OF POSITIVE ADAPTATION AND ADAPTATION PROBLEMS** (Continued)

Indicators of Positive Adaptation	Commonly Recurring Adaptation Problems
Self-Concept Mode: Physical Self	Self-Concept Mode: Physical Self
Positive body image	Body image disturbance
Effective sexual function	Sexual dysfunction
Psychic integrity with physical growth	Rape trauma syndrome
Adequate compensation for bodily changes	Loss
Effective coping strategies for loss	
Effective process of life closure	
Self-Concept Mode: Personal Self	Self-Concept Mode: Personal Self
Stable pattern of self-consistency	Anxiety
Effective integration of self-ideal	Powerlessness
Effective processes of moral-ethical-spiritual growth	Guilt
Functional self-esteem	Low-self-esteem
Effective coping strategies for threats to self	
Role Function Mode	Role Function Mode
Effective processes of role transition	Role transition
Integration of instrumental and expressive role behaviors	Role distance
Integration of primary, secondary, and tertiary roles	Role conflict
Stable pattern of role mastery	Role failure
Effective processes for coping with role changes	
Interdependence Mode	Interdependence Mode
Stable pattern of giving and receiving nurturing	Ineffective pattern of giving and receiving nurturing
Affectional adequacy	Ineffective pattern of aloneness and relating
Effective pattern of aloneness and relating	Separation anxiety
Effective coping strategies for separation and loneliness	Loneliness

Adapted from Roy, C., & Andrews, H.A. (1991). *The Roy adaptation model: The definitive statement* (pp. 38–39, 41–42). Norwalk, CT: Appleton & Lange, with permission.

The characteristic of equilibrium is addressed by Roy and Roberts (1981) in the following statement: "Helson's work points to adaptation as a dynamic state of equilibrium involving both heightened and lowered responses brought about by autonomic and cognitive processes triggered by internal and external stimuli" (p. 54).

Input, output, and feedback characteristics of systems model are also addressed by the Roy Adaptation Model. "Inputs for the person," Andrews and Roy (1991a) explained, "have been termed stimuli and may come externally from the environment (external stimuli) and internally from the self (internal stimuli). Certain stimuli pool to make up a specific input, the person's adaptation level" (p. 7). The outputs from the adaptive system are adaptive and ineffective responses. Andrews and Roy (1991a) explained that these responses "act as feedback or further input to the system, allowing the person to decide whether to increase or decrease efforts to cope with the stimuli" (pp. 7–8).

Characteristics of interaction models are also evident in the Roy Adaptation Model. The role function adaptive mode deals with the social integrity of the person. The characteristic of perception was incorporated in the discussion of the regulator and cognator mechanisms. In particular,

> Inputs to the regulator are transformed into perceptions. Perception is a process of the cognator. The responses following perception are feedback into both the cognator and regulator. (Roy & Roberts, 1981, p. 67)

Communication is not directly addressed by the Roy Adaptation Model. Role and self-concept are explicitly addressed through the adaptive modes of role function and self-concept. In fact, these modes were deliberately developed within the context of the interactionist viewpoint (Roy, 1989).

Meleis (1991) regarded the Roy Adaptation Model as an example of the outcomes school of thought and also categorized it as client-focused. Marriner-Tomey (1989) placed the model in the systems category. Barnum (1994) regarded the model as an example of her intervention category.

Content of the Model: Concepts

Person

"The recipient of nursing care," according to Andrews and Roy (1991a), "may be an individual, a family or group, a community, or society as a whole" (p. 6). Recipients of nursing care may be sick or well and may or may not be adapting positively (Roy, 1989).

The recipient of nursing care was specifically identified as an **adaptive system**. System is defined as "a set of parts connected to function as a whole for some purpose, and it does so by virtue of the interdependence of its parts" (Andrews & Roy, 1991a, p. 7). Adaptive "means that the human system has the capacity to adjust effectively to changes in the environment and, in turn, affects the environment" (Andrews & Roy, 1991a, p. 7).

The adaptive system is regarded as a holistic system. "Holistic pertains to the idea that the human system functions as a whole and is more than the mere sum of its parts" (Andrews & Roy, 1991a, pp. 6–7). The holistic adaptive system is regarded as an open system (Roy, 1984a).

The adaptive system has two major internal control processes, called the *regulator and cognator subsystems* (Andrews & Roy, 1991a). These subsystems are viewed as innate or acquired coping mechanisms used by the adaptive system to respond to changing internal and external environmental stimuli. Andrews and Roy (1991a) explained that "innate coping mechanisms are genetically determined or common to a species and are generally viewed as automatic processes; the person does not have to think about them . . . [whereas] acquired coping mechanisms are developed through processes such as learning" (p. 13).

The *regulator subsystem* "responds automatically through neural, chemical, and endocrine coping processes. Stimuli from the internal and external environment (through the senses) act as input to the nervous system and affect the fluid and electrolyte and endocrine systems. The information is channeled automatically in the appropriate manner and an automatic, unconscious response is produced" (Andrews & Roy, 1991a, p. 14). More specifically, "the internal and external stimuli are basically chemical or neural and act as inputs to the central nervous system and may be transduced into neural inputs. The spinal cord, brain stem, and autonomic reflexes act through effectors to produce automatic, unconscious effects on the body responses. The chemical stimuli in the circulation influence the endocrine glands to produce the appropriate hormone. The responsiveness of target organs or tissues then effects body responses. By some unknown process, the neural inputs are transformed into conscious perceptions in the brain. Eventually, this perception leads to psychomotor choices of response which activate a body response. These bodily responses, brought about through the chemical-neural-endocrine channels, are fed back as additional stimuli to the regulator" (Roy, 1984a, p. 31).

The *cognator subsystem* responds to inputs from external and internal stimuli that involve psychological, social, physical, and physiological factors, including regulator subsystem outputs. Andrews and Roy (1991a) explained that these stimuli are then processed "through four cognitive-emotive channels: perceptual/information processing, learning, judgment, and emotion" (p. 14). Elaborating, they stated, "Perceptual/information processing includes the activities of selective attention, coding, and memory. . . . Learning involves imitation, reinforcement, and insight whereas the judgment process encompasses such activities as problem solving and decision making. Through the person's emotions, defenses are used to seek relief from anxiety and to make affective appraisal and attachments" (p. 14).

Roy and Corliss (1993) went on to explain, "The cognitive-emotional processes of the cognator act within varying levels of consciousness as the person deals with internal and external states. [In contrast,] the neuro-chemical-endocrine processes of the regulator may be outside of consciousness, but provide the substrates of human conscious processes and actions" (p. 219).

Regulator and cognator activity is manifested through coping behavior in four **adaptive or response modes**. Behavior is regarded in its broadest sense as "internal or external actions and reactions under specified circumstances" (Andrews & Roy, 1991a, p. 12). The four adaptive modes of the Roy Adaptation Model are the *physiological mode*, the *self-concept mode*, the *role function mode*, and the *interdependence mode*. The regulator subsystem is related primarily to the physiological mode, and the cognator subsystem is related to all four modes (Roy & Roberts, 1981).

The four adaptive modes are predicated on the person's need for physiological integrity, psychic integrity, and social integrity. The *physiological mode* deals with the need for physiological integrity. This mode encompasses five basic physiological needs and four regulator processes. The physiological needs, hierarchically arranged, are oxygenation, nutrition, elimination, activity and rest, and protection. The regulator processes are the senses, fluids and electrolytes, neurological functions, and endocrine functions. "The physiological mode," Andrews and Roy (1991a) explained, "is associated with the way the person responds as a physical being to stimuli from the environment. Behavior in this mode is the manifestation of the physiological activities of all the cells, tissues, organs, and systems comprising the human body" (p. 15).

The *self-concept mode* focuses on the need for psychic integrity, that is, "the need to know who one is so that one can be or exist with a sense [of] unity" (Andrews & Roy, 1991a, p. 16). Self-concept is defined as "the composite of beliefs and feelings that a person holds about himself or herself at a given time" (Andrews & Roy, 1991a, p. 16). Self-concept is formed from internal perceptions and perceptions of others and directs the person's behavior. The self-concept mode encompasses perceptions of the physical and the personal self. The physical self deals with body sensation and body image. Body sensation refers to "how one feels and experiences oneself as a physical being," and body image refers to "how one views oneself physically and one's view of his or her appearance (Andrews, 1991b, p. 269). The personal self encompasses self-consistency, self-ideal, and the moral-ethical-spiritual self. Self-consistency refers to the striving "to maintain a consistent self-organization and thus to avoid disequilibrium" (Andrews, 1991b, p. 270). Self-ideal refers to "what one would like to be or is capable of doing" (Andrews 1991b, p. 271). The moral-ethical-spiritual self encompasses "one's belief system and an evaluation of who one is. . . . [and] that aspect of the personal self which functions as observer, standard-setter, dreamer, comparer, and most of all, evaluator of who this person says that he or she is" (Andrews, 1991b, pp. 270–271).

Andrews (1991b) explained that self-esteem, "the individual's perception of self-worth . . . [is] inherent in each component of the self-concept [mode]. . . . One's level of self-esteem reflects the self-concept and related behaviors give insight into adaptation in the self-concept mode" (pp. 270–272).

The role function mode emphasizes the need for social integrity, that is, "the need to know who one is in relation to others so that one can act" (Andrews & Roy, 1991a, p. 16). Roles are regarded as "the functioning units of society; . . . each role exists in relation to another [role]" (Andrews, 1991a, p. 348). Each role is associated with "a set of expectations about how a person behaves towards a person occupying the complementary position" (Andrews, 1991a, p. 348). People need to know who they are, that is, what roles they occupy, and the associated expectations about those roles so that they know how to act appropriately (Andrews, 1991a).

Roles are classified as primary, secondary, or tertiary. The primary role "determines the majority of behaviors engaged in by the person during a particular period of life. It is determined by age, sex, and developmental stage" (Andrews, 1991a, p. 349). An example of a primary role is a 53-year-old man who is in the developmental phase of generative adulthood. Secondary roles "are those that a person assumes to complete the tasks associated with a developmental stage and primary role. . . . Secondary roles are normally achieved positions as opposed to primary qualities and require specific role performance. They are typically stable and not readily relinquished since they are developed and mastered over a period of time" (Andrews, 1991a, p. 349). Examples of secondary roles are husband, artist, teacher.

Tertiary roles are "related primarily to secondary roles and represent ways in which individuals meet their role-associated obligations. . . . Tertiary roles are normally temporary in nature, freely chosen by the individual, and may include activities such as clubs or hobbies" (Andrews, 1991a, p. 349). An example is the role of Little League baseball coach associated with the secondary role of father.

Each role contains both instrumental and expressive components. The instrumental, or goal-oriented, component refers to "the actual physical performance of a behavior to achieve the goal of role mastery, [that is,] the demonstration of role behaviors that meet societal expectations" (Andrews, 1991a, pp. 348, 350). The expressive component refers to "the feelings, attitudes, likes, or dislikes that a person has about a role or about the performance of a role" (Andrews, 1991a, p. 348).

The interdependence mode also emphasizes the need for social integrity. Interdependence is "a way of maintaining integrity that involves the willingness and ability to love, respect, and value others, and to accept and respond to love, respect, and value given by others" (Roy, 1987c, p. 41). The giving of love, respect, and value in interdependent relationships is called contributive behavior and the receiving of love, respect, and value is called receptive behavior (Andrews & Roy, 1991a). The primary focus of the interdependence mode, according to Andrews and Roy (1991a), is affectional adequacy, defined as "the feeling of security in nurturing relationships" (p. 17). Significant others, "persons who are the most important to the individual," and support systems, "others contributing to the meeting of interdependence needs," are the two specific relationships of interest (Andrews & Roy, 1991a, p. 17).

Although the four modes are discussed separately, they are interrelated. In fact, "behavior in [one] mode may have an effect on or act as a stimulus for one or all of the other modes" (Andrews & Roy, 1991a, p. 17).

Environment

Andrews and Roy (1991a) defined **environment** as "all conditions, circumstances, and influences that surround and affect the development and behavior of the person" (p. 18). Environment is viewed as constantly changing and has internal and external components.

The internal and external environments, in the form of stimuli, are the inputs into the adaptive system. Following Helson (1964), Andrews and Roy (1991a) identified three classes of stimuli. The *focal stimulus* is "the internal or external stimulus most immediately confronting the person; the object or event that attracts one's attention" (p. 8). *Contextual stimuli* are "all other stimuli present in the situation that contribute to the effect of the focal stimulus. That is, . . . all the environmental factors that present to the person from within or without but which are not the center of the person's attention and/or energy. These factors will influence how the person can deal with the focal stimulus" (p. 9). The *residual stimuli* are "environmental factors within or without the person whose effects in the current situation are unclear. The person may not be aware of the influence of these factors, or it may not be clear to the observer that they are having an effect" (p. 9). More specifically, residual stimuli "are part of the person's interaction with the environment as the total cosmos, both elements within the person's awareness and those that are not, but are not easily analyzed as part of the current person-environment interaction [as focal and contextual stimuli]" (Roy & Corliss, 1993, p. 220). Residual stimuli become contextual stimuli or focal stimuli when their effects on the person are validated (Andrews & Roy, 1991b).

Roy and Corliss (1993) pointed out that the category of residual stimuli "is particularly compatible with [Roy's] philosophical assumptions about the person. . . . always being aware of a category for residual stimuli allows for the mystery in each person since each is unique within the common destiny and the nurse may not expect to know the other as the other knows self or is known by the Creator" (pp. 220–221).

The classification of a particular stimulus as focal, contextual, or residual changes as the situation changes. "What is focal at one time soon becomes contextual and what is contextual may slip far enough into the background to become residual, that is, just a possible influence" (Andrews & Roy, 1991a, p. 10).

Andrews and Roy (1991b) have identified categories of common stimuli, along with examples, that affect adaptation. The classification of any of these stimuli as focal, contextual, or residual depends on their influence on adaptation in a particular situation. The category of culture is exemplified by socioeconomic status, ethnicity, and the person's belief system. Examples for the category of family are structure and tasks. The developmental stage category is exemplified by age, sex, and tasks, as well as hereditary and genetic factors. Examples for the category of cognator effectiveness are perception, knowledge, and skill. The environmental category is exemplified by change in the internal or external environment, medical management, and the use of drugs, alcohol, and tobacco. Additional common stimuli fall into a category made up of relevant factors related to each of the four adaptive modes.

Person and Environment

"The person and environment are in constant interaction with each other" (Andrews & Roy, 1991a, p. 10). Consequently, further discussion of the environment requires consideration of that interaction:

> The changing environment stimulates the person to make adaptive responses. For human beings, life is never the same. It is constantly changing and presenting new challenges. The person has the ability to make new responses to these changing conditions. As the environment changes, the person has the opportunity to continue to grow, to develop, and to enhance the meaning of life for everyone. (Andrews & Roy, 1991a, p. 18)

The combined effects or pooling of the focal, contextual, and residual stimuli from the internal and external environments make up the person's **adaptation level**. Adaptation is regarded "as both a process and a state. As a process, it involves a systematic series of actions directed toward some end. . . . As a state, [it refers to] the condition of the person with respect to the environment. Taking time as a dimension of the environment, the person . . . may be viewed at a given time, and the state of adaptation may be described" (Artinian & Roy, 1990, p. 64). Adaptation level is "the constantly changing point that represents the person's ability to respond positively in a situation" (Andrews & Roy, 1991a, p. 10). The adaptation level depends on "the demands of the situation and the person's current internal conditions. . . . [More specifically,] ability to respond positively depends on all three types of stimuli and their current effect on the person" (Andrews & Roy, 1991a, p. 10).

Responses to environmental stimuli are adaptive or ineffective. **Adaptive responses** are "those that promote the integrity of the person in terms of the goals of adaptation: survival, growth, reproduction, and mastery" (Andrews & Roy, 1991a, p. 12). **Ineffective responses** are "those that neither promote integrity nor contribute to the goals of adaptation. That is, they may, in the immediate situation or if continued over a long time, threaten the person's survival, growth, reproduction, or mastery" (Andrews & Roy, 1991a, p. 12).

Roy (Artinian & Roy, 1990) has pointed out that she never intended that the goals of adaptation should be interpreted solely within a physiological context. Rather, she conceptualized these goals in a broader context. Reproduction, for example, "is not limited to a physiologic bringing forth of off-spring, but also is seen as generativity of other kinds, e.g., mentoring, producing works of art, and generating other accomplishments that actualize oneself" (p. 65).

Adaptive and ineffective responses occur for each component of each of the four adaptive modes. The responses, which are considered outputs from the adaptive system, are behaviors that reflect the activity of the regulator and cognator coping mechanisms. In a cyclical manner, the responses then act as feedback, which is further input for the system. Figure 9–1 illustrates the components of the person as an adaptive system. The diagram depicts the input of the focal, contextual, and residual stimuli, acting through the regulator and cognator coping mechanisms, to produce behavioral responses in the four interrelated adaptive modes.

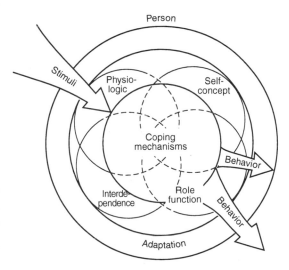

FIGURE 9–1. The person as an adaptive system. (From Roy, C., & Andrews, H.A. (1991). *The Roy adaptation model: The definitive statement* (p. 17). Norwalk, CT: Appleton & Lange, with permission.)

Adaptive behavioral responses, which promote the wholeness or integrity of the adaptive system, are depicted by the arrow that remains within the adaptation circle. Ineffective behavioral responses, which do not contribute to the wholeness or integrity of the adaptive system, are depicted by the arrow that extends beyond the adaptation circle.

Health

Health is defined as "a state and a process of being and becoming an integrated and whole person" (Andrews & Roy, 1991a, p. 19). "Being integrated," Roy (Artinian & Roy, 1990) explained, "is a state at any given point in time and may be described as such at that point in time. This state is reflective of the adaptation process. It is manifested by the wholeness and integration of physiologic components, self concept, role function, and interdependence" (p. 65). Roy (Artinian & Roy, 1990) went on to say, "Becoming is a process that is continuous and made up of the systematic series of actions directed toward some end. . . . This end [is] related to both individual goals and the purposefulness of human existence" (p. 65). A whole person, according to Andrews and Roy (1986), "is one with the highest possible fulfillment of human potential" (p. 8). They went on to explain that "a lack of integration [is] a lack of health" (p. 8).

The definition of health in the Roy Adaptation Model is linked to the interaction between the person and the environment, that is, to adaptation. Andrews and Roy (1991a) explained, "[The] person [is] described as an adaptive system constantly growing and developing within a changing environment. A person's health can be described as a reflection of this interaction or adaptation. . . . Health can be viewed in light of individual goals and the purposefulness of human existence. The fulfillment of one's purpose in life is reflected in becoming an integrated and whole person" (p. 19).

Roy and Corliss (1993) regard adaptation and health as "ongoing processes" (p. 221). They went on to explain that adaptation "is a process of promoting integrity, or one may also say that adaptation means interacting positively with the environment and thereby promoting health. One's health does not depend on the absence or presence of disease, rather it relates to use of the processes that lead to patterns of integrity of the person and the ability to move toward effective unity of the adaptive modes" (p. 221).

In recent publications, Roy (1987c; Artinian & Roy, 1990) has rejected her earlier conceptualization of health as a continuum from maximum wellness to maximum illness. In fact, she maintained that her view of health is not consistent with the notion of the health-illness continuum, because it "is a limited view and reflects a given point in time on a continuum" (1987c, p. 42). She noted that being and becoming integrated and whole may occur throughout life. Even "dying individuals are going through that process of final being and becoming where they are integrating themselves" (1987c, pp. 42–43). Now, Roy maintains that "it is more consistent with the model's scientific and philosophical assumptions to continue conceptual explication of the notion of health without reference to illness" (Artinian & Roy, 1990, p. 65).

Rather, it may be inferred that health is viewed as a dichotomy of adaptive and ineffective responses to the changing environment. This interpretation is supported by the definition of adaptive responses as those promoting integrity of the person and the definition of ineffective responses as those not contributing to integrity.

Nursing

Roy (1976a) defined nursing as "a theoretical system of knowledge which prescribes a process of analysis and action related to the care of the ill or potentially ill person" (p. 3). Furthermore, nursing is "a scientific discipline that is practice oriented" (Andrews & Roy, 1991b, p. 27). The Roy Adaptation Model stipulates that a nurse is needed "when unusual stresses or weakened coping mechanisms make the person's usual attempts to cope ineffective" (Roy & Roberts, 1981, p. 45).

Roy distinguished nursing from medicine by noting that medicine focuses on biological systems and the person's disease, whereas nursing focuses on the person as a total being who responds to internal and external environmental stimuli (Roy 1970; Roy & Roberts, 1981). This distinction is elaborated further by a comparison of the goals of medicine and nursing. The physician's goal is "to move the patient along the continuum from illness to health" (Roy, 1970, p. 43). The **goal of nursing** is the "*promotion of adaptation in each of the four [adaptive] modes*, thereby contributing to the person's health, quality of life, and dying with dignity" (Andrews & Roy, 1991a, p. 20). Furthermore, "nursing aims to increase the person's adaptive response and to decrease ineffective responses" (Roy, 1984a, p. 37).

Roy recognizes that "complete physical, mental, and social well-being, the common understanding of optimal health, is not possible for every person. It is the nurse's role to promote adaptation in situations of health and illness; to enhance the interaction of the person with [the] environment, thereby promoting health" (Andrews & Roy, 1991a, p. 20).

The goal of nursing was placed within the context of the overall goal of the health team in the following manner:

> The projected outcome [of nursing] is an adapted state in the patient which frees him to respond to other stimuli. This freeing of energy makes it possible for the goal of nursing to contribute to the overall goal of the health team, high-level wellness. When energy is freed from inadequate coping attempts, then it can promote healing and wellness. (Roy & Roberts, 1981, p. 45)

The Roy Adaptation Model includes a detailed **nursing process**, which is defined as "a problem-solving approach for gathering data, identifying the person's needs, selecting and implementing approaches for nursing care, and evaluating the outcomes of care being given" (Andrews & Roy, 1991b, p. 27). The nursing process encompasses six steps: *assessment of behavior, assessment of stimuli, nursing diagnosis, goal setting, intervention,* and *evaluation.*

Assessment of behavior involves collection of data regarding the person's observable and nonobservable behaviors. The behavior of particular interest to the nurse is that which "requires further adaptive response as a result of environmental changes straining the person's coping mechanisms" (Andrews & Roy, 1991b, p. 29). Behavior emanating from each of the four adaptive modes is considered. The methods of assessment include direct observation of behavior; objective measurement of behavior using appropriate tools, such as paper and pencil instruments and measures of physiological parameters; and interviewing to obtain subjective reports (Andrews & Roy, 1991b).

Once the data are collected, the nurse must judge whether the behavior is adaptive or ineffective. The judgment of adaptive or ineffective behavior takes the person's perception into account. "In making the initial judgment as to whether behavior is adaptive or ineffective, it is important that the nurse continually involve the person for whom she is caring. The person's perception of the effectiveness of the behavior is an integral consideration" (Andrews & Roy, 1991b, p. 32). Judgments are based on the person's individualized goals as well as on a comparison of the person's behavior with norms, established through research and cultural expectation, that signify adaptation. In the areas where norms have not been established, general signs of adaptation difficulty are used as a basis for comparison. These signs, according to Andrews and Roy (1991b), are identified as "pronounced regulator activity with cognator ineffectiveness" (p. 32). Some manifestations of pronounced regulator activity are increase in heart rate or blood pressure, tension, excitement, loss of appetite, and increase in serum cortisol. Manifestations of cognator ineffectiveness include faulty perceptual/information processing, ineffective learning, poor judgment, and inappropriate affect.

The first step of the nursing process ends and the second step begins with setting priorities for further assessment of behaviors. "The primary concern," according to Andrews and Roy (1991b), "would be the behaviors that are disrupting the person's integrity and not promoting adaptation" (p. 32). A more specific schema of priorities, which is based on the goals of the adaptive system, was offered by Roy (1984a). The first priority is behaviors that threaten the survival of the adaptive system; the second priority is behaviors that affect the growth of the adaptive system; the third priority is behaviors that affect the continuation of the human race or of society; and the fourth priority is behaviors that affect the attainment of full potential for the adaptive system.

The second step of the nursing process is *assessment of stimuli*. This step involves "the identification of internal and external stimuli that are influencing the behaviors" identified in the first step (Andrews & Roy, 1991b, p. 33). Ineffective behaviors are of interest because the nurse wants to change them to adaptive behaviors, and adaptive behaviors are of interest because the nurse wants to maintain or enhance them. Furthermore, "in situations where all presenting behaviors appear adaptive, it may be necessary to carry out [assessment of stimuli] to identify potential threats to that adaptation" (K. Des Rosiers, cited in Roy, 1984a, p. 51).

The assessment focuses on identification of the focal, contextual, and residual stimuli that influence the behaviors of interest and contribute to adaptive or ineffective responses. Stimuli are identified for each relevant behavior in the order of priority set at the end of the first nursing process step.

Logan (1990) maintained that "stimuli must be amenable to independent nurse functions" (p. 469). She contended that it would be inappropriate to label such factors as medical diagnoses and medical treatments as stimuli because these factors cannot be independently managed by nurses.

Roy (1984a) advocated continued participation of the person in the assessment of stimuli. She suggested using Orlando's (1961) deliberative nursing process to validate the relevant stimuli with the person. Accordingly, the nurse should share her ideas of influencing factors with the person and receive confirmation or discuss the person's perception of the situation until agreement is reached.

The third step of the Roy Adaptation Model nursing process is *nursing diagnosis*, which is defined as "a judgment process resulting in a statement conveying the person's adaptation status" (Andrews & Roy, 1991b, p. 37). Three approaches to nursing diagnosis are offered by Andrews and Roy (1991b): "(1) a statement of the behaviors within one mode with their most relevant influencing stimuli, (2) a summary label for behaviors in one mode with relevant stimuli, or (3) a label that summarizes a behavioral pattern when more than one mode is being affected by the same stimuli" (p. 37). Andrews and Roy (1991b) pointed out that each alternative has utility in particular situations. They regard the first two methods as the most appropriate ones to illustrate the typology of indicators of positive adaptation and the related adaptation problems (Table 9–1) but noted that the third method "is consistent with the efforts of the profession [of nursing] to develop a language of diagnosis whereby nurses can communicate regarding the unique services they provide" (p. 39).

The fourth step of the nursing process is *goal setting*, which is defined as "the establishment of clear statements of the behavioral outcomes of nursing care for the person" (Andrews & Roy, 1991b, p. 42). The goals for nursing care are established from the behavioral description of the person's situation developed through the first three steps of the nursing process. Goals are explicitly stated as short-term and long-term behavioral outcomes that are thought to promote adaptation. More specifically, "a goal statement should designate not only the behavior to be observed but the manner in which the behavior will change (as observed, measured, or subjectively reported), and the time frame in which the goal is to be attained" (Andrews & Roy, 1991b, p. 43). Goals may be stated for ineffective behaviors that are to be changed to adaptive behaviors and also for adaptive behaviors that should be maintained or enhanced. Andrews and Roy (1991b) underscored the importance of actively involving the person in the formation of behavioral goals if that is possible. "This involvement provides the nurse with the opportunity to explore the rationale behind certain goals and gives the person the chance to suggest goals and evaluate whether others are realistic. A person who is actively involved in the formulation of goals is more likely to be committed to attainment of [each] goal" (pp. 43–44).

The fifth step of the nursing process is *intervention*. This step involves management of relevant focal and contextual stimuli to achieve the stated goals for nursing care. Management encompasses "altering, increasing, decreasing, removing, or maintaining" relevant focal and/or contextual stimuli (Andrews & Roy, 1991b, p. 44). The focal stimulus is selected for management whenever possible because it is the primary influence on the behaviors of interest. If it is not possible to alter the focal stimulus, contextual stimuli are to be managed to raise the adaptation level. Andrews and Roy (1991b) advocated using the nursing judgment method outlined by McDonald and Harms (1966) as a basis for selection of which stimuli to change. They explained that in the McDonald and Harms method, "possible approaches are listed and the approach with the highest probability of attaining the goal is selected. In applying this method to the Roy model, the stimuli affecting specific behavior are listed. Next the consequences of changing each stimulus are identified together with the probability of their occurrence. The value of the consequence is judged as *desirable* or *undesirable*. This is accomplished in collaboration with the person, when possible and appropriate" (p. 45). Andrews and Roy (1991b) went on to say, "Once the most appropriate approach to nursing intervention has been selected, the nurse must determine and initiate the steps that will serve to alter the stimulus appropriately" (p. 46).

The sixth and final step of the nursing process is *evaluation* of the effectiveness of nursing intervention. The criterion for effectiveness of nursing intervention is whether the desired goal was attained, that is, whether the person exhibited adaptive behavior after the nursing intervention was performed. In particular, "The criterion for judging when the goal has been reached is generally any positive response made by the recipient to the stimuli present that frees energy for responses to other stimuli. This criterion must be applied to each specific instance of nursing intervention for which a special goal of adaptation has been set" (Roy, 1989, p. 109). The extent to which the behavior reflects the goals is determined by means of reassessment of behaviors, using the same skills of sensitive observation, measurement, and interview that were used in the first step of the nursing process.

If the goals are attained and if there is no threat that the behavior will become ineffective again, then that behavior may be deleted from nursing concern (Roy, 1984a). If, however, the goals are not attained, "the nurse must proceed to discover what went wrong. The goals may have been unrealistic or unacceptable to the person, the assessment data may have been inaccurate or incomplete, or the selected approaches may not have been carried out properly. The nurse returns to the first step of the nursing process to look closely at behaviors that continue to be ineffective and to try to further understand the situation" (Andrews & Roy, 1991b, p. 47). The end result of the sixth step is an update of the nursing care plan.

The Roy Adaptation Model nursing process is summarized in Table 9–2.

Content of the Model: Propositions

The metapardigm concepts of person, environment, and health are linked in the following statements:

> The changing environment stimulates the person to make adaptive responses. (Andrews & Roy, 1991a, p. 18)

> [The] person [is] described as an adaptive system constantly growing and developing within a changing environment. A person's health can be described as a reflection of this interaction or adaptation. (Andrews & Roy, 1991a, p. 19)

The metaparadigm concepts of person, health, and nursing are linked in the following statements:

> The goal of nursing [is] the promotion of adaptation in each of the four [adaptive] modes, thereby contributing to the person's health, quality of life, and dying with dignity. (Andrews & Roy, 1991a, p. 20)

> The goal of nursing intervention is to maintain and enhance adaptive behavior and to change ineffective behavior to adaptive. (Andrews & Roy, 1991b, p. 42)

The linkage of all four metaparadigm concepts are presented in this statement:

> It is the nurse's role to promote adaptation in situations of health and illness; to enhance the interaction of the person with [the] environment, thereby promoting adaptation. (Andrews & Roy, 1991a, p. 20)

EVALUATION OF ROY'S ADAPTATION MODEL

This section presents an evaluation of the Roy Adaptation Model. The evaluation is based on the results of the analysis of the conceptual model

TABLE 9–2. **SUMMARY OF THE NURSING PROCESS FOR THE ROY ADAPTATION MODEL**

I. Assessment of behaviors
   A. Methods used to collect data
      1. Observation
         a. Sight
         b. Sound
         c. Touch
         d. Taste
         e. Smell
      2. Objective measurement
         a. Paper and pencil instruments
         b. Measures of physiological parameters
      3. Interviews
   B. Behaviors to assess
      1. Physiological mode
         a. Oxygenation
         b. Nutrition
         c. Elimination
         d. Activity and rest
         e. Protection
         f. The senses
         g. Fluid and electrolytes
         h. Neurological functions
         i. Endocrine functions
      2. Self-concept mode
         a. Physical self
            (1) Body image
            (2) Body sensation
         b. Personal self
            (1) Self-consistency
            (2) Self-ideal
            (3) Moral-ethical-spiritual self
      3. Role function
         a. Primary role
            (1) Instrumental component(s)
            (2) Expressive component(s)
         b. Secondary roles
            (1) Instrumental component(s)
            (2) Expressive component(s)
         c. Tertiary roles
            (1) Instrumental component(s)
            (2) Expressive component(s)
      4. Interdependence mode
         a. Significant others
            (1) Contributive behavior
            (2) Receptive behavior
         b. Social support
            (1) Contributive behavior
            (2) Receptive behavior
   C. Judgment of behaviors
      1. Adaptive or ineffective responses
         a. Nurse's judgment
         b. Person's perception
      2. Criteria for judgment
         a. Person's individualized goals
         b. Comparison of behavior with norms signifying adaptation
         c. Regulator mechanism activity
         d. Cognator mechanism effectiveness

TABLE 9–2. **SUMMARY OF THE NURSING PROCESS FOR THE ROY ADAPTATION MODEL** (Continued)

II. Assessment of stimuli
  A. Criteria for priorities for further assessment of the person's behaviors
    1. Behaviors that threaten the survival of the individual, family, group, or community
    2. Behaviors that affect the growth of the individual, family, group, or community
    3. Behaviors that affect the continuation of the human race or of society
    4. Behaviors that affect the attainment of full potential for the individual or group
  B. Methods used to determine influence of stimuli
    1. Observation
    2. Objective measurement
    3. Interview
    4. Validate hunch about relevant stimuli with the person
  C. Stimuli
    1. Focal stimulus
    2. Contextual stimuli
      a. Culture
        (1) Socioeconomic status
        (2) Ethnicity
        (3) Belief system
      b. Family structure and tasks
      c. Developmental stage
        (1) Age
        (2) Sex
        (3) Tasks
        (4) Heredity
        (5) Genetic factors
      d. Integrity of adaptive modes
        (1) Physiological mode and disease pathology
        (2) Self-concept
        (3) Role function
        (4) Interdependence
      e. Cognator effectiveness
        (1) Perception
        (2) Knowledge
        (3) Skill
      f. Environmental considerations
        (1) Change in internal or external environment
        (2) Medical management
        (3) Use of drugs, alcohol, tobacco
    3. Residual stimuli
      a. Beliefs
      b. Attitudes
      c. Traits
      d. Cultural determinants
III. Nursing diagnosis
  A. Three approaches
    1. State behaviors within each adaptive mode and with their most relevant influencing stimuli
    2. Provide a summary label for behaviors in each adaptive mode with relevant stimuli
    3. Provide a label that summarizes a behavioral pattern across adaptive modes that is affected by the same stimuli
  B. Arrange diagnoses in order of priority using criteria in II.A.
IV. Goal setting
  A. Statement of behavioral outcomes of nursing intervention
  B. Determine that the person agrees with goal
V. Nursing Intervention
  A. Management of stimuli
    1. Alter stimuli

(Continued)

TABLE 9–2. **SUMMARY OF THE NURSING PROCESS
FOR THE ROY ADAPTATION MODEL** (Continued)

---

      2. Increase stimuli
      3. Decrease stimuli
      4. Remove stimuli
      5. Maintain stimuli
   B. Priorities
      1. Manage focal stimulus first if possible
      2. Manage contextual stimuli next
   C. Selection of nursing intervention approach
      1. List possible approaches
      2. Outline consequences of management of each stimulus
      3. Determine probability for each consequence
      4. Judge value of outcomes of each approach
      5. Share options with the person
      6. Select approach with highest probability of reaching valued goal
VI. Evaluation
   A. Methods used
      1. Observation
      2. Objective measurement
      3. Interview
   B. Criteria for judgment of effectiveness of nursing intervention
      1. Goal attained or not attained
      2. Person does or does not manifest behavior stated in goal

---

Constructed from Roy, C., & Andrews, H.A. (1991). *The Roy adaptation model: The definitive statement* (pp. 29–47). Norwalk, CT: Appleton & Lange.

as well as on publications by others who have used or commented on Roy's work.

Explication of Origins

Roy has explicated the origins of the Roy Adaptation Model clearly and concisely. She chronicled the development of the model over time and identified her motivation to formulate a conceptual model of nursing. Furthermore, she explicitly stated her philosophical claims in the form of scientific and philosophical assumptions about the person and values about the goal of nursing.

The statements that Roy (1989) labeled as scientific assumptions actually are propositions that define, describe, and link the concepts of the conceptual model. Strictly speaking, then, these statements are not assumptions upon which the model was based. The scientific assumptions as related by Roy and Corliss (1993) are, however, in the form of philosophical claims.

Roy assumes that people are integrated wholes capable of action, and she values the active participation of persons in their nursing care. She noted that although participation may not always be possible, as in the case of infants and unconscious or suicidal patients, the nurse "is constantly aware of the active responsibility of the patient to participate in his own care when he is able to do so" (Roy & Roberts, 1981, p. 47).

Roy acknowledged the nurses and other scholars whose works influenced her thinking. Moreover, she provided bibliographic citations to the works that were especially relevant and explained how each one contributed to the development of the Roy Adaptation Model.

Comprehensiveness of Content

Roy addressed each of the metaparadigm concepts explicitly and adequately for the level of abstraction of a conceptual model. Person is fully defined and described. Although some difficulty has been reported in distinguishing the adaptive mode to which a particular behavior belongs, especially in the self-concept, role function, and interdependence modes (Wagner, 1976), refinements in the Roy Adaptation Model have begun to clarify the focus of each adaptive mode. Roy (1987c) explained, "Through many revisions with input from educators, clinicians, and theory critics, the physiological mode has been reorganized, and can now be used for nursing assessment and the organization of curriculum content" (p. 39). She went on to say, "The content changes in the interdependence mode have been significant over the last couple of years. This allows interdependence to be distinguished from self-concept and role function" (p. 41).

Environment is defined sufficiently for a conceptual model. The distinction between the internal and external environments, however, is not always clear. Acknowledging this, Roy and Roberts (1981) commented: "Further clarification of environment as distinct from internal stimuli awaits additional theoretical work on the model" (p. 43). Additional work is also needed to describe the nature of environmental change. Further development of the concept of environment was undertaken by Randell, Poush-Tedrow, and Van Landingham (1982). Roy (1982) acknowledged that the introduction of the ideas of transaction and perception in their treatment of environment has expanded the conceptual model.

Health is clearly defined and is discussed in terms of adaptation, adaptation level, and adaptive and ineffective responses. Given that Roy (1987c) regarded the health-illness continuum as a limited viewpoint, it is not surprising that she gave no explicit definitions of wellness or illness. Although it is tempting to interpret adaptive responses as signifying wellness and ineffective responses as signifying illness, it is unclear whether Roy would agree with such an interpretation. Consequently, the exact meanings of the two types of responses with regard to health state need to be clarified to avoid confusion and misinterpretations.

Clarification is also required with regard to the use of the term illness in the vocabulary of the Roy Adaptation Model. A lack of consistency is noted between Roy's 1990 (Artinian & Roy, 1990) journal article and her 1991 text (Roy & Andrews, 1991). In the 1990 article, she stated that further explication of health should be "without reference to illness" (p. 65). Yet references to "situations of health and illness" (e.g., p. 20) appear in the 1991 text, which is regarded as "the definitive statement" about the model (p. xvii).

Another point about health that requires clarification is the connection between needs and responses. Roy (1987b) pointed out that the notion of needs was omitted from her 1984a discussion of the person as an adaptive system; yet she discussed and diagrammed the source of difficulty for the person as originating with a need excess or deficit in her 1989 book chapter. Furthermore, "identifying the person's needs" (p. 29) is part of the definition of the Roy Adaptation Model nursing process given in the 1991 Roy and Andrews text.

Still another point about health that requires clarification is the notion of the zone of adaptation. This term is included in the list of scientific assumptions, is diagrammed in Roy's 1989 book chapter, and is mentioned in the 1991 Roy and Andrews book (e.g., p. 29). The term is not, however, defined or described, and it is not listed in the index of the 1991 book.

The concept of nursing is defined and described clearly. The goal of nursing is articulated, and the nursing process is described in considerable detail. The Roy Adaptation Model nursing process is consistent with scientific findings on human behavior. A major concern in relation to the scientific basis of the Roy Adaptation Model, however, is the fact that the model was derived from Helson's (1964) work on adaptation, which was limited to investigation of the responses of the retina of the eye to environmental stimuli. The generalizability of Helson's findings to the whole person has not been firmly established. Thus, the credibility of the basic premise of the model—the person as an adaptive system—has not yet been supported.

Roy has consistently maintained that nursing science should provide the basis for the selection of behaviors to observe when assessing the adaptive system. Furthermore, judgments about the behaviors should be based on explicit criteria drawn from existing scientific knowledge, and interventions with the highest probability of empirically documented success should be selected.

The nursing process is dynamic in that the steps are "ongoing and simultaneous" (Andrews & Roy, 1991b, p. 29). Moreover, the results of the last step, evaluation, lead to the first step, assessment of behaviors, and subsequent updating of the nursing care plan.

Roy's insistence that the person be an active participant in the decision-making aspects of the nursing process attests to her concern for ethical standards of nursing practice. Indeed, "Collaboration with the person in each step of the nursing process is important. Individuals must be involved in observation of and decisions relative to their state of adaptation. They provide valuable insight that may assist the nurse in attempts to promote adaptation" (Andrews & Roy, 1991b, p. 28). Furthermore, the nursing process is consistent with the American Nurses' Association Standards of Practice (Roy & Roberts, 1981).

The Roy Adaptation Model is sufficiently comprehensive with regard to breadth of content. The model is equally applicable to individuals, families, groups, communities, or society as a whole in diverse situations of health and illness.

The comprehensiveness of the breadth of content of the Roy Adaptation Model is further supported by the direction it provides for research, education, administration, and practice. Rules for each area are being formulated.

Research, according to Roy (1988b), is directed toward the development of both basic nursing science and clinical nursing science. "The basic science of nursing focuses on human life processes as the core of knowledge to be developed. . . . The clinical science of nursing is based on the basic science of nursing as well as on the history and philosophy of nursing, which includes a strong ethical heritage. It [is directed toward the development of] substantive knowledge related to the diagnosis and treatment of the patterning of the life processes in wellness and traditional life situations, in chronic and acute illness, and particularly in life situations when the positive [adaptive] processes are threatened by health technologies and behaviorally induced health problems" (pp. 27–28).

Rules for Roy Adaptation Model–based research have been articulated by Fawcett and Downs (1992) and extended by Roy's comments about research. The phenomena to be studied include basic life processes and how nursing maintains or enhances adaptive responses or changes ineffective responses to adaptive responses in the areas of basic physiological needs and complex processes, self-concept, role function, and interdependence behaviors. Researchers are directed to study problems in adaptation to constantly changing environmental stimuli. The purpose of Roy Adaptation Model–based research is to describe how people adapt to environmental stimuli, explain how adaptive processes affect health, and predict the effects of nursing interventions on adaptive life processes and functioning.

Research subjects may be individuals or groups who are well or who have acute or chronic illnesses. Data can be gathered in any health care setting. Research is designed to yield basic knowledge about "the person and group as adaptive systems, their central processes, and modes [of adaptation]" (Artinian & Roy, 1990, p. 66), with emphasis on coping strategies that promote adaptation to constantly changing environmental stimuli. Research is also designed to yield clinical knowledge of the diagnosis of adaptive and ineffective responses and the effects of nursing intervention designed to promote adaptation (Artinian & Roy, 1990). Both qualitative and quantitative approaches can be used (Roy, 1991a). Research instruments should reflect the unique focus and intent of the Roy Adaptation Model. Indeed, Roy (Artinian & Roy, 1990) noted that although "some common tools measuring psychosocial or physiologic variables may be useful . . . they need content validity established within the context of the adaptation situation" (p. 6). Data analysis techniques encompass qualitative content analysis and nonparametric and parametric statistical procedures. Roy Adaptation Model–based research enhances understanding of the person's use of coping mechanisms and the role of nursing intervention in the promotion of adaptation to constantly changing environmental stimuli.

Rules for nursing education can be extracted from the content and focus of the Roy Adaptation Model and from Roy's publications. The distinctive focus of the curriculum is the responses of adaptive systems to constantly changing environmental stimuli. The purpose of nursing education is to prepare adaptation nurses by providing opportunities for students "to develop the knowledge of nursing science and the skills for nursing practice" (Roy, 1979b, p. 17).

The content of the curriculum is based on components of the Roy Adaptation Model (Roy, 1979b). The vertical strands of the curriculum focus on theory and practice. The theory strand encompasses content on the adapting person, health/illness, and stress/disruption. The practice strand emphasizes nursing management of environmental stimuli. The horizontal strands include the nursing process and student adaptation and leadership. The curricular sequence for a baccalaureate nursing program could begin with a sophomore year course that introduces the student to the content of the Roy Adaptation Model and the role of the nurse. The nursing process emphasizes identification of behaviors. Junior year courses would then focus on nursing science and medical science. The nursing process progresses to an emphasis on assessment of behavior and common stimuli and intervention using known approaches to the management of stimuli. Senior year courses would focus on nursing theory, nursing application, and issues in health care. The nursing process progresses to assessment of behavior and complex stimuli and creative approaches to the management of stimuli.

The Roy Adaptation Model is an appropriate curriculum guide for nursing problems offered by hospital-based schools of nursing, community colleges, and universities. Thus, the model may be used to guide curricula for diploma, associate degree, and baccalaureate and higher degree programs. Students would have to meet the requirements for admission to the relevant nursing program. Moreover, students must have the ability to adapt to a variety of stimuli in the educational environment. Camooso, Greene, and Reilly (1981) maintained that student adaptation is facilitated by "faculty and peer support and personal awareness of the factors involved" (p. 109).

Morales-Mann and Logan (1990) pointed out that teaching and learning strategies should be compatible with the Roy Adaptation Model. They strongly recommended that nursing process tools should incorporate the components of the model. In addition, they suggested that an introductory course could include such teaching strategies as exposing students to the views of experts in adjunctive disciplines and to the notions of general system theory before presenting the content of the Roy Adaptation Model, contracting with an adult client in the community to develop a nursing care plan that includes interventions to maintain health or correct existing problems, small group (15 or fewer students) seminars, group discussions, individual faculty-student consultations, and pen and paper tests.

Morales-Mann and Logan (1990) also recommended using the hospital record "as a source of information rather than a guide for care" (p. 146) when practice at the clinical agency is not based on the Roy Adaptation Model. Baldwin and Schaffer (1990) recommended the use of a continuing case study dealing with a fictional extended family throughout the academic year. Porth (1977) pointed out that the physiological mode content can be taught effectively by asking students to consider "why . . . the body need[s] to exhibit a particular set of physiological coping behaviors" (p. 782).

Rules for nursing administration were formulated by Fawcett, Botter, Burritt, Crossley, and Frink (1989) and extended by the work of Roy and Anway (1989). The distinctive focus and purpose of nursing in a clinical agency are provision of nursing services designed to promote patient adaptation in the physiological, self-concept, role function, and interdependence modes. The specific goal of nursing service management is "to ensure the most effective delivery of services to clients by adapting organization systems and their resources" (Roy & Anway, 1989, p. 78).

The collective nursing staff is viewed as an adaptive system in an environment of constantly changing internal and external conditions. The department of nursing or the entire health care institution also may be viewed as an adaptive system. Consequently, the nursing personnel, the department, and the institution must possess individual and collective abilities to adapt to the changing environmental conditions. Roy (1991b) advocated a differentiation of nursing personnel on the basis of knowledge of the Roy Adaptation Model, rather than by educational level or institutional definitions. The two levels of personnel are the general health care aide and the professional nurse. The aide has "public information, common sense, and basic instruction about persons and their needs related to the adaptive modes [that] can be turned to use in assisting professionals in providing care based on individual pattern maintenance" (pp. 37–38). Professional nurses are differentiated from aides and each other on the basis of their knowledge. At the first level, the professional nurse "may deal more specifically [than the aide] with developing patterns such as growth and development, eating, and sleeping" (p. 38). At the next level, the professional nurse is "prepared to deal with complex changes in patterns . . . [and] also could specialize in understanding given processes for particular populations" (p. 38). The highest level of professional nurse "conducts research related to the structure of knowledge and examines new patterns and processes that emerge in the evolving person-environment interactions," including societal processes that affect the health of entire populations (p. 38). The settings for nursing services encompass most types of clinical agencies and most specialty practice areas.

Management strategies emphasize promotion of staff, departmental, or institutional adaptation to constantly changing environmental stimuli. "The goal of the nurse manager," according to Roy and Anway (1989), "is to contain the stimulus within the organization's adaptive zone or in a positive sense, to broaden the range" (p. 83). In other words, the nurse manager strives to maintain or enhance the health of the organization. Roy and Anway (1989) noted that the managerial process emphasizes "planning, organizing, staffing, leading, and controlling. . . . Goal setting in management . . . is considered a key aspect of effective managerial activity" (p. 79). DiIorio (1989) added that the nurse manager assesses behaviors related to planning, organizing, staffing, leading, and controlling; identifies relevant focal, contextual, and residual stimuli; develops an administratively oriented nursing diagnosis; sets goals; intervenes by changing the focal stimulus, managing the contextual stimuli, and broadening the adaptation level; and evaluates the outcomes of intervention.

Rules for nursing practice stem from Roy's (1987a) view of nursing as a practice discipline and from the content of the Roy Adaptation Model. Roy commented, "As a practice discipline, nursing focuses on nursing's function of promoting adaptation, that is, nursing diagnoses, interventions, and outcomes for persons or groups. Nursing as a practice discipline can be seen from the point of view of the role of the nurse. Model-based practice helps look at how nursing models are taught. It sheds light on the content of nursing" (p. 44).

The purpose of nursing practice is to promote the person's adaptation in the physiological, self-concept, role function, and interdependence modes. "The nurse helps the person manage his or her environment, to effect appropriate adaptive responses" (Roy & Anway, 1989, p. 78). Clinical problems encompass adaptive and ineffective responses in the four adaptive modes (Table 9–1). Nursing practice extends from a focus on individuals to families and other groups, communities, and even to society. Legitimate recipients of nursing care may be sick or well and may or may not manifest specific adaptation problems. Settings for nursing practice include virtually every type of health care institution, people's homes, and the community at large.

The nursing process encompasses assessment of behavior in the four adaptive modes, assessment of focal, contextual, and residual stimuli, nursing diagnosis, goal setting, intervention, and evaluation. Nursing intervention takes the form of management of stimuli by altering, increasing, decreasing, removing, or maintaining the relevant focal and/or contextual stimuli. Intervention is judged to be effective when ineffective responses become adaptive or when previously adaptive responses remain adaptive. Nursing practice contributes to the well-being of individuals and collectives by maintaining or enhancing the level of adaptation.

Logical Congruence

The Roy Adaptation Model is generally logically congruent. Roy and Roberts (1981) began to translate the essentially reaction world view idea of adaptation to a view that is more in keeping with the reciprocal interaction world view. They stated, "This notion of adaptation does not negate the fact that humans do not merely respond to stimuli in the environment, but can take the initiative to change the environment" (p. 45). Elaborating, Roy and Corliss (1993) explained, "The use of the term stimuli sometimes has been misinterpreted as related to the framework of behaviorism. The language of behaviorism was in wide use during early stages of the Roy model development, however, it was clear from the beginning that Roy used the classes of stimuli to describe the complexity of the environment taken in by the person, and never referred to stimulus-response effects" (p. 220). Moreover, Roy and Corliss (1993) pointed out that the scientific assumptions of the Roy Adaptation Model "established belief in holism and in the person as the initiator of adaptive processes. The patterning of these processes in exchange with the environment allows one's adaptive abilities to provide the dynamic energy for health and effective living" (p. 217).

A logical inconsistency is noted, however, in Roy and Corliss's (1993) characterization of cognator processes as acting within "varying levels of consciousness" and regulator processes as "outside of consciousness" (p. 219). Without clarification, the term consciousness is associated with the reaction world view notions contained in psychoanalytic theory.

Sellers (1991) maintains that the Roy Adaptation Model "proposes a nursing philosophy of scientific realism and behaviorism" (p. 150). She went on to say that the model puts forth a conceptualization of the person that reflects "the mechanistic, deterministic, persistence world view . . . and a view of person as a passive, reactive participant in the human-environment relationship" (pp. 150–151). Her conclusions are in sharp contrast to those reached in this chapter, as noted in the section on world view. Furthermore, Roy (1988b) dismissed the charge that the conceptual model reflects a mechanistic view of the person and the environment. She explained that "the complexities and subtleties of the process whereby the person takes in and responds to the environment preclude such a behavioristic interpretation" of her use of the terms stimuli and behavior (p. 32). Moreover, adaptation "is far from being a passive process, because the adaptation level includes all the person's capabilities, hopes, dreams, aspirations, and motivations, in other words, all that makes the person constantly move toward greater mastery" (Artinian & Roy, 1990, p. 64).

Generation of Theory

The Roy Adaptation Model has generated a general **Theory of the Person as an Adaptive System** and individual theories of the four adaptive modes: the **Theory of the Physiological Mode**, the **Theory of the Self-Concept Mode**, the **Theory of the Role Function Mode**, and the **Theory of the Interdependence Mode** (Roy & Roberts, 1981). Roy (1984a, 1987a) pointed out that her distinctions between conceptual models and theories are based on form and function rather than on levels of abstraction, as is the case in this book. However, the work presented by Roy and Roberts (1981) clearly is directed toward development of middle-range theories as defined in this book.

The **Theory of the Person as an Adaptive System** considers the person holistically. The major concepts are system, adaptation, regulator subsystem, and cognator subsystem (Roy & Roberts, 1981). The regulator and cognator subsystems are explained in considerable detail through sets of propositions. Following are the basic regulator subsystem propositions:

> 1.1. Internal and external stimuli are basically chemical or neural; chemical stimuli may be transduced into neural inputs to the central nervous system.
>
> 1.2. Neural pathways to and from the central nervous system must be intact and functional if neural stimuli are to influence body responses.
>
> 2.1. Spinal cord, brainstem, and autonomic reflexes act through effectors to produce automatic, unconscious effects on the body responses.
>
> 3.1. The circulation must be intact for chemical stimuli to influence endocrine glands to produce the appropriate hormone.
>
> 3.2. Target organs and tissues must be able to respond to hormone levels to effect body responses.
>
> 4.1. Neural inputs are transformed into conscious perceptions in the brain (process unknown).
>
> 4.2. Increase in short-term or long-term memory will positively influence the effective choice of psychomotor response to neural input.
>
> 4.3. Effective choice of response, retained in long-term memory, will facilitate future effective choice of response.
>
> 4.4. The psychomotor response chosen will determine the effectors activated and the ultimate body response.
>
> 5.1. The body response resulting from regulator processes is fed back into the system. (Roy, personal communication, September 22, 1982; Roy & Roberts, 1981, p. 62)

Additional regulator subsystem propositions link the basic propositions. These linked propositions are:

The magnitude of the internal and external stimuli will positively influence the magnitude of the physiological response of an intact system. (1.1 through 2.1, 3.2, 4.4)

Intact neural pathways will positively influence neural output to effectors. (3.1 through 2.1, 4.4)

Chemical and neural inputs will influence normally responsive endocrine glands to hormonally influence target organs in a positive manner to maintain a state of dynamic equilibrium. (1.1 through 3.2)

The body's response to external and internal stimuli will alter those external and internal stimuli. (1.1 through 5.1)

The magnitude of the external and internal stimuli may be so great that the adaptive systems cannot return the body to a state of dynamic equilibrium. (1.1 through 5.1) (Roy & Roberts, 1981, p. 62)

The cognator subsystem propositions are:

1.1. The optimum amount and clarity of input of internal and external stimuli positively influences the adequacy of selective attention, coding, and memory.

1.2. The optimum amount and clarity of input of internal and external stimuli positively influences the adequacy of imitation, reinforcement, and insight.

1.3. The optimum amount and clarity of input of internal and external stimuli positively influences the adequacy of problem solving and decision making.

1.4. The optimum amount and clarity of input of internal and external stimuli positively influences the adequacy of defenses to seek relief, and affective appraisal and attachment.

2.1. Intact pathways and perceptual/information-processing apparatus positively influences the adequacy of selective attention, coding, and memory.

2.2. Intact pathways and learning apparatus positively influences imitation, reinforcement, and insight.

2.3. Intact pathways and judgment apparatus positively influences problem solving and decision making.

2.4. Intact pathways and emotional apparatus positively influences defenses to seek relief, and affective appraisal and attachment.

3.1. The higher the level of adequacy of all the cognator processes, the more effective the psychomotor choice of response.

4.1. The psychomotor response chosen will be activated through intact effectors.

5.1. Effector activity produces the response that is at an adaptive level determined by the total functioning of the cognator subsystem.

6.1. The level of adaptive responses to internal and external stimuli will alter those internal and external stimuli. (Roy & Roberts, 1981, p. 65)

The **Theory of the Physiological Mode** applies the propositions from the regulator subsystem to physiological needs. The theory encompasses adaptive and ineffective regulatory responses related to exercise and rest, nutrition, elimination, fluid and electrolytes, oxygen and circulation, temperature, the senses, and the endocrine system. Roy and Roberts

(1981) pointed out that by considering regulator activity, they avoided exploration of biological systems, which they viewed as the focus of medicine.

Roy and Roberts (1981) formulated one or more sample hypotheses for each component of the physiological mode. Each hypothesis was based on a deductive line of reasoning that proceeds from a general proposition (axiom) to a more specific proposition (theorem) to the hypothesis. The deductions for each component of the physiological mode are the following:

EXERCISE

> **Axiom:** The magnitude of the internal and external stimuli will positively influence the magnitude of the physiological response of an intact system.
> **Theorem:** The amount of mobility in the form of exercising positively influences the level of muscle integrity.
> **Hypothesis:** If the nurse helps the patient maintain muscle tone through proper exercising, the patient will experience fewer problems associated with immobility. (p. 90)

REST

> **Axiom:** The magnitude of the internal and external stimuli will positively influence the magnitude of the physiological response of an intact system.
> **Theorem:** The quality of uninterrupted REM sleep positively influences the patient's avoidance of REM sleep deprivation and dream deprivation.
> **Hypothesis:** If the nurse provides the patient with uninterrupted sleep where REM can be achieved, the patient will not experience sleep deprivation. (p. 91)

NUTRITION

> **Axiom:** The magnitude of the internal and external stimuli will positively influence the magnitude of the physiological response of an intact system.
> **Theorem$_1$:** The diet that is based on both biological needs and patient preference will positively influence the amount of dietary intake.
> **Hypothesis$_1$:** If the nurse assesses the patient's dietary needs in relation to his dietary preference, the patient will achieve an optimal level of nutritional intake. (pp. 109–110).
> **Axiom:** The magnitude of the internal and external stimuli will positively influence the magnitude of the physiological response of an intact system.
> **Theorem$_2$:** An environment conducive for eating will positively influence the level of anorexia or nausea.
> **Hypothesis$_2$:** If the nurse establishes an environment conducive for dietary intake, the patient will be less likely to experience anorexia or nausea. (p. 110)

ELIMINATION

Axiom: The magnitude of the internal and external stimuli will positively influence the magnitude of the physiological response of an intact system.

Theorem: The magnitude of internal and external stimuli will positively influence the level of urinary and intestinal elimination.

Hypothesis: If the nurse helps the patient achieve an optimal level of urinary and intestinal elimination, the patient's eliminatory system will perform at a higher level. (p. 129)

FLUIDS AND ELECTROLYTES

Axiom: The magnitude of the internal and external stimuli will positively influence the magnitude of the physiological response of an intact system.

Theorem: The level of hydration achieved will positively influence the level of fluid and electrolyte balance.

Hypothesis: If the nurse helps the patient maintain an optimal level of hydration, the patient will perform at a higher cellular level. (p. 156)

OXYGEN AND CIRCULATION

Axiom: The magnitude of the internal and external stimuli will positively influence the magnitude of the physiological response of an intact system.

Theorem: The level of alveolar-capillary exchange and perfusion will positively influence the level of oxygenation and circulatory balance.

Hypothesis: If the nurse helps the patient achieve an optimal level of oxygenation and circulation, the patient's alveolar-capillary system will perform at a higher level. (p. 181)

TEMPERATURE

Axiom: The magnitude of the internal and external stimuli will positively influence the magnitude of the physiological response of an intact system.

Theorem: The amount of input in the form of heat will positively influence the temperature regulatory system.

Hypothesis: If the nurse helps the patient maintain a temperature level for normal physiological functioning, the patient's cellular activity and body metabolism will perform at a more optimal level. (p. 190)

THE SENSES

Axiom: The magnitude of the internal and external stimuli will positively influence the magnitude of the physiological response of an intact system.

Theorem: The amount of sensory input via each sensory modality will positively influence the level of cortical arousal.

Hypothesis: If the nurse provides optimal sensory input, the patient will achieve an optimal level of cortical arousal. (p. 218)

ENDOCRINE SYSTEM

Axiom: Chemical and neural inputs will influence normally responsive endocrine glands to hormonally influence target organs in a positive manner to maintain a state of dynamic equilibrium.

Theorem: The amount of hormonal input and control will positively influence hormonal balance.

Hypothesis: If the nurse helps the patient maintain an optimal level of hormonal secretion, the patient will achieve a higher level of hormonal or endocrine balance. (p. 243)

The theories dealing with the psychosocial modes (self-concept, role function, and interdependence) consider these modes as systems "through which the regulator and cognator subsystems act to promote adaptation" (Roy & Roberts, 1981, p. 248). Each theory describes the relevant system in terms of its wholeness, subsystems, relation of parts, inputs, outputs, and self-regulation and control.

The following are propositions of the **Theory of the Self-Concept Mode**:

1.1. The positive quality of social experience in the form of others' appraisals positively influences the level of feelings of adequacy.

1.2. Adequacy of role taking positively influences the quality of input in the form of social experience.

1.3. The number of social rewards positively influences the quality of social experience.

1.4. Negative feedback in the form of performance compared with ideals leads to corrections in levels of feelings of adequacy.

1.5. Conflicts in input in the form of varying appraisals positively influences the amount of self-concept confusion experienced.

1.6. Confused self-concept leads to activation of mechanisms to reduce dissonance and maintain consistency.

1.7. Activity of mechanisms for reducing dissonance and maintaining consistency (e.g., choice) tends to lead to feelings of adequacy.

1.8. The level of feelings of adequacy positively influences the quality of presentation of self. (Roy & Roberts, 1981, p. 255)

Roy and Roberts (1981) offered the following deductive proposition set and a sample hypothesis as part of the **Theory of the Self-Concept Mode**:

Axiom$_1$: Adequacy of role taking positively influences the quality of input in the form of social experience.

Axiom$_2$: The positive quality of social experience positively influences the level of feelings of adequacy.

Theorem: Adequacy of role taking positively influences the level of feelings of adequacy.

Hypothesis: If the nurse helps the new mother to practice role taking, the mother will develop a higher level of feelings of adequacy. (p. 258)

Following are the propositions of the **Theory of the Role Function Mode**:

1.1. The amount of clarity of input in the form of role cues and cultural norms positively influences the adequacy of role taking.

1.2. Accuracy of perception positively influences the clarity of input in the form of role cues and cultural norms.

1.3. Adequacy of social learning positively influences the clarity of input in the form of role cues and cultural norms.

1.4. Negative feedback in the form of internal and external validations leads to corrections in adequacy of role taking.

1.5. Conflicts in input in the form of conflicting role sets positively influences the amount of role strain experienced.

1.6. Role strain leads to activation of mechanisms for reducing role strain and for articulating role sets.

1.7. Activity of mechanisms for reducing role strain and for articulating role sets (e.g., choice) leads to adequacy of role taking.

1.8. The level of adequacy of role taking positively influences the level of role mastery. (Roy & Roberts, 1981, p. 267)

Following are the deductive proposition set and sample hypothesis for the **Theory of the Role Function Mode**:

Axiom$_1$: The amount of clarity of input in the form of role cues positively influences the adequacy of role taking.

Axiom$_2$: The level of adequacy of role taking positively influences the level of role mastery.

Theorem: The amount of clarity of input in the form of role cues positively influences the level of role mastery.

Hypothesis: If the nurse orients the patient to the sick role, the patient will perform at a higher level of role mastery in the sick role. (Roy & Roberts, 1981, p. 270)

Following are the propositions for the **Theory of the Interdependence Mode**:

1.1. The balance and flexibility of coping style positively influences the adequacy of seeking nurturance and nurturing.

1.2. The optimum amount of environmental changes positively influences the adequacy of seeking nurturance and nurturing.

1.3. Clarity of feedback about self positively influences the balance and flexibility of coping style.

1.4. Clarity of validation regarding others positively influences the balance and flexibility of coping style.

1.5. Commonality and freedom of communication patterns positively influences the adequacy of seeking nurturance and nurturing.

1.6. The balance of dependency and aggressive drives positively influences the adequacy of seeking nurturance and nurturing.

1.7. Adequacy of seeking nurturance and nurturing positively influences interdependence. (Roy & Roberts, 1981, p. 277)

The following constitutes the deductive proposition set and sample hypothesis for the **Theory of the Interdependence Mode**:

Axiom$_1$: The optimum amount of environmental changes positively influences the adequacy of seeking nurturance and nurturing.

Axiom$_2$: Adequacy of seeking nurturance and nurturing positively influences interdependence.

Theorem: The optimum amount of environmental changes positively influences interdependence.

Hypothesis: If the nurse provides time and space for private family visits, the patient will demonstrate more appropriate attention-seeking behavior. (Roy & Roberts, 1981, p. 280)

The hypotheses derived from the propositions of each theory have not yet been tested empirically. However, Roy and Roberts (1981) recognized the need for a systematic program of research to test the sample hypotheses as well as other hypotheses that could be derived from the theories. They also recognized the need to further develop and test the general Theory of the Person as an Adaptive System. They commented, "We must look at the theory of the adaptive person to further explain the interrelatedness of the adaptive modes. In this process we must also search for multivariable and nonlinear relationships. Cognator and regulator processes must be studied to discover the proposed hierarchy of processes" (p. 289). Furthermore, as Roy and Roberts (1981) pointed out, nursing practice theory, or what Roy (1988b) now calls clinical science, must be developed within the context of the Roy Adaptation Model. That is, theories need to be formulated to explain and predict the effects of specific nursing interventions on the responses of individuals and groups.

The **Nursing Model of Cognitive Processing** has also been developed within the context of the Roy Adaptation Model (Roy, 1988a). The cognitive processing model, which is actually a rudimentary middle-range theory, focuses attention on the basic cognitive processes of arousal-attention, sensation-perception, coding-concept formation, memory, language, planning, and motor responses. The model proposes that the basic cognitive processes, which occur within the field of consciousness, are dependent on neurological and neurochemical functions. The model further proposes that cognitive processes are directed toward dealing with the focal stimulus of the immediate sensory experience, within the reference frame of contextual and residual stimuli in the form of the person's education and experience.

Other theory development work stemming from the Roy Adaptation Model includes the construction of explicit conceptual-theoretical-empirical structures for studies of preparation for cesarean childbirth (Fawcett, 1990), functional status in normal life situations and serious illness (Fawcett & Tulman, 1990; Samarel & Fawcett, 1992; Tulman & Fawcett, 1990a, 1990b), adaptation to chronic illness (Pollock, 1993), cross-cultural responses to pain (Calvillo & Flaskerud, 1993), and stress experiences of spouses of coronary artery bypass graft patients (Artinian, 1991, 1992).

Credibility

Social Utility

The utility of the Roy Adaptation Model for nursing research, education, administration, and practice is well documented. The conceptual model is being used by nurses throughout the United States and in other countries, including Canada and Switzerland (Roy, personal communication, May 15, 1982). In addition to Roy's own texts (Andrews & Roy, 1986; Roy, 1976b, 1984a; Roy & Andrews, 1991; Roy & Roberts, 1981), books related to the Roy Adaptation Model have been published by Randell et al. (1982), Rambo (1984), and Welsh and Clochesy (1990).

The Roy Adaptation Model encompasses an extensive vocabulary with several new words. Furthermore, even familiar words such as adaptation have been given new meanings in Roy's attempt to translate notions that reflect the reaction world view into ideas that reflect the reciprocal interaction world view. Consequently, considerable study is required to fully understand the unique focus and content of the Roy Adaptation Model. Roy (1991b) emphasized the need to study "development, interrelatedness, cultural, and other influences" on adaptive mode responses (p. 35). Andrews (1989) pointed out that "Conceptual clarity relative to the understanding of the essential elements of a nursing model is a particular challenge and of great importance if the conceptualization is to be effective in its application" (p. 139). She recommended detailed study of the content of the four adaptive modes and highlighted the importance of diagrams, such as Figure 9–1, to facilitate understanding of the various components of the Roy Adaptation Model.

Implementation of Roy Adaptation Model–based nursing practice is feasible. The human and material resources needed for implementation of the model at the clinical agency level are evident in the following descriptions of implementation projects.

Gray (1991) presented a comprehensive report of the strategies used for implementation of the Roy Adaptation Model at five Southern California hospitals. The hospitals ranged from a 100-bed proprietary hospital to a 248-bed nonprofit, community-owned hospital. Drawing from the Ingalls (1972) System of Management, Gray described the processes of climate setting, mutual planning, assessing needs, forming objectives, designing, implementing, and evaluating. Climate setting focuses on assessment of the physical, psychological, and organizational climate. She pointed out that "if a hospital waits for the perfect time to begin a change project, no change projects would ever be started" (p. 433). Planning should be carried out by all levels of nursing staff, along with the hospital personnel responsible for medical records, purchasing, central supply, social services, laboratories, x-ray, and respiratory therapy. Needs assessment encompasses the individual staff nurse, the nursing department, and the health care system as a whole. Gray (1991) underscored the importance of marketing the model-based nursing services to consumers as a method of contributing to the fiscal needs of the clinical agency.

Gray (1991) went on to point out that the overall objective of an implementation project dealing with the Roy Adaptation Model is "to improve the quality of patient care through the use of written care plans" (p. 437). More specific objectives should be developed for each nursing unit and individual staff nurses. Designing is a time-consuming but "exciting and professionally exhilarating" phase of implementation and is best accomplished through a committee structure (p. 439). Gray (1991) recommended establishment of a Standards of Practice Steering Committee and working committees on quality assurance, procedures and protocol, nursing process, professional development, and patient education.

Implementing, according to Gray (1991), is "the easiest step" if the previous phases were accomplished in an effective manner and if hospital personnel were adequately oriented to the model (p. 440). Evaluation is carried out continuously, from climate setting through implementation.

Mastal, Hammond, and Roberts (1982) cited the importance of a thorough analysis of the model, the heuristic value of a diagram to depict the relationships between the components of the model, and the pragmatic necessity of support from the agency administrators. They noted that funds for the necessary staff education can be allocated from the agency's continuing education budget. They added that if funds are not available, it may be possible to recruit one or more volunteers from the clinical agency and local schools of nursing to serve as implementation project staff.

Mastal et al. (1982) also noted the importance of the appointment of a project change team, as well as an introductory meeting of all personnel who would be involved in the change to model-based practice, including "float" staff. They commented that shared power, which involves group decision making and group problem solving, was especially effective as the implementation project progressed.

Dorsey and Purcell (1987) reported that remodeling a unit by removing the nursing station walls, which promoted increased nursing home resident-staff interaction, was a particularly important aspect of the implementation of Roy Adaptation Model–based nursing practice. They also noted the importance of comprehensive orientation and inservice programs for staff.

The importance of revising nursing documents so that they are consistent with the Roy Adaptation Model has been underscored by various authors (Jakocko & Sowden, 1986; Mastal et al., 1982; Rogers et al., 1991). Relevant documents include the agency's philosophy of nursing, mission statement, standards of practice, nursing history and assessment forms, nursing care plans, patient classification systems, computer information systems, job descriptions, performance appraisals, and quality monitoring tools.

Weiss, Hastings, Holly, and Craig's (1992) study of the implementation of the Roy Adaptation Model at Sharp Memorial Hospital in San Diego, California, revealed both facilitators and inhibitors to the integration of the model into nursing practice. Facilitators included prior experience with the model in an educational program, participation in the implementation project through shared governance councils, participation in career advancement programs, and ongoing continuing education. Inhibitors were resistance to change and lack of education about nursing models.

The application of the Roy Adaptation Model is feasible in many different clinical settings. However, Mason and Chandley (1990) noted that the lack of success in applying the model in special hospitals for the criminally insane "is due firstly to the limitation of adaptive responses in terms of the patient's goal due to the secure environment, and secondly, it creates a level of frustration when the 'treatment' values conflict with the social, political and legal values" (p. 671). Conversely, although she noted certain limitations in its use, Miller (1991) presented a largely successful application of the Roy Adaptation Model in the special hospital with which Mason is affiliated.

NURSING RESEARCH. The Roy Adaptation Model has proved useful as a guide for nursing research. A conference devoted to Roy Adaptation Model–based nursing research was sponsored by the Department of Nursing of William Paterson College of New Jersey in June 1989. Many doctoral dissertations and master's theses have been guided by the model. Those that could be identified through a search of *Dissertation Abstracts International* and *Master's Abstracts International* are listed in the bibliography at the end of this chapter.

Published full reports of research based on the Roy Adaptation Model include instrument development work, studies of patients' responses to diverse environmental stimuli, and studies of the effects of nursing interventions on patients' adaptation. Research instruments that have been derived from the Roy Adaptation Model include Ide's (1978) tool for measuring the self-perceived adaptation level of elderly clients, Roy's (1979a) tools to measure hospitalized patients' perception of powerlessness and their perceptions of their decision-making activities, and Lewis, Firsich, and Parsell's (1978, 1979) tool to measure health outcomes of nursing care for adult cancer patients receiving chemotherapy. In addition, Tulman et al. have developed questionnaires to measure functional status in diverse populations that are directly derived from the role function mode of the Roy Adaptation Model. The questionnaires include the Inventory of Functional Status-Antepartum (Tulman, Higgins, et al., 1991), the Inventory of Functional Status After Childbirth (Fawcett, Tulman, & Myers, 1988), the Inventory of Functional Status-Fathers (Tulman, Fawcett, & Weiss, 1993), the Inventory of Functional Status-Cancer (Tulman, Fawcett, & McEvoy, 1991), and the Inventory of Functional Status in the Elderly (Paier, in press). Furthermore, Roy and Corliss (1993) noted that instruments designed to measure cognitive adaptation processing are being developed.

Some studies have focused on descriptions of patients' responses to various environmental stimuli. Fawcett (1981b) classified mothers' and fathers' responses to the cesarean birth of their infants according to need deficits and excesses in each of the four adaptive modes. Kehoe (1981) identified and classified the needs of postpartum cesarean birth mothers in the four adaptive modes. Fawcett and Weiss (1993) extended the study of responses to cesarean birth to a cross-cultural sample of white, Hispanic, and Asian women. Tulman et al. have described changes in and correlates of the functional status of childbearing women during the postpartum (Tulman & Fawcett, 1988, 1990c; Tulman, Fawcett, Groblewski, & Silverman, 1990) and women with breast cancer (Tulman & Fawcett, 1993). Craig (1990) described the experiences encountered by spinal cord–injured women during pregnancy, highlighting their sense of powerlessness. Khanobdee, Sukratanachaiyakul, and Gay (1993) described the incidence of couvade symptoms in Thai expectant fathers. Norris, Campbell, and Brenkert (1982) described premature infants' responses, as measured by transcutaneous oxygen tension, to routine nursing procedures. Harrison, Leeper, and Yoon (1990) described preterm infants' responses, as measured by heart rate and arterial oxygen saturation level, to early parent touch.

Hunter (1991) measured the length of time needed to measure a stable axillary temperature in the neonate. Nyqvist and Sjoden (1993) reported the advice regarding breastfeeding given by Swedish mothers of infants in a neonatal intensive care unit. Broeder (1985) reported children's perceptions of isolation due to infectious diseases or immunodeficiency disorders. Germain (1984) described the common health problems of abused women and children who were residing in a shelter. Roy (1987d) described patients' responses to surgery for acoustic neuroma. Jackson et al. (1991; Frederickson, Jackson, Strauman, & Strauman, 1991) described patients' biopsychosocial responses to interleukin-2 therapy throughout the 15 days of treatment and at 1, 6, and 12 months post-treatment.

Strohmyer, Noroian, Patterson, and Carlin (1993) described the functional and psychosocial adaptation of adult survivors of multiple trauma who were at home 6 months after hospital discharge. Selman (1989) described the quality of life, as reflected in the four modes of adaptation, of men and women 12 to 24 months after total hip replacement. Leonard (1975) described psychiatric patients' attitudes toward nursing interventions. Pollock (1993) reported the results of her program of research dealing with patients' physiological and psychosocial responses to chronic illness.

Smith, Garvin, and Martinson (1983) identified the adaptive strengths of children with cancer and their parents. Gagliardi (1991) described the experiences of families with a child with Duchenne muscular dystrophy. Bradley and Williams (1990) identified the concerns of open heart surgery patients and their significant others during the preoperative in-hospital waiting period. Silva (1987b) identified the needs of spouses of surgical patients. Artinian (1991, 1992) described spouse adaptation, including life stressors, supports, perceptions of illness severity, role strain, stress symptoms, and marital quality during the mate's hospitalization for coronary artery bypass surgery, and 6 weeks and 1 year after discharge. Farkas (1981) identified problems in adaptation for elderly persons and their significant others. Smith et al. (1991) reported the family coping and family functioning scores of the caregivers of ventilator-dependent adults living at home. Hazlett (1989) found that home management of children requiring mechanical ventilation is medically safe and less costly when compared with prolonged hospitalization. The study also revealed that parental caregivers had both positive and negative psychosocial responses that would be amenable to nursing intervention in the discharge preparation and follow-up care periods.

Cheng and Williams (1989) examined the relationship of fraction of inspired oxygen levels and the number of hand ventilations to transcutaneous oxygen pressure in intubated very-low-birth-weight infants during chest physiotherapy. Christian (1993) found evidence of a relationship between the number and frequency of occurrence of symptoms of endometriosis and the severity of pain, as well as between the frequency and the number of symptoms, but no relationship between self-esteem and the number, frequency, or severity of the symptoms. Roy (1978b) explored the relationship between patients' adaptation to focal stimuli and their emotional feelings of distress during hospitalization and on the day before discharge. Phillips and Brown (1992) found that adaptation of rotating shiftworkers was related to circadian type, effects of the work environment, and coping style. McGill (1992) found evidence of a relationship between physical health and hope in elderly people with and without cancer. Preston and Dellasega (1990) found that elderly married women were in poorest health and the most vulnerable to stress when compared with elderly married men, unmarried women, and unmarried men. Baker (1993) reported that married stroke patients who completed a rehabilitation program had a higher level of functioning than their unmarried or widowed counterparts.

Calvillo and Flaskerud (1993) studied the correlates of the response to cholecystectomy pain, including culture, anxiety, physiological adaptation, self-esteem, self-coherence, sick role adaptation, and social support. They found that ethnic group membership (Anglo-American and Mexican-American) was not associated with pain response, but that there were negative relationships between anxiety and pain, self-esteem and pain, and self-coherence and pain. In contrast, no evidence of a relationship between sick role adaptation or social support and pain was found.

Lutjens (1992) reported that measures of nursing care, including hours of care and nursing diagnoses, explained most of the variance accounted for in length of hospital stay. Little variance was explained by either measures of medical condition or medical severity.

Other published studies have focused on the effects of various nursing interventions on patient adaptation. Nolan (1977) explored the relationship between nursing interventions in the operating room and postoperative patients' reports of the quality of their care. Bokinskie (1992) reported that care conferences that were focused on the nursing and environmental aspects of general care units reduced family members' anxiety when the patient was transferred from an intensive care unit to a general care unit. Guzzetta (1979) found that a formal cardiac teaching program improved male myocardial infarction patients' knowledge of illness and related health care issues. Campbell (1992) found that community-dwelling elderly persons who received an 8-week nursing intervention aimed at reinforcing positive-input thought patterns or craft classes experienced a reduction in depressive symptoms, whereas a control group experienced no change in depression scores. Francis, Turner, and Johnson (1985) and Calvert (1989) found that domestic animal visitation had beneficial effects on nursing home residents' adaptation responses. Meek (1993) reported that slow-stroke back massage promoted relaxation, as measured by blood pressure, heart rate, and skin temperature, in hospice clients.

Roy (1991a) reported the results of studies of head-injured patients designed to test her model of cognitive processing. One study was designed to describe cognitive processing in patients with minor and moderate head injuries. Findings indicated that cognitive processing scores improved over time and that "the pattern of information processing deficits is more pronounced for successive and planning functions than for simultaneous processing" (p. 453). Another study, which was designed to test a nursing intervention protocol for head-injured patients, revealed that the protocol was useful and that the experimental group demonstrated greater improvement than the control group on measures of cognitive processing.

Vicenzi and Thiel (1992) reported that a 2-hour safer sex educational module yielded changes in AIDS-related beliefs among college students but did not increase safer sex practices. Shannahan and Cottrell (1985) and Cottrell and Shannahan (1986, 1987) studied the effects of using a birth chair on duration of second-stage labor, as well as maternal and fetal outcomes. They found that the birth chair is a safe alternative delivery method, although maternal blood loss was increased when the birth chair was used and second-stage labor was not shorter than with the traditional delivery position. Fawcett and Burritt (1985) and Fawcett and Henklein (1987) reported the beneficial results of field tests of an antenatal education program designed to prepare expectant parents for unplanned cesarean childbirth. In contrast, Fawcett et al. (1993) reported that the antenatal education program did not have the expected beneficial effects across all four adaptive modes for the experimental group at 1 to 3 days and 6 weeks postpartum, when compared with the effects for a control group.

Gaberson (1991) reported that pilot study data revealed no differences in preoperative anxiety among groups of patients who listened to humorous audiotapes, tranquil music audiotapes, or no audiotapes. Komelasky (1990) reported that structured home nursing visits yielded no statistically significant effects on anxiety and retention of cardiopulmonary resuscitation knowledge in the parents of apnea-monitored infants when compared with a control group who did not receive the structured home nursing visits. Samarel, Fawcett, and Tulman (1993) reported that pilot study data revealed a trend toward decreased symptom distress but no other statistically significant effects for women with breast cancer who participated in a structured cancer support group (CSG) with coaching from a significant other when compared with women who participated in a CSG without coaching and with women who did not participate in a CSG. Printz-Feddersen (1990) found no differences in the burden experienced by the caregivers of stroke survivors who participated in a stroke club and those who did not.

A few studies have focused on the nurse as the study subject. Lynam and Miller (1992) compared nurses' and postpartum mothers' perceptions of the women's needs during preterm labor. Munn and Tichy (1987) reported their findings of nurses' perceptions of stressors in a pediatric intensive care unit. Kiikkala and Peitsi (1991) described the components of nursing care given to Finnish preschool children with minimal brain dysfunction. Hammond, Roberts, and Silva (1983) tested the contention of the Roy Adaptation Model that both first-level (behaviors) and second-level (stimuli) assessments are needed to make accurate nursing diagnoses. Their findings, which supported the hypothesis that nurses who used first-level assessment data would make as many accurate nursing diagnoses as those using both first- and second-level assessment, suggested that Roy's contention may be invalid. However, as Silva (1987a) pointed out, ". . . this conclusion must be tempered by the small sample size and the difficulty in operationally defining accurate nursing diagnoses" (p. 234). Leuze and McKenzie's (1987) findings supported the hypothesis that circulating nurses involved with patients who have had preoperative nursing assessments based on the Roy Adaptation Model would demonstrate increased knowledge of the patient's psychosocial needs over those nurses who were involved with patients who had routine preoperative assessments.

NURSING EDUCATION. The utility of the Roy Adaptation Model for nursing education is well documented. The early and widespread interest in using the model in educational programs is attested to by three conferences that were held for faculty members who planned to use or were already using the model as a basis for curriculum development in their schools. The first and second conferences were held at Alverno College in Milwaukee, Wisconsin, in 1978 and 1979. The third conference was held at Mount St. Mary's College in Los Angeles, California, in 1981. Currently, an annual conference is held at Mount St. Mary's College to recognize the leadership role of the College in initial development of the Roy Adaptation Model and to provide a forum for Roy Adaptation Model–based issues in education and practice (Wallace, 1993).

Roy (personal communication, May 15, 1982) provided a list of schools of nursing where she or a faculty member from Mount St. Mary's College "have made consultant visits and there is some evidence of follow-through with curriculum development." The nursing programs named were Cerritos Community College in Cerritos, California; Golden West College in Huntington Park, California; Mount St. Mary's College in Los Angeles, California; Point Loma College in San Diego, California; Harbor Community College in San Pedro, California; Wesley Passavant School of Nursing in Chicago, Illinois; Kansas State College in Pittsburg, Kansas; Maryland General Hospital in Baltimore, Maryland; Graceland College in Independence, Missouri; Northwest Missouri State University in Kirksville; William Patterson College in Wayne, New Jersey; Central State College in Edmond, Oklahoma; the University of Tulsa in Tulsa, Oklahoma; the University of Portland in Portland, Oregon; Widener University in Chester, Pennsylvania; Edinboro State College in Edinboro, Pennsylvania; Villa Maria College in Erie, Pennsylvania; Community College of Philadelphia, in Philadelphia, Pennsylvania; the University of Texas at Arlington and at Austin; Alverno College and Columbia Hospital in Milwaukee, Wisconsin; Royal Alexander Hospital in Edmonton and the University of Calgary in Calgary, both in Alberta, Canada; Health Sciences Centre in Winnipeg, Manitoba, Canada; Vanier College in Montreal, Québec, Canada; and École Génévoise D Infirmiére, Le Bon Secours, in Geneva, Switzerland. The model also is used as the basis for the first- and second-year nursing courses, as well as some third-year course work, in the baccalaureate program at the University of Ottawa in Ottawa, Ontario, Canada (Morales-Mann & Logan, 1990; Story & Ross, 1986).

Roy (1979b) described the nursing curriculum at Mount St. Mary's College in considerable detail. In other publications, she has noted that the use of the Roy Adaptation Model for curriculum construction originated at that college in 1970 (Roy, 1974, 1980, 1989).

Heinrich (1989) reported that the integration of the Roy Adaptation Model was begun at the University of Hartford in Hartford, Connecticut, in 1980. She identified three stages—upheaval, evolution, and integration—that both faculty and students passed through. The stage of upheaval was characterized by a "right-wrong struggle"; the stage of evolution, by "facing the conflict"; and the stage of integration, by "humor, creativity, and cooperative learning" (p. 4).

Mengel, Sherman, Nahigian, and Colman (1989) gave a detailed description of the ongoing experience of using the Roy Adaptation Model for the nursing curriculum at Community College of Philadelphia since 1978. They identified three periods of faculty evolution — excitement, reorganization, and acceptance. Elaborating, they explained, "In the period of excitement, we were naively overconfident that the revised curriculum would work. 'Why doesn't it work?' was the theme of the reorganization period. During reorganization we began to make changes to meet our needs. Finally, in the period of acceptance, we discovered that with further adaptations, a curriculum based on the Roy model does meet our needs" (p. 125).

Brower and Baker (1976) described the use of the Roy Adaptation Model in the geriatric nurse practitioner program at the University of Miami in Coral Gables, Florida. The four adaptive modes served as the organizing focus for the 10-month continuing education program. The authors contended that the adaptive modes permitted differentiation of nursing practice from medical practice. They explained, "If we conceptualize role function, self-concept, and interdependence as existing within the domain of nursing, and pathophysiology and treatment modalities as being domains shared by medicine and nursing and relevant to the physiological mode, we can formulate a nurse practitioner curriculum that provides for both overlap and distinction between the two roles" (p. 687).

Knowlton et al. (1983) described the development of a nursing curriculum based on the Roy Adaptation Model. They outlined the use of the model for various systems, including the family, groups, communities, and the health care system.

An interesting application of the model in nursing education was presented by Camooso, Greene, and Reilly (1981). The authors, who were graduate nursing students, described their adjustment to graduate school within the context of the four adaptive modes of Roy's model, citing adaptive and ineffective behaviors they exhibited throughout the master's degree program.

NURSING ADMINISTRATION. Roy (1987a) commented, "Implementing the [Roy Adaptation] model of nursing care in whole health care systems will require . . . expertise both in implementation and in evaluation of the outcomes. Some of the outcomes are important in relation to what the model does for nursing, such as increasing autonomy, accountability, and professionalism in general, and in changing relationships with other disciplines" (p. 44).

The utility of the Roy Adaptation Model for nursing service administration is documented. Roy and Anway (1989) adapted the model for nursing administration. The organizational modes of adaptation are the physical system, the role system, the interpersonal system, and the interdependence system. These systems adapt to internal and external environmental conditions through stabilizer and innovator central mechanisms. DiIorio (1989) described the application of the conceptual model to nursing administration. Furthermore, Roy and Martinez (1983) presented a conceptual framework for clinical specialist nursing practice based on the Roy Adaptation Model and systems notions.

Mastal et al. (1982) described the pilot phase of Roy Adaptation Model–based nursing practice at the National Hospital for Orthopaedics and Rehabilitation. Silva and Sorrell (1992) reported that the model was implemented throughout the hospital in 1981. Citing an October 1991 personal communication with A. Debisette, a unit director of nursing, they noted that "the model is still working well, and staff continue to see positive outcomes" (p. 20).

Torosian, Destefano, and Dietrick-Gallagher (1985) described the development of a day gynecologic chemotherapy unit at the Hospital of the University of Pennsylvania in Philadelphia. They used the Roy Adaptation Model as the basis for nursing interventions and identification of patient outcomes.

The Roy Adaptation Model serves as a basis for nursing practice at the Henry and Lucy Moses Division, Neurosurgical Nursing Unit of Montefiore Medical Center in New York City (Montefiore Medical Center, 1989; Studio Three, 1992); Providence Hospital in Oakland, California (Laros, 1977); Children's Hospital of Orange County in Orange, California (Jakocko & Sowden, 1986); Anaheim Memorial Hospital in Anaheim, California (Gray, 1991); South Coast Medical Center in Laguna Beach, California (Gray, 1991); Sharp Memorial Hospital in San Diego, California (Studio Three, 1992); the Nursing Home Care Unit at the Veterans Administration Medical Center in Roseburg, Oregon (Dorsey & Purcell, 1987); the Orthopaedic and Arthritic Hospital (Rogers et al., 1991) and Mount Sinai Hospital (Fitch et al., 1991) in Toronto, Ontario, Canada; and the Centre Hospitalier Pierre Janet in Hull, Québec, Canada (Robitaille-Tremblay, 1984).

Roy Adaptation Model–based nursing documentation has been described in several publications. Jakocko and Sowden (1986) described and displayed an admission history and assessment form for hospitalized children that is organized according to the four adaptive modes of the Roy Adaptation Model. Robitaille-Tremblay (1984) described and displayed a nursing history tool for psychiatric patients that is also organized according to the four adaptive modes. Rogers et al. (1991) displayed excerpts from Roy Adaptation Model–based job descriptions, standards for nursing care, and performance appraisal instruments.

Fawcett (1992) presented an outline for a Roy Adaptation Model–based nursing care plan. Peters (1993) briefly described the documentation forms used on a general medical unit of a hospital that used the model as a basis for nursing practice.

Starn and Niederhauser (1990) described their MCN Developmental/Diagnostic Model, which provides a format for nursing care plans for childrearing and childbearing families. They explained that the developmental component of the model is based on the Roy Adaptation Model.

Hinman (1983) described an assessment format, the Family Development/Nursing Intervention Identifier, for use with school-aged children and their families.

Laros (1977) used the Roy Adaptation Model to develop outcome criteria for patients with chronic obstructive pulmonary disease. The evaluation tool listed the criteria for each adaptive mode in a progressive sequence of days following admission to the hospital. Zarle (1987) described a model for planning continuing care following hospitalization that is based on the Roy Adaptation Model.

Riegel (1985) described a method of presenting intershift report based on the Roy Adaptation Model and the nursing process. She explained that the data for the report are organized according to the model components, including nursing diagnosis, stimuli, and adaptive mode responses.

NURSING PRACTICE. The Roy Adaptation Model has documented utility for nursing practice with patients across the lifespan and with various health problems and in various settings. Galligan (1979) formulated a Roy Adaptation Model–based nursing care plan for hospitalized children. A special feature of the care plan was its division into four stages; prehospitalization, preoperative state, postoperative stage, and discharge. Nash (1987) used the model to develop a nursing care plan for children with Kawasaki disease. Wright, Holcombe, Foote, and Piazza (1993) applied the model to the comprehensive care of an 8-year-old boy with acute lymphocytic leukemia.

Barnfather, Swain, and Erickson (1989) presented a Roy Adaptation Model–based nursing care plan for a 19-year-old college student. Roy (1971) described the application of the model to the nursing care of a diabetic teenager. Ellis (1991) identified the common adaptation problems and appropriate nursing interventions for adolescents with cancer.

Gerrish (1989) presented a detailed description of a Roy Adaptation Model–based assessment of a 25-year-old woman with Hodgkin's disease. Limandri (1986) described the use of the model for care of abused women.

Application of the Roy Adaptation Model to the nursing care of women and their partners during the childbearing period has received some attention. Sato (1986) described a Roy model-based nursing care plan for a pregnant woman. Stringer, Librizzi, and Weiner (1991) described nursing assessment and intervention for women undergoing genetic testing during pregnancy. Taylor (1993) developed a booklet for use by women experiencing preterm labor, which fully integrates the Roy Adaptation Model. Kehoe (1981) used the model to identify the nursing care needs of the postpartum cesarean mother. Fawcett (1981a) applied the model to the nursing care of cesarean fathers. Downey (1974) applied the model to the care of a 27-year-old Mexican-American woman who delivered an infant in respiratory distress. Sirignano (1987) described Roy Adaptation Model–based nursing care of patients experiencing cardiomyopathy during the peripartum period.

Janelli (1980) used the nursing process of the Roy Adaptation Model to describe nursing care for elderly people. Smith (1988) discussed the Roy model nursing process in relation to community-dwelling elderly individuals. Thornbury and King (1992) extended the discussion of the care of the elderly to those with Alzheimer's disease.

Wagner (1976) described the application of the Roy Adaptation Model in many acute care and outpatient settings. Hughes (1983) briefly described the use of the model in emergency nursing, Fawcett et al. (1992) explained its use as a guide for the care of patients in critical care units, and Hamner (1989) explained its use in coronary care units.

The Roy Adaptation Model has been used to develop nursing interventions designed to alleviate specific symptoms. Frederickson (1993) described Roy model-based nursing interventions designed to alleviate anxiety. She then presented case studies of a 34-year-old woman who underwent a craniotomy for the removal of a skull-based tumor and a 39-year-old man who had a myocardial infarction. Schmidt (1981) focused on the withdrawal behavior of people with schizophrenia.

Hamer (1991) used the Roy Adaptation Model as the basis for the application of music therapy for clients diagnosed with organic brain damage, mild-to-moderate mental retardation, and schizoaffective disorder. Although the effects of the music therapy could not be clearly distinguished from other therapy, improvements were noted in the clients' ego strength, socialization, activity levels, and psychotic symptoms. Kurek-Ovshinsky (1991) described Roy Adaptation Model-based group therapy for patients on a 15-bed acute inpatient psychiatric unit located in a metropolitan trauma center.

The Roy Adaptation Model has been used to guide the care of adults with various medical problems. Gordon (1974) used the Roy Adaptation Model nursing process format to guide the care of a 70-year-old male patient who had suffered a myocardial infarction. She described a nursing care plan that encompassed the first 2 days of the patient's care in the coronary care unit, structured according to the four adaptive modes. Other clinicians have outlined plans for holistic assessment and intervention for people with respiratory problems (Innes, 1992), diabetes (O'Reilly, 1989), renal disorders (Frank, 1988), hypernatremia (Aaronson & Seaman, 1989), alcoholism (McIver, 1987), osteoporosis (Doyle & Rajacich, 1991), and scleroderma (Crossfield, 1990).

Application of the Roy Adaptation Model to the nursing care of patients during the perioperative period has been the subject of several publications. Fox (1990) outlined the care required by patients waiting for surgery and applied the care plan to a woman scheduled for bilateral excision of breast lumps. West (1992) outlined the preoperative and postoperative nursing care of a 37-year-old woman who had a benign chest mass. Rogers (1991) and Jackson (1990) described Roy Adaptation Model –

based postanesthesia care. Roy (1971) described the nursing care of a postoperative patient who had had gynecological surgery. Hughes (1991) discussed the psychological problems experienced by patients following stomal surgery. Cardiff (1989) extended the use of the Roy Adaptation Model to the care of a patient who had had a heart transplant.

Giger, Bower, and Miller (1987) used the Roy Adaptation Model to guide care of a 23-year-old man who had been severely injured when he was thrown from and pinned under a farm mower. They developed a detailed nursing care plan that reflected the nursing process of the Roy Adaptation Model. DiMaria (1989) described Roy Adaptation Model–based care of patients who experienced multiple trauma. Summers (1991) presented a comprehensive discussion of the nursing care of burned patients from the initial resuscitative phase through the acute care phase and on to the rehabilitation phase. Piazza and Foote (1990) applied the Roy Adaptation Model to rehabilitation nursing practice and presented an example using a patient with a spinal cord injury.

Starr (1980) structured care of the dying client according to the Roy Adaptation Model. She emphasized the need to identify the clients' adaptive behaviors, relevant stimuli, and appropriate nursing interventions. Logan (1986) presented a comprehensive discussion of Roy model–based palliative nursing care.

The family members of hospitalized patients have been the focus of some Roy Adaptation Model–based practice applications. Miles and Carter (1983) developed a format for assessment of stress experienced by parents whose children are in intensive care units. Bawden, Ralph, and Herrick (1991) described psychoeducational group intervention designed to enhance the coping skills of the mothers of developmentally delayed children. Jay (1990) discussed the needs and nursing care of individuals who care for their terminally ill relatives. Logan (1988) discussed the assessment of the family members of terminally ill patients.

Roy (1983a, 1983b, 1983c) expanded her conceptual model to encompass nursing care of the family. She explained how the model could be used in the care of the expectant family and for a family that included an adolescent with diabetes. Whall (1986) reformulated and linked the theory of strategic family therapy with the Roy Adaptation Model to form a conceptual-theoretical structure for family therapy. deMontigny (1992a, 1992b) described the development, implementation, and evaluation of a nursing care plan for a family system. Dudek (1989) discussed the assessment of children with rickets and the children's parents.

Roy (1984b) and Hanchett (1990) extended the model for use in community health nursing. Schmitz (1980) applied the model in a community setting. She described the home nursing care of a family whose members included a 23-year-old mother, her 6-year-old son, 5-year-old twin daughters, a 2-month-old son, and the children's grandmother.

Social Congruence

The Roy Adaptation Model is generally congruent with societal expectations of nursing care. Consumers who expect to have input into their nursing care should find this model to be consistent with their views. Moreover, the model's emphasis on adaptation to a constantly changing environment is congruent with many people's perspective of the world today as a place of turmoil and rapid change. Indeed, Mastal et al. (1982) reported enhanced patient satisfaction and health outcomes as a result of the initial implementation of the Roy Adaptation Model at the National Hospital for Orthopaedics and Rehabilitation in Arlington, Virginia. In addition, Robitaille-Tremblay (1984; personal communication, August 4, 1982) reported that use of a Roy Adaptation Model–based nursing history tool for psychiatric patients enhanced the patients' satisfaction with care, quoting them as saying "It is the first time a professional has evaluated me so fully"; "I realize that most of my problems interrelate"; and "I have learned to know myself better than I have during any previous hospitalization." (1984, p. 28).

However, as with other conceptual models that include a focus on the well person, the Roy Adaptation Model may not be entirely congruent with some people's expectations of nursing care. This would be especially so when the nurse's action is directed toward reinforcement of already adaptive behaviors.

The Roy Adaptation Model is congruent with nurses', physicians', and hospital administrators' expectations for nursing care. Robitaille-Tremblay (1984) reported increased nurse satisfaction as the result of using a Roy Adaptation Model–based nursing history tool for psychiatric patients at Centre Hospitalier Pierre Janet. She noted that the tool "helped [nurses] get to know the patient more fully and to broaden their perspective in establishing priorities on the basis of identified stimuli. Some felt closer to the patient with whom the tool was used. One nurse stated, 'I have acquired more confidence in my independent role and I'm proud, very proud' " (p. 28). Nurses have also indicated their satisfaction with Roy Adaptation Model–based nursing practice by means of reduced turnover. In fact, Montefiore Medical Center in New York City realized a savings of approximately $300,000 in staff orientation costs due to the lack of resignations following the implementation of the model on the neurosurgical unit (K. Frederickson, cited in Studio Three, 1992).

Furthermore, Mastal et al. (1982) noted that the initial use of the model at the National Hospital for Orthopaedics and Rehabilitation led to enhanced professional nursing practice. Elaborating, they explained, "The staff has contributed to developing a tool that provides a way to assess the biopsychosocial status of patients. In planning for patient care, the nurses are not only meticulous about writing complete plans, but phrase existing patient problems in terms of nursing diagnoses, consistent with the concepts of the Adaptation Model" (p. 14).

Another indicator of enhanced professional practice at the National Hospital for Orthopaedics and Rehabilitation is the finding that an increased number of staff received baccalaureate and master's degrees after implementation of the Roy Adaptation Model (Silva & Sorrell, 1992). Moreover, physicians and hospital administrators have expressed their acceptance of the Roy Adaptation Model as an appropriate guide for nursing practice (Studio Three, 1992).

Social Significance

The social significance of the Roy Adaptation Model is beginning to be established. Anecdotal evidence regarding the impact of Roy Adaptation Model–based nursing care comes from Starn and Niederhauser (1990). They reported that several practicing nurses who used their Roy-based MCN Developmental/Diagnostic Model "were better able to identify problems [and] determine interventions more effectively" (p. 182).

Additional anecdotal evidence comes from Robitaille-Tremblay (personal communication, August 4, 1982), who commented that "Interestingly, patients stayed longer in the hospital" after a Roy Adaptation Model-based nursing history tool for psychiatric patients was implemented. She indicated that use of the tool led to more comprehensive assessments and nursing care plans. She went on to say that research is planned to determine whether there is a causal relationship between use of the tool and length of hospital stay. To date, no reports of this research have been located.

Empirical evidence comes from Hoch's (1987) research. She studied the effects of a treatment protocol derived from the Roy Adaptation Model on depression and life satisfaction in a sample of retired persons. She found that the Roy protocol group had lower depression scores and higher life satisfaction scores than a control group who received nursing intervention that was not based on an explicit conceptual model. Although the logical connection between depression and life satisfaction and the adaptive modes of the Roy Adaptation Model might be questioned, Hoch's study represents the beginning of the empirical work that is needed to determine the credibility of conceptual models of nursing.

Additional evidence, albeit mixed, comes from research that was based explicitly on propositions of the Roy Adaptation Model dealing with relationships between the adaptive modes or the effect of Roy-based interventions on adaptive mode responses.

Calvillo and Flaskerud (1993) carefully constructed a conceptual-theoretical-empirical structure to test the empirical adequacy of the Roy Adaptation Model. Their mixed findings for relationships between the adaptive modes, reviewed earlier in the social utility section on nursing research, revealed that "the empirical adequacy of the model as a whole could not be established" (p. 127).

Some experimental studies have revealed the expected adaptive responses to nursing interventions, others have yielded mixed findings, and still others have revealed no differences between the experimental and control conditions. Fawcett et al. (1993) concluded that their findings of no differences in outcomes between the experimental and control conditions of antenatal information about cesarean birth raised questions about the credibility of the Roy Adaptation Model. However, they pointed out that recent changes in childbirth education with regard to provision of cesarean birth information may have prevented an adequate test of the effects of increasing the contextual stimulus of information.

Additional Roy Adaptation Model–based research is warranted. Furthermore, sufficient research has been conducted to warrant a meta-analysis to determine the magnitude of effects and to identify design and other factors that might be contributing to the mixed findings (Rosenthal, 1991).

Contributions to the Discipline of Nursing

The Roy Adaptation Model makes a significant contribution to nursing knowledge by focusing attention on the nature of the person's adaptation to a changing environment. Roy's perspective of adaptation goes beyond that presented by other disciplines by placing it within the context of the person as a totality. Thus, the Roy Adaptation Model presents a distinctive view of the person, one that developed within the discipline of nursing.

Roy and others (e.g., Randell et al., 1982) have continued to develop the various concepts of the conceptual model, so that only a few gaps and omissions remain. Roy and Roberts' (1981) work to develop the Theory of the Person as an Adaptive System and the theories of the adaptive modes is especially noteworthy. This work has resulted in construction of the beginning of logically congruent conceptual-theoretical-empirical structures that can be used for nursing activities. The importance of the Theory of the Person as an Adaptive System to nursing was summarized by Roy and Roberts (1981). They stated, "Investigation of adaptive systems is evident in the literature of a number of fields including genetics, biology, physiology, physics, psychology, anthropology, and sociology. All of these approaches can be helpful in conceptualizing the adaptive system. Yet each approach views the person or the group from the perspective of that discipline. The nursing model directs that the nurse view the patient holistically. We need a theory of the holistic person as an adaptive system. Since the basic sciences do not provide nurses with a single working theory, the nurse using the adaptation model must create one for herself. This . . . is a beginning effort to do this—to create a theory of the holistic person as an adaptive system" (p. 49). Given the importance of this work, it is unfortunate that programs of research designed to systematically test propositions have not yet been developed.

Additional work is needed to fully establish the credibility of conceptual-theoretical-empirical structures derived from the Roy Adaptation Model. Gerrish's (1989) thoughtful evaluation of her use of the model in nursing practice represents a prototype clinical case study for credibility determination. Hoch's (1987) clinical study comparing the use of an explicit conceptual model of nursing with an implicit model is a prototype for more systematic credibility determination. More comprehensive case studies and clinical research that draw definitive conclusions regarding the credibility of the Roy Adaptation Model are needed.

In conclusion, the Roy Adaptation Model has been adopted enthusiastically by many nurse educators and clinicians. Although such enthusiasm about the model could result in its uncritical application, Roy has attempted to guard against this by pointing out areas of the model needing further clarification and development. She commented:

> As models and frameworks continue to make their contribution to nursing, conceptual clarification and other theoretical development will be done by the theorists and others. . . . A number of issues related to the concepts of the Roy adaptation [have been raised]. Although major changes in the model do not seem to be called for, a rethinking of some basic definitions and distinctions among the key concepts provides the stimulus for further theoretical and empirical growth. (Artinian & Roy, 1990, p. 66)

> Some assumptions about the model should be validated—for example, the assumption that the person has four modes of adaption. Assumed values, particularly the value concerning the uniqueness of nursing, need to be made more explicit, and perhaps should also be supported. The model's goal, patiency, source of difficulty, and intervention in terms of focus and mode are all replete with possibilities for further clarification. A particularly fruitful field for study is the patient's use of adaptive mechanisms and the nurse's support of these in each adaptive mode. (Roy, 1989, p. 113)

Further clarification and development of the Roy Adaptation Model and the Theory of the Person as an Adaptive System is being spearheaded by the Boston-Based Adaptation Research in Nursing Society. The purposes of the Society are to "advance nursing practice by developing basic and clinical nursing knowledge based on the Roy Adaptation Model, provide the scholarly colleagueship needed for knowledge development and research, enhance networks of dissemination or research for practice, and encourage scholars and facilitate programs of research" (Wallace, 1993, p. 308).

REFERENCES

Aaronson, L., & Seaman, L.P. (1989). Managing hypernatremia in fluid deficient elderly. *Journal of Gerontological Nursing*, 15(7), 29–34.

Abdellah, F.G., Beland, I., Martin A., & Matheney, R. (1960). *Patient-centered approaches to nursing*. New York Macmillan.

Andrews, H.A. (1989). Implementation of the Roy adaptation model: An application of education change research. In J.P. Riehl-Sisca, *Conceptual models for nursing practice* (3rd ed., pp. 133–148). Norwalk, CT: Appleton & Lange.

Andrews, H.A. (1991a). Overview of the role function mode. In C. Roy & H.A. Andrews, *The Roy adaptation model: The definitive statement* (pp. 347–361). Norwalk, CT: Appleton & Lange.

Andrews, H.A. (1991b). Overview of the self-concept mode. In C. Roy & H.A. Andrews, *The Roy adaptation model: The definitive statement* (pp. 269–279). Norwalk, CT: Appleton & Lange.

Andrews, H.A., & Roy, C. (1986). *Essentials of the Roy adaptation model.* Norwalk, CT: Appleton-Century-Crofts.

Andrews, H.A., & Roy, C. (1991a). Essentials of the Roy adaptation model. In Roy, C., & Andrews, H.C., *The Roy adaptation model: The definitive statement* (pp. 3–25). Norwalk, CT: Appleton & Lange.

Andrews, H.A., & Roy, C. (1991b). The nursing process according to the Roy adaptation model. In Roy, C., & Andrews, H.C., *The Roy adaptation model: The definitive statement* (pp. 27–54). Norwalk, CT: Appleton & Lange.

Artinian, N.T. (1991). Stress experience of spouses of patients having coronary artery bypass during hospitalization and 6 weeks after discharge. *Heart and Lung, 20,* 52–59.

Artinian, N.T. (1992). Spouse adaptation to mate's CABG surgery: 1-year follow-up. *American Journal of Critical Care, 1*(2), 36–42.

Artinian, N.T., & Roy, C. (1990). Strengthening the Roy adaptation model through conceptual clarification. Commentary [Artinian] and response [Roy]. *Nursing Science Quarterly, 3,* 60–66.

Baker, A.C. (1993). The spouse's positive effect on the stroke patient's recovery. *Rehabilitation Nursing, 18,* 30–33, 67–68.

Baldwin, J., & Schaffer, S. (1990). The continuing case study. *Nurse Educator, 15*(5), 6–9.

Barnfather, J.S., Swain, M.A.P., & Erickson, H.C. (1989). Evaluation of two assessment techniques for adaptation to stress. *Nursing Science Quarterly, 2,* 172–182.

Barnum, B.J.S. (1994). *Nursing theory: Analysis, application, evaluation* (4th ed.). Philadelphia: JB Lippincott.

Bawden, M., Ralph, J., & Herrick, C.A. (1991). Enhancing the coping skills of mothers with developmentally delayed children. *Journal of Child and Adolescent*

Psychiatric Mental Health Nursing, 4, 25–28.

Bertalanffy, L (1968). *General system theory.* New York: George Braziller.

Boas, G. (1957). *Dominant themes of modern philosophy.* New York: Ronald Press.

Bokinskie, J.C. (1992). Family conferences: A method to diminish transfer anxiety. *Journal of Neuroscience Nursing, 24,* 129–133.

Bradley, K.M. & Williams, D.M. (1990). A comparison of the preoperative concerns of open heart surgery patients and their significant others. *Journal of Cardiovascular Nursing, 5,* 43–53.

Broeder, J.L. (1985). School-age children's perceptions of isolation after hospital discharge. *Maternal-Child Nursing Journal, 14,* 153–174.

Brower, H.T.F., & Baker, B.J. (1976). Using the adaptation model in a practitioner curriculum. *Nursing Outlook, 24,* 686–689.

Calvert, M.M. (1989). Human-pet interaction and loneliness: A test of concepts from Roy's adaptation model. *Nursing Science Quarterly, 2,* 194–202.

Calvillo, E.R., & Flaskerud, J.H. (1993). The adequacy and scope of Roy's adaptation model to guide cross-cultural pain research. *Nursing Science Quarterly, 6,* 118–129.

Camooso, C., Greene, M., & Reilly, P. (1981). Students' adaptation according to Roy. *Nursing Outlook, 29,* 108–109.

Campbell, J.M. (1992). Treating depression in well older adults: Use of diaries in cognitive therapy. *Issues in Mental Health Nursing, 13,* 19–29.

Cardiff, J. (1989). Heartfelt care. *Nursing Times, 85*(3), 42–45.

Chardin, P.T. (1956). *Man's place in nature.* New York: Harper & Row.

Chardin, P.T. (1959). *The phenomenon of man.* New York: Harper & Row.

Chardin, P.T. (1965). *Hymn of the universe.* (S. Bartholomew, Trans.). New York: Harper & Row.

Cheng, M., & Williams, P.D. (1989). Oxygenation during chest physiotherapy of very-low-birth-weight infants: Relations among fraction of inspired oxygen levels, number of hand ventilations, and transcutaneous oxygen pressure. *Journal of Pediatric Nursing, 4,* 411–418.

Christian, A. (1993). The relationship between women's symptoms of endometriosis and self-esteem. *Journal of Obstetric, Gynecologic, and Neonatal Nursing, 22,* 370–376.

Coelho, G., Hamburg, D., & Adams, J. (Eds.).

(1974). *Coping and adaptation*. New York: Basic Books.

Cottrell, B., & Shannahan, M. (1986). Effect of the birth chair on duration of second stage labor and maternal outcome. *Nursing Research, 35*, 364–367.

Cottrell, B., & Shannahan, M. (1987). A comparison of fetal outcome in birth chair and delivery table births. *Research in Nursing and Health, 10*, 239–243.

Craig, D.I. (1990). The adaptation to pregnancy of spinal cord injured women. *Rehabilitation Nursing, 15*(1), 6–9.

Crossfield, T. (1990). Patients with scleroderma. *Nursing (London), 4*(10), 19–20.

DiIorio, C. (1989). Applying Roy's model to nursing administration. In B. Henry, M. DiVincenti, C. Arndt, & A. Marriner-Tomey (Eds.), *Dimensions of nursing administration: Theory, research, education, and practice* (pp. 89–104). Boston: Blackwell Scientific Publications.

DiMaria, R.A. (1989). Posttrauma responses: Potential for nursing. *Journal of Advanced Medical-Surgical Nursing, 2*(1), 41–48.

Dorsey, K., & Purcell, S. (1987). Translating a nursing theory into a nursing system. *Geriatric Nursing, 8*, 167–137.

Downey, C. (1974). Adaptation nursing applied to an obstetric patient. In J.P. Riehl & C. Roy, *Conceptual models for nursing practice* (pp. 151–159). New York: Appleton-Century-Crofts.

Doyle, R., & Rajacich, D. (1991). The Roy adaptation model: Health teaching about osteoporosis. *American Association of Occupational Health Nursing Journal, 39*, 508–512.

Dudek, G. (1989). Nursing update: Hypophosphatemic rickets. *Pediatric Nursing, 15*(1), 45–50.

Ellis, J.A. (1991). Coping with adolescent cancer: It's a matter of adaptation. *Journal of Pediatric Oncology Nursing, 8*, 10–17.

Ewing, A.C. (1951). *The fundamental questions of philosophy*. London: Routledge & Kegan Paul.

Farkas, L. (1981). Adaptation problems with nursing home application for elderly persons: An application of the Roy Adaptation Nursing Model. *Journal of Advanced Nursing, 8*, 363–368.

Fawcett, J. (1981a). Assessing and understanding the cesarean father. In C.F. Kehoe (Ed.), *The cesarean experience: Theoretical and clinical perspectives for nurses* (pp. 143–156). New York: Appleton-Century-Crofts.

Fawcett, J. (1981b). Needs of cesarean birth parents. *Journal of Obstetric, Gynecologic, and Neonatal Nursing, 10*, 371–376.

Fawcett, J. (1990). Preparation for caesarean childbirth: Derivation of a nursing intervention from the Roy adaptation model. *Journal of Advanced Nursing, 15*, 1418–1425.

Fawcett, J. (1992). Documentation using a conceptual model of nursing. *Nephrology Nursing Today, 2*(5), 1–8.

Fawcett, J., Archer, C.L., Becker, D., Brown, K.K., Gann, S., Wong, M.J., & Wurster, A.B. (1992). Guidelines for selecting a conceptual model of nursing: Focus on the individual patient. *Dimensions of Critical Care Nursing, 11*, 268–277.

Fawcett, J., Botter, M.L., Burritt, J., Crossley, J.D., & Frink, B.B. (1989). Conceptual models of nursing and organization theories. In B. Henry, M. DiVincenti, C. Arndt, & A. Marriner-Tomey (Eds.), *Dimensions of nursing administration: Theory, research, education, and practice* (pp. 143–154). Boston: Blackwell Scientific Publications.

Fawcett, J., & Burritt, J. (1985). An exploratory study of antenatal preparation for cesarean birth. *Journal of Obstetric, Gynecologic, and Neonatal Nursing, 14*, 224–230.

Fawcett, J., & Downs, F.S. (1992). *The relationship of theory and research* (2nd ed.). Philadelphia: FA Davis.

Fawcett, J., & Henklein, J. (1987). Antenatal education for cesarean birth: Extension of a field test. *Journal of Obstetric, Gynecologic, and Neonatal Nursing, 16*, 61–65.

Fawcett, J., Pollio, N., Tully, A., Baron, M., Henklein, J.C., & Jones, R.C. (1993). Effects of information on adaptation to cesarean birth. *Nursing Research, 42*, 49–53.

Fawcett, J., & Tulman, L. (1990). Building a programme of research from the Roy adaptation model of Nursing. *Journal of Advanced Nursing, 15*, 720–725.

Fawcett, J., Tulman, L., & Myers, S. (1988). Development of the Inventory of Functional Status after Childbirth. *Journal of Nurse-Midwifery, 33*, 252–260.

Fawcett, J., & Weiss, M.E. (1993). Cross-cultural adaptation to cesarean birth. *Western Journal of Nursing Research, 15*, 282–297.

Fitch, M., Rogers, M., Ross, E., Shea, H., Smith, I., & Tucker, D. (1991). Developing a plan to evaluate the use of nursing conceptual frameworks. *Canadian Journal of Nursing Administration, 4*(1), 22–28.

Fox, J.A. (1990). Bilateral breast lumps: A care plan in theatre using a stress adaptation model. *NATNews: British Journal of Theatre Nursing, 27*(11), 11–14.

Francis, G., Turner, J.T., & Johnson, S.B.

(1985). Domestic animal visitation as therapy with adult home residents. *International Journal of Nursing Studies, 22,* 201–206.

Frank, D.I. (1988). Psychosocial assessment of renal dialysis patients. *Journal of the American Nephrology Nurses Association, 15,* 207–232.

Frederickson, K. (1992). Research methodology and nursing science. *Nursing Science Quarterly, 5,* 150–151.

Frederickson, K. (1993). Using a nursing model to manage symptoms: Anxiety and the Roy adaptation model. *Holistic Nursing Practice, 7*(2), 36–42.

Frederickson, K., Jackson, B.S., Strauman, T., & Strauman, J. (1991). Testing hypotheses derived from the Roy adaptation model. *Nursing Science Quarterly, 4,* 168–174.

Gaberson, K.B. (1991). The effect of humorous distraction on preoperative anxiety. A pilot study. *Association of Operating Room Nurses Journal, 54,* 1258–1261, 1263–1264.

Gagliardi, B.A. (1991). The impact of Duchenne muscular dystrophy on families. *Orthopaedic Nursing, 10*(5), 41–49.

Galligan, A.C. (1979). Using Roy's concept of adaptation to care for young children. *American Journal of Maternal Child Nursing, 4,* 24–28.

Germain, C.P. (1984). Sheltering abused women: A nursing perspective. *Journal of Psychosocial Nursing, 22*(9), 24–31.

Gerrish, C. (1989). From theory to practice. *Nursing Times, 85*(35), 42–45.

Giger, J.A., Bower, C.A., & Miller, S.W. (1987). Roy Adaptation Model: ICU application. *Dimensions of Critical Care Nursing, 6,* 215–224.

Gordon, J. (1974). Nursing assessment and care plan for a cardiac patient. In J.P. Riehl & C. Roy, *Conceptual models for nursing practice* (pp. 144–151). New York: Appleton-Century-Crofts.

Gray, J. (1991). The Roy adaptation model in nursing practice. In C. Roy & H.A. Andrews, *The Roy adaptation model: The definitive statement* (pp. 429–443). Norwalk, CT: Appleton & Lange.

Guzzetta, C. (1979). Relationship between stress and learning. *Advances in Nursing Science, 1*(4), 35–49.

Hamer, B.A. (1991). Music therapy: Harmony for change. *Journal of Psychosocial Nursing and Mental Health Services, 29*(12), 5–7.

Hammond, H., Roberts, M., & Silva, M.

(1983, Spring). The effect of Roy's first level and second level assessment on nurses' determination of accurate nursing diagnoses. *Virginia Nurse,* 14–17.

Hamner, J.B. (1989). Applying the Roy adaptation model to the CCU. *Critical Care Nurse, 9*(3), 51–61.

Hanchett, E.S. (1990). Nursing models and community as client. *Nursing Science Quarterly, 3,* 67–72.

Harrison, L.L., Leeper, J.D., & Yoon, M. (1990). Effects of early parent touch on preterm infants' heart rates and arterial oxygen saturation levels. *Journal of Advanced Nursing, 15,* 877–885.

Hazlett, D.E. (1989). A study of pediatric home ventilator management: Medical, psychosocial, and financial aspects. *Journal of Pediatric Nursing, 4,* 284–294.

Heinrich, K. (1989). Growing pains: Faculty stages in adopting a nursing model. *Nurse Educator, 14*(1), 3–4, 29.

Helson, H. (1964). *Adaptation-level theory.* New York: Harper & Row.

Henderson, V. (1960). *Basic principles of nursing care.* London: International Council of Nurses.

Hinman, L.M. (1983). Focus on the school-aged child in family intervention. *Journal of School Health, 53,* 499–502.

Hoch, C.C. (1987). Assessing delivery of nursing care. *Journal of Gerontological Nursing, 13,* 10–17.

Hughes, A. (1991). Life with a stoma. *Nursing Times, 87*(25), 67–68.

Hughes, M.M. (1983). Nursing theories and emergency nursing. *Journal of Emergency Nursing, 9,* 95–97.

Hunter L.P. (1991). Measurement of axillary temperatures in neonates. *Western Journal of Nursing Research, 13,* 324–335.

Ide, B.A. (1978). SPAL: A tool for measuring self-perceived adaptation level appropriate for an elderly population. In E.E. Bauwens (Ed.), *Clinical nursing research: Its strategies and findings* (Monograph series 1978: Two, pp. 56–63). Indianapolis: Sigma Theta Tau.

Ingalls, J.D. (Ed.). (1972). *A trainer's guide to androgogy* (rev. ed.). Waltham, MA: Data Education, Inc.

Innes, M.H. (1992). Management of an inadequately ventilated patient. *British Journal of Nursing, 1,* 780–784.

Jackson, D.A. (1990). Roy in the postanesthesia care unit. *Journal of Post Anesthesia Nursing, 5,* 143–148.

Jackson, B.S., Strauman, J., Frederickson, K., & Strauman, T.J. (1991). Long-term biopsychosocial effects of interleukin-2 therapy. *Oncology Nursing Forum, 18,* 683–690.

Jakocko, M.T., & Sowden, L.A. (1986). The Roy adaptation model in nursing practice. In H.A. Andrews & C. Roy, *Essentials of the Roy adaptation model* (pp. 165–177). Norwalk, CT: Appleton & Lange.

Janelli, L. (1980). Utilizing Roy's adaptation model from a gerontological perspective. *Journal of Gerontological Nursing, 6,* 140–150.

Jay, P. (1990). Relatives caring for the terminally ill. *Nursing Standard, 5*(5), 30–32.

Kehoe, C.F. (1981). Identifying the nursing needs of the postpartum cesarean mother. In C.F. Kehoe (Ed.), *The cesarean experience: Theoretical and clinical perspectives for nurses* (pp. 85–141). New York: Appleton-Century-Crofts.

Khanobdee, C., Sukratanachaiyakul, V., & Gay, J.T. (1993). Couvade syndrome in expectant Thai fathers. *International Journal of Nursing Studies, 30,* 125–131.

Kiikkala, I., & Peitsi, T. (1991). The care of children with minimal brain dysfunction: A Roy adaptation analysis. *Journal of Pediatric Nursing, 6,* 290–292.

Knowlton, C., Goodwin, M., Moore, J., Alt-White, A., Guarino, S., & Pyne, H. (1983). Systems adaptation model for nursing for families, groups, and communities. *Journal of Nursing Education, 22,* 128–131.

Komelasky, A.L. (1990). The effect of home nursing visits on parental anxiety and CPR knowledge retention of parents of apnea-monitored infants. *Journal of Pediatric Nursing, 5,* 387–392.

Kurek-Ovshinsky, C. (1991). Group psychotherapy in an acute inpatient setting: Techniques that nourish self-esteem. *Issues in Mental Health Nursing, 12,* 81–88.

Laros, J. (1977). Deriving outcome criteria from a conceptual model. *Nursing Outlook, 25,* 333–336.

Lazarus, R.S., Averill, J.R., & Opton, E.M. Jr. (1974). The psychology of coping: Issues of research and assessment (pp. 249–315). In G.V. Coelho, D.A. Hamburg, & J.E. Adams (Eds.), *Coping and adaptation.* New York: Basic Books.

Leonard, C. (1975). Patient attitudes toward nursing interventions. *Nursing Research, 24,* 335–339.

Leuze, M., & McKenzie, J. (1987). Preoperative assessment using the Roy adaptation model. *Association of Operating Room Nurses Journal, 46,* 1122–1134.

Levine, M.E. (1966). Adaptation and assessment: A rationale for nursing intervention. *American Journal of Nursing, 66,* 2450–2453.

Lewis, F.M., Firsich, S.C., & Parsell, S. (1978). Development of reliable measures of patient health outcomes related to quality nursing care for chemotherapy patients. In J.C. Krueger, A.H. Nelson, & M.O. Wolanin, *Nursing research: Development, collaboration, and utilization* (pp. 225–228). Germantown, MD: Aspen.

Lewis, F.M., Firsich, S.C., & Parsell, S. (1979). Clinical tool development for adult chemotherapy patients: Process and content. *Cancer Nursing, 2,* 99–108.

Limandri, B. (1986). Research and practice with abused women: Use of the Roy adaptation model as an exploratory framework. *Advances in Nursing Science, 8*(4), 52–61.

Logan, M. (1986). Palliative care nursing: Applicability of the Roy model. *Journal of Palliative Care, 1*(2), 18–24.

Logan, M. (1988). Care of the terminally ill includes the family. *The Canadian Nurse, 84*(5), 30–33.

Logan, M. (1990). The Roy adaptation model: Are nursing diagnoses amenable to independent nurse functions? *Journal of Advanced Nursing, 15,* 468–470.

Lutjens, L.R.J. (1992). Derivation and testing of tenets of a theory of social organizations as adaptive systems. *Nursing Science Quarterly, 5,* 62–71.

Lynam, L.E., & Miller, M.A. (1992). Mothers' and nurses' perceptions of the needs of women experiencing preterm labor. *Journal of Obstetric, Gynecologic, and Neonatal Nursing, 21,* 126–136.

Marriner-Tomey, A. (1989). *Nursing theorists and their work* (2nd ed.). St. Louis: CV Mosby.

Mason, T., & Chandley, M. (1990). Nursing models in a special hospital: A critical analysis of efficacity. *Journal of Advanced Nursing, 15,* 667–673.

Mastal, M.F., Hammond, H., & Roberts, M.P. (1982). Theory into hospital practice: A pilot implementation. *Journal of Nursing Administration, 12*(6), 9–15.

McCain, R.F. (1965). Nursing by assessment-not intuition. *American Journal of Nursing, 65*(4), 82–84.

McDonald, F.J., & Harms, M. (1966). Theoretical model for an experimental curriculum. *Nursing Outlook, 14*(8), 48–51.

McGill, J.S. (1992). Functional status as it relates to hope in elders with and without cancer (Abstract). *Kentucky Nurse, 40*(4), 6.

McIver, M. (1987). Putting theory into practice. *The Canadian Nurse, 83*(10), 36–38.

Meek, S.S. (1993). Effects of slow stroke back massage on relaxation in hospice clients. *Image: Journal of Nursing Scholarship, 25*, 17–21.

Meleis, A.I. (1991). *Theoretical nursing: Development and progress* (2nd ed.). Philadelphia: JB Lippincott.

Mengel, A., Sherman, S., Nahigian, E., & Coleman, I. (1989). Adaptation of the Roy model in an educational setting. In J.P. Riehl-Sisca, *Conceptual models for nursing practice* (3rd ed., pp. 125–131). Norwalk, CT: Appleton & Lange.

Miles, M.S., & Carter, M.C. (1983). Assessing parental stress in intensive care units. *American Journal of Maternal Child Nursing, 8*, 354–359.

Miller, F. (1991). Using Roy's model in a special hospital. *Nursing Standard, 5*(27), 29–32.

Montefiore Medical Center. (1989). There's more at Montefiore. (Advertisement). *The New York Times*, November 19, 18.

deMontigney, F. (1992a). L'Intervention familiale selon Roy: La famille Joly: Cueillette et analyse des données. [Family intervention according to Roy]. *The Canadian Nurse, 88*(8), 41–45.

deMontigney, F. (1992b). L'Intervention familiale selon Roy: Planification, exécution et évaluation. [Family intervention according to Roy]. *The Canadian Nurse, 88*(9), 43–46.

Morales-Mann, E.T., & Logan, M. (1990). Implementing the Roy model: Challenges for nurse educators. *Journal of Advanced Nursing, 15*, 142–147.

Munn, V.A., & Tichy, A.M. (1987). Nurses' perceptions of stressors in pediatric intensive care. *Journal of Pediatric Nursing, 2*, 405–411.

Nash, D.J. (1987). Kawasaki disease: Application of the Roy adaptation model to determine interventions. *Journal of Pediatric Nursing, 2*, 308–315.

Nightingale, F. (1859). *Notes on nursing: What it is, and what it is not.* London: Harrison. Reprinted 1946. Philadelphia: JB Lippincott.

Nolan, M. (1977). Effects of nursing intervention in the operating room as recalled on the third postoperative day. In M.V. Batey (Ed.), *Communicating nursing research in the bicentennial year* (Vol. 9, pp. 41–50). Boulder, CO: Western Interstate Commission for Higher Education.

Norris, S., Campbell, L., & Brenkert, S.

(1982). Nursing procedures and alterations in transcutaneous oxygen tension in premature infants. *Nursing Research, 31*, 330–336.

Nyqvist, K.H., & Sjoden, P.O. (1993). Advice concerning breastfeeding from mothers of infants admitted to a neonatal intensive care unit: The Roy adaptation model as a conceptual structure. *Journal of Advanced Nursing, 18*, 54–63.

O'Reilly, M. (1989). Familiarity breeds acceptance. *Nursing Times, 85*(12), 29–30.

Orlando, I.J. (1961). *The dynamic nurse-patient relationship.* New York: GP Putnam's Sons.

Paier, G.S. (in press). Development and testing of an instrument to assess functional status in the elderly. *Dissertation Abstracts International.*

Peplau, H. (1952). *Interpersonal relations in nursing.* New York: GP Putnam's Sons.

Peters, V.J. (1993). Documentation using the Roy adaptation model. *American Nephrology Nurses Association Journal, 20*, 522.

Phillips, J.A., & Brown, K.C. (1992). Industrial workers on a rotating shift pattern: Adaptation and injury status. *American Association of Occupational Health Nurses Journal, 40*, 468–476.

Piazza, D., & Foote, A. (1990). Roy's adaptation model: A guide for rehabilitation nursing practice. *Rehabilitation Nursing, 15*, 254–259.

Pollock, S.E. (1993). Adaptation to chronic illness: A program of research for testing nursing theory. *Nursing Science Quarterly, 6*, 86–92.

Popper, K.R., & Eccles, J.C. (1981). *The self and its brain.* New York: Springer.

Porth, C.M. (1977). Physiological coping: A model for teaching pathophysiology. *Nursing Outlook, 25*, 781–784.

Preston, D.B., & Dellasega, C. (1990). Elderly women and stress. Does marriage make a difference? *Journal of Gerontological Nursing, 16*, 26–32.

Printz-Feddersen, V. (1990). Effect of group process on caregiver burden (Abstract). *Journal of Neuroscience Nursing, 22*, 50–51.

Rambo, B. (1984). *Adaptation nursing: Assessment and intervention.* Philadelphia: WB Saunders.

Randell, B., Poush Tedrow, M., & Van Landingham, J. (1982). *Adaptation nursing: The Roy conceptual model applied.* St. Louis: CV Mosby.

Riegel, B. (1985). A method of giving intershift report based on a conceptual model. *Focus on Critical Care, 12*(4), 12–18.

Riehl, J.P., & Roy, C. (1974). *Conceptual models for nursing practice.* New York: Appleton-Century-Crofts.

Riehl, J.P., & Roy, C. (1980). *Conceptual models for nursing practice* (2nd ed.). New York: Appleton-Century-Crofts.

Riehl-Sisca, J.P. (1989). *Conceptual models for nursing practice* (3rd ed.). Norwalk, CT: Appleton & Lange.

Robitaille-Tremblay, M. (1984). A data collection tool for the psychiatric nurse. *The Canadian Nurse, 80*(7), 26–28.

Rogers, E.J. (1991). Postanesthesia care of the cocaine abuser. *Journal of Post Anesthesia Nursing, 6,* 102–107.

Rogers, M., Paul, L.J., Clarke, J., MacKay, C., Potter, M., & Ward, W. (1991). The use of the Roy adaptation model in nursing administration. *Canadian Journal of Nursing Administration, 4*(2), 21–26.

Rosenthal, R. (1991). *Meta-analytic procedures for social research (rev. ed.).* Newbury Park, CA: Sage.

Roy, C. (1970). Adaptation: A conceptual framework for nursing. *Nursing Outlook, 18*(3), 42–45.

Roy, C. (1971). Adaptation: A basis for nursing practice. *Nursing Outlook, 19,* 254–257.

Roy, C. (1973). Adaptation: Implications for curriculum change. *Nursing Outlook, 21,* 163–168.

Roy, C. (1974). The Roy Adaptation Model. In J. P. Riehl & C. Roy, *Conceptual models for nursing practice* (pp. 135–144). New York: Appleton-Century-Crofts.

Roy, C. (1976a). Comment. *Nursing Outlook, 24,* 690–691.

Roy, C. (1976b). *Introduction to nursing: An adaptation model.* Englewood Cliffs, NJ: Prentice-Hall.

Roy, C. (1978a, December). *Adaptation model.* Paper presented at Second Annual Nurse Educator Conference, New York. (Cassette recording).

Roy, C. (1978b). The stress of hospital events: Measuring changes in level of stress. (Abstract). In *Communicating nursing research.* Vol. 11: *New approaches to communicating nursing research* (pp. 70–71). Boulder, CO: Western Interstate Commission for Higher Education.

Roy, C. (1979a). Health-illness (powerlessness) questionnaire and hospitalized patient decision making. In M.J. Ward & C.A. Lindeman (Eds.), *Instruments for measuring nursing practice and other health care variables* (Vol. 1, pp. 147–153). Hyattsville, MD: US Department of Health, Education, and Welfare.

Roy, C. (1979b). Relating nursing theory to education: A new era. *Nurse Educator, 4*(2), 16–21.

Roy, C. (1980). The Roy adaptation model. In J. P. Riehl & C. Roy, *Conceptual models for nursing practice* (2nd ed., pp. 179–188). New York: Appleton-Century-Crofts.

Roy, C. (1982). Foreword. In B. Randell, M. Poush Tedrow, & J. Van Landingham, *Adaptation nursing: The Roy conceptual model applied* (pp. vii–viii). St. Louis: CV Mosby.

Roy, C. (1983a). The expectant family: Analysis and application of the Roy Adaptation Model. In I.W. Clements & F.B. Roberts, *Family health: A theoretical approach to nursing care* (pp. 298–303). New York: John Wiley & Sons.

Roy, C. (1983b). The family in primary care: Analysis and application of the Roy adaptation model. In I.W. Clements & F.B. Roberts, *Family health: A theoretical approach to nursing care* (pp. 375–378). New York: John Wiley & Sons.

Roy, C. (1983c). Roy adaptation model. In I.W. Clements & F.B. Roberts, *Family health: A theoretical approach to nursing care* (pp. 255–278). New York: John Wiley & Sons.

Roy, C. (1984a). *Introduction to nursing: An adaptation model* (2nd ed.). Englewood Cliffs, NJ: Prentice-Hall.

Roy, C. (1984b). The Roy Adaptation Model: Applications in community health. In M.K. Asay & C.C. Ossler (Eds.), *Conceptual models of nursing: Applications in community health nursing: Proceedings of the Eighth Annual Community Health Nursing Conference* (pp. 51–73). Chapel Hill: Department of Public Health Nursing, School of Public Health, University of North Carolina.

Roy, C. (1987a). The influence of nursing models on clinical decision making II. In K.J. Hannah, M. Reimer, W.C. Mills, & S. Letourneau (Eds.), *Clinical judgment and decision making: The future with nursing diagnosis* (pp. 42–47). New York: John Wiley & Sons.

Roy, C. (1987b). Response to "Needs of spouses of surgical patients: A conceptualization within the Roy adaptation model." *Scholarly Inquiry for Nursing Practice, 1,* 45–50.

Roy, C. (1987c). Roy's adaptation model. In R.R. Parse, *Nursing science. Major paradigms, theories, and critiques* (pp. 35–45). Philadelphia: WB Saunders.

Roy, C. (1987d, May). *Roy's model.* Paper presented at the Nurse Theorist Conference, Pittsburgh, PA. (Cassette recording).

Roy, C. (1988a). Altered cognition: An information processing approach. In P.H. Mitchell, L.C. Hodges, M. Muwaswes, & C.A. Walleck (Eds.), *AANN's neuroscience nursing: Phenomenon and practice: Human responses to neurological health problems* (pp. 185–211). Norwalk, CT: Appleton & Lange.

Roy, C. (1988b). An explication of the philosophical assumptions of the Roy Adaptation Model. *Nursing Science Quarterly, 1,* 26–34.

Roy, C. (1988c). Sister Callista Roy. In T.M. Schorr & A. Zimmerman, *Making choices: Taking chances: Nurse leaders tell their stories* (pp. 291–298). St. Louis: CV Mosby.

Roy, C. (1989). The Roy adaptation model. In J.P. Riehl-Sisca, *Conceptual models for nursing practice* (3rd ed., pp. 105–114). Norwalk, CT: Appleton & Lange.

Roy, C. (1991a). The Roy adaptation model in nursing research. In C. Roy & H.A. Andrews, *The Roy adaptation model: The definitive statement* (pp. 445–458). Norwalk, CT: Appleton & Lange.

Roy, C. (1991b). Structure of knowledge: Paradigm, model, and research specifications for differentiated practice. In I.E. Goertzen (Ed.), *Differentiating nursing practice: Into the twenty-first century* (pp. 31–39). Kansas City, MO: American Academy of Nursing.

Roy, C. (1992). Vigor, variables, and vision: Commentary on Florence Nightingale. In F.N. Nightingale, *Notes on nursing: What it is, and what it is not* (Commemorative ed., pp. 63–71). Philadelphia: JB Lippincott.

Roy, C., & Andrews, H.A. (1991). *The Roy adaptation model: The definitive statement* Norwalk, CT: Appleton & Lange.

Roy, C., & Anway, J. (1989). Theories and hypotheses for nursing administration. In B. Henry, M. DiVincenti, C. Arndt, & A. Marriner-Tomey (Eds.), *Dimensions of nursing administration: Theory, research, education, and practice* (pp. 75–88). Boston: Blackwell Scientific Publications.

Roy, C., & Corliss, C.P. (1993). The Roy adaptation model: Theoretical update and knowledge for practice. In M.E. Parker (Ed.), *Patterns of nursing theories in practice* (pp. 215–229). New York: National League for Nursing.

Roy, C., & Martinez, C. (1983). A conceptual framework for CNS practice. In A. Hamric & J. Spross (Eds.), *The clinical nurse specialist in theory and practice* (pp. 3–20). New York: Grune & Stratton.

Roy, C., & Roberts, S.L. (1981). *Theory construction in nursing: An adaptation model.* Englewood Cliffs, NJ: Prentice-Hall.

Rush, J.E. (1981). *Towards a general theory of healing.* Washington, DC: University Press of America.

Samarel, N., & Fawcett, J. (1992). Enhancing adaptation to breast cancer: The addition of coaching to support groups. *Oncology Nursing Forum, 19,* 591–596.

Samarel, N., Fawcett, J., & Tulman, L. (1993). The effects of coaching in breast cancer support groups: A pilot study. *Oncology Nursing Forum, 20,* 795–798.

Sato, M.K. (1986). The Roy adaptation model. In P. Winstead-Fry (Ed.), *Case studies in nursing theory* (pp. 103–125). New York: National League for Nursing.

Schmidt, C.S. (1981). Withdrawal behavior of schizophrenics: Application of Roy's model. *Journal of Psychosocial Nursing and Mental Health Services, 19*(11), 26–33.

Schmitz, M. (1980). The Roy adaptation model: Application in a community setting. In J.P. Riehl & C. Roy, *Conceptual models for nursing practice* (2nd ed., pp. 193–206). New York: Appleton-Century-Crofts.

Sellers, S.C. (1991). A philosophical analysis of conceptual models of nursing. *Dissertation Abstracts International, 52,* 1937B. (University Microfilms No. AAC9126248).

Selman, S.W. (1989). Impact of total hip replacement on quality of life. *Orthopaedic Nursing, 8*(5), 43–49.

Shannahan, M., & Cottrell, B. (1985). Effect of the birth chair on duration of second stage labor, fetal outcome, and maternal blood loss. *Nursing Research, 34,* 89–92.

Silva, M.C. (1987a). Conceptual models of nursing. In J.J. Fitzpatrick & R.L. Taunton (Eds.), *Annual review of nursing research* (Vol. 5, pp. 229–246). New York: Springer.

Silva, M.C. (1987b). Needs of spouses of surgical patients: A conceptualization within the Roy adaptation model. *Scholarly Inquiry for Nursing Practice, 1,* 29–44.

Silva, M.C., & Sorrell, M.M. (1992). Testing of nursing theory: Critique and philosophical expansion. *Advances in Nursing Science, 14*(4), 12–23.

Sirignano, R.G. (1987). Peripartum cardiomyopathy: An application of the Roy adaptation model. *Journal of Cardiovascular Nursing, 2,* 24–32.

Smith, C., Garvis, M., & Martinson, I. (1983). Content analysis of interviews using nursing model: A look at parents adapting to the impact of childhood cancer. *Cancer Nursing, 6,* 269–275.

Smith, C.E., Mayer, L.S., Parkhurst, C., Perkins, S.B., & Pingleton, S.K. (1991). Adaptation in families with a member requiring mechanical ventilation at home. *Heart and Lung, 20,* 349–356.

Smith, M.C. (1988). Roy's adaptation model in practice. *Nursing Science Quarterly, 1,* 97–98.

Starn, J., & Niederhauser, V. (1990). An MCN model for nursing diagnosis to focus intervention. *American Journal of Maternal Child Nursing, 15,* 180–183.

Starr, S.L. (1980). Adaptation applied to the dying client. In J.P. Riehl & C. Roy, *Conceptual models for nursing practice* (2nd ed., pp. 189–192). New York: Appleton-Century-Crofts.

Story, E.L., & Ross, M.M. (1986). Family centered community health nursing and the Betty Neuman systems model. *Nursing Papers, 18*(2), 77–88.

Strickler, M., & LaSor, B. (1970). Concept of loss in crisis intervention. *Mental Hygiene, 54,* 301–305.

Stringer, M., Librizzi, R., & Weiner, S. (1991). Establishing a prenatal genetic diagnosis: The nurse's role. *American Journal of Maternal Child Nursing, 16,* 152–156.

Strohmyer, L.L., Noroian, E.L., Patterson, L.M., & Carlin, B.P. (1993). Adaptation six months after multiple trauma: A pilot study. *Journal of Neuroscience Nursing, 25,* 30–37.

Studio Three (1992). *The nurse theorists: Excellence in action–Callista Roy.* Athens, OH: Fuld Institute of Technology in Nursing Education.

Summers, T.M. (1991). Psychosocial support of the burned patient. *Critical Care Nursing Clinics of North America, 3,* 237–244.

Taylor, C. (1993). *The patient's guide to preterm labor.* Woodbury, NJ: Underwood-Memorial Hospital.

Thornburry, J.M., & King, L.D. (1992). The Roy adaptation model and care of persons with Alzheimer's disease. *Nursing Science Quarterly, 5,* 129–133.

Torosian, L.C., DeStefano, M., & Dietrick-Gallagher, M. (1985). Day gynecologic chemotherapy unit: An innovative approach to changing health care systems. *Cancer Nursing, 8,* 221–227.

Tulman, L., & Fawcett, J. (1988). Return of functional ability after childbirth. *Nursing Research, 37,* 77–81.

Tulman, L., & Fawcett, J. (1990a). A framework for studying functional status after diagnosis of breast cancer. *Cancer Nursing, 13,* 95–99.

Tulman, L., & Fawcett, J. (1990b). Functional status during pregnancy and the postpartum: A framework for research. *Image: Journal of Nursing Scholarship, 22,* 191–194.

Tulman, L., & Fawcett, J. (1990c). Maternal employment following childbirth. *Research in Nursing and Health, 13,* 181–188.

Tulman, L., & Fawcett, J. (1993). *Functional status following diagnosis of breast cancer: A pilot study.* Manuscript submitted for publication.

Tulman, L., Fawcett, J., Groblewski, L., & Silverman, L. (1990). Changes in functional status after childbirth. *Nursing Research, 39,* 70–75.

Tulman, L., Fawcett, J., & McEvoy, M.D. (1991). Development of the inventory of functional status-cancer. *Cancer Nursing, 14,* 254–260.

Tulman, L., Fawcett, J., & Weiss, M. (1993). The inventory of functional status-fathers: Development and psychometric testing. *Journal of Nurse-Midwifery, 38,* 117–123.

Tulman, L., Higgins, K., Fawcett, J., Nunno, C., Vansickel, C., Haas, M.B., Speca, M.M. (1991). The Inventory of functional status-antepartum period: Development and testing. *Journal of Nurse-Midwifery, 36,* 117–123.

Vicenzi, A.E., & Thiel, R. (1992). AIDS education on the college campus: Roy's adaptation model directs inquiry. *Public Health Nursing, 9,* 270–276.

Wagner, P. (1976). Testing the adaptation model in practice. *Nursing Outlook, 24,* 682–685.

Wallace, C.L. (1993). Resources for nursing theories in practice. In M.E. Parker (Ed.), *Patterns of nursing theories in practice* (pp. 301–311). New York: National League for Nursing.

Weiss, M.E., Hastings, W.J., Holly, D.C., & Craig, D.I. (1992). *Using the Roy model in nursing practice: Clinical nurses' perspectives.* Unpublished manuscript, Sharp Memorial Hospital, San Diego.

Welsh, M.D., & Clochesy, J.M. (Eds.). (1990). *Case studies in cardiovascular critical care nursing.* Rockville, MD: Aspen.

West, S. (1992). Number one priorities. *Nursing Times, 88*(17), 28–31.

Whall, A.L. (1986). Strategic family therapy: Nursing reformulations and applications.

In A.L. Whall, *Family therapy theory for nursing: Four approaches* (pp. 51–67). Norwalk, CT: Appleton-Century-Crofts.

Wright, P.S., Holcombe, J., Foote, A., & Piazza, D. (1993). The Roy adaptation model used as a guide for the nursing care of an 8-year-old child with leukemia. *Journal of Pediatric Oncology Nursing, 10,* 68–74.

Zarle, N.C. (1987). *Continuing care: The process and practice of discharge planning.* Rockville, MD: Aspen.

BIBLIOGRAPHY

PRIMARY SOURCES

Andrews, H.A., & Roy, C. (1986). *Essentials of the Roy adaptation model.* Norwalk, CT: Appleton-Century-Crofts.

Artinian, N.T., & Roy, C. (1990). Strengthening the Roy adaptation model through conceptual clarification. Commentary [Artinian] and response [Roy]. *Nursing Science Quarterly, 3,* 60–66.

Roy, C. (1970). Adaptation: A conceptual framework for nursing. *Nursing Outlook, 18,* 42–45.

Roy, C. (1971). Adaptation: A basis for nursing practice. *19,* 254–257.

Roy, C. (1973). Adaptation: Implications for curriculum change. *Nursing Outlook, 21,* 163–168.

Roy, C. (1974). The Roy adaptation model. In J.P. Riehl & C. Roy, *Conceptual models for nursing practice* (pp. 135–144). New York: Appleton-Century-Crofts.

Roy, C. (1976). *Introduction to nursing: An adaptation model.* Englewood Cliffs, NJ: Prentice-Hall.

Roy, C. (1979). Health-illness (powerlessness) questionnaire and hospitalized patient decision making. In M.J. Ward & C.A. Lindeman (Eds.), *Instruments for measuring nursing practice and other health care variables* (Vol. 1, pp. 147–153). Hyattsville, MD: US Department of Health, Education, and Welfare.

Roy, C. (1979). Relating nursing theory to education: A new era. *Nurse Educator, 4*(2), 16–21.

Roy, C. (1980). The Roy adaptation model. In J.P. Riehl & C. Roy, *Conceptual models for nursing practice* (2nd ed., pp. 179–188). New York: Appleton-Century-Crofts.

Roy, C. (1981). A systems model of nursing care and its effect on quality of human life. In G.E. Lasker (Ed.), *Applied systems and cybernetics.* Vol. 4. *System research in health care, biocybernetics and ecology* (pp. 1705–1714). New York: Pergamon Press.

Roy, C. (1983). Roy adaptation model. In I.W. Clements & F.B. Roberts, *Family health: A theoretical approach to nursing care* (pp. 255–278). New York: John Wiley & Sons.

Roy, C. (1983). The expectant family: Analysis and application of the Roy adaptation model. In I.W. Clements & F.B. Roberts, *Family health: A theoretical approach to nursing care* (pp. 298–303). New York: John Wiley & Sons.

Roy, C. (1983). The family in primary care: Analysis and application of the Roy adaptation model. In I.W. Clements & F.B. Roberts, *Family health: A theoretical approach to nursing care* (pp. 375–378). New York: John Wiley & Sons.

Roy, C. (1984). *Introduction to nursing: An adaptation model* (2nd ed.). Englewood Cliffs, NJ: Prentice-Hall.

Roy, C. (1984). The Roy adaptation model: Applications in community health. In M.K. Asay & C.C. Ossler (Eds.), *Conceptual models of nursing: Applications in community health nursing: Proceedings of the eighth annual community health nursing conference* (pp. 51–73). Chapel Hill: Department of Public Health Nursing, School of Public Health, University of North Carolina.

Roy, C. (1987). Roy's adaptation model. In R.R. Parse, *Nursing science: Major paradigms, theories, and critiques* (pp. 35–45). Philadelphia: WB Saunders.

Roy, C. (1987). The influence of nursing models on clinical decision making II. In K.J. Hannah, M. Reimer, W.C. Mills, & S. Letourneau (Eds.), *Clinical judgment and decision making: The future with nursing diagnosis* (pp. 42–47). New York: John Wiley & Sons.

Roy, C. (1988). Altered cognition: An information processing approach. In P.H. Mitchell, L.C. Hodges, M. Muwaswes, & C.A. Walleck (Eds.), *AANN's neuroscience nursing: Phenomenon and practice: Human responses to neurological health problems* (pp. 185–211). Norwalk, CT: Appleton & Lange.

Roy, C. (1988). An explication of the philosophical assumptions of the Roy adaptation model. *Nursing Science Quarterly, 1,* 26–34.

Roy, C. (1988). Sister Callista Roy. In T.M. Schorr & A. Zimmerman, *Making choices. Taking chances: Nurse leaders tell their* stories (pp. 291–298). St. Louis: CV Mosby.

Roy, C. (1989). The Roy adaptation model. In J.P. Riehl-Sisca, Conceptual models for nursing practice (3rd ed., pp. 105–114), Norwalk, CT: Appleton & Lange.

Roy, C. (1991). Structure of knowledge: Paradigm, model, and research specifications for differentiated practice. In I.E. Goertzen (Ed.), Differentiating nursing practice: Into the twenty-first century (pp. 31–39). Kansas City, MO: American Academy of Nursing.

Roy, C. (1992). Vigor, variables, and vision: Commentary on Florence Nightingale. In F.N. Nightingale, Notes on nursing: What it is, and what it is not (Commemorative ed., pp. 63–71). Philadelphia: JB Lippincott.

Roy, C., & Andrews, H.A.C. (1991). The Roy adaptation model: The definitive statement. Norwalk, CT: Appleton & Lange.

Roy, C., & Anway, J. (1989). Theories and hypotheses for nursing administration. In B. Henry, M. DiVincenti, C. Arndt, & A. Marriner-Tomey (Eds.), Dimensions of nursing administration: Theory, research, education, and practice (pp. 75–88). Boston: Blackwell Scientific Publications.

Roy, C., & Corliss, C.P. (1993). The Roy Adaptation Model: Theoretical update and knowledge for practice. In M.E. Parker (Ed.), Patterns of nursing theories in practice (pp. 215–229). New York: National League for Nursing.

Roy, C., & Martinez, C. (1983). A conceptual framework for CNS practice. In A. Hamric & J. Spross (Eds.), The clinical nurse specialist in theory and practice (pp. 3–20). New York: Grune & Stratton.

Roy, C., & Obloy, M. (1978). The practitioner movement-toward a science of nursing. American Journal of Nursing, 78, 1698–1702.

Roy, C., & Roberts, S.L. (1981). Theory construction in nursing: An adaptation model. Englewood Cliffs, NJ: Prentice-Hall.

COMMENTARY

Aggleton, P., & Chalmers, H. (1984). The Roy adaptation model. Nursing Times, 80(40), 45–48.

Blue, C.L., Brubaker, K.M., Fine, J.M., Kirsch, M.J., Papazian, K.R., & Riester, C.M. (1989). Sister Callista Roy: Adaptation model. In A. Marriner-Tomey, Nursing theorists and their work (2nd ed., pp. 325–344). St. Louis: CV Mosby.

Blue, C.L., Brubaker, K.M., Fine, J.M., Kirsch, M.J., Papazian, K.R., Riester, C.M., & Sobiech, M.A. (1994). Sister Callista Roy: Adaptation model. In A. Marriner-Tomey, Nursing theorists and their work (3rd ed., pp. 246–268). St. Louis: Mosby-Year Book.

Blue, C.L., Brubaker, K.M., Papazian, K.R., & Riester, C.M. (1986). Sister Callista Roy: Adaptation model. In A. Marriner, Nursing theorists and their work (pp. 297–312). St. Louis: CV Mosby.

Chavasse, J.M. (1987). A comparison of three models of nursing. Nurse Education Today, 7(4), 177–186.

Christensen, P.J., & Kenney, J.W. (1990). (Eds.). Nursing process: Application of conceptual models (3rd ed.). St. Louis: CV Mosby.

DeFeo, D.J. (1990). Change: A central concern of nursing. Nursing Science Quarterly, 3, 88–94.

Fitzpatrick, J.J., Whall, A.L., Johnston, R.L., & Floyd, J.A. (1982). Nursing models and their psychiatric mental health applications. Bowie, MD: Brady.

Frank, D.I., & Lang, A.R. (1990). Disturbances in sexual role performance of chronic alcoholics: An analysis using Roy's adaptation model. Issues in Mental Health Nursing, 11, 243–254.

Galbreath, J.G. (1980). Sister Callista Roy. In Nursing Theories Conference Group, Nursing theories: The base for professional nursing practice (pp. 199–212). Englewood Cliffs, NJ: Prentice-Hall.

Galbreath, J.G. (1985). Sister Callista Roy. In Nursing Theories Conference Group, Nursing theories: The base for professional nursing practice (2nd ed., pp. 300–318). Englewood Cliffs, NJ: Prentice-Hall.

Galbreath, J.G. (1990). Sister Callista Roy. In J.B. George (Ed.), Nursing theories: The base for professional nursing practice (3rd ed., pp. 231–258). Norwalk, CT: Appleton & Lange.

Germain, C.P. (1984). Power and powerlessness in the adult hospitalized cancer patient. In Proceedings of the 3rd International Conference on Cancer Nursing (pp. 158–162). Melbourne, Australia: The Cancer Institute/Peter MacCullum Hospital and the Royal Melbourne Hospital.

Giger, J.N., Davidhizar, R., & Millers, S.W. (1990). Nightingale and Roy: A comparison of nursing models. Today's OR Nurse, 12(4), 25–30.

Goodwin, J.O. (1980). A cross-cultural approach to integrating nursing theory and practice. Nurse Educator, 5(6), 15–20.

Grey, M., & Thurber, F.W. (1991). Adaptation to chronic illness in childhood: Diabetes mellitus. *Journal of Pediatric Nursing, 6*, 302–309.

Huch, M.H. (1987). A critique of the Roy adaptation model. In R.R. Parse, *Nursing science: Major paradigms, theories, and critiques* (pp. 47–66). Philadelphia: WB Saunders.

Jones, E.G., Badger, T.A., & Moore, I. (1992). Children's knowledge of internal anatomy: Conceptual orientation and review of research. *Journal of Pediatric Nursing, 7*, 262–268.

Karns, P.S. (1991). Building a foundation for spiritual care. *Journal of Christian Nursing, 8*(3), 10–13.

Kehoe, C.F., & Fawcett, J. (1981). An overview of the Roy adaptation model. In C.F. Kehoe (Ed.), *The cesarean experience: Theoretical and clinical perspectives for nurses* (pp. 79–83). New York: Appleton-Century-Crofts.

Limandri, B. Research and practice with abused women: Use of the Roy adaptation model as an exploratory framework. *Advances in Nursing Science, 8*(4), 52–61.

Lutjens, L.R.J. (1991). *Callista Roy: An adaptation model.* Newbury Park, CA: Sage.

Mastal, M.F., & Hammond, H. (1980). Analysis and expansion of the Roy adaptation model: A contribution to holistic nursing. *Advances in Nursing Science, 2*(4), 71–81.

McKinnon, N.C. (1991). Humanistic nursing: It can't stand up to scrutiny. *Nursing and Health Care, 12*, 414–416.

Meleis, A.I. (1991). *Theoretical nursing: Development and progress* (2nd ed.). Philadelphia: JB Lippincott.

Messner, R., & Smith, M.N. (1986). Neurofibromatosis: Relinquishing the masks: A quest for quality of life. *Journal of Advanced Nursing, 11*, 459–464.

Mitchell, G.J., & Pilkington, B. (1990). Theoretical approaches in nursing practice: A comparison of Roy and Parse. *Nursing Science Quarterly, 3*, 81–87.

Peddicord, K. (1991). Strategies for promoting stress reduction and relaxation. *Nursing Clinics of North America, 26*, 867–874.

Pioli, C.D., Sandor, J.K. (1989). The Roy adaptation model: An analysis. In J. P. Riehl-Sisca, *Conceptual models for nursing practice* (3rd ed., pp. 115–124). Norwalk, CT: Appleton & Lange.

Rafferty, C. (1987–1988). An apologist's theories for the nursing profession: Adaptation and art. *Nursing Forum, 23*, 124–126.

Taft, L.B. (1989). Conceptual analysis of agitation in the confused elderly. *Archives of Psychiatric Nursing, 3*, 102–107.

Tiedeman, M.E. (1983). The Roy adaptation model. In J.J. Fitzpatrick & A.L. Whall, *Conceptual models of nursing: Analysis and application* (pp. 157–180). Bowie, MD: Brady.

Tiedeman, M.E. (1989). The Roy adaptation model. In J.J. Fitzpatrick & A.L. Whall, *Conceptual models of nursing: Analysis and application* (2nd ed., pp. 185–204.). Norwalk, CT: Appleton & Lange.

Walker, J.M., & Campbell, S.M. (1989). Pain assessment, nursing models, and the nursing process. *Recent Advances in Nursing, 24*, 47–61.

Whall, A.L. (1986). Strategic family therapy: Nursing reformulations and applications. In A.L. Whall, *Family therapy theory for nursing: Four approaches* (pp. 51–67). Norwalk, CT: Appleton-Century-Crofts.

Varvaro, F. F. (1991). Women with coronary heart disease: An application of Roy's adaptation model. *Cardiovascular Nursing, 27*(6), 31–35.

RESEARCH

Artinian, N.T. (1991). Stress experience of spouses of patients having coronary artery bypass during hospitalization and 6 weeks after discharge. *Heart and Lung, 20*, 52–59.

Artinian, N.T. (1992). Spouse adaptation to mate's CBG surgery: 1-year follow-up. *American Journal of Critical Care, 1*(2), 36–42.

Baker, A.C. (1993). The spouse's positive effect on the stroke patient's recovery. *Rehabilitation Nursing, 18*, 30–33, 67–68.

Bokinskie, J.C. (1992). Family conferences: A method to diminish transfer anxiety. *Journal of Neuroscience Nursing, 24*, 129–133.

Bradley, K.M., & Williams, D.M. (1990). A comparison of the preoperative concerns of open heart surgery patients and their significant others. *Journal of Cardiovascular Nursing, 5*, 43–53.

Breslin, E.H., Roy, C., & Robinson, C.R. (1992). Physiological nursing research in dyspnea: A paradigm shift and a metaparadigm exemplar. *Scholarly Inquiry for Nursing Practice, 6*, 81–104.

Carrieri, V.K. (1992). Response to "Physiological nursing research in dyspnea: A paradigm shift and a metaparadigm exemplar." *Scholarly Inquiry for Nursing Practice, 6*, 105–109.

Broeder, J.L. (1985). School-age children's perceptions of isolation after hospital discharge. *Maternal-Child Nursing Journal*, *14*, 153–174.

Calvert, M.M. (1989). Human-pet interaction and loneliness: A test of concepts from Roy's adaptation model. *Nursing Science Quarterly*, *2*, 194–202.

Calvillo, E.R., & Flaskerud, J.H. (1993). The adequacy and scope of Roy's adaptation model to guide cross-cultural pain research. *Nursing Science Quarterly*, *6*, 118–129.

Campbell, J.M. (1992). Treating depression in well older adults: Use of diaries in cognitive therapy. *Issues in Mental Health Nursing*, *13*, 19–29.

Cheng, M., & Williams, P.D. (1989). Oxygenation during chest physiotherapy of very-low-birth-weight infants: Relations among fraction of inspired oxygen levels, number of hand ventilations, and transcutaneous oxygen pressure. *Journal of Pediatric Nursing*, *4*, 411–418.

Cottrell, B., & Shannahan, M. (1986). Effect of the birth chair on duration of second stage labor and maternal outcome. *Nursing Research*, *35*, 364–367.

Cottrell, B., & Shannahan, M. (1987). A comparison of fetal outcome in birth chair and delivery table births. *Research in Nursing and Health*, *10*, 239–243.

Craig, D.I. (1990). The adaptation to pregnancy of spinal cord injured women. *Rehabilitation Nursing*, *15*(1), 6–9.

Christian, A. (1993). The relationship between women's symptoms of endometriosis and self-esteem. *Journal of Obstetric, Gynecologic, and Neonatal Nursing*, *22*, 370–376.

Farkas, L. (1981). Adaptation problems with nursing home application for elderly persons: An application of the Roy Adaptation Nursing Model. *Journal of Advanced Nursing*, *8*, 363–368.

Fawcett, J. (1981). Needs of cesarean birth parents. *Journal of Obstetric, Gynecologic, and Neonatal Nursing*, *10*, 371–376.

Fawcett, J. (1990). Preparation for caesarean childbirth: Derivation of a nursing intervention from the Roy adaptation model. *Journal of Advanced Nursing*, *15*, 1418–1425.

Fawcett, J., & Burritt, J. (1985). An exploratory study of antenatal preparation for cesarean birth. *Journal of Obstetric, Gynecologic, and Neonatal Nursing*, *14*, 224–230.

Fawcett, J., & Henklein, J. (1987). Antenatal education for cesarean birth: Extension of a field test. *Journal of Obstetric, Gynecologic, and Neonatal Nursing*, *16*, 61–65.

Fawcett, J., Pollio, N., Tully, A., Baron, M., Henklein, J.C., & Jones, R.C. (1993). Effects of information on adaptation to cesarean birth. *Nursing Research*, *42*, 49–53.

Fawcett, J., & Tulman, L. (1990). Building a programme of research from the Roy adaptation model of nursing. *Journal of Advanced Nursing*, *15*, 720–725.

Fawcett, J., Tulman, L., & Myers, S. (1988). Development of the inventory of functional status after childbirth. *Journal of Nurse-Midwifery*, *33*, 252–260.

Fawcett, J., & Weiss, M.E. (1993). Cross-cultural adaptation to cesarean birth. *Western Journal of Nursing Research*, *15*, 282–297.

Francis, G., Turner, J.T., & Johnson, S.B. (1985). Domestic animal visitation as therapy with adult home residents. *International Journal of Nursing Studies*, *22*, 201–206.

Frederickson, K. (1992). Research methodology and nursing science. *Nursing Science Quarterly*, *5*, 150–151.

Frederickson, K., Jackson, B.S., Strauman, T., & Strauman, J. (1991). Testing hypotheses derived from the Roy adaptation model. *Nursing Science Quarterly*, *4*, 168–174.

Gaberson, K.B. (1991). The effect of humorous distraction on preoperative anxiety. A pilot study. *Association of Operating Room Nurses Journal*, *54*, 1258–1261, 1263–1264.

Gagliardi, B.A. (1991). The impact of Duchene muscular dystrophy on families. *Orthopaedic Nursing*, *10*(5), 41–49.

Germain, C.P. (1984). Sheltering abused women: A nursing perspective. *Journal of Psychosocial Nursing*, *22*(9), 24–31.

Guzzetta, C. (1979). Relationship between stress and learning. *Advances in Nursing Science*, *1*(4), 35–49.

Hammond, H., Roberts, M., & Silva, M. (1983, Spring). The effect of Roy's first level and second level assessment on nurses' determination of accurate nursing diagnoses. *Virginia Nurse*, 14–17.

Harrison, L.L., Leeper, J.D., & Yoon, M. (1990). Effects of early parent touch on preterm infants' heart rates and arterial oxygen saturation levels. *Journal of Advanced Nursing*, *15*, 877–885.

Hazlett, D.E. (1989). A study of pediatric home ventilator management: Medical, psychosocial, and financial aspects. *Journal of Pediatric Nursing*, *4*, 284–294.

Hoch, C.C. (1987). Assessing delivery of

nursing care. *Journal of Gerontological Nursing, 13*, 10–17.

Hunter, L.P. (1991). Measurement of axillary temperatures in neonates. *Western Journal of Nursing Research, 13*, 324–335.

Ide, B.A. (1978). SPAL: A tool for measuring self-perceived adaptation level appropriate for an elderly population. In E.E. Bauwens (Ed.), *Clinical nursing research: Its strategies and findings* (Monograph series 1978: Two, pp. 56–63). Indianapolis: Sigma Theta Tau.

Jackson, B.S., Strauman, J., Frederickson, K., & Strauman, T.J. (1991). Long-term biopsychosocial effects of interleukin-2 therapy. *Oncology Nursing Forum, 18*, 683–690.

Khanobdee, C., Sukratanachaiyakul, V., & Gay, J.T. (1993). Couvade syndrome in expectant Thai fathers. *International Journal of Nursing Studies, 30*, 125–131.

Kiikkala, I., & Peitsi, T. (1991). The care of children with minimal brain dysfunction: A Roy adaptation analysis: *Journal of Pediatric Nursing, 6*, 290–292.

Komelasky, A.L. (1990). The effect of home nursing visits on parental anxiety and CPR knowledge retention of parents of apnea-monitored infants. *Journal of Pediatric Nursing, 5*, 387–392.

Leonard, C. (1975). Patient attitudes toward nursing interventions. *Nursing Research, 24*, 335–339.

Leuze, M., & McKenzie, J. (1987). Preoperative assessment using the Roy adaptation model. *Association of Operating Room Nurses Journal, 46*, 1122–1134.

Lewis, F.M., Firsich, S.C., & Parsell, S. (1978). Development of reliable measures of patient health outcomes related to quality nursing care for chemotherapy patients. In J.C. Krueger, A.H. Nelson, & M.O. Wolanin, *Nursing research: Development, collaboration, and utilization* (pp. 225–228). Germantown, MD: Aspen.

Lewis, F.M., Firsich, S.C., & Parsell, S. (1979). Clinical tool development for adult chemotherapy patients: Process and content. *Cancer Nursing, 2*, 99–108.

Lutjens, L.R.J. (1991). Medical condition, nursing condition, nursing intensity, medical severity, and length of stay in hospitalized adults. *Nursing Administration Quarterly, 15*(2), 64–65.

Lutjens, L.R.J. (1992). Derivation and testing of tenets of a theory of social organizations as adaptive systems. *Nursing Science Quarterly, 5*, 62–71.

Lynam, L.E., & Miller, M.A. (1992). Mothers' and nurses' perceptions of the needs of women experiencing preterm labor. *Journal of Obstetric, Gynecologic, and Neonatal Nursing, 21*, 126–136.

McGill, J.S. (1992). Functional status as it relates to hope in elders with and without cancer. (Abstract). *Kentucky Nurse, 40*(4), 6.

Meek, S.S. (1993). Effects of slow stroke back massage on relaxation in hospice clients. *Image: Journal of Nursing Scholarship, 25*, 17–21.

Munn, V.A., & Tichy, A.M. (1987). Nurses' perceptions of stressors in pediatric intensive care. *Journal of Pediatric Nursing, 2*, 405–411.

Nolan, M. (1977). Effects of nursing intervention in the operating room as recalled on the third postoperative day. In M.V. Batey (Ed.), *Communicating nursing research in the bicentennial year* (Vol. 9, pp. 41–50). Boulder, CO: Western Interstate Commission for Higher Education.

Norris, S., Campbell, L., & Brenkert, S. (1982). Nursing procedures and alterations in transcutaneous oxygen tension in premature infants. *Nursing Research, 31*, 330–336.

Holloway, E., & King, I. (1983). Re: "What's going on here?" [Letter to the editor]. *Nursing Research, 32*, 319.

Berkemeyer, S.N., & Campbell, L.A. (1983). To the editor. [Letter to the editor]. *Nursing Research, 32*, 319–329.

Roy, C. (1983). To the editor. [Letter to the editor]. *Nursing Research, 32*, 320.

Nyqvist, K.H., & Sjoden, P.O. (1993). Advice concerning breastfeeding from mothers of infants admitted to a neonatal intensive care unit: The Roy adaptation model as a conceptual structure. *Journal of Advanced Nursing, 18*, 54–63.

Phillips, J.A., & Brown, K.C. (1992). Industrial workers on a rotating shift pattern: Adaptation and injury status. *American Association of Occupational Health Nurses Journal, 40*, 468–476.

Pollock, S.E. (1984). Adaptation to stress. *Texas Nursing, 58*(10), 12–13.

Pollock, S.E. (1984). The stress response. *Critical Care Quarterly, 6*(4), 1–14.

Pollock, S.E. (1986). Human responses to chronic illness: Physiologic and psychosocial adaptation. *Nursing Research, 35*, 90–95.

Pollock, S.E. (1989). Adaptive responses to diabetes mellitus. *Western Journal of Nursing Research, 11*, 265–280.

Pollock, S.E. (1989). The hardiness characteristic: A motivating factor in adaptation. *Advances in Nursing Science, 11*(2), 53–62.

Pollock, S.E. (1993). Adaptation to chronic illness: A program of research for testing nursing theory. *Nursing Science Quarterly, 6,* 86–92.

Preston, D.B., & Dellasega, C. (1990). Elderly women and stress: Does marriage make a difference? *Journal of Gerontological Nursing, 16,* 26–32.

Printz-Feddersen, V. (1990). Effect of group process on caregiver burden. (Abstract). *Journal of Neuroscience Nursing, 22,* 50–51.

Samarel, N., & Fawcett, J. (1992). Enhancing adaptation to breast cancer: The addition of coaching to support groups. *Oncology Nursing Forum, 19,* 591–596.

Samarel, N., Fawcett, J., & Tulman, L. (1993). The effects of coaching in breast cancer support groups: A pilot study. *Oncology Nursing Forum, 20,* 795–798.

Selman, S.W. (1989). Impact of total hip replacement on quality of life. *Orthopaedic Nursing, 8*(5), 43–49.

Shannahan, M., & Cottrell, B. (1985). Effect of the birth chair on duration of second stage labor, fetal outcome, and maternal blood loss. *Nursing Research, 34,* 89–92.

Silva, M.C. (1987). Needs of spouses of surgical patients: A conceptualization within the Roy adaptation model. *Scholarly Inquiry for Nursing Practice, 1,* 29–44.

Roy, C. (1987). Response to "Needs of spouses of surgical patients: A conceptualization within the Roy adaptation model." *Scholarly Inquiry for Nursing Practice, 1,* 45–50.

Smith, C., Garvis, M., & Martinson, I. (1983). Content analysis of interviews using nursing model: A look at parents adapting to the impact of childhood cancer. *Cancer Nursing, 6,* 269–275.

Smith, C.E., Mayer, L.S., Parkhurst, C., Perkins, S.B., & Pingleton, S.K. (1991). Adaptation in families with a member requiring mechanical ventilation at home. *Heart and Lung, 20,* 349–356.

Strohmyer, L.L., Noroian, E.L., Patterson, L.M., & Carlin, B.P. (1993). Adaptation six months after multiple trauma: A pilot study. *Journal of Neuroscience Nursing, 25,* 30–37.

Takahashi, J.J., & Bever, S.C. (1989). Preoperative nursing assessment: A research study. *Association of Operating Room Nurses Journal, 50,* 1022, 1024–1029, 1031–1032, 1034–1035.

Tulman, L., & Fawcett, J. (1988). Return of functional ability after childbirth. *Nursing Research, 37,* 77–81.

Tulman, L., & Fawcett, J. (1990). A framework for studying functional status after diagnosis of breast cancer. *Cancer Nursing, 13,* 95–99.

Tulman, L., & Fawcett, J. (1990). Functional status during pregnancy and the postpartum: A framework for research. *Image: Journal of Nursing Scholarship, 22,* 191–194.

Tulman, L., & Fawcett, J. (1990). Maternal employment following childbirth. *Research in Nursing and Health, 13,* 181–188.

Tulman, L., Fawcett, J., Groblewski, L., & Silverman, L. (1990). Changes in functional status after childbirth. *Nursing Research, 39,* 70–75.

Tulman, L., Fawcett, J., & McEvoy, M.D. (1991). Development of the inventory of functional status-cancer. *Cancer Nursing, 14,* 254–260.

Tulman, L., Fawcett, J., & Weiss, M. (1993). The inventory of functional status-fathers: Development and psychometric testing. *Journal of Nurse-Midwifery, 38,* 117–123.

Tulman, L., Higgins, K., Fawcett, J., Nunno, C., Vansickel, C., Haas, M.B., & Speca, M.M. (1991). The inventory of functional status-antepartum period: Development and testing. *Journal of Nurse-Midwifery, 36,* 117–123.

Vicenzi, A.E., & Thiel, R. (1992). AIDS education on the college campus: Roy's adaptation model directs inquiry. *Public Health Nursing, 9,* 270–276.

DOCTORAL DISSERTATIONS

Artinian, N.T. (1989). The stress process within the Roy adaptation framework: Sources, mediators and manifestations of stress in spouses of coronary artery bypass patients during hospitalization and six weeks post discharge. *Dissertation Abstracts International, 49,* 5225B.

Bean, C.A. (1988). Needs and stimuli influencing needs of adult cancer patients. *Dissertation Abstracts International, 48,* 2259B.

Beckerman, A. (1984). The impact of Roy's model of adaptation on nursing students' generation of patient data: A comparison study. *Dissertation Abstracts International, 45,* 513B.

Calvilo, E.R. (1992). Pain response in Mexican-American and white nonhispanic women. *Dissertation Abstracts International, 52,* 3524B.

Campbell-Heider, N. (1988). Patient adaptation to the hospital technological environment. *Dissertation Abstracts International, 49,* 1618B.

Cohen, B.J. (1980). The perception of patient adaptation to hemodialysis: A study of registered nurses and hemodialysis patients. *Dissertation Abstracts International, 41,* 129B–130B.

Collins, J.M. (1992). Functional health, social support, and morale of older women living alone in Appalachia. *Dissertation Abstracts International, 53,* 1781B.

Dahlen, R.A. (1980). Analysis of selected factors related to the elderly person's ability to adapt to visual prostheses following senile cataract surgery. *Dissertation Abstracts International, 41,* 894B.

Dobratz, M.C. (1991). Patterns of psychological adaptation in death and dying: A causal model and exploratory study. *Dissertation Abstracts International, 51,* 3320B.

Dow, K.H.M. (1993). An analysis of the experience of surviving and having children after breast cancer. *Dissertation Abstracts International, 53,* 5641B.

Edwards, M.R. (1992). Self-esteem, sense of mastery, and adequacy of prenatal care. *Dissertation Abstracts International, 53,* 768B.

Gilbert, C.M. (1991). A structured group nursing intervention for girls who have been sexually abused utilizing Roy's theory of the personal as an adaptive system. *Dissertation Abstracts International, 52,* 1350B.

Holcombe, J.K. (1986). Social support, perception of illness, and self-esteem of women with gynecologic cancer. *Dissertation Abstracts International, 47,* 1928B.

Holmes, J.L. (1983). An analysis of nurse supervisors' expressed levels of job stress as a key variable in discerning staff nurses' perceptions of the supervisory process. *Dissertation Abstracts International, 43,* 2873A.

Kiker, P.M. (1983). Role adequacy of pediatric outpatients undergoing surgery. *Dissertation Abstracts International, 44,* 1782B.

Lamb, M.A. (1991). Sexual adaptation of women treated for endometrial cancer. *Dissertation Abstracts International, 52,* 2994B.

Lavender, M.G. (1989). The relationship between maternal self esteem, work status, and sociodemographic characteristics and self esteem of the kindergarten child. *Dissertation Abstracts International, 49,* 5229B.

Lemr, M.A. (1991). Sexual adaptation of women treated for endometrial cancer. *Dissertation Abstracts International, 52,* 2994B.

Lutjens, L.R.J. (1991). Relationships between medical condition, nursing condition, nursing intensity, medical severity and length-of-stay in hospitalized medical-surgical adults using the theory of social organizations as adaptive systems. *Dissertation Abstracts International, 52,* 1354B.

McGill, J.S. (1992). Functional status as it relates to hope in elders with and without cancer. *Dissertation Abstracts International, 53,* 771B.

McRae, M.G. (1991). Adaptation to pregnancy and motherhood: Personality characteristics of primiparas age 30 years and older. *Dissertation Abstracts International, 51,* 3326B.

Modrcin-McCarthy, M.A.J. (1993). The physiological and behavioral effects of a gentle human touch nursing intervention on preterm infants. *Dissertation Abstracts International, 54,* 1336B.

Newman, A.M. (1991). The effect of the arthritis self-help course on arthritis self-efficacy, perceived social support, purpose and meaning in life, and arthritis impact in people with arthritis. *Dissertation Abstracts International, 52,* 2995B.

O'Leary, P.A. (1991). Family caregivers' log reports of sleep and activity behaviors of persons with Alzheimer's disease. *Dissertation Abstracts International, 51,* 4780B.

Paier, G.S. (in press). Development and testing of an instrument to assess functional status in the elderly. *Dissertation Abstracts International.*

Perkins, I. (1988). An analysis of relationships among interdependence in family caregivers and the elderly, caregiver burden, and adaptation of the homebound frail elderly. *Dissertation Abstracts International, 48,* 3250B–3251B.

Phillips, J.A. (1991). Adaptation and injury status of industrial workers on a rotating shift pattern. *Dissertation Abstracts International, 52,* 2995B.

Pittman, K.P. (1993). A Q-analysis of the enabling characteristics of chronically ill schoolage children for the promotion of personal wellness. *Dissertation Abstracts International, 5330,* 4593B.

Pollock, S. (1982). Level of adaptation: An analysis of stress factors that affect health status. *Dissertation Abstracts International, 41,* 4364B.

Pritzker, J.K. (1989). The development and formative evaluation of a psychoeducationally based program for post-mastectomy women. *Dissertation Abstracts International, 49,* 2547A.

Pruden, E.P.S. (1992). Roy adaptation model testing: Dyadic adaptation, social support, and loneliness in COPD dyads. *Dissertation Abstracts International, 52,* 6320B.

Rich, V.L. (1992). The use of personal, organizational, and coping resources in the prevention of staff nurse burnout: A test of a model. *Dissertation Abstracts International, 52,* 3532B.

Robinson, J.H. (1992). A description study of widows' grief responses, coping processes and social support within Roy's adaptation model. *Dissertation Abstracts International, 52,* 6320B.

Scherubel, J.C.M. (1986). Description of adaptation patterns following an acute cardiac event. *Dissertation Abstracts International, 46,* 2627B.

Schmidt, C.S. (1983). A comparison of the effectiveness of two nursing models in decreasing depression and increasing life satisfaction of retired individuals. *Dissertation Abstracts International, 43,* 2856B.

Shaffer, F.H. (1989). A comparison of maternal identity in younger and older primiparae during the third trimester of pregnancy. *Dissertation Abstracts International, 49,* 4236B.

Shuler, P.J. (1990). Physical and psychosocial adaptation, social isolation, loneliness, and self-concept of individuals with cancer. *Dissertation Abstracts International, 51,* 2289B.

Smith, B.J.A. (1990). Caregiver burden and adaptation in middle-aged daughters of dependent, elderly parents: A test of Roy's model. *Dissertation Abstracts International, 51,* 2290B.

Stein, P.R. (1992). Life events, self-esteem, and powerlessness among adolescents. *Dissertation Abstracts International, 52,* 5195B.

Stewart-Fahs, P.S. (1992). Effect of heparin injectate volume on pain and bruising using the Roy model. *Dissertation Abstracts International, 52,* 5195B.

Trentini, M. (1986). Nurses' decisions in dialysis patient care: An application of the Roy adaptation model. *Dissertation Abstracts International, 47,* 575B.

Weiss, M.E. (1991). The relationship between marital interdependence and adaptation to parenthood in primiparous couples. *Dissertation Abstracts International, 51,* 3783B.

Wilkerson, N.N. (1982). Effects of two preinstructional strategies on cognitive learning of the Roy adaptation model of nursing. *Dissertation Abstracts International, 43,* 1415A.

Wilson, F.S. (1984). The Roy adaptation model of nursing: Implications for baccalaureate nursing education. *Dissertation Abstracts International, 45,* 91A.

Zonka, B.J. (1980). The effects of a formal in-hospital patient education program on anxiety in postmyocardial infarction patients. *Dissertation Abstracts International, 41,* 1418A.

MASTER'S THESES

Andrews, H.A.C. (1987). Curricular implementation of the Roy adaptation model. *Dissertation Abstracts International, 48,* 1064A.

Berardy, S. (1991). Secondary post-traumatic stress disorder in Native Americans. *Master's Abstracts International, 30,* 432.

Bergin, M.A. (1986). Psychosocial responses of marital couples experiencing primary infertility. *Dissertation Abstracts International, 46,* 2197A.

Brown, G.J. (1990). The prevalence of elderly abuse: A descriptive survey of case management records. *Master's Abstracts International, 28,* 570.

Cheng, L-C. (1991). Social support related to the sleep pattern in Southern Taiwanese hospitalized adults. *Master's Abstracts International, 29,* 90.

Cornell, D.L. (1990). Patterns of anxiety with home parenteral antibiotic therapy. *Master's Abstracts International, 28,* 572.

Deruvao, S.L.S. (1993). Nursing diagnoses using Roy's adaptation model for persons with cancer receiving external bean radiation therapy. *Master's Abstracts International, 31,* 270.

Eves, L.M. (1993). Support for parents of developmentally disabled children: Effect on adaptation. *Master's Abstracts International, 31,* 271.

Ferraro, B.A. (1993). Unit size and nurses' quality of work life: An application of the Roy adaptation model. *Master's Abstracts International, 31,* 271.

Hampton, H.V. (1991). The impact of nursing case management on patients with a diagnosis of cerebrovascular accident: A retrospective study. *Master's Abstracts International, 29,* 643.

Hart, M.A. (1989). Rural parents' perception and management of fever in their school-age child. *Master's Abstracts International, 27,* 376.

Hughes, I.G. (1992). How registered nurses perceive their leadership preparedness and leadership skills. *Master's Abstracts International, 30,* 709.

Komara, C.A. (1992). Effects of music on fetal response. *Master's Abstracts International, 30,* 300.

Legault, F.M. (1991). Adaptation within the role function and self-concept modes among women during the postpartum period. *Master's Abstracts International, 29,* 439.

Miquel, L.J. (1990). The image of nursing: Prevalent perceptions among health care providers and consumers. *Master's Abstracts International, 28,* 579.

Moore, R.E. (1992). The effects of stress on critical care nurses versus noncritical care nurses. *Master's Abstracts International, 30,* 1296.

Neiterman, E.W. (1988). Assessment of parent's presence during anesthesia induction of children. *Master's Abstracts International, 26,* 109.

Novarro, J.T. (1992). A descriptive study of the motives, personal, and educational needs of adult women returning to school as practical nursing students. *Master's Abstracts International, 30,* 1297.

Nutten, S.C. (1989). Public program analysis: The relationship between staffing and quality of care in Michigan long term care facilities. *Master's Abstracts International, 27,* 379.

Nwoga, I.A.A. (1991). Adaptation to maternal roles, tasks, and behaviors by pregnant teenage girls. *Master's Abstracts International, 29,* 97.

O'Brien, C.S. (1992). A pilot study of perceived social adaptation of the elderly to the nursing home environment utilizing a mentorship program. *Master's Abstracts International, 30,* 1297.

Parlin, C.A. (1990). Physiological manifestations of human/animal interaction in the adult population over 55. *Master's Abstracts International, 28,* 113.

Perese, K. (1991). An application of Roy's adaptation model and home health care documentation. *Master's Abstracts International, 29,* 443.

Rebeschi, L.C. (1991). The Roy adaptation model: Curriculum to practice. *Master's Abstracts International, 29,* 267.

Rustic, D.L. (1993). A study of somatic symptomatology: Occurrence and severity as reported by international graduate students at Michigan State University. *Master's Abstracts International, 31,* 282.

Shrubsole, J.L. (1992). Mutual aid: Promoting adaptation in women with premenstrual syndrome. *Master's Abstracts International, 30,* 1301.

Smith, C.J. (1989). Cardiovascular responses in healthy males during basin bath, tub bath, and shower. *Master's Abstracts International, 27,* 103.

EDUCATION

Andrews, H.A. (1989). Implementation of the Roy adaptation model: An application of educational change research. In J.P. Riehl-Sisca, *Conceptual models for nursing practice* (3rd ed., pp. 133–148). Norwalk, CT: Appleton & Lange.

Baldwin, J., & Schaffer, S. (1990). The continuing case study. *Nurse Educator, 15*(5), 6–9.

Brower, H.T.F., & Baker, B.J. (1976). Using the adaptation model in a practitioner curriculum. *Nursing Outlook, 24,* 686–689.

Camooso, C., Greene, M., & Reilly, P. (1981). Students' adaptation according to Roy. *Nursing Outlook, 29,* 108–109.

Heinrich, K. (1989). Growing pains: Faculty stages in adopting a nursing model. *Nurse Educator, 14*(1), 3–4, 29.

Knowlton, C., Goodwin, M., Moore, J., Alt-White, A., Guarino, S., & Pyne, H. (1983). Systems adaptation model for nursing for families, groups and communities. *Journal of Nursing Education, 22,* 128–131.

Kurian, A. (1992). Effective teaching and its application in nursing. *Nursing Journal of India, 83,* 251–254.

Laschinger, H.S. (1990). Helping students apply a nursing conceptual framework in the clinical setting. *Nurse Educator, 15*(3), 20–24.

Mengel, A., Sherman, S., Nahigian, E., & Coleman, I. (1989). Adaptation of the Roy model in an educational setting. In J.P. Riehl-Sisca, *Conceptual models for nursing practice* (3rd ed., pp. 125–131). Norwalk, CT: Appleton & Lange.

Morales-Mann, E.T., & Logan, M. (1990). Implementing the Roy model: Challenges for nurse educators. *Journal of Advanced Nursing, 15,* 142–147.

Porth, C.M. (1977). Physiological coping: A model for teaching pathophysiology. *Nursing Outlook, 25,* 781–784.

Roy, C. (1976). Comment. *Nursing Outlook, 24,* 690–691.

Story, E.L., & Ross, M.M. (1986). Family centered community health nursing and the Betty Neuman systems model. *Nursing Papers, 18*(2), 77–88.

Wagner, P. (1976). Testing the adaptation model in practice. *Nursing Outlook, 24,* 682–685.

ADMINISTRATION

DiIorio, C. (1989). Applying Roy's model to nursing administration. In B. Henry, M.

DiVincenti, C. Arndt, & A. Marriner (Eds.), *Dimensions of nursing administration: Theory, research, education, and practice* (pp. 89–104). Boston: Blackwell Scientific Publications.

Dorsey, K., & Purcell, S. (1987). Translating a nursing theory into a nursing system. *Geriatric Nursing, 8,* 137–167.

Fawcett, J. (1992). Documentation using a conceptual model of nursing. *Nephrology Nursing Today, 2*(5), 1–8.

Fawcett, J., Botter, M.L., Burritt, J., Crossley, J.D., & Frink, B.B. (1989). Conceptual models of nursing and organization theories. In B. Henry, M. DiVincenti, C. Arndt, & A. Marriner (Eds.), *Dimensions of nursing administration: Theory, research, education, and practice* (pp. 143–154). Boston: Blackwell Scientific Publications.

Frederickson, K. (1991). Nursing theories — A basis for differentiated practice: Application of the Roy adaptation model in nursing practice. In I.E. Goertzen (Ed.), *Differentiating nursing practice: Into the twenty-first century* (pp. 41–44). Kansas City, MO: American Academy of Nursing.

Frederickson, K. (1993). Translating the Roy adaptation model into practice and research. In M.E. Parker (Ed.), *Patterns of nursing theories in practice* (pp. 230–238). New York: National League for Nursing.

Gray, J. (1991). The Roy adaptation model in nursing practice. In C. Roy & H.A. Andrews, *The Roy adaptation model: The definitive statement* (pp. 429–443). Norwalk, CT: Appleton & Lange.

Hinman, L.M. (1983). Focus on the school-aged child in family intervention. *Journal of School Health, 53,* 499–502.

Jakocko, M.T., & Sowden, L.A. (1986). The Roy adaptation model in nursing practice. In H.A. Andrews & C. Roy, *Essentials of the Roy adaptation model* (pp. 165–177). Norwalk, CT: Appleton & Lange.

Logan, M. (1990). The Roy adaptation model: Are nursing diagnoses amenable to independent nurse functions? *Journal of Advanced Nursing, 15,* 468–470.

Laros, J. (1977). Deriving outcome criteria from a conceptual model. *Nursing Outlook, 25,* 333–336.

Mason, T., & Chandley, M. (1990). Nursing models in a special hospital: A critical analysis of efficacity. *Journal of Advanced Nursing, 15,* 667–673.

Mastal, M.F., Hammond, H., & Roberts, M.P. (1982). Theory into hospital practice: A pilot implementation. *Journal of Nursing Administration, 12*(6), 9–15.

Peters, V.J. (1993). Documentation using the

Roy adaptation model. *American Nephrology Nurses Association Journal, 20,* 522.

Riegel, B. (1985). A method of giving intershift report based on a conceptual model. *Focus on Critical Care, 12*(4), 12–18.

Robitaille-Tremblay, M. (1984). A data collection tool for the psychiatric nurse. *The Canadian Nurse, 80*(7), 26–28.

Rogers, M., Paul, L.J., Clarke, J., MacKay, C., Potter, M., & Ward, W. (1991). The use of the Roy adaptation model in nursing administration. *Canadian Journal of Nursing Administration, 4*(2), 21–26.

Starn, J., & Niederhauser, V. (1990). An MCN model for nursing diagnosis to focus intervention. *American Journal of Maternal Child Nursing, 15,* 180–183.

Torosian, L.C., DeStefano, M., & Dietrick-Gallagher, M. (1985). Day gynecologic chemotherapy unit: An innovative approach to changing health care systems. *Cancer Nursing, 8,* 221–227.

Zarle, N.C. (1987). *Continuing care: The process and practice of discharge planning.* Rockville, MD: Aspen.

PRACTICE

Aaronson, L., & Seaman, L.P. (1989). Managing hypernatremia in fluid deficient elderly. *Journal of Gerontological Nursing, 15*(7), 29–34.

Barnfather, J.S., Swain, M.A.P., & Erickson, H.C. (1989). Evaluation of two assessment techniques for adaptation to stress. *Nursing Science Quarterly, 2,* 172–182.

Bawden, M., Ralph, J., & Herrick, C.A. (1991). Enhancing the coping skills of mothers with developmentally delayed children. *Journal of Child and Adolescent Psychiatric Mental Health Nursing, 4,* 25–28.

Caradus, A. (1991). Nursing theory and operating suite nursing practice. *ACORN Journal, 4*(2), 29–30, 32.

Cardiff, J. (1989). Heartfelt care. *Nursing Times, 85*(3), 42–45.

Crossfield, T. (1990). Patients with scleroderma. *Nursing (London), 4*(10), 19–20.

DiMaria, R.A. (1989). Posttrauma responses: Potential for nursing. *Journal of Advanced Medical-Surgical Nursing, 2*(1), 41–48.

Downey, C. (1974). Adaptation nursing applied to an obstetric patient. In J.P. Riehl & C. Roy, *Conceptual models for nursing practice* (pp. 151–159). New York: Appleton-Century-Crofts.

Doyle, R., & Rajacich, D. (1991). The Roy adaptation model: Health teaching about osteoporosis. *American Association of Oc-*

cupational Health Nursing Journal, 39, 508–512.

Dudek, G. (1989). Nursing update: Hypophosphatemic rickets. *Pediatric Nursing, 15*(1), 45–50.

Ellis, J.A. (1991). Coping with adolescent cancer: Its a matter of adaptation. *Journal of Pediatric Oncology Nursing, 8,* 10–17.

Fawcett, J. (1981). Assessing and understanding the cesarean father. In C.F. Kehoe (Ed.), *The cesarean experience: Theoretical and clinical perspectives for nurses* (pp. 143–156). New York: Appleton-Century-Crofts.

Fawcett, J., Archer, C.L., Becker, D., Brown, K.K., Gann, S., Wong, M.J., & Wurster, A.B. (1992). Guidelines for selecting a conceptual model of nursing: Focus on the individual patient. *Dimensions of Critical Care Nursing, 11,* 268–277.

Fox, J.A. (1990). Bilateral breast lumps: A care plan in theatre using a stress adaptation model. *NATNews: British Journal of Theatre Nursing, 27*(11), 11–14.

Galligan, A.C. (1979). Using Roy's concept of adaptation to care for young children. *American Journal of Maternal Child Nursing, 4,* 24–28.

Gerrish, C. (1989). From theory to practice. *Nursing Times, 85*(35), 42–45.

Giger, J.A., Bower, C.A., & Miller, S.W. (1987). Roy adaptation model: ICU application. *Dimensions of Critical Care Nursing, 6,* 215–224.

Gilbert, E., & Harmon, J. (1986). *High-risk pregnancy and delivery: Nursing perspectives.* St. Louis: CV Mosby.

Gordon, J. (1974). Nursing assessment and care plan for a cardiac patient. In J.P. Riehl & C. Roy, *Conceptual models for nursing practice* (pp. 144–151). New York: Appleton-Century-Crofts.

Hamer, B.A. (1991). Music therapy: Harmony for change. *Journal of Psychosocial Nursing and Mental Health Services, 29*(12), 5–7.

Hamner, J.B. (1989). Applying the Roy adaptation model to the CCU. *Critical Care Nurse, 9*(3), 51–61.

Hanchett, E.S. (1988). *Nursing frameworks and community as client: Bridging the gap.* Norwalk, CT: Appleton & Lange.

Hanchett, E.S. (1990). Nursing models and community as client. *Nursing Science Quarterly, 3,* 67–72.

Harvey, S. (1993). The genesis of a phenomenological approach to advanced nursing practice. *Journal of Advanced Nursing, 18,* 526–530.

Hughes, A. (1991). Life with a stoma. *Nursing Times, 87*(25), 67–68.

Hughes, M.M. (1983). Nursing theories and emergency nursing. *Journal of Emergency Nursing, 9,* 95–97.

Innes, M.H. (1992). Management of an inadequately ventilated patient. *British Journal of Nursing, 1,* 780–784.

Jackson, D.A. (1990). Roy in the postanesthesia care unit. *Journal of Post Anesthesia Nursing, 5,* 143–148.

Janelli, L. (1980). Utilizing Roy's adaptation model from a gerontological perspective. *Journal of Gerontological Nursing, 6,* 140–150.

Jay, P. (1990). Relatives caring for the terminally ill. *Nursing Standard, 5*(5), 30–32.

Kehoe, C.F. (1981). Identifying the nursing needs of the postpartum cesarean mother. In C.F. Kehoe (Ed.), *The cesarean experience: Theoretical and clinical perspectives for nurses* (pp. 85–141.). New York: Appleton-Century-Crofts.

Kurek-Ovshinsky, C. (1991). Group psychotherapy in an acute inpatient setting: Techniques that nourish self-esteem. *Issues in Mental Health Nursing, 12,* 81–88.

Logan, M. (1986). Palliative care nursing: Applicability of the Roy model. *Journal of Palliative Care, 1*(2), 18–24.

Logan, M. (1988). Care of the terminally ill includes the family. *The Canadian Nurse, 84*(5), 30–33.

McIver, M. (1987). Putting theory into practice. *The Canadian Nurse, 83*(10), 36–38.

deMontigney, F. (1992a). L'Intervention familiale selon Roy: La famille Joly: Cueillette et analyse des données. [Family intervention according to Roy]. *The Canadian Nurse, 88*(8), 41–45.

deMontigney, F. (1992b). L'Intervention familiale selon Roy: Planification, exécution et évaluation. [Family intervention according to Roy]. *The Canadian Nurse, 88*(9), 43–46.

Miles, M.S., & Carter, M.C. (1983). Assessing parental stress in intensive care units. *American Journal of Maternal Child Nursing, 8,* 354–359.

Miller, F. (1991). Using Roy's model in a special hospital. *Nursing Standard, 5*(27), 29–32.

Nash, D.J. (1987). Kawasaki disease: Application of the Roy adaptation model to determine interventions. *Journal of Pediatric Nursing, 2,* 308–315.

O'Reilly, M. (1989). Familiarity breeds acceptance. *Nursing Times, 85*(12), 29–30.

Piazza, D., & Foote, A. (1990). Roy's adaptation model: A guide for rehabilitation nursing practice. *Rehabilitation Nursing, 15,* 254–259.

Rambo, B. (1984). *Adaptation nursing: Assessment and intervention.* Philadelphia: WB Saunders.

Randell, B., Poush Tedrow, M., & Van Landingham, J. (1982). *Adaptation nursing: The Roy conceptual model applied.* St. Louis: CV Mosby.

Rogers, E.J. (1991). Postanesthesia care of the cocaine abuser. *Journal of Post Anesthesia Nursing, 6,* 102–107.

Sato, M.K. (1986). The Roy adaptation model. In P. Winstead-Fry (Ed.), *Case studies in nursing theory* (pp. 103–125). New York: National League for Nursing.

Schmidt, C.S. (1981). Withdrawal behavior of schizophrenics: Application of Roy's model. *Journal of Psychosocial Nursing and Mental Health Services, 19*(11), 26–33.

Schmitz, M. (1980). The Roy adaptation model: Application in a community setting. In J.P. Riehl & C. Roy, *Conceptual models for nursing practice* (2nd ed., pp. 193–206). New York: Appleton-Century-Crofts.

Sirignano, R.G. (1987). Peripartum cardiomyopathy: An application of the Roy adaptation model. *Journal of Cardiovascular Nursing, 2,* 24–32.

Smith, M.C. (1988). Roy's adaptation model in practice. *Nursing Science Quarterly, 1,* 97–98.

Starr, S.L. (1980). Adaptation applied to the dying client. In J.P. Riehl & C. Roy, *Conceptual models for nursing practice* (2nd ed., pp. 189–192). New York: Appleton-Century-Crofts.

Stringer, M., Librizzi, R., & Weiner, S. (1991). Establishing a prenatal genetic diagnosis: The nurse's role. *American Journal of Maternal Child Nursing, 16,* 152–156.

Summers, T.M. (1991). Psychosocial support of the burned patient. *Critical Care Nursing Clinics of North America, 3,* 237–244.

Thornbury, J.M., & King, L.D. (1992). The Roy adaptation model and care of persons with Alzheimer's disease. *Nursing Science Quarterly, 5,* 129–133.

Welsh, M.D., & Clochesy, J.M. (Eds.). (1990). *Case studies in cardiovascular critical care nursing.* Rockville, MD: Aspen.

West, S. (1992). Number one priorities. *Nursing Times, 88*(17), 28–31.

Wright, P.S., Holcombe, J., Foote, A., & Piazza, D. (1993). The Roy adaptation model used as a guide for the nursing care of an 8-year-old child with leukemia. *Journal of Pediatric Oncology Nursing, 10,* 68–74.

CHAPTER 10

Implementing Conceptual Models in Nursing Practice

This chapter presents a discussion of the substantive and process elements of the implementation of conceptual models of nursing in the real world of clinical practice. The chapter begins with a discussion of the value of using an explicit nursing perspective to guide nursing practice. The chapter continues with an explanation of the substantive elements of implementing conceptual model–based nursing practice that emphasizes the translation of the components of the structural hierarchy of contemporary nursing knowledge into conceptual-theoretical-empirical systems of nursing knowledge for nursing practice. Next, the process elements of implementing conceptual model-based nursing practice are discussed, including identification of the eight phases of implementation and a description of the perspective transformation that nurses experience when they adopt an explicit conceptual model as a guide for nursing practice. The chapter concludes with a discussion of directions for future work with conceptual-theoretical-empirical systems of nursing knowledge in nursing practice.

The key terms used in this chapter are listed below. Each term is defined and described in the chapter.

KEY TERMS

VALUE OF CONCEPTUAL MODEL–
 BASED NURSING PRACTICE
SUBSTANTIVE ELEMENTS OF
 IMPLEMENTING CONCEPTUAL
 MODEL–BASED NURSING
 PRACTICE

Translation of the Metaparadigm of
 Nursing
 Care Recipient
 Environment of the Care Recipient
 Health State of the Care Recipient
 Nursing Processes

Translation of Philosophies
   ANA Code of Ethics
   Patient's Bill of Rights
   Philosophy of the Nursing
     Department
Translation of the Conceptual
   Model, Theories, and Empirical
   Indicators
   Clinical Specialty Knowledge
   Nursing Care Delivery Systems
   Standards for Nursing Practice
   Assessment Formats
   Diagnostic Taxonomies
   Intervention Protocols
   Evaluation Criteria
PROCESS ELEMENTS OF
   IMPLEMENTING CONCEPTUAL
   MODEL – BASED NURSING
   PRACTICE
First Phase: Idea or Vision
Second Phase: Formation of Task
   Force for Feasibility Study
Third Phase: Planning Committee

Fourth Phase: Review of Documents
   and Long-Range Plan
Fifth Phase: Selection and
   Development of Conceptual-
   Theoretical-Empirical System of
   Nursing Knowledge
Sixth Phase: Education of the
   Nursing Staff
Seventh Phase: Demonstration Sites
Eighth Phase: Institution-Wide
   Implementation and Evaluation of
   Outcomes
Perspective Transformation
   Stability
   Dissonance
   Confusion
   Dwelling with Uncertainty
   Saturation
   Synthesis
   Resolution
   Reconceptualization
   Return to Stability
DIRECTIONS FOR THE FUTURE

THE VALUE OF CONCEPTUAL MODEL-BASED NURSING PRACTICE

The number of nurses throughout the world who recognize the **value of conceptual model–based nursing practice** is rapidly increasing. Indeed, Cash's (1990) claim that "there is no central core that can distinguish nursing theoretically from a number of other occupational activities" (p. 255) is readily offset by many claims to the contrary. Clearly, his claim fails to take into account the contributions made by explicit conceptual models of nursing to the articulation of practice that is distinctively *nursing*. As Chalmers (cited in Chalmers, Kershaw, Melia, & Kendrich, 1990) pointed out, "Nursing models have provided what many would argue is a much needed alternative knowledge base from which nurses can practice in an informed way. An alternative, that is, to the medical model which for so many years has dominated many aspects of health care" (p. 34). Nursing models also provide an alternative to the institutional model of practice, in which "the most salient values [are] efficiency, standardized care, rules, and regulations" (Rogers, 1989, p. 113). The institutional model, moreover, typically upholds, reinforces, and supports the medical model (Grossman & Hooton, 1993).

In fact, conceptual models of nursing provide explicit frames of reference for *professional nursing practice* by delineating the scope of nursing practice and by identifying who the care recipient is, what the relevant environment is, what aspects of health are to be considered, and what the steps and substance of the nursing process are. As such, conceptual models of nursing move the practice of nursing away from that driven by a medical or institutional model and, therefore, foster autonomy from medicine and a coherent purpose of practice (Bélanger, 1991; Bridges, 1991; Ingram, 1991). Furthermore, conceptual models specify innovative goals for nursing practice and introduce ideas that are designed to improve practice (Lindsay, 1990) by facilitating the identification of relevant information, reducing the fragmentation of care, and improving the coordination of care (Chalmers, cited in Chalmers et al., 1990). In particular, conceptual models provide a nursing knowledge base that has a positive effect on practice "by enabling well-coordinated care to take place, by providing a basis for the justification of care actions and by enabling nurses to *talk nursing*" (Chalmers, cited in Chalmers et al., 1990, p. 34) and to *think nursing* (Perry, 1985).

Hayne (1992), moreover, pointed out that although some clinicians hold the "unfortunate view [that conceptual models] are the inventions and predictions only of scholars and academics [that have] little significance for their own practice environments," many other clinicians recognize the beneficial effects of conceptual models on practice (p. 105). Indeed, conceptual model–based nursing practice "help[s] nurses better communicate what they do" (Neff, 1991, p. 534) and why they do it.

The importance of communicating what nursing is and what nurses do was underscored by Feeg (1989), who identified the following three reasons for implementing conceptual model–based nursing practice:

1. In this time of information saturation and rapid change, we know it is not valuable to focus on every detail and, therefore, we need [conceptual models] to help guide our judgments in new situations.

2. In this time of technological overdrive, we need a holistic orientation to remind us of our caring perspective.

3. In this time of professional territoriality, it has become even more important to understand our identity in nursing and operationalize our practice from a . . . knowledge base. (p. 450)

Another reason for implementing conceptual model–based nursing practice highlights the need for the discipline of nursing to be clear about its mission in the current climate of health care reform that is taking place in the United States and other countries:

4. In this time of health care reform, it is crucial that we explicate *what we know and why we do what we do*. In other words, it is crucial that we communicate our nursing knowledge and explain how that knowledge governs the actions we perform on behalf of or in conjunction with people who require health care.

Johnson (1990) noted that although individual clinicians and nursing departments take risks when the decision is made to implement conceptual model–based nursing practice, the rewards far outweigh the risks. She stated:

> To openly use a nursing model is risk-taking behavior for the individual nurse. For a nursing department to adopt one of these models for unit or institution use is risk-taking behavior of an even higher order. The reward for such risk-taking for the individual practitioner lies in the great satisfaction gained from being able to specify explicit concrete nursing goals in the care of patients and from documenting the actual achievement of the desired outcomes. The reward for the nursing department is having a rational, cohesive, and comprehensive basis for the development of standards of nursing practice, for the evaluation of practitioners, and for the documentation of the contribution of nursing to patient welfare. (p. 32)

Anecdotal and empirical evidence is accumulating that additional rewards of conceptual model–based nursing practice include reduced staff nurse turnover (Fernandez, Brennan, Alvarez, & Duffy, 1990; K. Frederickson, cited in Studio Three, 1992; Scherer, 1988), more rapid movement from novice to expert nurse (Field, 1989), and increased patient satisfaction (Scherer, 1988).

Furthermore, as the use of conceptual models moves nursing practice from a base of implicit knowledge to explicit nursing knowledge, both nurses and the recipients of nursing care are empowered. Indeed, "[nursing] knowledge is power" (Orr, 1991, p. 218), which can, as Lister (1991) and Malin and Teasdale (1991) pointed out, be used to empower recipients of health care to fully participate in decisions about that care. The challenge, then, is to help each nurse to adopt an explicit nursing model and each health care institution to implement conceptual model–based nursing practice.

IMPLEMENTING CONCEPTUAL MODEL–BASED NURSING PRACTICE

The implementation of conceptual model–based nursing practice requires considerable thought, careful planning, and commitment to a long-term project that typically involves much change in the form and scope of nursing practice. Recommendations regarding the **substantive elements** and the **process elements** of implementation are discussed in the text that follows. These recommendations are based on an integration of published descriptions of successful projects that were designed to implement specific conceptual models in nursing practice settings (e.g., Byrne-Coker & Schreiber, 1990a, 1990b; Capers, O'Brien, Quinn, Kelly, & Fenerty, 1985; Caramanica & Thibodeau, 1987; Cox, 1991; Dee, 1990; Ference, 1989; Fitch et al., 1991; Gray, 1991; Nunn & Marriner-Tomey, 1989). Additional citations to informative publications, as well as citations to publications that present strategies for implementing particular conceptual models of nursing, are given in the bibliography at the end of this chapter.

Although the discussion in this chapter focuses on implementing conceptual model–based nursing practice in nursing departments within larger health care institutions, the substantive and process elements are equally applicable to clinicians and practitioners in private or group practices and to free-standing nursing organizations. The substantive and process elements also are applicable for nursing education, where the emphasis is on using conceptual models to guide curriculum construction and teaching students to base nursing practice on one or more explicit conceptual models of nursing.

Substantive Elements

The **substantive elements of implementing conceptual model–based nursing practice** involve the translation of the components of the structural hierarchy of contemporary nursing knowledge for the real world of clinical nursing practice (Figure 10–1). The components of the structural

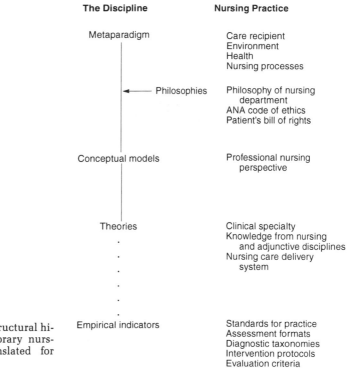

FIGURE 10–1. The structural hierarchy of contemporary nursing knowledge translated for nursing practice.

The Discipline | Nursing Practice

Metaparadigm — Care recipient / Environment / Health / Nursing processes

Philosophies — Philosophy of nursing department / ANA code of ethics / Patient's bill of rights

Conceptual models — Professional nursing perspective

Theories — Clinical specialty / Knowledge from nursing and adjunctive disciplines / Nursing care delivery system

Empirical indicators — Standards for practice / Assessment formats / Diagnostic taxonomies / Intervention protocols / Evaluation criteria hierarchy, which are the metaparadigm, philosophies, conceptual models, theories, and empirical indicators, were described in detail in Chapter 1 of this book. Successful implementation of conceptual model–based nursing practice requires consideration of each component of the structural hierarchy as it relates to the particular nursing department and health care institution.

Translating the Metaparadigm Concepts for Nursing Practice

The first substantive element of implementing conceptual model–based nursing practice is the *translation of the metaparadigm of* nursing, which identifies the phenomena of interest to the discipline of nursing, for nursing practice in a particular health care institution. When translated, the concepts of the metaparadigm become the care recipient, who may be an individual, a family, or a community; the environment of the care recipient, including significant others, physical surroundings, and the nursing care setting; the health state of the care recipient; and the nursing processes used.

The mission statement of each health care institution identifies the particular characteristics and health states of the population of care recipients served by that institution. For example, a general children's hospital provides care for children with various health problems, whereas a children's rehabilitation hospital provides care only to children with health problems requiring intensive inpatient or outpatient rehabilitation. Similarly, a large inner city tertiary medical center provides care to all residents of the city and to persons referred from other locations, whereas a small community hospital typically serves only the members of the immediate community.

The limitations imposed by the mission of the institution on the population of care recipients served and types of health problems considered, as well as the structural design of the institution, have an influence on the relevant environments of care recipients and the scope of the nursing process. For example, the physical structure of units may require nursing care to be provided in large open wards or in private rooms. Moreover, direct assessment of care recipients' home resources and frequent direct contact with family members may be impossible if the care recipients have been referred from distant communities. In addition, nursing activities that emphasize primary prevention and health promotion may be more limited in an institution whose mission is trauma care than in an institution whose mission is ambulatory care.

Translating the Philosophy for Nursing Practice

The second substantive element is the *translation of philosophies* for nursing practice. When translated for nursing practice, the philosophy refers to statements that reflect beliefs and values about nursing as a discipline and a profession; the beliefs and values held by a particular health care institution about the care recipient and health care; and the beliefs and values of the nurses who work in the institution about the care recipient, the environment, health, and nursing processes. Philosophical statements about the discipline and the profession of nursing appear in the American Nurses' Association (ANA) Code of Ethics, and philosophical statements about care recipients and health care appear in the Patient's Bill of Rights. The philosophy of the nursing department of each health care institution typically incorporates relevant notions from the ANA Code of Ethics and the Patient's Bill of Rights and further articulates the nurses' particular beliefs and values.

Translating the Conceptual Model, Theories, and Empirical Indicators into a Professional Practice Model

The third substantive element of implementing conceptual model–based nursing practice is the *translation of the conceptual model, theories, and empirical indicators* into a formal conceptual-theoretical-empirical system of nursing knowledge for nursing practice. Conceptual-theoretical-empirical systems of nursing knowledge are created when the conceptual model of nursing is linked with relevant theories and appropriate empirical indicators. Conceptual-theoretical-empirical systems of nursing knowledge may be considered comprehensive professional practice models that go beyond the governance structures (Zelauskas & Howes, 1992) or structural relationships and communication channels (Stenglein et al., 1993) of nursing departments.

The conceptual models of nursing include Johnson's Behavioral System Model, King's General Systems Framework, Levine's Conservation Model, Neuman's Systems Model, Orem's Self-Care Framework, Rogers' Science of Unitary Human Beings, and Roy's Adaptation Model. Each of these nursing models was discussed in detail in previous chapters of this book.

The process of selecting the conceptual model that will provide the professional practice perspective is discussed later in this chapter. Suffice it to say here that the conceptual model of nursing that is selected must be appropriate for the population of care recipients served by the health care institution and congruent with the philosophy of the nursing department. Once the conceptual model is selected, theories from nursing and adjunctive disciplines that address the specific knowledge required for the care of the population of care recipients served by the health care institution have to be identified. These theories represent clinical specialty knowledge and may differ from unit to unit in a general purpose agency, depending on the population of care recipients served. More specifically, the knowledge sought for linkage with the conceptual model is in the form of relatively specific and concrete descriptions, explanations, and predictions about elements of nursing practice that come from nursing research and research in such adjunctive disciplines as physiology, biochemistry, nutrition, pharmacology, sociology, psychology, and education.

Additional knowledge that must be linked with the conceptual model comes from <u>nursing care delivery systems</u>. Systems or models of nursing care delivery or patient care delivery actually are theories about such methods used to provide patient care services as team nursing, primary nursing, case management, and managed care (Manthey, 1990; Rafferty, 1992; Zander, 1990). The theories of nursing care delivery address only the way in which nursing care is organized and delivered to the care recipient; they do not provide the substance of that nursing care (Brazen, 1992). The substance comes from the conceptual model and clinical specialty knowledge.

The recognition of the need to link theories with conceptual models reflects an understanding of the different functions of conceptual models and theories. As Aggleton and Chalmers (1990) explained, "While it is reasonable to expect a model of nursing to provide general guidelines for intervention, it is unlikely that [the model] will give detailed guidance on the precise ways in which nurses can act. It is crucial for the model to have this kind of emphasis, since it alerts nurses to the need to look elsewhere to find out more about a particular issue. Indeed, it is probably undesirable for a model to go beyond advocating certain broad principles of intervention. This way, nurses will be encouraged to make use of up-to-date studies to inform practice" (p. 42). In fact, the results of studies represent the theories that further specify the general parameters of assessment, planning, intervention, and evaluation that are provided by the conceptual model.

Empirical indicators are selected after the conceptual model and relevant theories have been selected. When translated for nursing practice, empirical indicators refer to such actual documents as <u>standards for nursing practice</u>, <u>assessment formats</u>, <u>diagnostic taxonomies</u>, <u>intervention protocols</u>, and <u>evaluation criteria</u>.

Process Elements

The **process elements of implementing conceptual model–based nursing practice** encompass eight phases of implementation and a transformation in nurses' perspectives of what nursing is and what nurses do.

Phases of Implementation

The *first phase* of the implementation of conceptual model–based nursing practice is an *idea or vision* of what nursing practice can be. The idea may be put forth by one or more staff nurses, clinical specialists, or nurse managers, or by the nurse executive. Regardless of who initiates the idea, it is crucial that both administrators and staff are willing to at least consider a new approach to the practice of nursing in the health care institution. Moreover, a spirit of adventure and risk-taking on the part of administrators and staff, as well as a high tolerance for ambiguity and resistance to change, will greatly facilitate the continuation of the implementation project.

The *second phase* is the *formation of a task force to determine the feasibility* of implementing conceptual model–based nursing practice. Indeed, much time can be saved and much frustration can be avoided if the originators of the idea of conceptual model–based practice would conduct a feasibility study in the form of an initial assessment of the practice climate to determine if it is conducive to using an explicit conceptual model (Capers, 1986; Gray, 1991). The task force should include key nursing personnel, including the nurse executive or designée and a representative from each category of nursing personnel who work in the health care institution. The feasibility study questionnaire, which should be sent to all nursing personnel, should focus on the physical, psychological, and organizational climate for change to a new way of practicing nursing (Gray, 1991).

Implementation proceeds to the *third phase* if the results of the feasibility study reveal a favorable climate for conceptual model–based nursing practice. The third phase encompasses formation of a *planning committee* and the development of a *long-range plan or formal action plan*.

The *planning committee* may include the original task force members and/or other interested nurses. The committee should also include representatives from other organizational units of the health care institution, such as the institution administrator or designée, and representatives from medicine, social work, dietetics, physical therapy, occupational therapy, respiratory therapy, and other relevant departments. Although such a broad membership may seem cumbersome, it is important that all individuals who will be affected by the change in nursing practice be directly involved in that change. Subcommittees can be formed to carry out various tasks involved in planning and implementing conceptual model–based nursing practice. In addition, the planning committee may include a consultant who is an expert in the content of conceptual models of nursing and the process of implementing conceptual model–based nursing practice. Although one or more nurses within the health care institution may have such expertise, a nurse consultant who has no formal tie to the institution frequently is more effective in moving the implementation project forward.

The *long-range plan* should contain a specific time line for actions and the human and material resources required. More specifically, the plan should address:

- The outcomes that are anticipated from use of the conceptual model
- The nursing personnel who will use the model
- The identification of subsequent phases of implementation and the time required for each phase
- The financial resources that are needed and those that are available

The decision to implement conceptual model–based nursing practice typically is undertaken in response to the quest for a way to articulate the substance and scope of professional nursing practice to other health care disciplines and the public and to improve the conditions and outcomes of nursing practice. Consequently, one anticipated outcome of conceptual model–based nursing practice is enhanced understanding of the role of nursing in health care by administrators, physicians, social workers, dietitians, physical therapists, occupational therapists, respiratory therapists, and other health care team members, as well as by the population of care recipients who is served by the institution. Another anticipated outcome is increased nursing staff satisfaction with the conditions and outcomes of nursing practice through an explicit focus on and identification of nursing problems and actions, as well as through enhanced communication and documentation (Fitch et al., 1991). Still another anticipated outcome is increased satisfaction of patients and their families with the nursing care received.

Other more specific outcomes that are relevant to a particular health care institution may be formulated as the long-range plan is developed. For example, a computerized documentation system or a patient classification system based on the conceptual model may be a desired outcome. In fact, such an outcome may be the catalyst for the implementation of conceptual model–based nursing practice. Still other outcomes are tied to the particular conceptual model selected. For example, anticipated outcomes from the use of Orem's Self-Care Framework include enhanced patient self-care agency and enhanced family dependent-care agency.

Conceptual model–based nursing practice is most effective when all categories of nursing personnel, from aides through the nurse executive, use the designated conceptual model to guide their nursing activities. The conceptual model can be adapted to the particular focus of each person's activities. For example, nurse managers and the nurse executive may use a version of the conceptual model that is adapted for administration, whereas the nurse aides, practical nurses, registered nurses, and clinical specialists will use the version of the model that directly addresses nursing practice. The depth of use and the scope of phenomena addressed within the context of the particular conceptual model will vary according to the educational level and concomitant knowledge of each category of nursing personnel (Cox, 1991).

As the long-range plan develops, additional phases of planning and implementing conceptual model–based nursing practice need to be identified, along with the estimated time for each phase. The typical implementation project proceeds through five more phases, that is, phases four, five, six, seven, and eight. Each of those phases is discussed in the following text.

The eight phases of an implementation project require at least 27 to 36 months. The first five phases take approximately 9 to 12 months. The sixth phase takes at least another 6 months. The seventh and eighth phases require an additional 12 to 18 months and may require even more time. Consequently, the decision to implement conceptual model–based nursing practice in a health care institution involves not only the willingness to do so but also the motivation to continue a long-term project.

The actual cost of implementing conceptual model–based nursing practice has not yet been fully addressed in the nursing or health care literature. Costs most likely will vary from institution to institution depending on the staff's existing knowledge of conceptual models, existing staff development resources, extent of change in documentation, and the like. Categories of costs include but are not limited to consultation fees, printing of all documents, staff orientation and development, and data analysis. Some cost categories represent existing budget items, but others represent new items. For example, most health care institutions already allocate funds for staff orientation and development, but few regularly allocate funds for consultation from nurse experts. Consequently, the nurse executive must be prepared to negotiate with the finance officer and the institution administrator for the supplemental funds that will be needed to sustain the implementation project. In addition, the nurse executive may apply to federal agencies, foundations, or other extramural sources for funding (Capers et al., 1985).

The *fourth phase* is a *review of documents* that serve as a base for nursing practice. In particular, the mission statement of the health care institution and the philosophy of the nursing department should be reviewed at this point in the implementation process. The written mission statement of the health care institution should be examined to determine its congruence with the actual situation. As the statement is examined, the opportunity for all members of the health care team to reaffirm their commitment to a particular population of care recipients is provided. The opportunity to discuss changes in the population of care recipients served is, of course, also provided.

Next, the philosophy of the nursing department should be reviewed to determine if it reflects current beliefs about nursing held by the members of the discipline at large as well as by the nurses at the health care institution where the implementation project is taking place. In fact, the implementation project may act as a catalyst for reaffirmation or revision of the nursing department's current philosophy of nursing care.

A comprehensive review of the current philosophy could take the form of a survey of all nursing personnel, which seeks to elicit each nurse's beliefs and values about care recipients, their environments and health, and nursing processes. The review also could be in the form of a request that all nursing personnel comment on the current philosophy. Regardless of the approach taken, the result should be a document that articulates a philosophy representing the beliefs and values of those nurses who are responsible for the nursing care of the population of care recipients served by the health care institution.

Moreover, as Johns (1989) noted, the philosophy of the nursing department "must be relevant to the context of where the care is carried out . . . [as well as] to how nursing organizes the delivery of care on the unit and the relationship nursing has with medicine and the organization in general" (p. 3). He pointed out that the document may go through successive drafts until both the philosophical content and the language in which it is expressed are clearly understood and accepted by all nursing personnel (Johns, 1990).

The *fifth phase* is the *selection of a conceptual model and development of a formal conceptual-theoretical-empirical system of nursing knowledge.* The process of *selecting a conceptual model* should proceed through the following four steps:

1. Thoroughly analyze and evaluate several conceptual models of nursing.

2. Compare the content of each conceptual model with the mission statement of the health care institution to determine if the model is appropriate for use with the population of care recipients served.

3. Determine if the philosophical claims undergirding each conceptual model are congruent with the philosophy of the nursing department.

4. Select the conceptual model that most closely matches the mission of the health care institution and the philosophy of the nursing department.

Chapters 3 through 9 of this book contain thorough analyses and evaluations of Johnson's Behavioral System Model, King's General Systems Framework, Levine's Conservation Model, Neuman's Systems Model, Orem's Self-Care Framework, Rogers' Science of Unitary Human Beings, and Roy's Adaptation Model. Reading these chapters, along with the primary source material for each conceptual model, provides the foundation for the selection of the conceptual model.

The next step is the comparison of the content of various conceptual models with the mission statement of the institution, with particular attention given to whether that content will lead to nursing actions that are appropriate for the population of care recipients served by that institution. Next, the fit of the underlying philosophical claims of each conceptual model with the philosophy of the nursing department should be determined.

The literature associated with the seven conceptual models included in this book suggests that each model is appropriate in a wide range of nursing specialties and for many different populations of care recipients. Aggleton and Chalmers (1985) noted that the literature "might encourage some nurses to feel that it does not really matter which model of nursing is chosen to inform nursing practice within a particular care setting" (p. 39). They also noted that that literature might "encourage the view that choosing between models is something one does intuitively, as an act of personal preference. Even worse, it might encourage some nurses to feel that all their everyday problems might be eliminated were they to make the 'right choice' in selecting a particular model for use across a care setting" (p. 39).

Critical appraisals of the literature have not yet revealed the extent to which the fit of the conceptual model to particular populations of care recipients might have been forced. In fact, the issue of forced fit has not yet been addressed in the literature. Furthermore, little attention has been given to the extent to which a particular conceptual model is modified by an individual or group to fit a given situation (C.P. Germain, personal communication, October 21, 1987). Although modifications certainly are acceptable, they should be acknowledged, and serious consideration should be given to renaming the conceptual model to indicate that modifications have been made. Clearly, systematic exploration of the nursing clinical specialty practice implications of various conceptual models, coupled with more practical experience with each model in a variety of settings, is required.

Although pluralism in conceptual models is currently advocated (Kristjanson, Tamblyn, & Kuypers, 1987; Nagle & Mitchell, 1991; Story & Ross, 1986), it is recommended that just one nursing model be initially selected for use on all nursing units of a health care institution. Health care institutions that serve just one particular population of care recipients or encompass just one clinical specialty area should not have difficulty using one conceptual model to guide all nursing practice activities. General purpose agencies, however, may encounter difficulties if the conceptual model selected does not readily guide practice for all nursing specialty areas and all populations of care recipients served. However, use of more than one conceptual model within an agency may pose problems for a nurse who works on different units as well as for care recipients who are moved from unit to unit as their health states change.

Schmieding (1984) claimed that adopting a single conceptual model for nursing practice in a health care institution "can help nurses work together for quality nursing care" (p. 759). Furthermore, "Without commitment to one [conceptual model] the confusion remains; attitudes, values, and beliefs about nursing vary from one nurse to another and the delivery of care is left to the whim of the moment, one day demanding patient self-care and the next placing the patient back in a dependent and passive role" (Mascord, 1988/1989, p. 15). Moreover, all of the successful implementation projects that have been reported in the literature focused on just one conceptual model of nursing.

Once a conceptual model has been selected, work can proceed to *development of a formal conceptual-theoretical-empirical system of nursing knowledge* by selecting relevant clinical specialty knowledge and a theory of nursing care delivery and developing a methodology for nursing practice. As noted earlier in this chapter, clinical specialty knowledge is in the form of nursing theories and theories from adjunctive disciplines that address particular aspects of nursing care for particular populations of care recipients. These theories can be found in textbooks, clinical specialty journals, and research journals.

A system or theory of nursing care delivery also needs to be selected. Inasmuch as conceptual model–based nursing practice virtually mandates individualized patient care, the care delivery system should facilitate this type of care. Primary nursing has been recommended as a particularly appropriate system of care delivery for conceptual model–based nursing practice (Shea et al., 1989; Walsh, 1989). Another appropriate system of care delivery is nursing case management (Ethridge, 1991).

The methodology for nursing practice is represented by empirical indicators in the form of the documents and technology used to guide and direct nursing care, to record observations and results of interventions, and to describe and evaluate nursing job performance. In other words, the methodology encompasses the standards for nursing care, department and unit objectives, nursing care plans, patient data base and classification tools, flow sheets, Kardex forms, computer information systems, quality assurance tools, nursing job descriptions and performance appraisal tools, and other relevant documents and technologies (Fawcett, 1992; Fitch et al., 1991; Laurie-Shaw & Ives, 1988). Each existing document and all current technology must be reviewed for its congruence with the conceptual model and revised as necessary. Although revisions frequently are needed and although the work may seem overwhelming at the outset, the importance of having documents and technologies that are congruent with the conceptual model cannot be overemphasized. In fact, this congruence may be regarded as the *sine qua non* of conceptual model–based nursing practice.

The need seems obvious for revisions in or development of new documents and technology that have a direct influence on nursing practice, such as standards for care, nursing care plans, and patient classification systems, so that they are congruent with the conceptual model. The need to revise job descriptions and performance appraisal tools so that they, too, are congruent with the conceptual model may not be as obvious. Yet as Laurie-Shaw and Ives (1988) pointed out, these documents should acknowledge the use of the conceptual model and "reinforce the importance of operationalizing the nursing standards of the department" (p. 18).

The *sixth phase* is the *education of the nursing staff* for conceptual model – based practice. Education may occur through participation in staff development or continuing education seminars, workshops, retreats, discussion groups, unit conferences, and nursing grand rounds; formal courses offered by local colleges; and independent study. Ongoing educational activities should be made available to the current nursing staff and other members of the health care team as well as to individuals who join the institution as the implementation project proceeds.

Educational programs should contain information about the content of the conceptual model and realistic examples of the use of the model in nursing practice. Initially, the consultant and other nurses who have experience with conceptual model – based nursing practice may act as preceptors to the staff. As the staff becomes proficient, they can take over the preceptor role during the orientation of new employees.

The *seventh phase* encompasses the designation of certain nursing units to serve as *demonstration sites* and the implementation of conceptual model – based practice on those units. In fact, participants in many implementation projects credit their success to careful phasing-in of conceptual model – based practice through demonstration projects on pilot units prior to implementing the conceptual model on all of the nursing units. Implementation of conceptual model – based nursing practice appears to be most successful when the procedures are "tailored to the particular style and variables of each nursing unit" (Laurie-Shaw & Ives, 1988, p. 19). The seventh phase also includes evaluation of the results of conceptual model – based nursing practice on the pilot units, with emphasis on the refinement of nursing documents and procedures for implementation.

The *eighth phase* is the *institution-wide implementation* of conceptual model – based nursing practice and the *evaluation of outcomes*. This phase requires continuing attention to the education of current staff and the orientation of new staff with regard to conceptual model – based nursing practice, as well as ongoing monitoring of and refinements in the implementation procedures. As previously noted, procedures for implementation should take the characteristics of each unit into account.

Evaluation of administrative, nurse, and patient outcomes should be done periodically throughout the eighth phase "to capture the flow and timing of the change [in outcomes]" (Fitch et al., 1991, p. 25). The evaluation should also include documentation of environmental factors that might influence nurse and patient outcomes, such as a major organizational change or changes in leadership within nursing or the larger institution (Fitch et al., 1991). Other environmental factors to consider include changes in institutional accreditation criteria and changes in standards developed by national and international nursing organizations.

Conclusions drawn from the evaluation of administrative, nurse, and patient outcomes should be in the form of statements regarding the credibility of the conceptual model. As explained in Chapter 2 of this book, the credibility of a conceptual model is determined by examining the extent to which that model is a useful guide for nursing practice in particular situations (social utility); is compatible with expectations of care recipients, the community, and the health care system for nursing practice (social congruence); and leads to beneficial effects on the health status of care recipients (social significance).

Perspective Transformation

The successful implementation of conceptual model–based nursing practice requires recognition of the fact that each nurse and the health care institution as a whole need time to evolve from the use of individual, implicit frames of reference for nursing practice to an explicit conceptual model. The process that occurs during the period of evolution is referred to as *perspective transformation*. Drawing from Mezirow's (1975, 1978) early work in the development of adult learning theory, Rogers (1989) explained that perspective transformation is based on the assumption that "individuals have a personal paradigm or meaning perspective that structures the way in which they existentially experience, interpret, and understand their world" (p. 112). She went on to define and describe perspective transformation as the process "whereby the assumptions, values, and beliefs that constitute a given meaning perspective come to consciousness, are reflected upon, and are critically analyzed. The process involves gradually taking on a new perspective along with the corresponding assumptions, values, and beliefs. The new perspective gives rise to fundamental structural changes in the way individuals see themselves and their relationships with others, leading to a reinterpretation of their personal, social, or occupational worlds" (p. 112).

Thus, the process of perspective transformation when conceptual model–based nursing practice is implemented in a health care institution involves the shift from one meaning perspective about nursing and nursing practice to another, from one way "of viewing and being with human beings" to another (Nagle & Mitchell, 1991, p. 22). Inasmuch as clinical practice that is not based on an explicit conceptual model is based on an implicit, private image of nursing (Reilly, 1975), the shift in meaning perspective is from a private image of nursing to a public image, that is, to an explicit "professional meaning perspective" (Rogers, 1989, p. 113).

Rogers (1989, 1992), a Canadian nurse who is not related to the author of the Science of Unitary Human Beings, commented that her work as a consultant to clinical agencies that were implementing conceptual model–based nursing practice revealed that the cognitive and emotional aspects of perspective transformation represent "dramatic individual change for every nurse" (1989, p. 112). Moreover, she underscored the

FIGURE 10-2. Learning a conceptual model of nursing: phases of the transformation process. (From Rogers, M. (1992 February-April): *Transformative learning: Understanding and facilitating nurses' learning of nursing conceptual frameworks.* Presented at Sigma Theta Tau Conferences on Improving Practice and Education Through Theory. February-April, Chicago, IL; Pittsburgh, PA; Wilkes-Barre, PA; © 1991 Martha Rogers with permission.)

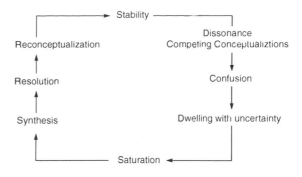

importance of recognizing, appreciating, and acknowledging that during the process of perspective transformation, each nurse evolves from feeling "a [profound] sense of loss followed by an ultimate sense of liberation and empowerment" (1992, p. 23). Clearly, as Nagle and Mitchell (1991) pointed out, perspective transformation requires considerable effort and a strong commitment to change.

Perspective transformation encompasses the nine phases depicted in Figure 10-2: stability, dissonance, confusion, dwelling with uncertainty, saturation, synthesis, resolution, reconceptualization, and return to stability (Rogers, 1992). The prevailing period of stability is disrupted when the idea of implementing conceptual model-based nursing practice is introduced. Dissonance occurs as the nurses begin to examine their private images or meaning perspectives in light of the challenge to adopt a public, professional one. As the nurses begin to learn the content of the conceptual model that is to be implemented, they see the discrepancies between the current way of practice and what nursing practice could be. A phase of confusion follows. As the nurses struggle to learn more about the conceptual model and its implications for practice, they find themselves "lying in limbo between [meaning] perspectives" (Rogers, 1992, p. 22). Throughout the phases of dissonance and confusion, the nurses frequently feel anxious, angry, and unable to think. Rogers (1992) explained that these distressing emotions "seem to arise out of the grieving of a loss of an intimate part of the self. The existing meaning perspective no longer makes sense, yet the new perspective is not sufficiently internalized to provide resolution" (p. 22).

The phase of confusion is followed by the phase of dwelling with uncertainty. At this point, each nurse acknowledges that his or her confusion "is not a result of some personal inadequacy" (Rogers, 1992, p. 22). As a consequence, anxiety is replaced by a "feeling of freedom to critically examine old ways and explore the new [meaning] perspective" (Rogers, 1992, p. 22). The phase of dwelling with uncertainty is spent immersed in information that frequently seems obscure and irrelevant. It is a time of "wallowing in the obscure while waiting for moments of coherence that lead to unity of thought" (Smith, 1988, p. 3).

The phase of <u>saturation</u> occurs when the nurses "feel that they cannot think about or learn anything more about the nursing conceptual [model]" (Rogers, 1992, p. 22). The phase does not represent resistance but rather "the need to separate from the difficult process of transformation, [which] is part of the natural ebb and flow of the learning experience" (Rogers, 1992, p. 22).

The phase of <u>synthesis</u> occurs as insights render the content of the conceptual model coherent and meaningful. The formerly obscure conceptual model–based nursing practice becomes clear and worthy of the implementation effort. Increasing tension is followed by exhilaration as insights illuminate the connections between the content of the conceptual model and its use in nursing practice (Rogers, 1992; Smith, 1988). "These insights," Smith (1988) explained, "are moments of coherence, flashes of unity, as though suddenly the fog lifts and clarity prevails. These moments of coherence push one beyond to deepened levels of understanding" (p. 3).

The phase of <u>resolution</u> is characterized by "a feeling of comfort with the new nursing conceptual [model]. The feelings of dissonance and discontent . . . are resolved and the anxiety is dissipated" (Rogers, 1992, p. 23). During this phase, "Nurses describe themselves as changed, as seeing the world differently and feeling a distinct sense of empowerment" (Rogers, 1992, p. 23).

The phase of <u>reconceptualization</u> occurs as the nurses consciously reconceptualize nursing practice using the new meaning perspective, that is, the conceptual model (Rogers, 1992). During this phase, the nurses compare the activities of practice, from patient assessment through shift reports, according to the old and new meaning perspectives and change those activities so that they are in keeping with the new perspective. The final phase, <u>return to stability</u>, occurs when the new meaning perspective prevails, that is, when nursing practice is based on an explicit conceptual model of nursing.

STRATEGIES TO FACILITATE PERSPECTIVE TRANSFORMATION. Rogers (1989) identified several strategies that can be used to facilitate perspective transformation as conceptual model–based nursing practice is being implemented in a health care institution. These strategies are especially effective during the early phases of perspective transformation, when the nurses are experiencing a move from their implicit, private images of nursing to a shared perspective in the form of an explicit conceptual model.

One strategy is to use analogies to facilitate understanding of the term "conceptual model." Such analogies as chair or book can be used for conceptual, and the analogy of a model home or model airplane can be used for model. Rogers (1989) noted that the act of conceptualizing can be demystified "by stating that it is not a process reserved for intellectuals, but rather a cognitive process of all humans that begins in infancy as a baby puts together all the pieces to form the concept of mother" (p. 114).

Two other strategies are directed toward identification of the nurses' existing private images of nursing practice. One of those strategies is to ask each nurse to list words that reflect his or her view of nursing practice. Similarly, each nurse could be asked to depict his or her view of nursing practice in drawings or collages of photographs. Another strategy is to ask each nurse to present a detailed description of a recent interaction with a patient. Regardless of the strategy selected, group discussion is then used to extract each nurse's underlying perspective of nursing practice from the words, pictures, or descriptions of interactions.

Once the nurses have gained a clear understanding of their private images, they need to be helped to explore the difference between nursing practice as it is now and as it should be, between real and ideal nursing practice. This can be accomplished through the use of provocative strategies. One provocative strategy is to raise questions about how such situations as childbirth and death are managed and how they ought to be managed. Another strategy is to ask the nurses to describe what is unique about nursing practice or what they would do if they did not have to carry out physicians' orders.

Rogers (1989) pointed out that as the nurses become aware of the differences between the real and the ideal, they experience a cognitive dissonance or discomfort that comes from "the awareness of the 'what is' versus 'what should be'" (p. 115). She went on to point out,

> Most nurses hold in the back of their minds a clear image of the ideal nurse and ideal practice. Much of the ideal image was learned in their educational programs and sustained, if at all, by collegial interaction with other nurses or mentors who shared the same image. It also appears that while many nurses have a clear sense of the ideal, they have had to sublimate that image to accommodate a system which does not share the same image. Many nurses can describe their feelings of loss as they let go of the ideal and came to accept the real. [Consequently,] nurses need to rekindle an image of the ideal, the what could be or should be [that is represented by the conceptual model]. More importantly, nurses need to experience a sense of powerfulness to realize the ideal vision. Empowerment of nurses through discussion of the value and importance of nursing knowledge, acts, and processes is essential. (pp. 115–116)

Rogers (1989) concluded by noting that when cognitive dissonance "has been experienced by nurses both individually or collectively, then perspective transformation can occur and a climate for the implementation of a nursing conceptual [model] will have been created" (p. 116).

Subsequent stages of perspective transformation and the implementation of conceptual model–based nursing practice are facilitated by constant reinforcement. Accordingly, all nursing activities at the health care institution should be tied to the conceptual model in a systematic manner. The novice user of a conceptual model should not become discouraged if initial experiences with the model seem forced or awkward. Adoption of an explicit conceptual model does require restructuring the nurse's way of thinking about nursing situations and use of a new vocabulary. However, repeated use of the conceptual model should lead to more systematic and organized endeavors. Regarding this, Broncatello (1980) commented, "The nurse's consistent use of any model for the interpretation of observable client data is most definitely not an easy task. Much like the development of any habitual behavior, it initially requires thought, discipline and the gradual evolvement of a mind set of what is important to observe within the guidelines of the model. As is true of most habits, however, it makes decision making less complicated" (p. 23).

DIRECTIONS FOR THE FUTURE

The future of the discipline of nursing depends at least in part on social and political factors that can be influenced by the explicit articulation of a distinctive body of nursing knowledge. The development and testing of this knowledge in the form of conceptual-theoretical-empirical structures can best be advanced through the combined efforts of nursing service and nursing education. **Directions for the future** are, therefore, discussed in terms of the contributions that can be made by the service and educational sectors of the discipline of nursing.

Contributions from Nursing Service

The extensive review of the nursing literature undertaken for this book revealed increasing attention to the explication and testing of the conceptual-theoretical-empirical structures that guide nursing research but little attention to the development of such structures for nursing practice. If nursing is to continue to advance as a discipline and to claim its rightful place in the health care arena, the articulation and testing of formal conceptual-theoretical-empirical systems of nursing knowledge for nursing practice must be a major priority of all nurses and the nursing departments of all health care institutions. Efforts should be concentrated on articulating formal conceptual-theoretical-empirical structures for specific populations of care recipients and determining the credibility of these structures by formal research projects, as well as by systematic analysis of data obtained from quality assurance reviews, staff satisfaction surveys, and patient satisfaction surveys.

Contributions from Nursing Education

Furthermore, the implementation of conceptual model–based nursing practice in health care institutions would be greatly facilitated and the emotional and cognitive difficulties inherent in perspective transformation might be reduced or eliminated if the process of learning and applying explicit conceptual model were taught in an explicit manner in nursing education programs. The curricula of many schools of nursing in the United States and other countries are already based on one or more conceptual models. Moreover, most schools offer at least one required or elective course dealing with conceptual models. Yet little attention is paid to the process underlying the learning of any conceptual model and the process of using a conceptual model to guide nursing practice. It is, therefore, recommended that relevant courses include content on the substantive and process elements of implementing conceptual model–based nursing practice that were identified in this chapter.

In addition, faculty and clinical specialists who fully understand the elements of implementing conceptual model–based nursing practice must act as partners and be role models for students. Indeed, Grossman and Hooton (1993) maintained that only when "the skills and knowledge base of teachers from the university and [clinical specialists from] service sectors [are] virtually indistinguishable . . . can students and staff . . . experience a professional world based on knowledge, inquiry and social relevance" (p. 871).

CONCLUSION

This chapter identified the major substantive and process elements involved in the implementation of conceptual model–based nursing practice. The beliefs that conceptual models of nursing, rather than medical or institutional models, are the proper guides for nursing practice and that nursing practice should be guided by explicit conceptual models, rather than implicit private images, have permeated the discussion. This author is convinced that the discipline of nursing can survive and advance only if nurses celebrate their own heritage and acknowledge their own knowledge base by adopting explicit conceptual models of nursing to guide their activities. Whether the conceptual model selected by each nurse is one of the existing public models or one of his or her own design does not matter; what does matter is that the conceptual model chosen be explicit and open to public scrutiny to determine its credibility.

REFERENCES

Aggleton, P., & Chalmers, H. (1985). Critical examination. *Nursing Times*, *81*(14), 38–39.

Aggleton, P., & Chalmers, H. (1990). Model future. *Nursing Times*, *86*(3), 41–43.

Bélanger, P. (1991). Nursing models—A major step towards professional autonomy. *AARN Newsletter*, *48*(8), 13.

Brazen, L. (1992). Project 2000: The difference between conceptual models, practice models. *Association of Operating Room Nurses Journal*, *56*, 840–842, 844.

Bridges, J. (1991). Working with doctors: Distinct from medicine. *Nursing Times*, *87*(27), 42–43.

Broncatello, K.F. (1980). Auger in action:

Application of the model. *Advances in Nursing Science, 2*(2), 13–23.

Byrne-Coker, E., & Schreiber, R. (1990a). Implementing King's conceptual framework at the bedside. In M.E. Parker (Ed.), *Nursing theories in practice*, (pp. 85–102). New York: National League for Nursing.

Byrne-Coker, E., & Schreiber, R. (1990b). King at the bedside. *The Canadian Nurse, 86*(1), 24–26.

Capers, C.F. (1986). Some basic facts about models, nursing conceptualizations, and nursing theories. *Journal of Continuing Education, 16,* 149–154.

Capers, C.F., O'Brien, C., Quinn, R., Kelly, R., & Fenerty, A. (1985). The Neuman systems model in practice: Planning phase. *Journal of Nursing Administration, 15*(5), 29–39.

Caramanica, L., & Thibodeau, J. (1987). Nursing philosophy and the selection of a model for practice. *Nursing Management, 10*(10), 71.

Cash, K. (1990). Nursing models and the idea of nursing. *International Journal of Nursing Studies, 27,* 249–256.

Chalmers, H., Kershaw, B., Melia, K., & Kendrich, M. (1990). Nursing models: Enhancing or inhibiting practice? *Nursing Standard, 5*(11), 34–40.

Cox, Sr. R.A. (1991). A tradition of caring: Use of Levine's model in long-term care. In K.M. Schaefer & J.B. Pond (Eds.), *Levine's conservation model: A framework for nursing practice* (pp. 179–197). Philadelphia: FA Davis.

Dee, V. (1990). Implementation of the Johnson model: One hospital's experience. In M.E. Parker (Ed.), *Nursing theories in practice* (pp. 33–44). New York: National League for Nursing.

Ethridge, P. (1991). A nursing HMO: Carondelet St. Mary's experience. *Nursing Management, 22*(7), 22–27.

Fawcett, J. (1992). Conceptual models and nursing practice: The reciprocal relationship. *Journal of Advanced Nursing, 17,* 224–228.

Feeg, V. (1989). From the editor: Is theory application merely an intellectual exercise? *Pediatric Nursing, 15,* 450.

Ference, H.M. (1989). Nursing science theories and administration. In B. Henry, C. Arndt, M. DiVincenti, & A. Marriner-Tomey (Eds.), *Dimensions of nursing administration: Theory, research, education, and practice* (pp. 121–131). Boston: Blackwell Scientific Publications.

Fernandez, R., Brennan, M.L., Alvarez, A., & Duffy, M.R. (1990). Theory-based practice:

A model for nurse retention. *Nursing Administration Quarterly, 12*(4), 47–53.

Field, P.A. (1989). Brenda, Beth, and Susan: Three approaches to health promotion. *The Canadian Nurse, 85*(5), 20–24.

Fitch, M., Rogers, M., Ross, E., Shea, H., Smith, I., & Tucker, D. (1991). Developing a plan to evaluate the use of nursing conceptual frameworks. *Canadian Journal of Nursing Administration, 4*(1), 22–28.

Gray, J. (1991). The Roy adaptation model in nursing practice. In C. Roy & H.A. Andrews, *The Roy adaptation model: The definitive statement* (pp. 429–443). Norwalk, CT: Appleton & Lange.

Grossman, M., & Hooton, M. (1993). The significance of the relationship between a discipline and its practice. *Journal of Advanced Nursing, 18,* 866–872.

Hayne, Y. (1992). The current status and future significance of nursing as a discipline. *Journal of Advanced Nursing, 17,* 104–107.

Ingram, R. (1991). Why does nursing need theory? *Journal of Advanced Nursing, 16,* 350–353.

Johns, C. (1989). Developing a philosophy. *Nursing Practice, 3*(1), 2–4.

Johns, C. (1990). Developing a philosophy (Part 2). *Nursing Practice, 3*(2), 2–6.

Johnson, D.E. (1990). The behavioral system model for nursing. In M.E. Parker (Ed.), *Nursing theories in practice* (pp. 23–32). New York: National League for Nursing.

Kristjanson, L.J., Tamblyn, R., & Kuypers, J.A. (1987). A model to guide development and application of multiple nursing theories. *Journal of Advanced Nursing, 12,* 523–529.

Laurie-Shaw, B., & Ives, S.M. (1988). Implementing Orem's self-care deficit theory: Part II—Adopting a conceptual framework of nursing. *Canadian Journal of Nursing Administration, 1*(2), 16–19.

Lindsay, B. (1990). The gap between theory and practice. *Nursing Standard, 5*(4), 34–35.

Lister, P. (1991). Approaching models of nursing from a postmodernist perspective. *Journal of Advanced Nursing, 16,* 206–212.

Malin, N., & Teasdale, K. (1991). Caring versus empowerment: Considerations for nursing practice. *Journal of Advanced Nursing, 16,* 657–662.

Manthey, M. (1990). Definitions and basic elements of a patient care delivery system with an emphasis on primary nursing. In G.G. Mayer, M.J. Madden, & E. Lawrenz

(Eds.), *Patient care delivery models* (pp. 201–211). Rockville, MD: Aspen.

Mascord, P. (1988/1989). Five days: Five nursing theories. *Australian Journal of Advanced Nursing, 6*(2), 13–15.

Mezirow, J. (1975). *Education for perspective transformation: Women's re-entry programs in community colleges.* New York: Center for Adult Education, Teachers College, Columbia University.

Mezirow, J. (1978). Perspective transformation. *Adult Education, 28,* 100–110.

Nagle, L.M., & Mitchell, G.J. (1991). Theoretic diversity: Evolving paradigmatic issues in research and practice. *Advances in Nursing Science, 14*(1), 17–25.

Neff, M. (1991). President's message: The future of our profession from the eyes of today. *American Nephrology Nurses Association Journal, 18,* 534.

Nunn, D., & Marriner-Tomey, A. (1989). Applying Orem's model in nursing administration. In B. Henry, C. Arndt, M. DiVincenti, & A. Marriner-Tomey (Eds.), *Dimensions of nursing administration: Theory, research, education, practice* (pp. 63–67). Boston: Blackwell Scientific Publications.

Orr, J. (1991). Knowledge is power. *Health Visitor, 64,* 218.

Perry, J. (1985). Has the discipline of nursing developed to the stage where nurses do "think nursing"? *Journal of Advanced Nursing, 10,* 31–37.

Rafferty, D. (1992). Team and primary nursing. *Senior Nurse, 12*(1), 31–34, 39.

Reilly, D.E. (1975). Why a conceptual framework? *Nursing Outlook, 23,* 566–569.

Rogers, M.E. (1989). Creating a climate for the implementation of a nursing conceptual framework. *Journal of Continuing Education in Nursing, 20,* 112–116.

Rogers, M.E. (1992, February-April). *Transformative learning: Understanding and facilitating nurses' learning of nursing conceptual frameworks.* Paper presented at Sigma Theta Tau Conferences, "Improving Practice and Education Through Theory." Chicago, IL; Pittsburgh, PA; Wilkes-Barre, PA.

Scherer, P. (1988). Hospitals that attract (and keep) nurses. *American Journal of Nursing, 88,* 34–40.

Schmieding, N.J. (1984). Putting Orlando's theory into practice. *American Journal of Nursing, 84,* 759–761.

Shea, H., Rogers, M., Ross, E., Tucker, D., Fitch, M., & Smith, I., (1989). Implementation of nursing conceptual models: Observations of a multi-site research team. *Canadian Journal of Nursing Administration, 2*(1), 15–20.

Smith, M.J. (1988). Wallowing while waiting. *Nursing Science Quarterly, 1,* 3.

Stenglein, E., Doepke, C., Hall, J., Lochmer, L., Piersol, L., Szalapski, J., Vanderbilt, D., & Winston, P.B. (1993). Transforming beliefs into action: A professional practice model. *Aspen's Advisor for Nurse Executives, 8*(6), 1, 4–5, 8.

Story, E.L., & Ross, M.M. (1986). Family centered community health nursing and the Betty Neuman Systems Model. *Nursing Papers, 18*(2), 77–78.

Studio Three. (1992). *The Nurse Theorists: Excellence in Action — Callista Roy.* Athens, OH: Fuld Institute of Technology in Nursing Education.

Walsh, M. (1989). Nursing models: Model example. *Nursing Standard, 3*(22), 22–24.

Zander, K. (1990). Managed care and nursing case management. In G.G. Mayer, M.J. Madden, & E. Lawrenz (Eds.), *Patient care delivery models* (pp. 37–61). Rockville, MD: Aspen.

Zelauskas, B., & Howes, D.G. (1992). The effects of implementing a professional practice model. *Journal of Nursing Administration, 22*(7/8), 18–23.

BIBLIOGRAPHY

COMMENTARY: THE VALUE OF CONCEPTUAL MODELS OF NURSING

Adam, E.T. (1975). A conceptual model for nursing. *The Canadian Nurse, 7*(9), 40–41.

Antrobus, S. (1993). Nursing's nature and boundaries. *Senior Nurse, 13*(2), 46–50.

Armentrout, G. (1993). A comparison of the medical model and the wellness model: The importance of knowing the difference. *Holistic Nursing Practice, 7*(4), 57–62.

Baldwin, S. (1983). Nursing models in special hospital settings. *Journal of Advanced Nursing, 8,* 473–476.

Bélanger, P. (1991). Nursing models — A major step towards professional autonomy. *AARN Newsletter, 48*(8), 13.

Bridges, J. (1991). Working with doctors: Distinct from medicine. *Nursing Times*, *87*(27), 42–43.

Cash, K. (1990). Nursing models and the idea of nursing. *International Journal of Nursing Studies*, *27*, 249–256.

Cessario, L. (1987). Utilization of board gaming for conceptual models of nursing. *Journal of Nursing Education*, *26*, 167–169.

Chalmers, H., Kershaw, B., Melia, K., & Kendrich, M. (1990). Nursing models: Enhancing or inhibiting practice? *Nursing Standard*, *5*(11), 34–40.

Cruickshank, C.N. (1992). Creating your own conceptual framework. *The Canadian Nurse*, *88*(2), 31–32.

Derstine, J.B., & Mandzak-McCarron, K. (1990). Theory-based practice in the workplace: The next step. *Rehabilitation Nursing*, *15*, 138–139.

DeSocio, J., & Sebastian, L. (1988). Toward a theoretical model for clinical nursing practice at Menningers. *The Kansas Nurse*, *63*(12), 4–5.

Draper, J. (1992). The impact of nursing models. *Senior Nurse*, *12*(3), 38–39.

Fawcett, J. (1992). Conceptual models and nursing practice: The reciprocal relationship. *Journal of Advanced Nursing*, *17*, 224–228.

Draper, P. (1993). A critique of Fawcett's "Conceptual models and nursing practice: The reciprocal relationship." *Journal of Advanced Nursing*, *18*, 558–564.

Fernandez, R., Brennan, M.L., Alvarez, A., & Duffy, M.R. (1990). Theory-based practice: A model for nurse retention. *Nursing Administration Quarterly*, *12*(4), 47–53.

Field, L., & Winslow, E.H. (1985). Moving to a nursing model. *American Journal of Nursing*, *85*, 1100–1101.

Field, P.A. (1989). Brenda, Beth, and Susan: Three approaches to health promotion. *The Canadian Nurse*, *85*(5), 20–24.

Fitzpatrick, J.J., & Whall, A.L. (1984). Should nursing models be used in psychiatric nursing practice? *Journal of Psychosocial Nursing and Mental Health Services*, *22*(6), 44–45.

Folbrook, P. (1992). Assessing needs and planning actions. *Senior Nurse*, *12*(1), 42–43.

Freda, M.C. (1991). Home care for preterm birth prevention: Is nursing monitoring the interventions? *American Journal of Maternal Child Nursing*, *16*, 9–14.

Frissell, S. (1988). So many models, so much confusion. *Nursing Administration Quarterly*, *12*(2), 13–17.

Grossman, M., & Hooton, M. (1993). The significance of the relationship between a discipline and its practice. *Journal of Advanced Nursing*, *18*, 866–872.

Hayne, Y. (1992). The current status and future significance of nursing as a discipline. *Journal of Advanced Nursing*, *17*, 104–107.

Hils-Williams, J. (1985). Conceptual models —A framework for nursing practice. *Emphasis: Nursing*, *1*(2), 77–83.

Hodgson, R. (1992). A nursing muse. *British Journal of Nursing*, *1*, 330–333.

Ingram, R. (1991). Why does nursing need theory? *Journal of Advanced Nursing*, *16*, 350–353.

Kenny, T. (1992). Nursing models fail in practice. *British Journal of Nursing*, *2*, 133–136.

Kinney, M. (1984). Nursing models. *Focus on Critical Care*, *11*(6), 5–6.

Kristjanson, L.J., Tamblyn, R., & Kuypers, J.A. (1987). A model to guide development and application of multiple nursing theories. *Journal of Advanced Nursing*, *12*, 523–529.

Lewis, T. (1988). Leaping the chasm between nursing theory and practice. *Journal of Professional Nursing*, *13*, 345–351.

Lindsey, B. (1990). The gap between theory and practice. *Nursing Standard*, *5*(4), 34–35.

Lister, P. (1991). Approaching models of nursing from a postmodernist perspective. *Journal of Advanced Nursing*, *16*, 206–212.

Malin, N., & Teasdale, K. (1991). Caring versus empowerment: Considerations for nursing practice. *Journal of Advanced Nursing*, *16*, 657–662.

Mascord, P. (1988/1989). Five days: Five nursing theories. *Australian Journal of Advanced Nursing*, *6*(2), 13–15.

McCaugherty, D. (1992). Theoretical shift. *Nursing Times*, *88*(41), 66.

Moore, S. (1990). Thoughts on the discipline of nursing as we approach the year 2000. *Journal of Advanced Nursing*, *15*, 822–825.

Muller-Smith, P.A. (1992). When paradigms shift. *Journal of Post Anesthesia Nursing*, *7*, 278–280.

Nagle, L.M., & Mitchell, G.J. (1991). Theoretic diversity: Evolving paradigmatic issues in research and practice. *Advances in Nursing Science*, *14*(1), 17–25.

Neff, M. (1991). President's message: The future of our profession from the eyes of today. *American Nephrology Nurses Association Journal*, *18*, 534.

Orr, J. (1991). Knowledge is power. *Health Visitor*, *64*, 218.

Perry, J. (1985). Has the discipline of nursing developed to the stage where nurses do "think nursing?" *Journal of Advanced Nursing*, *10*, 31–37.

Powell, J.H. (1989). The reflective practitioner in nursing. *Journal of Advanced Nursing*, *14*, 824–832.

Rapley, P., & Robertson, J. (1990). Justifying nursing practice: The scientific rationale. *Nurse Education Today*, *10*, 233–236.

Speedy, S. (1989). Theory-practice debate: Setting the scene. *Australian Journal of Advanced Nursing*, *6*(3), 12–20.

IMPLEMENTING CONCEPTUAL MODEL-BASED NURSING PRACTICE: SUBSTANTIVE ELEMENTS

Brazen, L. Project 2000: The difference between conceptual models, practice models. *Association of Operating Room Nurses Journal*, *56*, 840–842, 844.

Fawcett, J., Botter, M.L., Burritt, J., Crossley, J.D., & Fink, B.B. (1989). Conceptual models of nursing and organization theories. In B. Henry, M. DiVincenti, C. Arndt, & A. Marriner (Eds.), *Dimensions of nursing administration: Theory, research, education, and practice* (pp. 143–154). Boston: Blackwell Scientific Publications.

Girard, N. (1993). Nursing care delivery models. *Association of Operating Room Nurses Journal*, *57*, 481–488.

Manthey, M. (1990). Definitions and basic elements of a patient care delivery system with an emphasis on primary nursing. In G.G. Mayer, M.I. Madden, & E. Lawrenz (Eds.), *Patient care delivery models* (pp. 201–211). Rockville, MD: Aspen.

Manthey, M. (1991). Delivery systems and practice models: A dynamic balance. *Nursing Management*, *22*(1), 28–30.

Mark, B.A. (1992). Characteristics of nursing practice models. *Journal of Nursing Administration*, *22*(11), 57–63.

Martin, L., & Glasper, A. (1986). Core plans: Nursing models and the nursing process in action. *Nurse Practitioner*, *1*, 268–273.

Quayhagen, M.P., & Roth, P.A. (1989). From models to measures in assessment of mature families. *Journal of Professional Nursing*, *5*, 144–151.

Rafferty, D. (1992). Team and primary nursing. *Senior Nurse*, *12*(1), 31–34, 39.

Redfern, S.J., & Norman, I.J. (1990). Measuring the quality of nursing care: A consideration of different approaches. *Journal of Advanced Nursing*, *15*, 1260–1271.

Stenglein, E., Doepke, C., & Hall, J. (1993).

Transforming beliefs into action: A professional practice model. *Aspen's Advisor for Nurse Executives*, *6*(1), 4–5, 8.

Waters, K. (1986). Editorial. *Nurse Practitioner*, *1*, 201.

Williams, B.S. (1991). The utility of nursing theory in nursing case management practice. *Nursing Administration Quarterly*, *15*(3), 60–65.

Zander, K. (1990). Managed care and nursing case management. In G.G. Mayer, M.J. Madden, & E. Lawrenz (Eds.), *Patient care delivery models* (pp. 37–61). Rockville, MD: Aspen.

Zelauskas, B., & Howes, D.G. (1992). The effects of implementing a professional practice model. *Journal of Nursing Administration*, *22*(7/8), 18–23.

IMPLEMENTING CONCEPTUAL MODEL-BASED NURSING PRACTICE: PROCESS ELEMENTS

Aggleton, P., & Chalmers, H. (1986). Model choice. *Senior Nurse*, *5*(5/6), 18–20.

Ali, L. (1990). Clinical nursing assessment: Models in accident and emergency. *Nursing Standard*, *5*(3), 33–35.

Capers, C.F. (1986). Some basic facts about models, nursing conceptualizations, and nursing theories. *Journal of Continuing Education*, *16*, 149–154.

Clifford, C. (1989). An experience of transition from a medical model to a nursing model in nursing education. *Nurse Education Today*, *9*, 413–418.

Duff, V. (1989). Perspective transformation: The challenge for the RN in the baccalaureate program. *Journal of Nursing Education*, *28*(1), 38–39.

Haddon, R. (1991). The implications of shifting paradigms. *Aspen's Advisor for Nurse Executives*, *6*(22), 1, 3–6.

Hawkett, S. (1991). A gap which must be bridged: Nurses' attitudes to theory and practice. *Professional Nurse*, *6*, 166, 168–170.

Hoch, C.C. (1987). Assessing delivery of nursing care. *Journal of Gerontological Nursing*, *13*, 10–17.

Holzemer, W.L. (1992). Linking primary health care and self-care through case management. *International Nursing Review*, *39*, 83–89.

Hughes, E., & Anderson, C.L. (1993). How to implement a different structure of nursing care delivery. *Perspectives*, *17*(2), 9–16.

Johns, C. (1989). Developing a philosophy. *Nursing Practice*, *3*(1), 2–4.

Johns, C. (1990). Developing a philosophy—Part 2. *Nursing Practice*, *3*(2), 2–6.

Johnston, N., & Baumann, A. (1992). A process oriented approach: Selecting a nursing model for psychiatric nursing. *Journal of Psychosocial Nursing and Mental Health Services, 30*(4), 7–12.

Lashinger, H.S. (1991). Nurses' attitudes about nursing models in practice. *Journal of Nursing Administration, 21*(10), 12, 15, 18.

MacVicar, B., & Swan, J. (1992). Mental health: Theory into practice. *Nursing Times, 88*(12), 38–40.

McKenna, H.P. (1989). The selection by ward managers of an appropriate nursing model for long-stay psychiatric patient care. *Journal of Advanced Nursing, 14,* 762–775.

McKenna, H.P. (1990). The perception of psychiatric-hospital ward sisters/charge nurses towards nursing models. *Journal of Advanced Nursing, 15,* 1319–1325.

McKenna, H.P. (1990). Which model? *Nursing Times, 86*(25), 50–52.

Mezirow, J. (1975). *Education for perspective transformation: Women's re-entry programs in community colleges.* New York: Center for Adult Education, Teachers College, Columbia University.

Mezirow, J. (1978). Perspective transformation. *Adult Education, 28,* 100–110.

Nevin-Haas, M. (1992). Checking the fit. *The Canadian Nurse, 88*(2), 33–34.

Ouellet, L., Rogers, R., & Gibson, C. (1989). Guidelines for selecting a nursing model for practice. *Canadian Journal of Nursing Administration, 2*(3), 5, 8–9, 15.

Pearson, A. (1989). Therapeutic nursing—Transforming models and theories into action. *Nurse Education Today, 24,* 123–151.

Rogers, M.E. (1989). Creating a climate for the implementation of a nursing conceptual framework. *Journal of Continuing Education in Nursing, 20,* 112–116.

Sbaih, L.C. (1992). Finding a model that fits. *Professional Nurse, 7,* 566–569.

Schlentz, M.D. (1993). The minimum data set and the levels of prevention in the long-term care facility. *Geriatric Nursing, 14,* 79–83.

Shea, H., Rogers, M., Ross, E., Tucker, D., Fitch, M., & Smith, I. (1989). Implementation of nursing conceptual models: Observations of a multi-site research team. *Canadian Journal of Nursing Administration, 2*(1), 15–20.

Smith, M.C. (1991). Evaluating nursing theory-based practice. *Nursing Science Quarterly, 4,* 98–99.

Smith, M.J. (1988). Wallowing while waiting. *Nursing Science Quarterly, 1,* 3.

Walsh, M. (1989). Nursing models: Model example. *Nursing Standard, 3*(22), 22–24.

IMPLEMENTING JOHNSON'S BEHAVIORAL SYSTEM MODEL

Auger, J.A., & Dee, V. (1983). A patient classification system based on the behavioral system model of nursing: Part 1. *Journal of Nursing Administration, 13*(4), 38–43.

Dee, V. (1990). Implementation of the Johnson model: One hospital's experience. In M.E. Parker (Ed.), *Nursing theories in practice* (pp. 33–44). New York: National League for Nursing.

Dee, V., & Auger, J.A. (1983). A patient classification system based on the behavioral system model of nursing: Part 2. *Journal of Nursing Administration, 13*(5), 18–23.

Derdiarian, A.K. (1983). An instrument for theory and research using the behavioral systems model for nursing: The cancer patient—Part I. *Nursing Research, 32,* 196–201.

Derdiarian, A.K. (1988). Sensitivity of the Derdiarian behavioral system model instrument to age, site, and stage of cancer: A preliminary validation study. *Scholarly Inquiry for Nursing Practice, 2,* 103–121.

Holaday, B. (1989). Response to "Sensitivity of the Derdiarian behavioral system model instrument to age, site, and stage of cancer: A preliminary validation study." *Scholarly Inquiry for Nursing Practice, 2,* 123–125.

Derdiarian, A.K. (1990). Effects of using systematic assessment instruments on patient and nurse satisfaction with nursing care. *Oncology Nursing Forum, 17,* 95–101.

Derdiarian, A.K. (1991). Effects of using a nursing model-based assessment instrument on quality of nursing care. *Nursing Administration Quarterly, 15*(3), 1–16.

Derdiarian, A.K., & Forsythe, A.B. (1983). An instrument for theory and research using the behavioral systems model for nursing: The cancer patient—Part II. *Nursing Research, 32,* 260–266.

Derdiarian, A.K., & Schobel, D. (1990). Comprehensive assessment of AIDS patients using the behavioral systems model for nursing practice instrument. *Journal of Advanced Nursing, 15,* 436–446.

Glennin, C.G. (1974). Formulation of standards of nursing practice using a nursing model. In J.P. Riehl & C. Roy, *Conceptual models for nursing practice* (pp. 234–246). New York: Appleton-Century-Crofts. Reprinted in J.P. Riehl & C. Roy (1980). *Conceptual models for nursing practice* (2nd ed., pp. 290–301). New York: Appleton-Century-Crofts.

Majesky, S.J., Brester, M.H., & Nishio, K.T. (1978). Development of a research tool: Patient indicators of nursing care. *Nursing Research, 27,* 365–371.

IMPLEMENTING KING'S GENERAL SYSTEMS FRAMEWORK

Byrne-Coker, E., Fradley, T., Harris, J., Tomarchio, D., Chan, V., & Caron, C. (1990). Implementing nursing diagnoses within the context of King's conceptual framework. *Nursing Diagnosis, 1,* 107–114.

Byrne-Coker, E., & Schreiber, R. (1990). Implementing King's conceptual framework at the bedside. In M.E. Parker (Ed.), *Nursing theories in practice* (pp. 85–102). New York: National League for Nursing.

Byrne-Coker, E., & Schreiber, R. (1990). King at the bedside. *The Canadian Nurse, 86*(1), 24–26.

Elberson, K. (1989). Applying King's model to nursing administration. In B. Henry, M. DiVincenti, C. Arndt, & A. Marriner (Eds.), *Dimensions of nursing administration: Theory, research, education, and practice* (pp. 47–53). Boston: Blackwell Scientific Publications.

Messmer, P.R. (1992). Implementing theory based nursing practice. *Florida Nurse, 40*(3), 8.

Schreiber, R. (1991). Psychiatric assessment —"à la King." *Nursing Management, 22*(5), 90–94.

West, P. (1991). Theory implementation: A challenging journey. *Canadian Journal of Nursing Administration, 4*(1), 29–30.

IMPLEMENTING LEVINE'S CONSERVATION MODEL

Cox, R.A., Sr. (1991). A tradition of caring: Use of Levine's model in long-term care. In K.M. Schaefer & J.B. Pond (Eds.), *Levine's conservation model: A framework for nursing practice* (pp. 179–197). Philadelphia: FA Davis.

Lynn-McHale, D.J., & Smith, A. (1991). Comprehensive assessment of families of the critically ill. *AACN Clinical Issues in Critical Care Nursing, 2,* 195–209.

McCall, B.H. (1991). Neurological intensive monitoring system: Unit assessment tool. In K.M. Schaefer & J.B. Pond (Eds.), *Levine's conservation model: A framework for nursing practice* (pp. 83–90). Philadelphia: FA Davis.

Taylor, J.W. (1974). Measuring the outcomes of nursing care. *Nursing Clinics of North America, 9,* 337–340.

Taylor, J.W. (1987). Organizing data for nursing diagnoses using conservation principles. In A.M. McLane (Ed.), *Classification of nursing diagnoses: Proceedings of the seventh conference: North American Nursing Diagnosis Association* (pp. 103–111). St. Louis: CV Mosby.

Taylor, J.W. (1989). Levine's conservation principles: Using the model for nursing diagnosis in a neurological setting. In J.P. Riehl-Sisca, *Conceptual models for nursing practice* (3rd ed., pp. 349–358). Norwalk, CT: Appleton & Lange.

IMPLEMENTING NEUMAN'S SYSTEMS MODEL

Bowman, G.E. (1982). The Neuman assessment tool adapted for child day-care centers. In B. Neuman, *The Neuman systems model: Application to nursing education and practice.* (pp. 324–334). Norwalk, CT: Appleton-Century-Crofts.

Breckenridge, D.M., Cupit, M.C., & Raimondo, J.M. (1982). Systematic nursing assessment tool for the CAPD client. *Nephrology Nurse,* (January/February), 24, 26–27, 30–31.

Burke, M.E., Sr., Capers, C.F., O'Connell, R.K., Quinn, R.M., & Sinnott, M. (1989). Neuman-based nursing practice in a hospital setting. In B. Neuman, *The Neuman systems model* (2nd ed., pp. 423–444). Norwalk, CT: Appleton & Lange.

Capers, C.F. (1986). Some basic facts about models, nursing conceptualizations, and nursing theories. *Journal of Continuing Education, 16,* 149–154.

Capers, C.F., & Kelly, R. (1987). Neuman nursing process: A model of holistic care. *Holistic Nursing Practice, 1*(3), 19–26.

Capers, C.F., O'Brien, C., Quinn, R., Kelly, R., & Fenerty, A. (1985). The Neuman systems model in practice: Planning phase. *Journal of Nursing Administration, 15*(5), 29–39.

Caramanica, L., & Thibodeau, J. (1987). Nursing philosophy and the selection of a model for practice. *Nursing Management, 10*(10), 71.

Flannery, J. (1991). FAMLI-RESCUE: A family assessment tool for use by neuroscience nurses in the acute care setting. *Journal of Neuroscience Nursing, 23,* 111–115.

Hinton-Walker, P., & Raborn, M. (1989). Application of the Neuman model in nursing administration and practice. In B. Henry, C. Arndt, M. DiVincenti, & A. Marriner-

Tomey (Eds.), *Dimensions of nursing administration: Theory, research, education, and practice* (pp. 711–723). Boston: Blackwell Scientific Publications.

Mayers, M.A., & Watson, A.B. (1982). Nursing care plans and the Neuman systems model: In B. Neuman, *The Neuman systems model: Application to nursing education and practice* (pp. 69–84). Norwalk, CT: Appleton-Century-Crofts.

Mischke-Berkey, K., & Hanson, S.M.H. (1991). *Pocket guide to family assessment and intervention*. St. Louis: Mosby-Year Book.

Mischke-Berkey, K., Warner, P., & Hanson, S. (1989). Family health assessment and intervention. In P.J. Bomar (Ed.), *Nurses and family health promotion: Concepts, assessment, and interventions* (pp. 115–154). Baltimore: Williams & Wilkins.

Moynihan, M.M. (1990) Implementation of the Neuman systems model in an acute care nursing department. In M.E. Parker (Ed.), *Nursing theories in practice* (pp. 263–273). New York: National League for Nursing.

Neal, M.C. (1982). Nursing care plans and the Neuman Systems Model: II. In B. Neuman, *The Neuman systems model: Application to nursing education and practice* (pp. 85–93). Norwalk, CT: Appleton-Century-Crofts.

Quayhagen, M.P., & Roth, P.A. (1989). From models to measures in assessment of mature families. *Journal of Professional Nursing, 5,* 144–151.

Schlentz, M.D. (1993). The minimum data set and the levels of prevention in the long-term care facility. *Geriatric Nursing, 14,* 79–83.

IMPLEMENTING OREM'S SELF-CARE FRAMEWORK

Allison, S.E. (1985). Structuring nursing practice based on Orem's theory of nursing: A nurse administrator's perspective. In J. Riehl-Sisca, *The science and art of self-care* (pp. 225–235). Norwalk, CT: Appleton-Century-Crofts.

Angeles, D.M. (1991). An Orem-based NICU orientation checklist. *Neonatal Network, 9*(7), 43–48.

Avery, P. (1992). Self-care in the hospital setting: The Prince Henry Hospital experience. *Lamp, 49*(2), 26–28.

Bliss-Holtz, J., McLaughlin, K., & Taylor, S.G. (1990). Validating nursing theory for use within a computerized nursing information system. *Advances in Nursing Science, 13*(2), 46–52.

Bliss-Holtz, J., Taylor, S.G., & McLaughlin, K. (1992). Nursing theory as a base for a computerized nursing information system. *Nursing Science Quarterly, 5,* 124–128.

Bliss-Holtz, J., Taylor, S.G., McLaughlin, K., Sayers, P., & Nickle, L. (1992). Development of a computerized information system based on self-care deficit nursing theory. In J.M. Arnold & G.A. Pearson, *Computer applications in nursing education and practice* (pp. 87–93). New York: National League for Nursing.

Clinton, J.F., Denyes, M.J., Goodwin, J.O., & Koto, E.M. (1977). Developing criterion measures of nursing care: Case study of a process. *Journal of Nursing Administration, 7*(7), 41–45.

Del Togno-Armanasco, V., Olivas, G.S., & Harter, S. (1989). Developing an integrated nursing case management model. *Nursing Management, 20*(10), 26–29.

Feldsine, F. (1982). Options for transition into practice: Nursing process orientation program. *Journal of New York State Nurses' Association, 13,* 11–16.

Fernandez, R., & Wheeler, J.I. (1990). Organizing a nursing system through theory-based practice. In G.G. Mayer, M.J. Madden, & E. Lawrenz (Eds.), *Patient care delivery models* (pp. 63–83). Rockville, MD: Aspen.

Fridgen, R., & Nelson, S. (1992). Teaching tool for renal transplant recipients using Orem's self-care model. *CANNT Journal, 2*(3), 18–26.

Fukuda, N. (1990). Outcome standards for the client with chronic congestive heart failure. *Journal of Cardiovascular Nursing, 4*(3), 59–70.

Gallant, B.W., & McLane, A.M. (1979). Outcome criteria: A process for validation at the unit level. *Journal of Nursing Administration, 9*(1), 14–21.

Hageman, P., & Ventura, M. (1981). Utilizing patient outcome criteria to measure the effects of a medication teaching regimen. *Western Journal of Nursing Research, 3,* 25–33.

Harman, L., Wabin, D., MacInnis, L., Baird, D., Mattiuzzi, D., & Savage, P. (1989). Developing clinical decision-making skills in staff nurses: An educational program. *Journal of Continuing Education in Nursing, 20,* 102–106.

Hooten, S.L. (1992). Education of staff nurses to practice within a conceptual framework. *Nursing Administration Quarterly, 16*(3), 34–35.

Horn, B.J., & Swain, M.A. (1976). An approach to development of criterion measures for quality patient care. In Issues in evaluation research (pp. 74–82). Kansas City: American Nurses Association.

Horn, B.J., & Swain, M.A. (1977). Development of criterion measures of nursing care (Vols. 1–2, NTIS Nos. PB–267 004 and PB-267 005). Ann Arbor, MI: University of Michigan.

Kitson, A.L. (1986). Indicators of quality in nursing care—An alternative approach. Journal of Advanced Nursing, 11, 133–144.

Laurie-Shaw, B., & Ives, S.M. (1988). Implementing Orem's self-care deficit theory: Part I—Selecting a framework and planning for implementation. Canadian Journal of Nursing Administration, 1(1), 9–12.

Laurie-Shaw, B., & Ives, S.M. (1988). Implementing Orem's self-care deficit theory: Part II—Adopting a conceptual framework of nursing. Canadian Journal of Nursing Administration, 1(2), 16–19.

Leatt, P., Bay, K.S., & Stinson, S.M. (1981). An instrument for assessing and classifying patients by type of care. Nursing Research, 30, 145–150.

Loveland-Cherry, C., Whall, A., Griswold, E., Bronneville, R., & Pagé, G. (1985). A nursing protocol based on Orem's self-care model: Application with aftercare clients. In J. Riehl-Sisca, The science and art of self-care (pp. 285–297). Norwalk, CT: Appleton-Century-Crofts.

McLaughlin, K., Taylor, S., Bliss-Holtz, J., Sayers, P., & Nickle, L. (1990). Shaping the future: The marriage of nursing theory and informatics. Computers in Nursing, 8, 174–179.

Nunn, D., & Marriner-Tomey, A. (1989). Applying Orem's model in nursing administration. In B. Henry, C. Arndt, M. DiVincenti, & A. Marriner-Tomey (Eds.), Dimensions of nursing administration: Theory, research, education, practice (pp. 63–67). Boston: Blackwell Scientific Publications.

Padilla, G.V., & Grant, M.M. (1982). Quality assurance programme for nursing. Journal of Advanced Nursing, 7, 135–145.

Paternostro, I. (1992). Developing theory-based software for nurses, by nurses. Nursing Administration Quarterly, 16(3), 33–34.

Roach, K.G., & Woods, H.B. (1993). Implementing cooperative care on an acute care medical unit. Clinical Nurse Specialist, 7, 26–29.

Romine, S. (1986). Applying Orem's theory of self-care to staff development. Journal of Nursing Staff Development, 2(2), 77–79.

Rossow-Sebring, J., Carrieri, V., & Seward, H. (1992). Effect of Orem's model on nurse attitudes and charting behavior. Journal of Nursing Staff Development, 8, 207–212.

Scherer, P. (1988). Hospitals that attract (and keep) nurses. American Journal of Nursing, 88, 34–40.

Taylor, S.G. (1987). A model for nursing diagnosis and clinical decision making using Orem's self-care deficit theory of nursing. In K.J. Hannah, M. Reimer, W.C. Mills, & S. Letourneau (Eds.), Clinical judgment and decision making: The future with nursing diagnosis (pp. 84–86). New York: John Wiley & Sons.

Taylor, S.G. (1991). The structure of nursing diagnoses from Orem's theory. Nursing Science Quarterly, 4, 24–32.

IMPLEMENTING ROGERS' SCIENCE OF UNITARY HUMAN BEINGS

Alligood, M.R. (1989). Applying Rogers' model to nursing administration: Emphasis on environment, health. In B. Henry, C. Arndt, M. DiVincenti, & A. Marriner-Tomey (Eds.), Dimensions of nursing administration: Theory, research, education, and practice. (pp. 105–111). Boston: Blackwell Scientific Publications.

Caroselli-Dervan, C. (1990). Visionary opportunities for knowledge development in nursing administration. In E.A.M. Barrett (Ed.), Visions of Rogers' science based nursing (pp. 151–158). New York: National League for Nursing.

Rizzo, J.A. (1990). Nursing service as an energy field: A response to "Visionary opportunities for knowledge development in nursing administration." In E.A.M. Barrett (Ed.), Visions of Rogers' science based nursing (pp. 159–164). New York: National League for Nursing.

Decker, K. (1989). Theory in action. The geriatric assessment team. Journal of Gerontological Nursing, 15(10), 25–28.

Ference, H.M. (1989). Nursing science theories and administration. In B. Henry, C. Arndt, M. DiVincenti, & A. Marriner-Tomey (Eds.), Dimensions of nursing administration: Theory, research, education, and practice (pp. 121–131). Boston: Blackwell Scientific Publications.

Garon, M. (1991). Assessment and management of pain in the home care setting: Application of Rogers' science of unitary human beings. Holistic Nursing Practice, 6(1), 47–57.

Gueldner, S.H. (1989). Applying Rogers' model to nursing administration: Emphasis on client and nursing. In B. Henry, C. Arndt, M. DiVincenti, & A. Marriner-

Tomey (Eds.), *Dimensions of nursing administration: Theory, research, education, and practice* (pp. 113–119). Boston: Blackwell Scientific Publications.

Hanchett, E.S. (1979). *Community health assessment: A conceptual tool kit.* New York: John Wiley & Sons.

IMPLEMENTING ROY'S ADAPTATION MODEL

DiIorio, C. (1989). Applying Roy's model to nursing administration. In B. Henry, M. DiVincenti, C. Arndt, & A. Marriner (Eds.), *Dimensions of nursing administration: Theory, research, education, and practice* (pp. 89–104). Boston: Blackwell Scientific Publications.

Dorsey, K., & Purcell, S. (1987). Translating a nursing theory into a nursing system. *Geriatric Nursing, 8,* 136–137.

Fawcett, J. (1992). Documentation using a conceptual model of nursing. *Nephrology Nursing Today, 2*(5), 1–8.

Frederickson, K. (1993). Translating the Roy Adaptation Model into practice and research. In M.E. Parker (Ed.), *Patterns of nursing theories in practice* (pp. 230–238). New York: National League for Nursing.

Gray, J. (1991). The Roy adaptation model in nursing practice. In C. Roy & H.A. Andrews, *The Roy adaptation model: The definitive statement* (pp. 429–443). Norwalk, CT: Appleton & Lange.

Jakocko, M.T., & Sowden, L.A. (1986). The Roy adaptation model in nursing practice. In H. A. Andrews & C. Roy, *Essentials of the Roy adaptation model* (pp. 165–177). Norwalk, CT: Appleton & Lange.

Laros, J. (1977). Deriving outcome criteria from a conceptual model. *Nursing Outlook, 25,* 333–336.

Mastal, M.F., Hammond, H., & Roberts, M.P. (1982). Theory into hospital practice: A pilot implementation. *Journal of Nursing Administration, 12*(6), 9–15.

Peters, V.J. (1993). Documentation using the Roy adaptation model. *American Nephrology Nurses Association Journal, 20,* 522.

Riegel, B. (1985). A method of giving intershift report based on a conceptual model. *Focus on Critical Care, 12*(4), 12–18.

Robitaille-Tremblay, M. (1984). A data collection tool for the psychiatric nurse. *The Canadian Nurse, 80*(7), 26–28.

Rogers, M., Paul, L.J., Clarke, J., MacKay, C., Potter, M., & Ward, W. (1991). The use of the Roy adaptation model in nursing administration. *Canadian Journal of Nursing Administration, 4*(2), 21–26.

Resources for Conceptual Models of Nursing

AUDIO PRODUCTIONS

The Second Annual Nurse Educator Conference

Audio tapes available from Teach 'em, Inc., 160 E. Illinois Street, Chicago, IL 60611. (Tapes are no longer available from the distributor.)

Audio tapes of the papers presented at the Nurse Educator Conference held in New York, New York, in December 1978. Presentations are by Johnson, King, Levine, Orem, Rogers, Roy, Leininger, Newman, and Paterson and Zderad. A presentation by Dickoff and James was also taped.

Nurse Theorist Conference

Audio tapes available from Kennedy Recordings, RR5, Edmonton, Alberta, Canada T5P 4B7.

Audio tapes of the papers presented at the Nurse Theorist Conference held in Edmonton, Alberta, Canada, in August 1984. Presenters include King, Levine, Rogers, Roy, and Newman.

Nursing Theory in Action

Audio tapes available from Kennedy Recordings, RR5, Edmonton, Alberta, Canada T5P 4B7.

Audio tapes of the papers and concurrent sessions on applications to practice, research, and education presented at the Nursing Theory in Action Conference held in Edmonton, Alberta, Canada, in August 1985. Presenters include King, Levine, Neuman, Orem (presented by S. Taylor), Rogers, Roy, Newman, and Parse. In addition, a presentation on the Roper/Logan/Tierney Framework also is available.

Nursing Theory Congress, 1986

Audio tapes available from Audio Archives International, 100 West Beaver Creek, Unit 18, Richmond Hill, Ontario, Canada L4B 1H4.

Audio tapes of the papers and concurrent sessions on applications to practice, research, and education presented at the Nursing Theory Congress, "Theoretical Pluralism: Direction for a Practice Discipline," held in Toronto, Ontario, Canada in August 1986. Presentations are by King, Levine, Neuman, Rogers, Roy, Holaday (Johnson's model), Taylor (Orem's framework), Parse, Allen (a developmental health model), Kritek (nursing diagnosis), Dickoff and James (theoretical pluralism), and McGee (criteria for selection and use of a nursing model for practice).

Nursing Theory Congress, 1988

Audio tapes available from Audio Archives International, 100 West Beaver Creek, Unit 18, Richmond Hill, Ontario, Canada L4B 1H4.

Audio tapes of the papers presented at the Nursing Theory Congress, "From Theory to Practice," held in Toronto, Ontario, Canada in August 1988. Presentations are by Parse (nursing science as a basis for research and practice), Watson (one or many models), Henderson (historical perspective), Lindeman (elitism or realism of nursing theory), Moccia (emerging world views), Gordon (nursing diagnosis), and Kritek (agendas for the future). In addition, a panel presentation on the impact of nursing theory on the profession is moderated by Kritek. Concurrent sessions focus on the application of nursing models and theories to practice, education, research, and quality assurance and administration.

VIDEO PRODUCTIONS

The Nurse Theorists: Portraits of Excellence

Video tapes available from Fuld Institute for Technology in Nursing Education, 5 Depot Street, Athens, OH 45701.

A series of video tapes, funded by the Helene Fuld Health Trust and produced by Studio Three of Samuel Merritt College of Nursing in Oakland, California, depicting the major events and incidents in the lives of 16 nurse theorists. Interviews are conducted by Jacqueline Fawcett. The series includes separate video tapes of Johnson, King, Levine, Neuman, Orem, Rogers, Roy, Leininger, Newman, Orlando, Parse, Peplau, Watson, Rubin, Henderson, and Nightingale.

The Nurse Theorists: Excellence in Action

Video tapes available from Fuld Institute for Technology in Nursing Education, 5 Depot Street, Athens, OH 45701.

A series of video tapes, funded by the Helene Fuld Health Trust and produced by Studio Three of Samuel Merritt College of Nursing in Oakland, California, depicting the implementation of the works of nurse theorists in nursing practice. To date, the series includes separate video tapes of the application of Orem's Self-Care Framework and Roy's Adaptation Model.

Nursing Theory: A Circle of Knowledge

Video tape available from National League for Nursing, 350 Hudson Street, New York, NY 10014.

Patricia Moccia interviews several nurse theorists, including Orem, Rogers, Roy, Watson, Henderson, and Benner. The discussion emphasizes philosophy of science.

A Conversation on Caring with Jean Watson and Janet Quinn

Video tape available from National League for Nursing, 350 Hudson Street, New York, NY 10014.

Video tape of Patricia Moccia's interviews with Jean Watson and Janet Quinn. Watson and Quinn discuss their views of human caring and health. Coverage includes the Denver Nursing Project in Human Caring, which focuses on individuals with AIDS, and Quinn's Senior Citizen's Therapeutic Touch Education Program.

Teaching the Self-Care Deficit Nursing Theory

Video tapes available from Media Sales, Biomedical Communications, University of British Columbia, 2194 Health Sciences Mall, Room B-32, Vancouver, British Columbia, Canada V6T 1Z3.

Eight video tapes, which were produced by the Vancouver Health Department, explain the content and use of Orem's Self-Care Framework in clinical nursing practice. A *Teaching Manual* and a *Facilitators' Manual* are included with the package of video tapes. The package is designed for use by individuals or groups.

Care with a Concept

Video tape available from Health Sciences Consortium, 201 Cedar Court, Chapel Hill, NC 27514.

Mary Hale and Gates Rhodes of the University of Pennsylvania School of Nursing produced this video tape documenting the use of Orem's Self-Care Framework at Children's Seashore House when it was located in Atlantic City, New Jersey.

Care Plans That Work

Video tape available from St. Clare Hospital Video Productions, Department No. BB, 515 22nd Avenue, Monroe, WI 53566.

An instructional video that demonstrates the use of Orem's Self-Care Framework and Roy's Adaptation Model to guide nursing care planning.

AUDIO AND VIDEO PRODUCTIONS

Nurse Theorist Conference, 1985

Audio and video tapes available from Veranda Communications, Inc., 1200 Delor Avenue, Louisville, KY 40217.

Audio and video tapes from the 1985 Nurse Theorist Conference sponsored by Discovery International, Inc. Audio-taped presentations are by King, Orem, Rogers, Roy and Parse, followed by critiques of each model or theory. In addition, Peplau presents a historical overview of nursing science, and a panel presentation features all conference speakers. Video tapes are available for the presentations by Orem and Peplau, as well as for the panel presentation.

Nurse Theorist Conference, 1987

Audio and video tapes available from Veranda Communications, Inc., 1200 Delor Avenue, Louisville, KY 40217.

Audio and video tapes from the 1987 Nurse Theorist Conference sponsored by Discovery International, Inc. Presentations are by King, Rogers, Roy, Parse, and Watson. In addition, Peplau presents a paper on the art and science of nursing, Schlotfeldt presents a paper on nursing science in the twenty-first century, and a panel presentation features all conference speakers. Audio tapes are also available of the small group sessions led by King, Rogers, Roy, Parse, and Watson.

Nurse Theorist Conference, 1989

Audio and video tapes available from Veranda Communications, Inc., 1200 Delor Avenue, Louisville, KY 40217.

Audio and video tapes from the 1989 Nurse Theorist Conference sponsored by Discovery International, Inc. Presentations are by King, Neuman, Rogers, and Parse. In addition, Meleis presents a paper on being and becoming healthy, Pender presents a paper on expression of health through beliefs and actions, and a panel presentation features all conference speakers.

Nurse Theorist Conference, 1993

Audio and video tapes available from Veranda Communications, Inc., 1200 Delor Avenue, Louisville, KY 40217.

Audio and video tapes from the 1993 Nurse Theorist Conference sponsored by Discovery International, Inc. Presentations are by Leininger,

King, Parse, Peplau, and Rogers. In addition, M.C. Smith, C. Forchuk, G.J. Mitchell, and J. Chapman present a session on nursing theory-based research and practice in Canada, and a panel presentation features all conference speakers.

National Nursing Theory Conference, 1990

Audio tapes available from Convention Recorders, 5401 Linda Vista Road, Suite C, San Diego, CA 92110.

Video tapes available from UCLA Neuropsychiatric Institute and Hospital, Nursing Department, 760 Westwood Plaza, Room 17-364, Los Angeles, CA 90024-1759.

Audio tapes of the papers presented at the National Nursing Theory Conference held at the University of California-Los Angeles Neuropsychiatric Institute and Hospital in September 1990. Presentations are by Flaskerud, Fawcett, and Meleis, as well as by numerous nurses who report the results of their use of the works of Johnson, Neuman, Orem, Rogers, Roy, and Parse. In addition, both audio and video tapes of a panel presentation featuring the nurse theorists, which is moderated by Randell, are available.

COMPUTER SEARCH STRATEGIES

Cumulative Index to Nursing and Allied Health Literature (CINAHL)

CINAHL may be accessed via on-line BRS Colleague, CD-ROMs available at libraries, and other databases. The following headings yield the most relevant citations for specific *conceptual models of nursing* when searching CINAHL:

Johnson Behavioral System Model
King Open Systems Model
Levine Conservation Model
Neuman Systems Model
Orem Self-Care Model
Rogers' Science of Unitary Human Beings
Roy Adaptation Model

Citations for general literature about conceptual models and theories can be obtained using the following headings:

Nursing Models, Theoretical
Conceptual Framework
Nursing Theory

Before 1988, the most relevant citations for specific conceptual models of nursing in the CINAHL database can be located by using the subject headings listed below. The same subject headings can be used to locate citations for general materials about nursing models and theories.

Models, Theoretical
Nursing Theory

MEDLINE

MEDLINE may be accessed via on-line Grateful Med, BRS Colleague, CD-ROMs available at libraries, and other databases. The following subject headings yield the most relevant citations for *conceptual models of nursing* when searching MEDLINE:

Nursing Models
Nursing Theories

Dissertation Abstracts International (DAI)

DAI, which also includes Master's Abstracts, may be accessed via on-line BRS Colleague, CD-ROMs available at libraries, and other databases. The following subject headings yield the most relevant citations for *conceptual models of nursing* when searching DAI:

Johnson Behavioral System Model
King and Transaction
King and Interaction
Levine and Conservation
Neuman Systems Model
Orem and Self-Care
Martha Rogers
Unitary Human Beings
Roy Adaptation Model
Roy and Adaptation

Sigma Theta Tau International Directory of Nurse Researchers

The Sigma Theta Tau International Directory of Nurse Researchers is available on-line via the Virginia Henderson International Nursing Library. The Directory and other research-oriented databases provided by the Library contain information on both completed and ongoing research.

Contact Sigma Theta Tau International, 550 W. North Street, Indianapolis, IN 46209–0209, (317) 634-8171 for instructions on access to the on-line databases.

The subject headings for *conceptual models of nursing* are:

Johnson Behavioral System
King Interacting System

Levine Conservation
Neuman Systems
Orem Self Care
Rogers Science of Unitary Human Beings
Roy Adaptation Model

A discussion of computer and hand searches is given in Johnson, E.D. (1989). In search of applications of nursing theories: The Nursing Citation Index. *Bulletin of the Medical Library Association, 77,* 176–184.

SOCIETIES FOR CONCEPTUAL MODELS OF NURSING

The Neuman Systems Model Trustees Group, Inc.

PO Box 488
Beverly, OH 45715

International Orem Society for Nursing Science and Scholarship

Dr. Susan Taylor, Treasurer
School of Nursing
University of Missouri–Columbia
Columbia, MO 65211

Society of Rogerian Scholars, Inc.

Canal Street Station
PO Box 1195
New York, NY 10013–0867

Boston-Based Adaptation Research in Nursing Society

Boston College School of Nursing
211 Cushing Hall
Chestnut Hill, MA 02167

Index

A *t* following a page number indicates a table; an *f* following a page number indicates a figure.

Accelerating Evolution, Theory of, 399–400
Achievement behavioral subsystem, 76, 77
Action
  as component of nursing process, 128, 128t
Action (behavior)
  as structural component, 78
Activities of Daily Living (ADL) Self-Care Scale, 323
Activity and rest
  as physiological need, 446t, 451
Adaptation, 172–173, 176. *See also* Adaptive *entries*; Roy Adaptation Model
  adaptation level, 454–456
    adaptive responses, 455–456, 455f
    ineffective responses, 455, 455f
  mechanistic theory of, 223
  zone of, 466
Adaptation Model. *See* Roy Adaptation Model
Adaptive change, patterns of, 181–183
Adaptive system, recipient as, 14, 449–453
  adaptive/response modes, 451–453, 455f
  cognator subsystem, 450–451, 473
  regulator subsystem, 450, 472–478
Adaptive/response modes, 451–453, 455f
  interdependence mode, 452–453, 455–456, 455f
  physiological mode, 451, 455f
  role function mode, 452, 455f
  self-concept mode, 451–452, 455f
Administration. *See* Nursing service administration
Adolescents
  alcohol abuse, 335
  chronically ill, 323
Affiliative (attachment) behavioral subsystem, 75, 76
Aggressive behavioral subsystem, 76, 77
Agreement
  in transaction model, 128
AIDS
  environmental patterning, 410
  nurses' attitudes, 328

patients and their beliefs, 94
students' knowledge vs. practices, 484
Allison, Sarah E., 287
Altzheimer-type dementia, 324
American Association of Critical Care Nurses, 146
American Nurses' Association
  Code of Ethics, 523
  Psychiatric/Mental Health Standards of Nursing Practice, 206
  Standards of Practice, 467
Analysis of conceptual models, 52–55, 53t
  content, 54–55
  content, comprehensiveness of, 56–57
  of Behavioral System Model, 68–85
  of Conservation Model, 166–191
  of General Systems Framework, 110–131
  of Neuman Systems Model, 218–237
  of Roy Adaptation Model, 438–461
  of Science of Unitary Human Beings, 376–391
  of Self-Care Framework, 287–387
  origins, 52, 53t, 54
  unique focus, 54–55
Anarchy of disease, 183
Animal visitation, 484
Appraisal of Self-Care Agency Scale, 322–323
Artificial boundaries, 130
ASA-A and ASA-B. *See* Appraisal of Self-Care Agency Scale
Assessment
  as nursing action, 7
  assessment phase of nursing process, 128
Assessment formats
  as empirical indicators, 524
Assessment of behavior, 458, 462t
Assessment of stimuli, 459, 463t
Assumptions of
  Behavioral System Model, 69–70
  Conservation Model, 167–168
  General Systems Framework, 113, 114–115
  Neuman Systems Model, 220–221

Assumptions of—*Continued*
  Roy Adaptation Model
    philosophical assumptions, 441–442
    scientific assumptions, 439–440
  Science of Unitary Human Beings, 378
  Self-Care Framework, 280–285
Attachment (affiliative) behavioral
    subsystem, 75, 76
Attainment of goal
  in transaction model, 128
Attitudes Toward Nurse Impairment
    Inventory, 90
Attribution
  as shared theory, 26
Auditory system, 180
Authority
  in social system, 124
Awareness phase of implementation, 404

Backscheider, Joan E., 287
Balmat, Cora S., 287
Basic orienting system, 180
Battered women, 324
Behavior
  assessment of, 458, 462t
  behavior (action), as functional
    component, 78
  in reaction world view, 15
  in reciprocal interaction world view, 16
  restorative behavior, 87
Behavioral Capabilities Scale for Older
    Adults, 93
Behavioral Observation-Validation Form,
    90
Behavioral system balance and stability
  orderly behavior, 79
  predictable behavior, 79
  purposeful behavior, 79
Behavioral System Model, 67–107
  analysis of, 68–85
  behavioral system balance and stability,
    79–80
    orderly behavior, 79
    predictable behavior, 79
    purposeful behavior, 79
  behavioral system disorders, types of, 74
  concepts, 75–84
  content, 75–85
  content, comprehensiveness of, 85–89
  contributions to discipline of nursing,
    99–100
  credibility, 91–99
  diagnostic classification schemes, 81,
    82t, 83
    internal subsystem problems, 81, 82t
    intersystem problems, 82t, 83
  environment, 78–79
  evaluation of, 85–100
  health, 79–80

historical evolution and motivation,
    68–69
  implementation of, 92
  influences from other scholars, 72–73
  logical congruence of, 89–90
  nursing, 80–84, 86–87
    administration, 89, 95–97
    diagnostic and treatment process,
      81–84, 82–83t
    education, 88–89, 94–95
    goal of nursing, 70, 80
    nursing service administration, 89
    practice, 89, 97
    research, 88, 92–94
  origins of model, 68–74, 85
  person, 74, 75–76, 86
  philosophical claims, 69–71
    assumptions, 69–70
    premises, 70
    propositions, 84–85
  social congruence, 97–98
  social significance, 98–99
  social utility in nursing, 91–97
    research, 92–94
  strategies of knowledge development,
    71–73
  subsystems, 75–77
    functional requirements, 77
    structural requirements, 77–78
  theory, generation of, 90–91
  unique focus, 74–75
  value system, 70–71, 92
  world view, 73
Beliefs
  of Conservation Model, 168
  of General Systems Framework, 113, 114
Bernard, Claude, 176
Biggs Elderly Self-Care Assessment Tool
    (BESCAT), 323
Borderline personality disorder, 410
Body image, 93
  in personal system, 121
Borrowed nursing theories, 26
Boston-Based Adaptation Research in
    Nursing Society, 495
Boundary, 118, 174–175, 224, 278–279
  artificial boundaries, 130
  boundary permeability, 75, 224
  exterior boundaries, 142
  in Behavioral System Model, 74–75
  in systems approach, 20
  interior boundaries, 142
Buddhism, 380

Cancer patients, 98, 147, 153
  cancer survivors' needs, 246
  children, 334, 482
  self-care behaviors, 325

support groups, 485
visitors of, 93–94
Canonical correlation, 395
Cardiac rehabilitation patients, 146
Care recipient and translation of
metaparadigm, 522
Care-by-Parents units, 335
Caring
as suggested nursing concept, 11–13
Categories of nursing knowledge. See
Nursing knowledge
Causality, 378
mechanistic causality, 381
Central core of client/client system, 226,
226f
Change
in General Systems Framework, 117, 126
in other models, 73, 174–175, 222–223,
288–289, 380–381, 444–445
in reaction world view, 15
in systems approach, 19
Change world view, 15
Chaos theory, 391
Children
cancer, 334, 482
child health, 147, 150, 204–205, 253
chronically ill, 146
developmentally disabled, 206
hospitalized, 489
infections, 246
safety knowledge and seat belts, 327
self-care agency, 325–326
sexual abuse, 335
studies of, 94
Choice
as functional component, 78
Clairvoyance, 400
Client(s), 220
as term for person, 8–9
category of nursing knowledge, 23, 23t
client domain, 9
client-focused category of models, 75, 224
client-nurse domain, 9
client/client system, 225–227, 226f, 229
central core, 226, 226f
community as, 225
family as, 225
individual as, 225
social issues as, 225
nursing client, as concept, 10
Clinical nursing practice, 34–35. See also
Nursing practice and process
Clinical specialty knowledge, 523–524, 530
Closed system, 19
Code of Ethics of ANA, 521f, 523
Cognator subsystems, 450–451, 473
Cognitive dissonance during perspective
transformation, 535
Cognitive Processing, Nursing Model of, 478
Collins, Mary B., 287

Comatose patients, 150
Communication
in interaction approach, 21–22
in interpersonal system, 119, 122, 123
in Theory of Goal Attainment, 139
learning roles and, 22
Community, 411
as client system, 225, 254
community health nursing, 97, 151, 252,
254, 328, 335, 491
factors in environment, 295–296
Comprehensiveness of content of models,
56–57
Behavioral System Model, 85–89
conceptual model, 1
Conservation Model, 192–197
General Systems Framework, 132–138
Neuman Systems Model, 238–241
Roy Adaptation Model, 465–471
Science of Unitary Human Beings,
392–411
Self-Care Framework, 308–315
Computers
computer-assisted learning, 250
nursing documentation, 333
taxonomy of nursing diagnoses, 251
Concept Formalization in Nursing (NDCG),
279
Concepts
central concepts of nursing, 7
definition and usage, 2
metaparadigm and, 7–8
of Behavioral System Model, 75–84
of Conservation Model, 175–188
of General Systems Framework, 120–126
of Neuman Systems Model, 225–235
of Roy Adaptation Model, 449–461
of Science of Unitary Human Beings,
383–390
of Self-Care Framework, 290–306
Conceptual environment, 178
Conceptual framework
as synonym for conceptual model, 2
Conceptual models. See also Analysis of
conceptual models; Conceptual-
theoretical-empirical systems;
Evaluation of conceptual models;
Implementing conceptual models;
Metaparadigm(s); Philosophies
as distinct from theories, 27–29
basics, 2–3
concepts, definition and usage, 2
contemporary nursing knowledge and,
1–50
cross-cultural applications, 152
defined, 2, 27
descriptive and correlational studies, 93,
246
difference from "model" in other usages,
29

Conceptual models—*Continued*
  empirical indicators and, 6*f*, 29–30
  framework for analysis and evaluation,
    52, 53*t*
  functions and requirements, 3–4, 6–7
  hierarchy of knowledge and, 6*f*
  historical evolution of, 4–5
  importance in advancing nursing, 5
  instruments for measurement of, 93
  metaparadigm and, 6*f*, 13–14
  nursing models historical evolution, 4–5
  propositions, definition and usage, 2
  synonyms for, 2
  testing of, steps involved, 28–29
  theories and, 27–29
  translating into practice model, 521*f*, 522
  value of models, 518–520
  vocabulary of, 2–3
Conceptual Models for Nursing Practice
    (Riehl and Roy), 68, 218, 376, 438
Conceptual system
  as synonym for conceptual model, 2
Conceptual-theoretical-empirical systems,
    30–35, 61–62
  clinical nursing practice as, 34–35
  logical congruence and, 30–31
  nursing administration as, 33–34
    rules for approach, 33–34
  nursing education as, 32–33
  nursing research as, 31–32
    rules for theory generation and
      testing, 32
  social significance and, 61–62
Conflict, 75, 118, 173, 224, 445
  in systems approach, 20
Confusion phase of perspective
    transformation, 533, 533*f*
Congruence
  Nadler-Tushman Congruence Model, 90
Congruence. *See* Logical congruence
Conservation
  category of nursing knowledge, 23*t*, 24
Conservation Model, 165–215
  adaptation, 172–173, 176, 178–180
  analysis of, 166–172, 166–191
  assumptions, 167–168
  beliefs, 168
  concepts, 175–188
  conservation principles, 186–188,
      189–190*t*, 195*t*
    energy, 187, 189*t*, 195*t*, 200
    personal integrity, 187–188, 189*t*,
      195*t*, 200
    social integrity, 188, 190*t*, 195*t*
    structural integrity, 187, 189*t*, 195*t*, 201
  content, 175–191
  content, comprehensiveness of, 192–197
  contributions to discipline of nursing,
      207–208
  credibility, 200–208

environment, 176–178
  external environment, 177–178
  internal environment, 176–177
  person and, 178–181
evaluation of, 191–208
external environment
  conceptual, 178
  operational, 177–178
  perceptual, 177
health, 181–183
historical evolution and motivation,
    166–167
holism, 167
homeorrhesis, 174, 176–177, 181
homeostasis, 174, 176–177, 181
influences from other scholars, 170–171
internal environment
  homeorrhesis, 174, 176–177, 181
  homeostasis, 174, 176–177, 181
intervention/action, 185–188, 189–190*t*
  supportive, 185
  therapeutic, 185
keeping together function, 184, 188
logical congruence, 198
nursing, 183–191
  administration, 196–197, 203–204
  education, 196, 202–203
  goal of nursing, 183
  nursing process, 183–188, 186*t*,
    189–190*t*
  practice, 197, 204–205
  research, 194–196, 201–202
organismic responses, 179–180
  fight or flight, 179–180
  inflammatory-immune response, 180
  perceptual awareness, 180
  stress response, 180
origins of, 166–172, 191–92
perceptual systems, 180
person, 167–168, 175–176
person and environment, 178–181
philosophical claims, 167–170
propositions, 188, 191
social congruence, 205–206
social significance, 206–207
social utility, 200–205
strategies for knowledge development,
    170
theory, generation of, 198–200
  Theory of Redundancy, 199
  Theory of Therapeutic Intention,
    198–199
trophicognosis, 184–185, 186*t*
  observation, 184–185
  provocative facts, 185
  testable hypothesis, 185
unique focus, 172–175
wellness, 182
wholeness, 171, 172–173, 175, 187, 193
world view, 171–172

Conservation Model: A Framework for Nursing Practice (Levine), 200
Conservation principles
  of energy, 186–187, 189t, 195t
  of personal integrity, 187, 189–190t, 195t
  of social integrity, 188, 190t, 195t
  of structural integrity, 187, 189t, 195t
  variables that represent, 195, 195t
Consumer-centric advocacy, 412
Content of conceptual models. *See also* Comprehensiveness of content of models
  analysis of, 55
  of Behavioral System Model, 75–85
  of Conservation Model, 175–191
  of General Systems Framework, 120–126
  of Neuman Systems Model, 225–237
  of Roy Adaptation Model, 449–461
  of Science of Unitary Human Beings, 383–391
  of Self-Care Framework, 290–307
Contextual stimuli, 453–454
Continuing nursing education, 148, 250
Contractual relationship, 298–299
Contributions to discipline of nursing
  Behavioral System Model, 99–100
  Conservation Model, 207–208
  evaluation of, 62
  General Systems Framework, 154
  Neuman Systems Model, 256
  Roy Adaptation Model, 494–495
  Science of Unitary Human Beings, 413–415
  Self-Care Framework, 339–340
Contributive behavior, 453
Control
  in social system, 124–125
Controlling operations, 306
Coping
  as borrowed theory, 26
  coping mechanisms, 444, 455t
  in interpersonal system, 122, 123
  in Theory of Goal Attainment, 149
Correlation
  canonical correlation, 395
  correlational and descriptive studies, 93, 246
Cost of implementing models, 527
Couvade, 408, 482
Created-environment, 228, 232
Credibility of conceptual models, 58–62
  of Behavioral System Model, 91–99
  of Conservation Model, 200–208
  of General Systems Framework, 143–154
  of Neuman Systems Model, 243–356
  of Roy Adaptation Model, 479–494
  of Science of Unitary Human Beings, 403–413
  of Self-Care Framework, 319–340
  social congruence, 60

social significance, 60–62
social utility, 59–60
Crews, Judy, 287
Criterion-Referenced Measure of Goal Attainment Tool, 129, 140
Cross-cultural applications of models, 152, 324, 336
Culture care diversity and universality, theory of, 25
Curriculum development, 94–95, 147–148, 202
  Neuman Systems Model and, 240–241, 248–250
  Roy Adaptation Model, 468–469, 486–487
  Self-Care Framework and, 311–313, 329

Danger Assessment instrument, 324
Data analysis techniques, 394–395
DBSM (Derdiarian Behavioral System Model) instruments, 93, 96
Dealing with Nurse Impairment Questionnaire, 90
Decision making
  in social system, 124
Deductive reasoning, 72, 170, 221, 240, 379, 442
Defense
  flexible line of, 225–226
  normal line of, 226–227
Déjà vu, 400
Deliberate action, nursing as, 281, 288
Deliberative mutual patterning, 390
Deliberative nursing process, theory of, 25
Demographic Pain Data Form, 90
Demonstration sites phase of implementation, 531
Dependency behavioral subsystem, 76
Dependent Care Agency questionnaire, 323
Dependent-care, 291
Dependent-care agent, 291, 304
Dependent-care deficit, 293, 295
Dependent-care systems, 304
Derdiarian Behavioral System Model (DBSM) instrument, 93, 96
Descriptive and correlational studies, 93
Development
  as model and category of knowledge, 17–19, 19t, 289–290, 316, 382
Developmental self-care requisites, 293, 294t
Developmental variable, 225
Diagnostic classification schemes, 81, 82t, 83
  internal subsystem problems, 81, 82t
  intersystem problems, 82t, 83
Diagnostic taxonomies
  as empirical indicators, 524
Dialysis patients, 251

Disciplinary matrix
  as synonym for conceptual model, 2
Disease, 296
  anarchy of disease, 183
  as patterns of adaptive change, 181–183
Dissonance phase of perspective
      transformation, 533, 533f
  cognitive dissonance during, 535
Disturbance
  in transaction model, 128
Documents
  adaptation and development of, 530–531
  computerization of, 333
  review during implementation, 480, 488,
      527–528
Domain
  of nursing, 127, 278–279
    identification in metapardigm, 6
    propositions as central, 7–8
  of nursing knowledge, 10, 34
  proposed metaparadigm concepts
    client domain, 9
    client-nurse domain, 9
    environment domain, 10
    practice domain, 9–10
Domestic animal visitation, 484
Drive (goal)
  as structural component, 77–78
Duration of implementation phases, 527
Dwelling with uncertainty phase of
      perspective transformation,
      533–534, 533f
Dynamic equilibrium, 224
Dynamic life experiences, as health, 126

Education, nursing
  computer-assisted learning, 250
  continuing nursing education, 148, 250
  in Behavioral System Model, 88–89,
      94–95
  in Conservation Model, 196, 202–203
  in General Systems Framework,
      135–137, 147–148
  in Neuman Systems Model, 240–241,
      248–250
  in Roy Adaptation Model, 468–469,
      485–487
  in Science of Unitary Human Beings,
      395–397, 408–409
  in Self-Care Framework, 31–32,
      311–313, 329
  nursing knowledge and, 32–33
Education of nursing staff phase of
      implementation, 531
Educational Revolution in Nursing
      (Rogers), 377
Elderly patients, 150–151, 200–201, 409,
      490
  confusion in, 202

Elimination
  as physiological need, 446t, 451
  hypothesis about, 475
Eliminative behavioral subsystem, 76–77
Emergency department care, 206, 490
Empirical indicators, 6f, 29–30
  conceptual models and, 6f, 29–30
  hierarchy of knowledge and, 6f
  translation to nursing practice, 521f, 524
  use of, 29
Endocrine function
  as regulator process, 447t, 451
Endocrine system
  hypothesis about, 475
Energy, conservation principle of,
      186–187, 189t, 195t, 200
Energy fields, 378, 380–381, 383–386
  as category of nursing knowledge, 23,
      23t, 174–175
  environmental energy field, 380–381,
      383–386
  group energy fields, 385
  human energy field, 380–381, 383–386
Enhancement
  category of nursing knowledge, 23t, 24
Entropy, 19, 230, 238
  illness as, 223
Environment
  as central concept of metaparadigm, 7, 10
    rejected as concept, 12
  community factors in, 295–296
  contextual stimuli, 453–454
  created-environment, 228, 232
  definition depends on model, 14
  environment domain, 10
  environmental contexts, as nursing
      concept, 11
  environmental energy field, 383–386
  environmental patterning, 410
  environmental regulators, 86
  external environment, 125–126, 173,
      176–178, 228
  family factors in, 295
  in Behavioral System Model, 74, 78–79,
      86
  in Conservation Model, 176–178
    conceptual environment, 178
    operational environment, 177–178
    perceptual environment, 177
  in General Systems Framework, 118,
      125–126, 132–133
  in Neuman Systems Model, 227–229
  in Roy Adaptation Model, 453–54,
      465
  in Science of Unitary Human Beings,
      383–386
  in Self-Care Framework, 295–296
  internal environment, 125–126, 173,
      176–178, 228
  of care recipient, and translation of

metaparadigm, 522
residual stimuli, 453–454
Epilepsy patient, 203
Epistemic claims of philosophies, 15
Equilibrium, 119, 449
  compared to steady state, 20
  dynamic equilibrium, 224, 238
  in systems approach, 20
Erikson, E. H., 175
Essentials of the Roy Adaptation Model
  (Andrews and Roy), 438
Ethical claims of philosophies, 14–15
Ethical standards, 134, 169, 309, 393
Ethology, 72
Evaluation
  as nursing action, 7
  in diagnostic and treatment process, 83t,
    84
  in nursing process, 460–461, 464t
Evaluation criteria
  as empirical indicators, 524
Evaluation of conceptual models
  content, comprehensiveness of, 56–57
  contributions to discipline of nursing, 62
  credibility, 58–62
    social congruence, 60
    social significance, 60–62
    social utility, 59–60
  logical congruence, 57–58
  of Behavioral System Model, 85–100
  of Conservation Model, 191–208
  of General Systems Framework, 131–154
  of Neuman Systems Model, 237–256
  of Roy Adaptation Model, 461–495
  of Science of Unitary Human Beings,
    391–415
  of Self-Care Framework, 307–340
  origins, explication of, 56
  questions to ask, 53t, 55–62
  theory, generation of, 58
  unique focus, 54–55
Evaluation phase of nursing process, 129,
    188
Evolution of conceptual models. *See*
    Historical evolution and motivation
    of conceptual models
Exercise
  hypothesis about, 474
Existentialism, 394
Expert reinforcement phase of
    implementation, 404
Explicit from implicit framework, 5
Exploitation, 30
Exploration of means
  in transaction model, 128
*Explorations on Martha Rogers' Science of
    Unitary Human Beings* (Malinski,
    ed.), 376, 403
Expressive component of role, 452
Exterior boundaries

in Theory of Goal Attainment, 142
External environment, 125–126, 173, 228,
    453
Extrapersonal stressors, 229

Family, 151, 254, 407–408, 411, 483, 491
  as client system, 225
  Care-by-Parents units, 335
  factors in environment, 295
  family assessment tool, 203–204
  family health, 147
  family therapy, 151
  family-centered nursing care, 97
  involvement in care giving, 330
  needs when DNR order, 245
  needs with chronically ill children, 146
Family Development/Nursing Intervention
    Identifier, 489
Family Needs Assessment Tool, 146
FAMLI-RESCUE, 251
Feedback, 75, 119, 128t, 173–174, 224
  in systems approach, 20
Field pattern(ing), 383–384, 385t
Fight or flight mechanism, 179–180
Flexible line of defense, 225–226
Fluids and electrolytes
  as regulator process, 447t, 451
  hypothesis about, 475
Focal stimuli, 453–454
Framework of nursing
  implicit to explicit, 5
Freud, Sigmund, 138
Functional requirements, 77
  change structural components, 83
  fulfillment of, as management, 83
Functioning in social roles, as health, 122

Gate control theory of pain, 90
General system theory, 72–73, 111–112,
    222, 238
General Systems Framework, 109–163
  analysis of, 110–131
  assumptions, 113, 114–115
  beliefs, 113, 114
  boundaries of Theory of Goal
    Attainment, 142
  concepts, 120–126
  content, 120–131
  content, comprehensiveness of, 132–138
  contributions to discipline of nursing, 154
  credibility, 143–154
  environment, 118, 125–26
    external environment, 125–126
    internal environment, 125–126
  evaluation of, 131–154
  health, 118, 126
  historical evolution and motivation,
    110–112

General Systems Framework—*Continued*
  hypotheses of, 141–142
  implementation, 144–145, 149, 153
  influences from other scholars, 116–117
  interaction-transaction process model,
      128–130, 128*f*
  interpersonal systems, 120, 122–123, 125*f*
  logical congruence, 138
  nursing, 126–131
    education, 135–137, 147–148
    goal of nursing, 127
    nursing service administration, 137,
        148–149
    practice, 127–130, 137–138, 150–151
    process, 127–30
    research, 134–135, 145–147
  organization, as major concept, 124
  origins of, 110–117, 132
  person, 120–125, 125*f*, 132
  personal systems, 120–122, 125*f*
  philosophical claims, 112–15
  physiological modes, 446–447*t*, 451
  propositions, 113–114, 130–131, 141
  social congruence, 151–153
  social significance, 153–154
  social systems, 120, 123–125, 125*f*
  social utility, 143–151
  strategies of knowledge development,
      115–116
  theory, generation of, 139–143
  unique focus, 117–120
  world view, 117
General Theory of Nursing Administration,
    286, 286–287, 319
Generation of theory. *See* Theory,
    generation of
Goal attainment
  in transaction model, 128
Goal Attainment, Theory of, 26, 139–143.
    See also General Systems Framework
Goal (drive)
  as structural component, 77–78
Goal of nursing
  Behavioral System Model, 70, 80
  Conservation Model, 183
  definition depends on model, 14
  General Systems Framework, 127
  Neuman Systems Model, 231
  Roy Adaptation Model, 442, 457
  Science of Unitary Human Beings,
      387–388
  Self-Care Framework, 298
Goal setting, 459–460, 463–464*t*
Goal-oriented (instrumental) component of
    role, 452
Goal-Oriented Nursing Record (GONR),
    129–130, 131*t*, 134, 138, 149–151
  GONR data base, 129–130, 131*t*
God
  as nursing concept, 10

GONR. *See* Goal-Oriented Nursing Record
Grand theories, 24–25
  examples of, 25
Group energy fields, 385
Growth and development
  in personal system, 121
  in Theory of Goal Attainment, 139
*Guides for Developing Curricula for the
    Education of Practical Nurses*
    (Orem), 279

Haptic system, 180
Hassenplug, Lulu Wolfe, 72, 222
Health
  as central concept of metaparadigm, 7, 10
    rejected as concept, 10, 12
  as living energy, 230
  as patterns of adaptive change, 181–183
  characteristics of, 126
  definition depends on model, 14
  dynamic life experiences as, 126
  functioning in social roles as, 122
  in Behavioral System Model, 79–80, 86
  in Conservation Model, 181–183
  in General Systems Framework, 117,
      118, 126, 133, 140
  in Neuman Systems Model, 229–231
  in Roy Adaptation Model, 456–457,
      465–466
  in Science of Unitary Human Beings,
      383–384, 391, 392
  in Self-Care Framework, 296–297, 308
  of care recipient and metaparadigm
      translation, 522
Health as expanding consciousness, theory
    of, 25, 401
Health and disease patterns of adaptive
    change, 181–183
Health Education Questionnaire, 332
Health and nursing
  as metaparadigm proposition, 7
Health patterning, as psychotherapy, 411
Health-deviation self-care requisites, 293,
    294–295*t*
Helicy, principle of, 383, 385–386, 391,
    396, 402
Helson, Harry, 438, 449
HES (Human Energy Systems) Model,
    402–403
Historical evolution and motivation of
    models, 52
  Behavioral System Model, 68–69
  Conservation Model, 166–167
  General Systems Framework, 110–112
  Neuman Systems Model, 218–219
  Roy Adaptation Model, 438–439
  Science of Unitary Human Beings,
      376–377
  Self-Care Framework, 278–280

Holism (wholism), 117, 219, 288, 450
  holistic world view, 379–380
  in reciprocal interaction world view, 16
Homeless, nursing care of, 205, 207, 324,
    335
Homeodynamics, principles of, 377,
    385–386, 404
  helicy, 383, 385–386, 391, 396, 402
  integrality, 382, 385–386, 395, 402
  resonancy, 383, 385, 396, 402
Homeorrhesis, 174, 176–177, 181
Homeostasis, 174, 176–177, 181, 224, 238
Human becoming, theory of, 25, 401
Human care
  as nursing concept, 11–13
Human caring, theory of, 25
Human energy field, 380–381, 383–386
Human Energy Field Assessment Form, 406
Human Field Image Metaphor Scale, 406
Human Field Motion Test, 406
Human Field Motion, Theory of, 402
Human interaction subscale, 129
Humanism, principle of, 15, 441–442
Humanistic category of nursing knowledge,
    23, 23t, 290
Husserlian phenomenology, 394
Hypotheses
  of components of physiological mode,
    474–476
  of General Systems Framework, 141–142
  testable, 185

Idea (vision) phase of implemention,
    524–525
Identifiable state, 383
Identification, 30
Illness, 80, 126, 230–231, 297, 386,
    456–457, 465–466
  as entropy, 223
Imagery, 389, 394, 400, 407, 411
Impaired nurses, 93
  Attitudes Toward Nurse Impairment
    Inventory, 90
  Dealing with Nurse Impairment
    Questionnaire, 90
Implementation phase of nursing process,
    129
Implementing conceptual models in
    nursing practice, 517–546. See also
    Process elements of implementing
    models; Substantive elements of
    implementing models
  cost of implementing, 527
  duration of phases, 527
  future directions, 536–537
    nursing education contributions,
    536–537
    nursing service contributions, 536
  of Behavioral System Model, 92

of Conservation Model, 200–201
of General Systems Framework,
    144–145, 149, 153
of Neuman Systems Model, 244–245
of Roy Adaptation Model, 479–481,
    486–489
of Science of Unitary Human Beings,
    403–405, 411
of Self-Care Framework, 319–322
reasons for implementing, 519
rewards of implementing, 520
risks of implementing, 520
value of models, 518–520
Implicit to explicit framework, 5
Individual
  as client system, 225
Inductive reasoning, 72, 221, 240, 442–443
Ineffective responses, 455, 455f
Inflammatory-immune response, 180
Ingestive behavioral subsystem, 76
Insight (Lonergan), 287
Institution-wide implementation/
    evaluation phase of implementation,
    531–532
Instrumental (goal-oriented) component of
    role, 452
Integrality, principle of, 382, 385–386, 395,
    396, 402
Interacting Systems Framework, 109
Interaction
  as concept, 10
  category of nursing knowledge, 20–21,
    22t
    major characteristics of, 21
  in interpersonal system, 122
  in Theory of Goal Attainment, 139
  interacting variables
    developmental, 225
    physiological, 225
    psychological, 225
    sociocultural, 225
    spiritual, 225
  interaction models, 119, 122
    interaction-transaction process model,
    128–130, 128f
Interactive-integrative world view, 15
Interdependence adaptative/response
    mode, 448t, 452–453, 455–456, 455f
  contributive behavior, 453
  receptive behavior, 453
  significant others, 453
  supportive systems, 453
Interdependence Mode, Theory of, 472,
    477–478
Interior boundaries
  in Theory of Goal Attainment, 142
Internal environment, 125–126, 173,
    176–178, 228, 453
  homeorrhesis, 174, 176–177, 181
  homeostasis, 174, 176–177, 181

Internal subsystem problems, 81, 82t
International in scope
  as requirement of metaparadigm, 6-7
International Neuman Systems Model
  Symposia, 243
International Orem Society for Nursing
  Science and Scholarship, 340
Interpersonal component of nursing
  practice, 299
Interpersonal relations
  as concept, 10
  theory of, 25, 29-30
Interpersonal stressors, 228-229
Interpersonal systems, 120, 122-123, 125f
Intersystem problems, 82t, 83
Intervention, 460
  as category of nursing knowledge,
    23-24, 23t, 75
  as nursing action, 7
  intervention/action, 185-188, 189-190t
    supportive, 185
    therapeutic, 185
  protocols, as empirical indicators, 524
Intrapersonal stressors, 228
Introduction to Clinical Nursing (Levine),
  166, 199
Introduction to Nursing: An Adaptation
  Model (Roy), 438
An Introduction to the Theoretical Basis of
  Nursing (Rogers), 376, 408
Inventories of Functional Status, 481-482

JFFA-J (Johnson Model First-Level Family
  Assessment Tool), 93
Johnson, Dorothy E., 67, 438, 443. See also
  Behavioral System Model
Johnson Model First-Level Family
  Assessment Tool (JFFA-J), 93
Judgement
  in transaction model, 128, 128t

Keeping together function, 184, 188
King, Imogene M., 109. See also General
  Systems Framework
Kinlein, M. Lucille, 287
Knowledge. See Strategies for knowledge
  development
Koertvelyessy, Audrey, 242-243

Labeling
  as nursing action, 7
Labor and delivery, 202
Lapniewski, Janina B., 287
Laughing at oneself, 406
Learning, concept of, 122
Legitimate patients/nurses (professional,

not legal, term), 241, 298, 310, 313,
  470
Levine, Myra E., 165. See also
  Conservation Model
Life, sanctity of, 168
Life Perspective Rhythm Model, 402
Lines of resistance, 226f, 227
Locus of control
  as borrowed theory, 26
  external locus of control, 152, 154
Logical congruence of models, 30-31
  evaluation of, 57-58
  of Behavioral System Model, 89-90
  of Conservation Model, 198
  of General Systems Framework and, 138
  of Neuman Systems Model, 242
  of Roy Adaptation Model, 471-472
  of Science of Unitary Human Beings, 399
  of Self-Care Framework, 315-316
  reformulation or translation of, 57-58
Lonergan, B. J. F., 287
Long-range plan in implementation,
  525-526

McCarthy, Sheila M., 287
Madhyamika-Prasangika school of Tibetan
  Buddhism, 380
Malatesta, Melba Anger, 287
Man
  as original concept of nursing, 8, 10
Management of nursing problems, 82-83t,
  83-84
Management strategies, 470
Managerial tasks and work operations,
  313-314
Martha E. Rogers: Eighty Years of
  Excellence (Barrett and Malinski,
  eds.), 403
Martha E. Rogers: Her Life and Her Work
  (Barrett and Malinski, eds.), 403
MCN Developmental/Diagnostic Model,
  488, 493
MDS RAPS (Minimum Data Set Resident
  Assessment Protocol Summary), 252
Mechanistic causality, 381
Mechanistic theory of
  stress and adaptation, 223
Mechanistic world view, 15
Medicine (discipline of)
  differentiated from nursing, 5, 69, 87,
    297, 412, 457
Meditative modalities, 400
Metaparadigm(s), 5-14, 6f. See also
  Nursing metaparadigm
  central concepts of, 7
  conceptual models and, 6f, 13-14
  defined, 5
  function and requirements, 6-7

hierarchy of knowledge and, 6f
propositions of, 7
translation to nursing practice, 521f, 522
Methods of helping, 302–303t, 304
Meyer, Burton, 443
Middle-range theories, 25–26
    distinct from conceptual models, 27–29
    examples of, 25
    testing of, 29
Milieu interne, 176
Minimum Data Set Resident Assessment
        Protocol Summary (MDS RAPS), 252
Mission statement of facility, 522, 528–529
Moral-ethical-spiritual self, 451–452
Motivation for conceptual models. See
        Historical evolution and motivation
        of conceptual models
Movement subscale, 129
Movement therapy, 389, 407
MS-Related Symptom Checklist, 323
Multivariate analysis, 395
Music therapy, 490
Mutual Exploration of the Healing
        Human . . . instrument, 406
Mutual goal setting, 152
    in transaction model, 128

Nadler-Tushman Congruence Model, 90
NANDA (North American Nursing
        Diagnosis Association), 96, 129
National League of Nursing, 8, 10
National Rogerian Conferences, 403
Needs
    category of nursing knowledge, 22–23,
        23t, 290
Negentropy, 19, 230, 238
Nettleton, Joan, 287
Neuman, Betty, 217. See also Neuman
        System Model
Neuman Systems Model, 3, 217–275
    analysis of, 218–237
    assumptions, basic, 220–221
    boundaries, 224
    client/client system, 222, 225–227, 226f
        central core, 226, 226f
        community as, 225
        family as, 225
        individual as, 225
        social issues as, 225
    concepts, 225–235
    content, 225–237
    content, comprehensiveness of, 238–241
    contributions to discipline of nursing, 256
    credibility, 243–356
    entropy, 230, 238
    environment, 224, 227–229
    evaluation of, 237–256
    flexible line of defense, 225–226

health, 229–231
    as living energy, 230
    optimal client system stability,
        229–230
historical evolution and motivation,
        218–219
implementation of, 244–245
influences from other scholars, 222
interacting variables, 225
lines of resistance, 227
logical congruence, 242
negentropy, 230, 238
Neuman Systems Model Trustee Group,
        239, 256
Neuman Wheel, 241
normal line of defense, 226–227
nursing, 231–235
    administration, 241, 250–251
    diagnosis, 232
    education, 240–241, 248–250
    goal of nursing, 231
    Nursing Process Format, 231–234,
        234–235t, 241–242
    practice, 241–242, 252–254
    Prevention as Intervention, Format
        and Theory of, 233–234, 235t,
        242–243
    research, 239–240, 245–248
    origins of, 218–223, 237–238
    person, 223, 225–227
    person and environment, 229
    philosophical claims, 219–221
    philosophical statements, 221
    prevention as intervention, 233, 235t,
        242–243
    propositions, 236–237, 238
    social congruence, 254–255
    social significance, 255–256
    social utility, 243–254
    strategies for knowledge development,
        221
    stressors, 228–229
    theory, generation of, 242–243
    Theory of Optimal Client System
        Stability, 242
    Theory of Prevention as Intervention,
        233–234, 235t, 242–243
    unique focus, 223–224
    wellness, 223, 229–231
    wholism, 239
    world view, 222–223
The Neuman Systems Model: Application
        to Nursing Education and Practice
        (Neuman), 218, 238, 243
Neuman Systems Model Trustee Group,
        239, 256
Neuman Systems-Management Tool,
        250–251
Neurological function
    as regulator process, 447t, 451

Neurological patients, 203
Nightingale, Florence, 4, 8, 68–69, 72, 171, 377, 443–444
Noninvasive modalities, 389–390, 407
Nonrepeating rhythmicities, 378, 383
Normal line of defense, 226–227, 226*f*
North American Nursing Diagnosis Association (NANDA), 96, 129, 332
Nurse impairment. *See under* Nurses
Nurses. *See also* Nursing *entries*
    as study subjects, 247, 328, 485
    attitudes about AIDS, 328
    impaired nurses, 93
    Attitudes Toward Nurse Impairment Inventory, 90
    Dealing with Nurse Impairment Questionnaire, 90
    smoking rates and quitting, 146, 247–248
Nursing: Concepts of Practice (Orem), 279, 280, 308
Nursing. *See also other* Nursing *entries*
    as central concept of metaparadigm, 7
        suggested elimination of term, 9, 12
    as deliberate action, 281, 288
    as learned profession, 387
    as science and art, 387
    definition depends on model, 14
    differentiated from medicine, 5, 69, 87, 297, 412, 457
    in Behavioral System Model, 80–84, 86–87
    in Conservation Model, 183–191
    in General Systems Framework, 126–131, 133
    in Neuman Systems Model, 231–235
    in Roy Adaptation Model, 457–461
    in Science of Unitary Human Beings, 387–390, 392
    in Self-Care Framework, 297–306
    major ideas about, 112
    nursing system design, 302, 302–303*t*, 304
    preventive nursing, 98, 194, 205, 255, 337
    quality of, 96, 149–150, 203, 332–333, 480
Nursing actions, 7
Nursing acts
    as proposed metaparadigm concept, 9
Nursing administration. *See* Nursing service administration
Nursing agency (of individual nurses), 296
Nursing audits, 149–150
Nursing client
    as concept, 10
Nursing Development Conference Group, 4, 279–280, 287, 308
Nursing diagnosis, 130, 232, 459, 463*t*
    computerized taxonomy for, 251
    levels of, 299–300, 300–301*t*
    self-care and, 299–300, 300–301*t*
    system for, 96

Nursing diagnostic and treatment process, 81–84, 82–83*t*
    diagnostic classification schemes, 81–83, 82*t*
    evaluation, 83*t*, 84
    management of problems, 82–83*t*, 83–84
    problem determination, 81, 82*t*
Nursing domain. *See* Domain of nursing
Nursing education. *See* Education, nursing
Nursing goals (vs. goals of nursing), 232
Nursing knowledge. *See also* Conceptual-theoretical-empirical systems
    categories of, 17–24, 19*t*, 21*t*, 22*t*, 23*t*
        client-focused, 23, 23*t*
        conservation, 23*t*, 24
        developmental, 17–19, 19*t*, 289–290, 316, 382
        energy fields, 23, 23*t*
        enhancement, 23*t*, 24
        humanistic, 23, 23*t*
        interaction, 20–21, 22*t*
        intervention, 23–24, 23*t*
        needs, 22–23, 23*t*
        nursing therapeutics, 23, 23*t*
        outcomes, 22–23, 23*t*
        person-environment-focused, 23, 23*t*
        substitution, 23*t*, 24
        sustenance, 23*t*, 24
        systems, 19–20, 21*t*
    clinical specialty knowledge, 523–524
    conceptual models and, 1–50
    empirical indicators, 6*f*, 29–30
    structural hierarchy of, 6*f*
    theories, 6*f*, 24–29
        borrowed, 26
        defined, 24
        grand theories, 24–25
        middle-range theories, 25–26
        shared, 26
        unique, 26
Nursing metaparadigm, 7–8
    alternative metaparadigms, 8–13
    central concepts of
        environment, 7
        health, 7
        nursing, 7
        person, 7
    propositions of, 7
Nursing Model of Cognitive Processing, 478
Nursing outcomes, 232–233, 478
Nursing practice and process. *See also* Implementing conceptual models in nursing practice
    as concept, 10
    as conceptual-theoretical-empirical system, 31–32
    assessment phase of, 128
    evaluation phase of, 129
    implementation phase of, 129

Neuman nursing process format,
231–234, 234–235t, 241
nursing knowledge and, 34–35
of Behavioral System Model, 81–84,
82–83t, 89, 97
of Conservation Model, 183–188, 186t,
189–190t, 197, 204–205
of General Systems Framework,
127–130, 137–138, 150–151
of Neuman Systems Model, 231–234,
234–235t, 241–242, 252–254
of Roy Adaptation Model, 458–461,
462–464t, 464–464t, 466–467,
470–471, 489–491
of Science of Unitary Human Beings,
388–390, 398–405, 409–410
of Self-Care Framework, 298–306,
300–301t, 302–303t, 305t, 308–309,
314–315, 333–336
planning phase of, 128
professional nursing practice, 519
rules for specifying domain, 34
Nursing prescription, 302
Nursing process. See Nursing practice and
process
Nursing research. See Research, nursing
Nursing service administration
General Theory of Nursing
Administration, 286, 286–287, 319
in Behavioral System Model, 89, 95–97
in Conservation Model, 183–188, 186t,
189–190t, 196–197, 203–204
in General Systems Framework, 137,
148–149
in Neuman Systems Model, 241, 250–251
in Roy Adaptation Model, 469–470,
487–489
in Science of Unitary Human Beings,
397–398, 409
in Self-Care Framework, 313–314,
329–333
managerial tasks and work operations,
313–314
nursing knowledge and, 33–34
rules for structure and management,
33–34
Nursing system design, 302–304, 302–303t
partly compensatory nursing system,
302, 303t, 304
supportive-educative nursing system,
302, 303t, 304
wholly compensatory nursing system,
302, 302–303t, 304
Nursing System, Theory of. See under
Self-Care Framework
Nursing therapeutics
as concept, 10
category of nursing knowledge, 23, 23t,
174, 290

Nurturance
as functional requirement, 77
Nutrition
as physiological need, 446t, 451
hypotheses about, 474
nutritional status, assessment of, 253

Observation, 184–185
Ontological claims of philosophies, 14–15
Open system, 19, 77, 118, 173–174, 223, 230
Open Systems Model, 109
Openness, 383–384
Operational environment, 177–178
Optimal Client System Stability, Theory
of, 242
Optimal wellness, 230
Orderly behavior, 79
Orem, Dorothea, 277, 287, 443. See also
Self-Care Framework
Organicism world view, 15
Organismic responses, 179–180
fight or flight, 179–180
inflammatory-immune response, 180
perceptual awareness, 180
stress responses, 180
Organization, as concept, 124
Orientation, 30
Origins of
Behavioral System Model, 68–74, 85
conceptual models, 52–54
analysis of, 52, 53t, 54
explication for evaluation, 53t, 56
Conservation Model, 166–172, 191–192
General Systems Framework, 110–17,
132
Neuman Systems Model, 218–223,
237–238
Roy Adaptation Model, 438–445,
464–465
Science of Unitary Human Beings,
376–381, 391
Self-Care Framework, 278–288, 307–308
Outcome
category of nursing knowledge, 22–23,
23t, 75, 174
Oxygenation
as physiological need, 446t, 451
Oxygenation and circualtion
hypothesis about, 475

Pain management, 204, 245, 328, 410
Pandimensionality, 379, 383, 385
Paradigm
as synonym for conceptual model, 2
totality paradigm, 138
Paranormal Phenomenona, Theory of,
400–401

Participatory management, 398

Particulate-deterministic world view, 15

Partly compensatory nursing system, 302, 303t, 304

Patient Classification Instrument (PCI), 93

Patient classification system, 332

Patient Indicators of Nursing Care Instrument, 93, 96

Patient's Bill of Rights, 521f, 523

Pattern, 383–385, 385t

  defined, 384

  deliberative mutual patterning, 390, 399

  environmental patterning, 410

  field pattern(ing), 383–384, 385t

  health patterning, as psychotherapy, 411

  pattern manifestation appraisal, 388–390, 399

PCI (Patient Classification Instrument), 93

Peer reinforcement phase of implementation, 405

Perception

  as concept, 10

  in interaction approach, 21

  in personal system, 119, 120–121

  in Theory of Goal Attainment, 139

  in transaction model, 128, 128t

Perceptual awareness systems

  auditory, 180

  basic orienting, 180

  haptic, 180

  taste-smell system, 180

  visual, 180

Perceptual environment, 177

Persistence world view, 15, 73, 222–223, 288

Person

  as central concept of metaparadigm, 7

    rejected as concept, 12

  as energy field, 14, 383–386

  as self-care agent, 14, 291

  care recipient and metaparadigm translation, 522

  definition depends on model, 14

  in reaction world view, 15

  in reciprocal interaction world view, 16

  in the models

    Behavioral System Model, 74, 75–78, 86

    Conservation Model and, 167–168, 175–176

    General Systems Framework, 120–125, 125f, 132

    Neuman Systems Model, 223, 225–227

    Roy Adaptation Model, 444, 445, 449–454, 465

    Science of Unitary Human Beings, 383–391, 392, 403–404

    Self-Care Framework, 290–295, 308

  rejected as concept, 12

Person as an Adaptive System, Theory of, 472–473, 478, 494–495

Person and environment

  adaptation level, 454

  adaptive responses, 455–456, 455f

  as metaparadigm proposition, 7

  energy fields, 383–386

    environmental energy field, 383–386

    group energy fields, 385

    human energy field, 380–381, 383–386

  ineffective responses, 455

  in Conservation Model, 178–181

  in Neuman Systems Model, 229

  in Roy Adaptation Model, 454–456

  in Science of Unitary Human Beings, 383–386

  interaction as category of nursing knowledge, 23, 23t

  interaction in reciprocal interaction world view, 16

  openness, 383–384

  pandimensionality, 383, 385

  pattern, 383–385, 385t

Person, environment, and health

  as metaparadigm proposition, 454

Person and health

  as metaparadigm proposition, 7

Personal hygiene subscale, 129

Personal integrity, conservation principle of, 187, 189–190t, 195t, 200

Personal self

  as self-concept mode, 441, 448t

Personal space

  in Theory of Goal Attainment, 139

Personal structural analysis, 394

Personal systems, 120–122, 125f

Perspective transformation during implementation, 532–536, 533f

  phases of, 533–534, 533f

  strategies to facilitate, 534–536

Perspective-neutral

  as requirement of metaparadigm, 6

Phenomenology, 394

Philosophical assumptions, 441–442

Philosophical claims of

  Behavioral System Model, 69–71

  Conservation Model, 167–170

  General Systems Framework, 112–15

  Neuman Systems Model, 219–221

  Roy Adaptation Model, 439–442

  Science of Unitary Human Beings, 378–379

  Self-Care Framework, 280–286

Philosophical statements as propositions, 238

Philosophies, 14–24

  defined, 14

  epistemic claims of, 15

  ethical claims of, 14–15

hierarchy of knowledge and, 6f, 14–24
ontological claims of, 14–15
translating for nursing practice, 521f,
    522–523
world views, 15–17
    reaction, 15, 15t, 223
    reciprocal interaction, 15–16, 16t, 73,
        117, 171–172, 222–223, 288
    simultaneous action, 16–17, 17t, 380
Philosophy. See Philosophies
Physical self
    as self-concept mode, 448, 451
Physiological adaptive/response mode,
    451, 455f
    basic physiological needs, 451
    regulator processes, 451, 472–478
Physiological Mode, Theory of, 472,
    473–476
Physiological modes, 446–447t, 451, 455t
Physiological variable, 225
Planning
    as nursing action, 7
Planning committee/action plan phase of
    implementation, 525–527
    long-range plan, 525–526
Planning of case management, 305
Planning phase of nursing process, 128
Pluralism in conceptual models and
    implementation, 529–530
Power, 402, 422
    in social system, 124
    participatory management and, 398
    power components of self-care, 291–292,
        322
    shared power, 480
Power as Knowing Participation in Change
    Test, 406
Practice domain
    as proposed metaparadigm concept, 9–10
Precognition, 400
Predictable behavior, 79
Premises
    of Behavioral System Model, 70
Pressure ulcers, 201
Prevention or alleviation of suffering,
    168–169
Prevention as intervention format, 233,
    235t, 242–243, 246–247
    primary/secondary/tertiary prevention,
        233, 235t
Prevention as Intervention, Format and
    Theory of, 233–234, 235t
Preventive nursing, 98, 194, 205, 255,
    337
    prevention as negative concept, 388
Primary prevention, 233, 235t, 236
Primary role, 452
Problem determination, 81, 82t
Problem Oriented Medical Record, 129

Process elements of implementing models,
    524–536
    demonstration sites, 531
    education of nursing staff, 531
    idea or vision, 524–525
    institution-wide implementation and
        evaluation, 531–532
    perspective transformation during
        implementation, 532–536, 533f
    phases of, 533–534, 533f
    strategies to facilitate, 534–536
    planning committee/action plan,
        525–527
    cost of implementing, 527
    duration of phases, 527
    long-range plan, 525–526
    review of documents, 480, 488, 527–528
    selection/development phase, 528–531
        forced fit and, 529
        mission statement and, 528–529
        pluralism in conceptual models and,
            529–530
        steps of, 528
    task force, 525
Professional and case management
    operations of nursing practice,
    299–306
Professional nursing practice
    educational requirements, 88–89,
        395–397, 397, 411, 469–470, 519
Propositions. See also Propositions of
    definition and usage, 2
    essential propositions of nursing, 7–8
    as domain of nursing, 7
    philosophical statements as, 238
Propositions of
    Behavioral System Model, 84–85
    conceptual models, 7
    Conservation Model, 188, 191
    General Systems Framework, 113–114,
        130–131, 141
    Neuman Systems Model, 236–237
    nursing metaparadigm, 7
    Roy Adaptation Model, 461
    Science of Unitary Human Beings,
        390–391
    Self-Care Framework, 306–307
    Theory of Goal Attainment, 143
    Theory of Nursing Systems, 318–319
    Theory of Self-Care, 316–317
    Theory of Self-Care Deficit, 317–318
Protection
    as functional requirement, 77
    as physiological need, 446t, 451
Provocative facts, 185
Psychiatric patients, 151, 206, 246, 324,
    330, 338
    borderline personality disorder, 410
Psychological variable, 225

Q-sort, 394
Quality assurance, 96, 149–150, 203,
    332–333, 480

Rauckhorst, Louise Hartnett, 287
Reaction
    as component of nursing process, 128,
        128t
Reaction world view, 15, 15t, 89, 223
    behavior in, 15
    change in, 15
    person in, 15
    stability in, 15
    translation into reaction world view, 479
Readiness phase of implementation, 404
Reasoning, inductive and deductive, 72,
        170, 221, 240, 286–287, 379, 442–443
Reasons for implementing conceptual
        models, 519
Receptive behavior, 453
Reciprocal interaction world view
    change of behavior in, 16
    description of, 15–16, 16t
    models based on, 73, 117, 171–172,
        222–223, 288, 315
    person in, 16
    person-environment interaction in, 16
    translation from reaction world view, 479
Reconcepualization phase of perspective
        transformation, 533f, 534
Reconstitution, 231
Redundancy, 179–180
Redundancy, Theory of, 199
Reformulation or translation of models,
        57–58, 521f, 523
Regulator subsystems, 450, 472–478
Regulatory care operations, 305, 305t
Relationship Form, 29
Research, nursing
    in Behavioral System Model, 88, 92–94
    in Conservation Model, 194–196,
        201–202
    in the models General Systems
        Framework, 134–135, 145–147
    in Neuman Systems Model, 239–240,
        245–248
    in Roy Adaptation Model, 467–468,
        481–485
    in Science of Unitary Human Beings,
        393–395, 405–408
    in Self-Care Framework, 310–311,
        322–329
    nursing knowledge and, 31–32
    rules for theory generation and testing,
        32
Residual stimuli, 453–454
Resolution, 30
    phase of perspective transformation,
        533f, 534

Resonancy, principle of, 383, 385, 396, 402
Rest
    hypothesis about, 474
Restorative behavior, 87
Return to stability phase of perspective
        transformation, 533f, 534
Reveille in Nursing (Rogers), 377
Review of documents phase of
        implementation, 527–528
Rewards of implementing conceptual
        models, 52
Rhythmical Correlates of Change, Theory
        of, 400
Rhythmicities, nonrepeating, 378, 383
Risks of implementing conceptual models,
        520
Robinson, Connie, 443
Rogerian Nursing Science News, 415
Rogers, Martha E., 375, 443. *See also*
        Martha E. Rogers entries; Science of
        Unitary Human Beings
Rogers' Scientific Art of Nursing Practice
        (Madrid and Barrett, eds.), 403
Role function mode, 448, 452, 455t
Role Function Mode, Theory of, 472, 477
Role(s)
    as concept, 10
    classification of, 452
    communication and, 22
    expressive component of, 452
    in interaction approach, 22
    in interpersonal system, 119, 122, 123
    in Theory of Goal Attainment, 139
    instrumental (goal-oriented) component
        of, 452
Roy, Sister Callista, 437. *See also* Roy
        Adaptation Model
Roy Adaptation Model, 2, 4, 437–516
    adaptation indicators and problems of,
        445, 446–448t
    adaptation level, 2, 454–456
    adaptive responses, 455–456, 455f
    adaptive system, recipient as, 449–453
        adaptive/response modes, 446–447t,
            451–453, 455t
        cognator subsystem, 450–451, 473
        regulator subsystem, 450, 472–478
    analysis of, 438–461
    assessment of behavior, 458, 462t
    assessment of stimuli, 459, 463t
    assumptions
        philosophical assumptions, 441–442
        scientific assumptions, 439–440, 464
    change, 444–445
    cognator subsystems, 450–451, 473
    concepts, 449–461
    content, 449–461
    content, comprehensiveness of, 465–471
    contributions to discipline of nursing,
        494–495

coping, 444
credibility, 479–494
curriculum development, 468–469,
    486–487
environment, 445, 453–454, 465
    contextual stimuli, 453–454
    focal stimuli, 453–454
    residual stimuli, 453–454
evaluation, in nursing process, 460–461,
    464t
evaluation of, 461–495
focal stimuli, 453–454
goal setting, 459–460, 463–464t
health, 456–457, 465–466
historical evolution and motivation,
    438–439
humanism, principle of, 15, 441
illness, 456–457, 465–466
implementation of, 479–481, 486–489
ineffective responses, 455, 455f
influences from other scholars,
    443–444
interdependence mode, 448t, 452–453,
    455t
intervention, 460
logical congruence, 471–472
nursing, 457–461, 466
    administration, 469–470, 487–489
    education, 468–469, 485–487
    goal of nursing, 442, 457
    nursing diagnosis, 459, 463t
    practice, 470–471, 489–491
    process, 458–461, 462–464t, 466–467,
        470–471
    research, 467–468, 481–485
origins of model, 438–445, 464–465
person, 444, 445, 449–454, 465
    adaptation level, 454
person and environment, 454–456
philosophical claims, 439–442
    philosophical assumptions, 441–442
    scientific assumptions, 439–441, 464
physiological modes, 446–448t, 451, 455t
    hypotheses of, 474–476
propositions
    of cognator subsystem, 473
    of conceptual model, 461
    of regulator subsystems, 472–473,
        473–476, 477–478
regulator subsystems, 450, 472–478
role function mode, 448, 452, 455t
self-concept adaptative/response mode,
    448t, 451–452, 455f
social congruence, 492–493
social significance, 493–494
social utility, 470–491
stimuli, classes of
    contextual, 453–454
    focal, 453–454
    residual, 453–454

strategies for knowledge development,
    442–443
theory, generation of, 472–478
    Nursing Model of Cognitive
        Processing, 478
    Theory of the Interdependence Mode,
        472, 477–478
    Theory of the Person as an Adaptive
        System, 472–473, 478, 494–495
    Theory of the Physiological Mode, 472,
        473–476
    Theory of the Role Function Mode,
        472, 477
    Theory of the Self-Concept Mode,
        472, 476
unique focus, 445–449
veritivity, principle of, 441, 442
world view, 444–445
zone of adaptation, 466
The Roy Adaptation Model: The Definitive
    Statement (Roy and Andrews), 438

Sanctity of life, 168
Saturation phase of perspective
    transformation, 533f, 534
Sayers, Patricia, 333
SCAT (Self-Care Assessment Tool), 323
Science of Unitary Human Beings, 375–436
    analysis of, 376–391
    application, levels and phases of, 404–405
    assumptions of, 378
    change, 380–381
    concepts, 383–386, 383–390
    content, 383–391
    content, comprehensiveness of, 392–411
    contributions to discipline of nursing,
        413–415
    credibility, 403–413
    disease, 386
    energy fields, 378, 380, 381, 383–386
        environmental, 383–386
        group, 385
        human, 383–386
    environment, 383–386
    environmental patterning, 410
    ethical standards, 393
    evaluation of, 391–415
    field pattern, 383
    health, 383–384, 391, 392
    helicy, principle of, 383, 385–386, 391,
        396, 402
    historical evolution and motivation,
        376–377
    holistic world view, 379–380
    homeodynamics, principles of, 377,
        385–386, 404
        helicy, 383, 385–386, 391, 396, 402
        integrality, 382, 385–386, 395, 402
        resonancy, 383, 385, 396, 402

Human Energy Systems (HES) Model,
    402–403
illness, 386
imagery, as noninvasive modality, 389,
    407
implementation of, 403–405, 441
influences from other scholars, 379
integrality, principle of, 382, 385–386,
    395, 402
logical congruence, 399
noninvasive modalities, 389–390, 407
nonrepeating rhythmicities, 378, 383
nursing, 387–390, 392
    administration, 397–398, 409
    as learned profession, 387
    as science and art, 387
    education, 395–397, 408–409
    goal of nursing, 387–388
    nursing process, 388–390
    practice, 398–405, 409–410
    research, 393–395, 405–408
openness, 383–384
origins, 376–381, 391
pandimensionality, 379, 383, 385
pattern, 383–385, 385t
    defined, 384
    deliberative mutual patterning, 390,
        399
    field pattern(ing), 383–384, 385t
    pattern manifestation appraisal,
        388–389, 399
person, 383–391, 392, 403–404
person and environment, 383–386
philosophical claims, 378–379
power, 402
propositions, 390–391
resonancy, principle of, 383, 385, 396,
    402
social congruence, 411–412
social significance, 412–413
social utility, 403–411
strategies of knowledge development,
    379
theory, generation of, 399–403
    Life Perspective Rhythm Model, 402
    Theory of Accelerating Evolution,
        399–400
    Theory of Health as Expanding
        Consciousness, 401
    Theory of Human Becoming, 401
    Theory of Human Field Motion, 402
    Theory of Paranormal Phenomenona,
        400–401
    Theory of Rhythmical Correlates of
        Change, 400
therapeutic touch, 389, 400–401, 406,
    407, 410, 411, 413
unique focus, 381–383
wellness, 386
world view, 379–381

Scientific Art of Nursing Practice (Rogers),
    403
Scientific assumptions, 439–440, 464
Secondary roles, 452
Secondary prevention, 233, 235t, 236
Selection/development phase of
        implementation, 528–531
    forced fit and, 529
    misssion statement and, 528–529
    pluralism in conceptual models and,
        529–530
    steps of, 528
Self. See also Self- entries
    in personal system, 121
    in Theory of Goal Attainment, 139
Self-Care Deficit Nursing Theory
        Newsletter, 340
Self-Care Deficit Theory. See also Self-Care
        Framework
Self-Care Framework, 3, 277–374
    analysis of, 287–387
    Appraisal of Self–Care Agency Scale,
        322–323
    assumptions of, 280–285
    basic conditioning factors for self–care,
        292
    concepts, 290–306
    content, 290–307
    content, comprehensiveness of, 308–
        315
    contributions to discipline of nursing,
        339–340
    controlling, 306
    credibility, 319–340
    dependent-care, 291
    dependent-care agent, 291, 304
    dependent-care deficit, 293, 295
    dependent-care systems, 304
    disease, 296
    environment, 295–296, 308
    ethical standards, 308
    evaluation of, 307–340
    General Theory of Nursing
        Administration, 286, 319
        presuppositions of, 286
    health, 296–297, 308
    historical evolution and motivation,
        278–280
    identifiable state, 383
    illness, 297
    implementation of, 320–322
    influences from other scholars, 287–288
    logical congruence, 315–316
    methods of helping, 302–303t, 304
    nursing, 297–306, 308
        administration, 313–314, 329–333
        as deliberate action, 281, 288
        diagnosis, 299–300, 300–301t
        education, 311–313, 329
        goal of nursing agency, 298

nursing agency, 296
nursing system design, 302, 302–303t,
   304
practice, 298–306, 300–301t,
   302–303t, 305t, 308–309, 314–315,
   333–336
research, 310–311, 322–329
origins of, 278–288, 307–308
person, 290–295, 308
philosophical claims, 280–286
planning, 305
power components of self–care,
   291–292, 322
premises of, 282–283, 284
professional and case management
   operations of nursing practice,
   299–306
propositions, 306–307
regulatory care, 305, 305t
self-care
   defined, 290
   self-care agent, 291, 325–326
   self-care deficit, 293, 295
   self-care requisites, 284–285
Self-Care Agency Questionnaire, 322
Self-Care Assessment Tool (SCAT),
   323
social congruence, 336–338
social significance, 338–339
social utility, 319–336
strategies for knowledge development,
   286–287
technological component of nursing
   practice, 299–306
   controlling, 306
   nursing diagnosis, 299–300, 300–301t
   nursing prescription, 302
   nursing system design, 302–304,
      302–303t
   planning, 305
   regulatory care, 305, 305t
theory, generation of, 316–319
Theory of Nursing System, 26, 277, 286,
   307, 318–319
   presuppositions of, 286
   propositions of, 286, 318
Theory of Self-Care, 26, 277, 285, 307,
   316–317
   presuppositions of, 285
   propositions of, 316–317
Theory of Self-Care Deficit, 26, 277,
   285–286, 307, 317–318
   presuppositions of, 285–386
   propositions of, 317–318
therapeutic self-care demand, 292–295,
   294–295t
   developmental self-care requisites,
      293, 294t
   health-deviation self-care requisites,
      293, 294–295t

universal self-care requisites, 292–293,
   294t
unique focus, 288–290
well-being, 296, 308
world view, 288
Self-Care Institute, 340
The Self-Care Manual for Patients (Kyle
   and Pitzer), 337
Self-Care, Theory of. See under Self–Care
   Framework
Self-concept, 119. See also other
   Self–concept entries
   in interaction approach, 21–22
Self-concept adaptative/response mode,
   451–452, 455f
   personal self, 451
   physical self, 451
Self-Concept Mode, Theory of, 472, 476
Self-concept modes, 448t, 451–452
Self-consistency, 451
Self-efficacy
   as borrowed (almost shared) theory, 26
Self-esteem, 452
Self-ideal, 451
Self-Management Inventory, 311
Self-transcendence, 402
Selye, Hans, 138, 198, 242
Senses, the
   as regulator mode, 447t, 451
   hypothesis about, 475
Set
   as structural component, 78
Sexual abuse of children, 335
Sexual behavioral subsystem, 76, 77
Shared nursing theories, 26
Shared power, 480
Side effect management techniques
   (SEMT), 327–328
Significant others, 453
Simultaneity world view, 15
Simultaneous action world view, 16–17,
   17t, 380
Smoking
   nurses' attempts to quit, 146
SOAP format, 129
Social acts and relationships
   in interaction approach, 21
Social component of nursing practice,
   298–299
Social congruence
   conceptual models and, 60
   of Behavioral System Model, 97–98
   of Conservation Model, 205–206
   of General Systems Framework, 151–
      153
   of Neuman Systems Model, 254–255
   of Roy Adaptation Model, 492–493
   of Science of Unitary Human Beings,
      411–412
   of Self-Care Framework, 336–338

Social integrity, conservation principle of, 188, 190t, 195t
Social issues
  as client system, 225
Social psychology, 118
Social significance, 60–62
  of Behavioral System Model and, 98–99
  of Conservation Model, 206–207
  of General Systems Framework, 153–154
  of Neuman Systems Model, 255–256
  of Roy Adaptation Model, 493–494
  of Science of Unitary Human Beings, 412–413
  of Self-Care Framework, 338–339
Social system(s)
  as concept, 10
  of General Systems Framework, 120, 123–125, 125f
Social utility
  conceptual models and, 59–60
  of Behavioral System Model, 91–97
  of Conservation Model, 200–205
  of General Systems Framework, 143–151
  of Neuman Systems Model, 243–254
  of Roy Adaptation Model, 470–491
  of Science of Unitary Human Beings, 403–411
  of Self-Care Framework, 319–336
Society
  as original concept of nursing, 8
Society of Rogerian Scholars, 414–415
Sociocultural variable, 225
Space
  in personal system, 121
  in Theory of Goal Attainment, 139
Spiritual varible, 225
Squaires, Marjorie, 222
Stability, 75, 223, 224
  in reaction world view, 15
Stability phase of perspective transformation, 533, 533f
  return to stability phase, 533f, 534
Standards for nursing practice
  as empirical indicators, 524
Status
  in social system, 124
Steady state, 75, 119, 173, 224, 238
  compared to equilibrium, 20
  in systems approach, 20
Stimulation
  as functional requirement, 77
Stimuli
  assessment of, 459, 463t
  classes of
    contextual, 453–454
    focal, 453–454
    residual, 453–454
Strain, 75, 118, 174, 224, 445
  in systems approach, 20

Strategies for knowledge development
  Behavioral System Model, 71–72
  Conservation Model, 170
  General Systems Framework, 115–116
  Neuman Systems Model, 221
  Roy Adaptation Model, 442–443
  Self-Care Framework, 286–287
  Science of Unitary Human Beings, 379
Strategies to facilitate perspective transformation, 534–536
St. Denis, Helen A., 287
Stress, 75, 118, 174, 224, 445
  as borrowed theory, 26
  in interpersonal system, 122, 123, 139
  in systems approach, 20
  in Theory of Goal Attainment, 139
  mechanistic theory of, 223
  stress response, 180
  stressors, 228–229
    extrapersonal stressors, 229
    interpersonal stressors, 228–229
    intrapersonal stressors, 228
Structural hierarchy of nursing knowledge, 5, 6f
Structural integrity, conservation principle of, 187, 189t, 200
Substantive elements of implementing models, 520, 521–524, 521f
  translating conceptual model, 521f, 523
  translating empirical indicators, 521f, 524
  translating metaparadigm concepts, 521f, 522
  translating philosophy, 521f, 522–523
  translating theories, 521f, 523–524
Substitution category of nursing knowledge, 23t, 24, 290
Suffering, prevention or alleviation of, 168–169
Supportive intervention/action, 185
Supportive systems, 453
Supportive-educative nursing system, 302, 303t, 304
Sustenance
  category of nursing knowledge, 23t, 24
Symbolic interactionism, 21, 118, 173
Synchrony Scale, 403
Synthesis phase of perspective transformation, 533f, 534
System theory, general, 72–73, 111–112
Systems
  category of nursing knowledge, 19–20, 21t
  change and, 19
  closed system, 19
  open system, 19, 77, 118, 173–174
Systems analysis, 111
Systems models, 223. See also Neuman Systems Model

Task force phase of implemention, 525
Taste-smell system, 180
Technical nursing practice
  requirements, 88–89
Technological component of nursing
    practice, 299–306
  controlling, 306
  nursing diagnosis, 299–300, 300–301t
  nursing prescription, 302
  nursing system design, 302–304,
    302–303t
  planning, 305
  regulatory care, 305, 305t
Telepathy (mental), 400
Temperature
  hypothesis about, 475
Temporal Experience Scales (TES), 406
Tension, 75, 118, 174, 224, 445
  in systems approach, 20
Tertiary prevention, 233, 235t, 236
Tertiary roles, 452
TES (Temporal Experience Scales), 406
Testable hypothesis, 185
Testing of
  conceptual models, steps involved, 28–29
  theories, steps involved, 29
Testing phase of implementation, 404
Theoretical subconstruction, 27
Theories, 6f, 24–29
  as distinct from conceptual model, 27–
    29
  borrowed, 26
  conceptual models and, 27–29
  defined, 24, 27
  grand theories, 24–25
    examples of, 25
  hierarchy of nursing knowledge and, 6f,
    24–29
  middle-range theories, 25–26
    examples of, 25
    testing of, 28–29
  rules for generation and testing, 32
  shared, 26
  translating into practice model, 423–524,
    521f
  unique, 26–27
Theory Construction in Nursing: An
    Adaptation Model (Roy and
    Roberts), 438
Theory formalization, 27
Theory, generation of, 58
  Behavioral System Model, 90–91
  Conservation Model, 198–200
  General Systems Framework, 139–143
  Neuman Systems Model, 242–243
  Roy Adaptation Model, 472–478
  Science of Unitary Human Beings,
    399–403
  Self-Care Framework, 316–319

A Theory of Nursing: Systems, Concepts,
    Process (King), 110
Therapeutic Intention, Theory of, 198–199
Therapeutic intervention/action, 185
Therapeutic self-care demand, 292–295,
    294–295t
  developmental self-care requisites, 293,
    294t
  health-deviation self-care requisites,
    293, 294–295t
  universal self-care requisites, 292–293,
    294t
Therapeutic touch, 389, 400–401, 406,
    407, 410, 411, 413
Tibetan Buddhism, 380
Time
  in personal system, 121
  in Theory of Goal Attainment, 139
Time Dragging Scale, 406
Time Racing Scale, 406
Timelessness Scale, 406
Totality paradigm, 138
Totality world view, 15
Toward a Theory of Nursing (King), 110
Transaction
  in interpersonal system, 122, 123
  in Theory of Goal Attainment, 139
  in transaction model, 128, 128t
  interaction-transaction model, 128,
    128–130, 128t
  operational definition of, 140
Transitions
  as concept, 10
Translation to nursing practice
  conceptual models, 57–58, 521f, 523
  empirical indicators, 521f, 524
  metaparadigm concepts, 521f, 522
    mission statement and, 522
  philosophy, 521f, 522–523
  theories, 521f, 523–524
    clinical specialty knowledge and,
      523–524
Trophicognosis, 184–185, 186t
  observation, 184–185
  provocative facts, 185
  testable hypothesis, 185

Uncertainty, dwelling with, phase of
    perspective transformation,
    533–534, 533f
Unique focus of
  Behavioral System Model, 74–75
  conceptual models, 54–55
  Conservation Model, 172–175
  General Systems Framework, 117–120
  Neuman Systems Model, 223–224
  Roy Adaptation Model, 445–449

Unique focus of—*Continued*
  Science of Unitary Human Beings,
    381–383
  Self-Care Framework, 288–290
Unique nursing theories, 26–27
Unitary-transformative world view, 15
Universal self-care requisites, 292–293,
    294t

Value of conceptual models, 518–520
Value system
  of Behavioral System Model, 70–71, 92
  of Conservation Model, 193
Variances from wellness, 231
Veritivity, principle of, 441, 442
Virtual reality, as noninvasive modality,
    390
Vision (idea) phase of implemention,
    524–525
*Visions: The Journal of Rogerian Nursing
    Science*, 403, 415
Visions of Rogers' Science-Based Nursing
    (Barrett, ed.), 376, 403
Visitors
  of cancer patients, 93–94
Visual system, 180
Vocabulary of conceptual models, 2–3

Well-being, 296
  well-being (health), as nursing concept,
    11
Well-Being Index, 402–403

Wellness, 80, 182, 219, 383
  in Neuman Systems Model, 223, 229–231
  optimal wellness, 230
Wholeness, 171, 172–173, 175, 182, 187, 193
Wholly compensatory nursing system, 302,
    302– 303t, 304
World view(s), 15–17
  of Behavioral System Model, 73
  of Conservation Model, 171–172
  of General Systems Framework, 117
  of Neuman Systems Model, 222–223
  of Roy Adaptation Model, 444–445
  of Science of Unitary Human Beings,
    379–381
  of Self-Care Framework, 288
  reaction world view, 15, 15t, 73, 90, 223
  reciprocal interaction world view,
    15–16, 16t, 73, 89, 117, 171–172,
    222–223, 288, 444
  simultaneous action world view, 16–17,
    17t, 380
  various world views
    change and persistence, 15
    interactive-integrative, 15
    mechanistic and organistic, 15
    particulate-deterministic, 15
    totality and simultaneity, 15
    unitary-transformative, 15

Young, Rae Jean, 222

Zone of adaptation, 466